OBESITY AND DIABETES

CONTEMPORARY DIABETES

ARISTIDIS VEVES, MD
SERIES EDITOR

The Diabetic Foot: *Second Edition,* edited by *Aristidis Veves, MD, John M. Giurini, DPM, and Frank W. LoGerfo, MD, 2006*

The Diabetic Kidney, edited by *Pedro Cortes, MD and Carl Erik Mogensen, MD, 2006*

Obesity and Diabetes, edited by *Christos S. Mantzoros, MD, 2006*

OBESITY AND DIABETES

Edited by

CHRISTOS S. MANTZOROS, MD, DSc

Division of Endocrinology, Diabetes & Metabolism,
Beth Israel Deaconess Medical Center,
Harvard Medical School,
Boston, MA

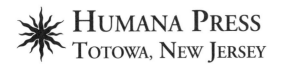

HUMANA PRESS
TOTOWA, NEW JERSEY

© 2006 Humana Press Inc.
999 Riverview Drive, Suite 208
Totowa, New Jersey 07512

www.humanapress.com

Production Editor: Tracy Catanese

Cover design by Patricia F. Cleary

For additional copies, pricing for bulk purchases, and/or information about other Humana titles, contact Humana at the above address or at any of the following numbers: Tel.: 973-256-1699; Fax: 973-256-8341, E-mail: orders@humanapr.com; or visit our Website: www.humanapress.com

This publication is printed on acid-free paper. ∞
ANSI Z39.48-1984 (American National Standards Institute) Permanence of Paper for Printed Library Materials.

Printed in the United States of America. 10 9 8 7 6 5 4 3 2 1

Library of Congress Cataloging-in-Publication Data

e-ISBN 1-59259-985-0

Obesity and diabetes / edited by Christos S. Mantzoros.
       p. ; cm. -- (Contemporary diabetes)
  Includes bibliographical references and index.
  ISBN 1-58829-538-9 (alk. paper)
 1. Diabetes. 2. Obesity. 3. Diabetes--Complications. 4. Obesity--Complications.
  [DNLM: 1. Diabetes Complications--complications. 2. Diabetes
Mellitus--physiopathology. 3. Obesity--complications. 4. Obesity--physiopathology. WK 835 O12 2005]
I. Mantzoros, Christos S. II.
Series.
  RC660.O24 2005
  616.3'98--dc22
                                                                                    2005016101

DEDICATION

To my parents and teachers;
    without them, this work would never have been possible,
and to my students and patients;
    without them, this work would never have had real meaning.

SERIES EDITOR'S INTRODUCTION

It is common knowledge that diabetes has become, over the last few decades, one of the most important public health problems. This is mainly the result of the explosive increase in the number of people who are diagnosed with type 2 diabetes in every part of the world and in almost every society, whether they have limited or advanced resources. As a matter of fact, it is the developing countries that present themselves with the highest rate of increase in diabetes. It is also not surprising that the increase in type 2 diabetes is accompanied by and related to the increase in obesity, which in some countries, like the United States, tends to be at an epidemic level. The terms "diabesity" and "metabolic syndrome" are recent additions to the medical dictionary, and they refer to new conditions that were described during the last 20 yr.

The management of diabetes and the complications that are associated with it, such as cardiovascular disease, neuropathy, retinopathy, and renal disease, is one of the main challenges of medicine in this century. It has long become obvious that this task cannot be achieved by the efforts of one discipline, which traditionally has been endocrinology, but will require a multidisciplinary approach that includes the services of numerous health professionals, such as the primary care physician, the endocrinologist, the specialist nurse, the dietitian, the exercise physiologist, the cardiologist, the podiatrist, and the vascular surgeon, to name only a few. In addition, the financial burden of the management of both diabetes and obesity is very high, and in some cases prohibitive, even in advanced societies that can afford to allocate considerable recourses for this purpose.

Education of the health professionals who are involved in the management of diabetes is probably one of the most important priorities. In that sense, I feel very excited and privileged that Humana Press has asked me to be the editor of its Contemporary Diabetes series. I hope that our collaboration will lead to the publication of high-quality books that will be edited by scientists who are world leaders in this field. It is our hope that these books will have a significant impact in the management of a condition that can affect the lives of so many people.

I am proud to present *Obesity and Diabetes*, the first book in the new series, which was edited by Dr. Chris Mantzoros, MD. Dr. Mantzoros, a friend and compatriot of mine who also works in the same institution with me, is a world leader in the field of obesity and its links to diabetes. In this volume, he has managed to bring together all of the authorities in diabetes and obesity to produce a high-quality book. I have no doubt that his work can be a major contribution and help the medical community to manage these conditions.

Aristidis Veves, MD
Series Editor

PREFACE

Obesity and diabetes are reaching epidemic proportions in developed countries in the 21st century while, at the same time, they are also becoming disturbingly more prevalent in developing countries. In the United States alone, one-third of the population is obese and another third is overweight, more than 10 million people have been diagnosed with diabetes mellitus, and another 5 million remain undiagnosed. Similar numbers have been reported in other Western nations as well. Because these disease states are closely linked with the development of serious complications, including cardiovascular disease and several malignancies, their impact from a public health perspective is enormous and continues to increase. As the population ages and becomes more sedentary, the morbidity and mortality associated with obesity and diabetes will continue to escalate.

Thus, it is imperative to focus our research efforts on trying to understand the etiology of obesity and diabetes as well as the mechanisms underlying the development of the complications associated with these conditions. It is also critically important to focus our public health efforts on the prevention and our clinical efforts on the treatment of these disease states. *Obesity and Diabetes* furthers these goals by presenting a comprehensive review of both the research and clinical aspects of obesity and diabetes to scientists and practicing clinicians alike.

Part I (Chapters 1 and 2) is a review of the history and epidemiology of these conditions. Part II (Chapters 3–7) focuses on the genetics and pathophysiology of obesity and diabetes, reviewing known mechanisms and interactions. In Part III (Chapters 8–23), the diagnosis, clinical manifestations, and complications associated with obesity and diabetes are discussed in detail. Finally, Part IV (Chapters 24–31) presents state-of-the-art approaches (lifestyle and pharmacological) to the treatment of these conditions.

I am indebted to the many people, all leading experts in their respective fields, who have contributed to *Obesity and Diabetes*. I certainly hope that our efforts will not only serve as a stimulus for further research in this increasingly important field of medicine, but also provide cutting-edge and clinically vital information to our students and practicing colleagues that will enhance the quality of care that we provide to our patients.

Christos Mantzoros, MD, DSc

CONTENTS

CONTRIBUTORS

MARTIN J. ABRAHAMSON, MD • *Division of Endocrinology, Diabetes, and Metabolism, Beth Israel Deaconess Medical Center, Harvard Medical School, Boston, MA*

HANS-OLOV ADAMI, MD, PhD • *Department of Medical Epidemiology and Biostatistics, Karolinska Institutet, Stockholm, Sweden*

ERIC S. BACHMAN MD, PhD • *Pharmacology Group, Merck Research Laboratories, Boston, MA*

MARY ANN BANERJI, MD • *Division of Endocrinology, SUNY Downstate Medical Center, Brooklyn, NY*

DIANA BARB, MD • *Division of Endocrinology, Diabetes & Metabolism, Beth Israel Deaconess Medical Center, Harvard Medical School, Boston, MA*

GEORGE L. BLACKBURN, MD, PhD • *Division of Nutrition, Beth Israel Deaconess Medical Center, Harvard Medical School, Boston, MA*

SUSANN BLÜHER, MD • *Hospital for Children and Adolescents, University of Leipzig, Germany*

GEORGE A. BRAY, MD • *Clinical Research, Pennington Biomedical Research Center, Baton Rouge, LA*

STEPHEN A. BRIETZKE, MD • *Department of Internal Medicine, Health Sciences Center, Columbia, MO*

ROCHELLE L. CHAIKEN, MD • *Vice President, Worldwide Medical Cardiovascular, Metabolic, and Endocrine Diseases, New York, NY*

JEAN L. CHAN, MD • *Division of Endocrinology, Diabetes & Metabolism, Beth Israel Deaconess Medical Center, Harvard Medical School, Boston, MA*

THANH L. DINH, DPM • *Division of Podiatry, Beth Israel Deaconess Medical Center, Harvard Medical School, Boston, MA*

JODY DUSHAY, MD • *Department of Medicine, Beth Israel Deaconess Medical Center, Harvard Medical School, Boston, MA*

ROY FREEMAN, MD • *Department of Neurology, Beth Israel Deaconess Medical Center, Harvard Medical School, Boston, MA*

DAVID W. GARDNER, MD • *Department of Internal Medicine, Health Sciences Center, Columbia, MO*

AYMAN GENEIDY, MD • *Fletcher Allen Health Care, University of Vermont College of Medicine, Burlington, VT*

ALLEN HAMDAN, MD • *Division of Vascular Surgery, Beth Israel Deaconess Medical Center, Harvard Medical School, Boston, MA*

OSAMA HAMDY, MD, PhD • *Clinical Research, Joslin Diabetes Center, Harvard Medical School, Boston, MA*

EDWARD S. HORTON, MD • *Clinical Research, Joslin Diabetes Center, Harvard Medical School, Boston, MA*

FRANK B. HU, MD, PhD • *Department of Nutrition, Harvard School of Public Health, Boston, MA*

GEORGE KARANASTASIS, MD • *Division of Endocrinology, Diabetes & Metabolism, Beth Israel Deaconess Medical Center, Harvard Medical School, Boston, MA*

ADOLF W. KARCHMER, MD • *Division of Infectious Diseases, Beth Israel Deaconess Medical Center, Harvard Medical School, Boston, MA*

IOSIF KELESIDIS, MD • *Division of Endocrinology, Diabetes & Metabolism, Beth Israel Deaconess Medical Center, Harvard Medical School, Boston, MA*

THEODOROS KELESIDIS, MD • *Division of Endocrinology, Diabetes & Metabolism, Beth Israel Deaconess Medical Center, Harvard Medical School, Boston, MA*

WIELAND KIESS, MD • *Hospital for Children and Adolescents, University of Leipzig, Germany*

SUSANNA C. LARSSON, LicMedSci • *Division of Nutritional Epidemiology, The National Institute of Environmental Medicine, Karolinska Institutet, Stockholm, Sweden*

EMILIA P. LIAO, MD • *Division of Endocrinology, Department of Medicine, Beth Israel Hospital, New York, NY*

CHRISTOS S. MANTZOROS, MD, DSc • *Division of Endocrinology, Diabetes & Metabolism, Beth Israel Deaconess Medical Center, Harvard Medical School, Boston, MA*

JOAN W. MILLER, MD • *Massachusetts Eye and Ear Infirmary, Harvard Medical School, Boston, MA*

EDWARD C. MUN, MD • *Department of Surgery, Beth Israel Deaconess Medical Center, Harvard Medical School, Boston, MA*

SATISH N. NADIG, MD • *Department of Surgery, Beth Israel Deaconess Medical Center, Harvard Medical School, Boston, MA*

RACHEL NARDIN, MD • *Department of Neurology, Beth Israel Deaconess Medical Center, Harvard Medical School, Boston, MA*

J. PETER OETTGEN, MD • *Division of Cardiology, Beth Israel Deaconess Medical Center, Harvard Medical School, Boston, MA*

LEONID PORETSKY, MD • *Division of Endocrinology, Department of Medicine, Beth Israel Hospital, New York, NY*

VASSILIKI POULAKI, MD, PhD • *Retina Research Laboratory, Massachusetts Eye and Ear Infirmary, Harvard Medical School, Boston, MA*

DONNA H. RYAN, MD • *Office of Associate Executive Director for Clinical Research, Pennington Biomedical Research Center, Baton Rouge, LA*

DESPINA SANOUDOU, PhD • *Department of Genetics, Children's Hospital, Harvard Medical School, Boston, MA*

BENJAMIN E. SCHNEIDER MD • *Department of Surgery, Beth Israel Deaconess Medical Center, Harvard Medical School, Boston, MA, and Department of Molecular Biology, Foundation for Biomedical Research of the Academy of Athens, Athens, Greece*

GREESHMA K. SHETTY, MD • *Division of Endocrinology, Diabetes and Metabolism, Beth Israel Deaconess Medical Center, Harvard Medical School, Boston, MA*

KENNETH J. SNOW, MD • *Adult Diabetes, Joslin Diabetes Center, Harvard Medical School, Boston, MA*

RICHARD SOLOMON, MD • *University of Vermont College of Medicine, Fletcher Allen Health Care, Burlington, VT*

GEETHA R. SOODINI, MD • *Clinical Research, Joslin Diabetes Center, Harvard Medical School, Boston, MA*

JAMES R. SOWERS, MD • *Department of Internal Medicine, Health Sciences Center, Columbia, MO*

VIOLETA STOYNEVA, BS • *Division of Endocrinology, Diabetes and Metabolism, Beth Israel Deaconess Medical Center, Harvard Medical School, Boston, MA*

ANJANETTE S. TAN, MD • *Department of Internal Medicine, Health Sciences Center, Columbia, MO*

SOTIRIOS TSIODRAS, MD • *Division of Infectious Diseases, Beth Israel Deaconess Medical Center, Harvard Medical School, Boston, MA*

ARISTIDIS VEVES, MD • *Joslin-Beth Israel Deaconess Foot Center, Harvard Medical School, Boston, MA*

ALICJA WOLK, DrMedSci • *Division of Nutritional Epidemiology, The National Institute of Environmental Medicine, Karolinska Institutet, Stockholm, Sweden*

I HISTORY AND EPIDEMIOLOGY

1

Obesity and Diabetes

The Historical Events Marking the Evolution of the Understanding of the Pathophysiology and Treatment of Two Related Diseases

George Karanastasis, MD
and Christos S. Mantzoros, MD, DSc

INTRODUCTION

Throughout history, man has shown a keen interest in understanding the mechanisms that sustain our existence and the relentless attempts of pathology to hinder our survival. Obesity, in the simplest of descriptions the result of an imbalance of energy intake and energy expenditure (EE), has been viewed in a multitude of differing ways throughout the centuries. At an early point in history when starvation was so prevalent, obesity was regarded as the aesthetic ideal. In today's society of affluence, however, the continual projection of a slender image through the media and the morbidity and mortality associated with this disease have likened obesity to an unyielding plague.

In the same respect, another disease entity, one that was originally identified as an obscure syndrome of excessive thirst despite copious fluid intake, has also attracted considerable attention throughout the history of investigative medicine. Now a disease with an ever-increasing prevalence, diabetes has been a topic of intense research and

From: *Contemporary Diabetes: Obesity and Diabetes*
Edited by: C. S. Mantzoros © Humana Press Inc., Totowa, NJ

exploration throughout the evolution of medicine and, more recently, has come to be recognized as a comorbidity of obesity.

Although physicians had made great efforts in understanding both diseases, breakthroughs were not significant enough to result in effective therapy until the early twentieth century. Previous to that point in history, the prognosis of a patient suffering from obesity and/or diabetes was largely similar to one of 3000 yr ago. It has been through the rapid progression in knowledge obtained about these illnesses in the last century that a correlation between the two has been established and effective treatment strategies have emerged.

The purpose of this chapter is to outline the evolution of our understanding of the pathophysiology and treatment of these two disease states originally regarded as unrelated phenomena and their later association following extensive probing into their causes. Thus, we provide separate descriptions of obesity and diabetes in an interleaved pattern until that point in history where a relationship between the two was established. Then we continue with a combined discussion of scientific milestones in the history of these two associated diseases.

THE ORIGINS OF OBESITY AND DIABETES

Obesity

The first descriptions of obesity date back to the Paleolithic Stone Age (approx 25,000 yr ago), as illustrated by the discovery and excavation of a series of artifacts spread across Europe. These artifacts, of various height and composition, depict obese women with pendulous breasts, the most famous of these being the Venus of Willendorf. They serve not only as proof of the presence of obesity, but perhaps as a symbol of the projected ideal of health and fertility, a state that so sparingly existed in that era *(1)*. Through the Neolithic period (8000 BC to 5500 BC) and into the Charcolithic age (3000 BC), several more artifacts, coined "Mother Goddesses," depicting women exhibiting exaggerated breasts, bellies, and hips were uncovered.

Continuing into the era of Egyptian medicine, it is evident from the Ebers Papyrus and the Edwin Smith Papyrus *(2)*, an even older document written sometime between 2500 and 2000 BC, that Egyptians were oblivious neither to the phenomenon of excessive body weight nor to the association with certain social classes in which it commonly existed. It would be inaccurate to conclude that, in those times, being obese was only a "commodity" of the rich, but it is clear from studies of royal mummies that obesity had earned a firm place among the more fortunate. This variation is readily apparent in artistic engravings set in stone that portray situations such as a grossly obese harpist playing before Prince Aki *(3)*, and a fat man enjoying food presented to him by his lean servants in Mereruka's tomb (reviewed in ref. *4*)

Obesity was also of interest in the medicine practiced in other parts of the world. The early Chinese attempted to treat it using a technique of inserting needles into the flesh, currently widely known as acupuncture. They applied this approach to obese individuals by placing the needle into the pinna of the ear in hopes of reducing appetite and causing body weight and size to decrease (reviewed in ref. *4*).

Considered by many the offspring of Chinese tradition, Tibetan medicine followed up on its ancestors' ideology that overeating was the cause of obesity and the only defense one had in the face of this problem was to decrease energy intake. As described in an ancient text entitled *The Four Tantras*, the Tibetans acknowledged the fact that "overeating . . . causes illness and shortens life span" *(5)*. The realization was made that a catabolic state was imperative in the fight against this unwavering condition. Their treatment strategies, however, would eventually prove far too inadequate; to mention a few: "The vigorous massage of the body with pea flour counteracts phlegm diseases and obesity. . . . The gullet, hair compress and flesh of a wolf remedy goiters, dropsy, and obesity" *(6)*.

Diabetes

The clinical syndrome of diabetes also shares the deep roots of obesity in the prehistoric era despite being clearly documented at a much later time. The first evidence of diabetes was recorded in the Egyptian Papyrus written in 1500 BC and was discovered by Egyptologist Georg Ebers in AD 1862 during the excavation of an ancient grave in Thebes. It was within this document that a condition of "too great emptying of urine" was noted, perhaps a reference to the syndrome of diabetes (reviewed in ref. *7*). Coinciding in time with the discovery of Ebers, physicians in India, through their observations of the attraction of flies and ants to diabetic urine, essentially developed the first crude clinical test for its diagnosis. They named the condition *madhumeha* (honey urine) and recognized that patients suffering from this disease exhibited polyuria and relentless polydipsia (reviewed in ref. *7*).

THE CLASSICAL AGES (500 BC TO AD 100)

Obesity

During the times of Greco-Roman medicine, the understanding and characterization of obesity as a serious disease evolved to a great extent. Hippocrates made the astute observation that "sudden death is more common in those who are naturally fat than in the lean" *(8)*. Also documented in his writings was the correlation among an inordinate body mass, infertility, and oligomennorhea in those affected by this condition. Hippocrates was as serious in his treatment approach of obesity as he was with the study of the other end of the energy homeostasis spectrum, anorexia, noting that "extreme diets leading to anorexia are of equal peril as those leading to obesity" *(9)*. He recognized that a state of starvation was just as dangerous as obesity itself and that weight loss should not be attempted by total caloric restriction. Hippocrates suggested that

> *Obese people and those desiring to lose weight should perform hard work before food. Meals should be taken after exertion and while still panting from fatigue and with no other refreshment before meals except only wine, diluted and slightly cold. Their meals should be prepared with a sesame or seasoning and other similar substances and be of a fatty natures as people get thus, satiated with little food. They should, moreover, eat only once a day and take no baths and sleep on a hard bed and walk naked as long as possible. (10)*

In addition to diet and lifestyle modification, the first operations dedicated to weight reduction date back to this point in history. Essentially, these were crude methods of tissue removal whereby anesthesia would be achieved through the administration of "sleeping potions," followed by the removal of large quantities of adipose tissue from the body *(11)*.

Galen, a highly regarded Greek physician of the Roman times, went as far as to characterize obesity as "moderate" and "immoderate," the former being somewhat of a variation of a normal condition, and the latter carrying with it considerable morbidity and mortality.

Diabetes

In 230 BC, Apollonius of Memphis was the first person to refer to the clinical presentation of this state as "diabetes," a Greek term literally translated as "to pass through." Based on the Greeks' observation of such profuse urine output, they incorrectly attributed this disease to kidney pathology. It was only later that they went on to describe this clinical scenario in full.

Aulus Cornelius Celsus made the first thorough clinical description of the disease in his eight-volume work entitled "De medicina." In the second century AD, the syndrome of diabetes mellitus was further differentiated from its polyuric equivalent, diabetes insipidus, by the Greek physician Aretaus of Cappadocia, who partially described its etiology, observing that it consisted of a series of events following acute illness, injury, or emotional stress. He wrote:

> *Diabetes is a dreadful affliction, not very frequent among men, being a melting down of the flesh and limbs into urine. The patients never stop making water and the flow is incessant, like the opening of aqueducts. Life is short, unpleasant and painful, thirst unquenchable, drinking excessive and disproportionate to the large quantity of urine, for yet more urine is passed. . . . . If for a while they abstain from drinking, their mouths become parched and their bodies dry; the viscera seem scorched up, the patients are affected by nausea, restlessness and a burning thirst, and within a short time they expire. (12)*

THE SCIENTIFIC ERA (AD 1500 TO PRESENT)

The Scientific Era was essentially built on the time-honored principles of Hippocrates, a historic figure considered to be the founding father of modern medicine. By abandoning the spiritual approach to sickness and following his example of evidence-based medicine through the application of scientific principles, men continued to make great headway not only regarding science but in the field of medicine as a whole. Later, tools such as the mechanical watch and the magnifying glass, along with the invention of movable type and printing by Steven Guttenberg, allowed physicians and scientists to gage their theories more effectively and communicate them more efficiently to others. Out of this interaction grew the method of experimentation and hypothesis falsification that provides the theoretical framework of the Scientific Era *(13)*.

Obesity

The Scientific Era marked the onset of the partitioning of medicine into its respective scientific disciplines. Andreas Vesalius published the first modern atlas of human anatomy in 1543, allowing others, including Nicholas Bonetus, to follow in his footsteps. The latter was the first man to perform dissections on obese individuals describing the presence of enormous amounts of fat *(14)*. The birth of histology enabled Theodor Schwann and his colleague Matthias Schleiden to develop the cell theory in 1839. The physicians David L. Hoggan and William Hassal recognized shortly thereafter that similar to other cells in the body, the fat cell was the basic unit responsible for altered body composition and that obesity was associated with the presence of a large amount of these fat cells *(15,16)*.

Subsequently, the development of physiology made possible the application of Gallileo's principle "Measure what can be measured, and make measurable what cannot be measured" to the problem of obesity (reviewed in ref. *4*). Santorio created the weighing scale in 1614, allowing physicians to appreciate the extent of obesity by accurately measuring body weight and using it as a longitudinal marker of improvement or deterioration.

The understanding of obesity was further significantly impacted by the physiological studies of the gastrointestinal (GI) tract and digestion. In 1752, Rene Reamur isolated gastric juice from a bird and demonstrated its digestive effect on food, a finding that was later confirmed by Lazzaro Spallanzani. François Magendie and his student Claude Bernard discovered the central role of the pancreas in this mechanism and thus further clarified the digestive process (reviewed in ref. *7*).

The contribution of chemistry to the study of obesity was made possible by the efforts of Lavoiser in the eighteenth century, which served as the basis for the laws of the conservation of mass and energy. These principles, along with Max Rubner's conception of the law of surface area, paved the way for the creation of the first human calorimeter by Atwater and Rosa in 1896. These measurements of EE and overall metabolic rate would later have an important impact on the study of obesity.

Diabetes

The beginning of the Scientific Era proved to be an important period in the study of diabetes as well. It was Aureolus Theophrastus Bombast von Hohenheim, best known as Paracelsus, who first observed that diabetic urine formed a white residue on evaporation. Although the content of the urine was initially incorrectly attributed to salt accumulation, this observation proved to be on the right path in terms of uncovering the presence of a dissolved substance in this disease. Initially, it was believed that salty urine residues were related to similar depositions in the kidneys that were in turn responsible for the perceived thirst in subjects with this affliction, polyuria being the end result of this phenomenon *(17)*. In 1674, the English anatomist and physician Thomas Willis published his scientific work in the area of pharmacology in Oxford entitled *Pharmaceutice rationalis*. Within this text he described the sweet taste of diabetic urine. Willis acknowledged that diabetes had been rare in classical times

> *but in our age, given to good fellowship and gusling down chiefly of unalloyed wine, we meet with examples and instances enough, I may say daily, of this disease . . . wherefore the urine of the sick is wonderfully sweet, or hath an honied taste. . . . As to what belongs the cure, it seems a most hard thing in this disease to draw propositions for curing, for that its cause lies so deeply hid, and hath its origin so deep and remote. (18)*

Thomas Sydenham later hypothesized that diabetes arose from an error in metabolism and was the first to challenge previous opinions of kidney deposits as a probable cause. Matthew Dobson, a British physiologist working out of Liverpool, would later publish a more concrete description of his predecessors' theories identifying the syrupy substance in urine to be sugar and concluding that it circulated in the bloodstream, rather than was formed directly by the kidney, thus establishing the concept of hyperglycemia. Shortly thereafter, Dr. John Rollo became the first physician to attribute the amount of glycosuria to the foods that one ate. He was also among the first doctors to address this condition as diabetes mellitus (the latter word coming from the Greek, meaning honey) in order to distinguish it from other diseases that exhibited copious urine output devoid of sugar, such as diabetes insipidus (as cited in ref. 7). Finally, toward the end of the eighteenth century, it was Thomas Cawley who discovered a link between pancreatic injury and diabetes. On postmortem examination, he noticed tissue damage and calculus formation of the pancreas in patients who had died of this disease (19). At that time, Cawley could not be certain if these findings were the cause of diabetes or a pathological feature of the disease itself. It would take nearly an additional century for the pancreas's role in diabetes to become clearly established.

TWO CENTURIES OF RAPID DEVELOPMENT: THE PATH TOWARD A TREATMENT

Treatment of Diabetes

It may not be an exaggeration to suggest that the science and practice of medicine gained more during the nineteenth century than in all of the previous centuries combined. With Von Fehling's development of a method to measure glucose in urine, the latter became one of the diagnostic criteria of diabetes (20). In addition, the famous French physiologist Claude Bernard discovered the storage of carbohydrates in the liver as glycogen and the technique of pancreatic ligation, a procedure that would later be used to isolate the active substance of this gland (insulin) and prove that it is responsible for carbohydrate metabolism. He was also able to attribute the role of glucose control not only to the pancreas itself but to the central nervous system (CNS) as well. By stimulating the motor nuclei of the vagal nerve with the use of a needle, Bernard demonstrated a transient induction of hyperglycemia and glycosuria in rabbits (21).

Paul Langerhans, a doctoral student working in Berlin, would bring science one step closer to the localization of the pancreatic product responsible for glucose regulation. In 1869, he recognized a clear demarcation between collections of cells from the rest of the gland (22). His discovery would later lead Edouard Laguesse, in 1893, to suggest the endocrine nature of this heap of cells, which he named "the islets of Langerhans," in recognition of his predecessor's discovery.

That same year, Edouard Hedon would prove the physiological importance of these islets by demonstrating that incomplete pancreatectomy failed to produce the symptoms of diabetes. Following total pancreatic extraction, the ensuing polyuric and polydipsic symptoms were interpreted as strengthening the evidence that the absence of a discrete component of the gland (now known to be the islets) was responsible for the development of diabetes.

Treatment of Obesity

Much like in the case of diabetes, great progress continued to be made regarding obesity. The ability of biochemical studies to illustrate the basic building blocks of our bodies coupled with the understanding of energy intake and EE still, to this day, serve as the basis of the etiology, prevention, and treatment of obesity.

As mentioned previously, several recommendations had been repeatedly made throughout history having the common notion that food restriction and physical activity were the key to a leaner body. For example, in 1825, Brillat-Savarin attributed obesity to both the inclinations and eating habits of an individual: "[A] *double cause of obesity results from too much sleep combined with too little exercise. . . . The final cause of obesity is excess, whether in eating or drinking*" (23).

In addition to "natural" methods of therapy, the development of pharmacology advocated a chemical approach to this problem. The thyroid gland was recognized to have a catabolic effect in the scheme of metabolism and thyroid extracts were thus used to "melt away the fat" *(24)*.

Further application of drugs in the treatment of obesity followed the discovery of the slimming effects of aniline dyes. It was recognized that workers in chemical factories who came in contact with these substances on a daily basis experienced significant weight loss *(25)*. The use of these medications was later discouraged, however, following the realization of inherent side effects such as cataracts and neuropathy *(25)*. In the 1930s, the weight-reducing effects of amphetamines were identified during their use in the treatment of narcolepsy *(26)*. Thus, they became another class of drugs advocated for the management of obesity, but their popularity quickly faded owing to their addictive properties.

Consequently, in the beginning of the twentieth century, the potential neural etiology of obesity attracted the interest of several scientists. Physicians such as Joseph François Felix Babinski and Alfred Frohlich noted a link between the development of obesity and basal brain tumors. According to the specific location affected, increased or decreased appetite was noted, which eventually led to Stellar's hypothalamic dual center hypothesis in 1954 *(27)*. This theory established the ventromedial hypothalamus as the satiety center, with lesions in this location resulting in the development of obesity, whereas the lateral hypothalamus was proposed to be the antagonistic hunger center, which was responsible for weight loss in the presence of a structural abnormality *(27)*.

Unable to attribute the cause of obesity to hypothalamic lesions in the vast majority of subjects, however, physicians turned their attention toward CNS function including the autonomic nervous system. In 1979, Bray and York *(28)* postulated the autonomic hypothesis, which attributed the development of this disease to an imbalance of sympathetic and parasympathetic activity. They suggested that in the presence of ventromedial hypothalamic lesions, the vagal response to feeding was greatly exaggerated, leading to hyperinsulinemia. The anabolic effects of insulin coupled with a lack of lipolysis and thermogenesis owing to suppressed sympathetic activity was thought to be a key determinant of weight gain *(28)*. These findings have been central to the development of ideas that were later translated into the discovery of drugs such as adrenergic-serotonergic reuptake inhibitors and the study of GI tract–CNS peptide interactions as they pertain to the development of obesity. Furthermore, these findings have directed physicians toward a combined neural and endocrine etiology of this disease and have opened the door to an exciting new field of research.

Owing to the lack of effective and safe medications, however, surgery has continued to play an important role in the treatment of obesity. As mentioned previously, the procedures employed in the days of the first obesity surgeries shared the common goal of contemporary surgeries—to rid the body of excess fat. These operations evolved from crude methods of tissue removal to more sophisticated interventions based on the physiology of the digestive process. Up until the 1970s, gastric bypass was the main procedure employed, which served to inhibit the absorption of food by diverting it to the large bowel, altogether "bypassing" the small intestine. These procedures were abandoned because of side effects, including diarrhea, infections, and serious metabolic disturbances. The palliative and not etiological nature of this treatment approach was made evident by experiments creating corrective reanastomosis of the intestine, after which all the weight previously lost was gained once more *(29)*. Today's surgical procedures involve the reduction of the stomach's capacity to store food, thus inducing satiety after relatively smaller meals. First developed by Mason and Ito *(30)*, these gastric reduction procedures are becoming the mainstay of therapy in the surgical treatment of obesity, providing a safe and controlled method of caloric restriction.

RECENT DISCOVERIES THAT HAVE REVOLUTIONIZED THE APPROACH TO DIABETES AND OBESITY

The third decade of the 20th century would mark investigators' triumphs in finally isolating insulin, an accomplishment that stands unequivocally as one of the greatest milestones in the history of diabetes. Through techniques developed by physicians such as Claude Bernard and Oskar Minkowski, Frederick Grant Banting and Charles H. Best used the pancreatic duct ligation procedure to successfully isolate insulin for its use in the treatment of diabetes.

Banting, having studied previous publications of a pancreatic product as a viable treatment method for diabetes, gained interest in this disease. After communicating his aspirations to J. J. R. Macleod, a physiology professor at the University of Toronto, Macleod was enticed to provide Banting with a designated facility to carry out his work; research subjects; and a student helper, Charles H. Best, who was awarded this great honor following the victory of a coin toss over another willing student. James B. Collip, a prominent biochemist, would later join their group to assist in the extraction and purification of insulin.

Nearly 6 mo later, on January 11, 1922, the final product of their extensive labor was put to trial on Leonard Thompson, a 14-yr-old patient with diabetes in Toronto General Hospital. Their first attempt proved disappointing: the boy's symptoms not only failed to abate but were further exacerbated by abscesses formed at the sites of injection. Following the administration of a second, more purified injection 12 d later, however, the team made history with the resolution of the boy's symptoms, dissolution of ketonuria, and initiation of weight gain. They named the therapeutic substance "isletin," which they later changed to "insulin" *(31)*.

In recognition of their achievements Macleod and Banting were awarded the Nobel Prize in 1923 for the discovery of insulin. Rightfully so, Macleod and Banting shared the award with Best and Collip, acknowledging their contributions to this breakthrough *(17)*.

Later, the development of more sensitive techniques for the quantification of physiologically important substances in biological fluids revolutionized research of not only diabetes, but also endocrinology as a whole. More specifically, in 1959, Rosalyn Yalow and her colleague Salomon A. Berson formulated a concept that, although in essence relatively simple, was at that time considered iconoclastic. They speculated that antibodies against human antigens can be created and that these antibodies competing for available binding sites on either endogenous circulating antigens or exogenously added in known quantities could be used as a method of measuring the concentration of ligands of interest. This technique, now widely known as radioimmunoassay, was initially used to quantify insulin. The results of subsequent insulin measurements in samples from patients with diabetes clearly demonstrated for the first time that diabetic symptoms were not always dependent on the absence of this hormone. Further studies would later lead to the classification of diabetes into two principal types: one mainly related to insulin deficiency, the other with insulin resistance (accompanied by hyperinsulinemia). Subsequent applications of the same concept in the development of enzyme-linked immunosorbert assays and immunoradiometric assays have proven to be of paramount importance in the study of diabetes and obesity.

RECENT ADVANCES IN GENETICS CREATE A RESURGENCE OF INTEREST IN OBESITY AND DIABETES RESEARCH

The intensification of research in genetics and biology in recent years made it possible to discover several genes related to obesity and diabetes, which, in turn, resulted in an explosion of research in these areas. In 1992, S. J. Bultman discovered the first gene linked to obesity, the *agouti* gene, in an overweight mouse model with yellow fur (the yellow obese mouse) *(32)*. We subsequently learned that the *agouti* gene is expressed in many tissues, leading to the production of a 131 amino acid long peptide called the *agouti*-related peptide *(32)*, which blocks the action of α-melanocyte-stimulating hormone at the level of the melanocortin receptor, thus leading to both yellow fur and hyperphagia/obesity *(32)*.

The second gene identified in association with obesity was the *ob* gene, which was discovered in 1994 by Zhang et al. *(33)*, who utilized the technique of positional cloning of the *ob/ob* mouse model of obesity. Genetic defects of this gene are now known to be responsible for the abnormal translation of the protein leptin (from the Greek *leptos*, meaning thin), whose physiological role is to communicate the availability of peripheral energy stores to the CNS. The deficiency of leptin (owing to the *ob* gene mutation) as a determining factor in the development of obesity was proven by weight loss observed following its exogenous administration in *ob/ob* mice *(34)*. However, it was later realized that "garden variety" obesity in humans is a leptin-resistant and not a leptin-deficient state *(35)*.

Continued research efforts geared toward the development of medications for the treatment of obesity have led to the exploration of potential causes of leptin resistance and the discovery of proteins acting as negative regulators downstream of the leptin receptor *(36)*. In addition, some of these negative regulators of leptin were identified as inhibitors of insulin signal transduction *(37)*. As the molecular pathways responsible for energy homeostasis are mapped, extensive research efforts that could exploit these new discoveries are under way in attempts to treat obesity and insulin resistance as well as prevent the onset of diabetes *(38)*. The scientific community is enthusiastic that in the near future these research efforts will lead to the discovery of new pharmaceutical agents that will eventually offer tangible benefits to the enlarging segment of society that strives to decrease body weight and control associated comorbidities.

The discovery of leptin has essentially revived a new field of research. Moreover, it soon altered researchers' perception of adipose tissue from that of an inactive storage depot of energy to that of an active endocrine organ. Furthermore, it changed the perception of obesity from that of a condition related to lack of "willpower" to that of a biological problem with strong genetic and environmental determinants. These findings are currently leading physicians to take a multifaceted approach to the problem of obesity, giving increasing importance to the genetic and neuroendocrine aspects of the disease in addition to evaluating and modifying diet and lifestyle habits.

CONCLUSIONS

The incidence of obesity and diabetes is becoming increasingly prevalent at an alarming rate as the world embraces a Westernized lifestyle. Never before has there been a greater need to spread awareness of the risk factors associated with these diseases and to coordinate medical progress with cultural modification. Through the continuous exploration of the biological mechanisms underlying these illnesses, researchers can hope to offer, in the near future, new treatment and prevention strategies for these prevalent disease states.

REFERENCES

1. Beller AS. Fat & Thin: A Natural History of Obesity. Farrar, Straus & Giroux, New York, 1977.
2. Breasted JH. The Edwin Smith Surgical Papyrus: Published in facsimile and hieroglyphic transliteration with translation and commentary in two volumes by James Henry Breasted. Special Edition. The Univ. of Chicago-Oriental Institute Publications, Birmingham, 1984, pp. 596.
3. Reeves C. Egyptian Medicine. Shire Publications, Buckinghamshire, 1992.
4. Bray GA. Historical framework for the development of ideas about obesity. In: Bray GA, Bouchard C, James WPT, eds. Handbook of Obesity. Marcel Dekker, New York, 1998.
5. Parfionovitch Y, Dorje G, Meyer F. Illustrations to the Blue Beryl Treatise of Sangye Gyamtso (1653–1705). Harry N. Abrams, New York, 1992.
6. Darby WJ, Ghalioungui P, Grevetti L. Food: The Gift of Osiris. Academic, London, 1977.
7. Zajak J, Shrestha A, Poretsky L. The main events in the history of diabetes mellitus. In: Poretsky L, ed. Principles of Diabetes Mellitus. Kluwer Academic, Boston, 2002.
8. Lypourlis D. Aphorisms 44. In: Hippokrates. Zitros Publications, 2000, pp. 177.
9. Lypourlis D. Aphorisms 4. In: Hippokrates. Zitros Publications, 2000, pp. 163.
10. Precope J. Hippocrates on Diet and Hygiene. Zeno, London, 1952.
11. Preuss J. Biblical and Talmudic Medicine (translated and edited by Rosner F, MD). Hebrew Publishing, New York, 1978.
12. Medvei VC. The Greco-Roman period. The history of clinical endocrinology: a comprehensive account of endocrinology from earliest times to the present day. Parthenon, New York, 1993; pp. 34, 37.
13. Beaujouan G. Motives and opportunities for science in the medieval universities. In: Crombe AC, ed. Scientific Change: Historical Studies in the Intellectual, Social and Technical Conditions for Scientific Discovery and Technical Invention from Antiquity to Present. Basic Books, 1963; pp. 232–234.
14. Bonetus T. Sepulchretum, sive anatomia practica, ex cadaveribus morbo denatis, proponenes historias omnium humani corporis affectum. Sumptibus Leonardi Chouet, Geneva, 1679.
15. Hoggan G, Hogan FE. On the development and retrogression of the fat cell. J R Microscope Soc 1879;2:353.
16. Hassal A. Observations on the development of the fat vesicle. Lancet 1849;1:63, 64.
17. Medvei VC. The history of clinical endocrinology: a comprehensive account of endocrinology from earliest times to the present day. In: Story of Insulin. Parthenon, New York, 1993; pp. 249–251, 253–256.
18 Willis T. Pharmaceutica Rationalessive Diatriba de Medicamentorium Operationitus in Humano Corpore. In: Oxoniae. London, 1674.
19. Medvei VC. The history of clinical endocrinology: a comprehensive account of endocrinology from earliest times to the present day. In: The 16th century and the Renaissance. Parthenon, New York, 1993; pp. 55, 56.
20. Medvei VC. The history of clinical endocrinology: a comprehensive account of endocrinology from the earliest times to the present day. In: The 18th century and the beginning of the 19th century. Parthenon, New York, 1993, pp. 97.
21. Bernard C. Lecons de Physiologie. Bailliere, Paris, 1855.
22. Langerhans P. Beitrage zur mikroskopischen Anatomie der Bauchspeicheldruse. Gustave Lange, Berlin, 1869.
23. Brillat-Savarin. The Physiology of Taste or, Meditations on Transcendental Gastronomy (translated from the French by Fisher MFK; drawings and color lithographs by Thiebaud W). Arion, San Francisco, 1994.
24. Sajous CE, de M. The Internal Secretion and the Principles of Medicine, 7th ed. FA Davis, Philadelphia, 1916.
25. Ehrlich P, Hata S. Die experimentelle chemotherapie der spirillosen. Julius Springer, Berlin, 1910.
26. Lesses MF, Myerson A. Human autonomic pharmacology. XVI. Benzedrine sulfate as an aid in the treatment of obesity. N Engl J Med 1938;218:119–124.

27. Stellar E. The physiology of motivation: 1954. Psychol Rev 1994;101(2):301–311.
28. Bray GA, York DA. Hypothalamic and genetic obesity in experimental animals: an autonomic and endocrine hypothesis. Physiol Rev 1979;59(3):719–809.
29. Payne JH, DeWind LT, Commons RR. Metabolic observations in patients with jejunocolic shunts. Am J Surg 1963;106:273–289.
30. Mason EE, Ito C. Gastric bypass. Ann Surg 1969;170(3):329–339.
31. Bliss M. Triumph. The Discovery of Insulin. University of Chicago Press, Chicago, 1990; pp. 112, 113, 120, 121, 127.
32. Bultman SJ, Michaud EJ, Woychik RP. Molecular characterization of the mouse agouti locus. Cell 1992;71(7):1195–1204.
33. Zhang Y, Proenca R, Maffei M, Barone M, Leopold L, Friedman JM. Positional cloning of the mouse obese gene and its human homologue. Nature 1994;372(6505):425–432.
34. Halaas JL, Gajiwala KS, Maffei M, et al. Weight-reducing effects of the plasma protein encoded by the obese gene. Science 1995;269(5223):543–546.
35. Considine RV, Considine EL, Williams CJ, et al. Evidence against either a premature stop codon or the absence of obese gene mRNA in human obesity. J Clin Invest 1995;95(6):2986–2988.
36. Bjorbaek C, El Haschimi K, Frantz JD, Flier JS. The role of SOCS-3 in leptin signaling and leptin resistance. J Biol Chem 1999;274(42):30,059–30,065.
37. Rui L, Yuan M, Frantz D, Shoelson S, White MF. SOCS-1 and SOCS-3 block insulin signaling by ubiquitin-mediated degradation of IRS1 and IRS2. J Biol Chem 2002;277(44):42,394–42,398.
38. Zhang ZY, Lee SY. PTP1B inhibitors as potential therapeutics in the treatment of type 2 diabetes and obesity. Expert Opin Invest Drugs 2003;12(2):223–233.

2

Epidemiology of Obesity and Diabetes
Prevalence and Trends

Susanna C. Larsson, LicMedSci
and Alicja Wolk, DrMedSci

CONTENTS

INTRODUCTION

Overweight and obesity have reached epidemic proportions globally along with an adoption of a westernized lifestyle characterized by a combination of excessive food intake and inadequate physical activity. In the United States, the prevalence of obesity doubled during the past two decades, and currently 30% of the US adult population is classified as obese. An additional 35% of US adults are overweight but not obese. Children and adolescents are not immune to the epidemic. Among US children and adolescents, 16% are overweight and an additional 15% are at risk of overweight.

The dramatic rise in the prevalence of obesity and changes in lifestyle-related factors such as a reduction in physical activity have been accompanied by alarming increases in the incidence and prevalence of type 2 diabetes. It has been estimated that the total number of adults with diabetes (mainly type 2 diabetes) will approximately double between 2000 and 2030, from 171 million to 366 million *(1)*. The epidemic proportions of the disease are particularly noticeable in indigenous populations that have undergone rapid acculturation from their traditional lifestyles.

Considering the tremendous economic and human costs associated with obesity and diabetes, public health intervention programs aiming at preventing these two diseases are urgently needed.

From: *Contemporary Diabetes: Obesity and Diabetes*
Edited by: C. S. Mantzoros © Humana Press Inc., Totowa, NJ

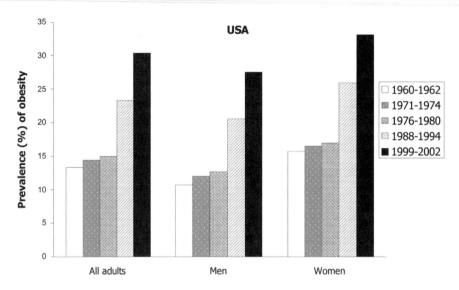

Fig. 1. Time trends in prevalence (%) of obesity (body mass index $\geq$ 30.0 kg/m^2) in adults (ages 20–74 yr) in the United States, 1960–2002. The data are from NHES I (1960–1962) and NHANES (1971–1974, 1976–1980, 1988–1994, 1999–2002) *(3,4)*.

This chapter presents the prevalence, secular trends, and geographic distribution of overweight, obesity, and diabetes in adults, children, and adolescents in the Unites States and in other developed countries as well as in developing countries. In addition, it briefly summarizes the epidemiological literature on obesity, weight gain, weight loss, and physical activity in relation to the risk of developing diabetes.

PREVALENCE AND TRENDS OF OBESITY IN ADULTS

Overweight in adults has been defined as a body mass index ([BMI]; the weight in kilograms divided by the square of height in meters) of 25.0–29.9 kg/m^2 and obesity as a BMI of 30.0 kg/m^2 or higher, in accordance with World Health Organization (WHO) recommendations *(2)*. Even though the same classifications for overweight and obesity have been used in the studies summarized here, these studies may not be directly comparable because of differences in methods (measured or self-reported weights and heights) and periods of data collection (secular trends). Other issues include representativeness of samples (limited geographic area or national, urban, or rural), sample size, age, and sex.

United States, Canada, and Latin America

Estimates of the prevalence and time trends of obesity in the United States are based on data from the National Health and Nutrition Examination Survey (NHANES), which includes nationally representative samples of the US civilian noninstitutionalized population. The surveys include the first National Health Examination Survey (NHES I); the first, second, and third NHANES surveys; and a continuous survey that began in 1999 *(3,4)*. Height and weight were measured in a mobile examination center using standardized techniques and equipment. As shown in Fig. 1, the prevalence of obesity among adults ages 20–76 yr was relatively constant from 1960 to 1980, then increased steeply. Comparison of the period 1976–1980 with 1999–2002, reveals that the prevalence of overweight (BMI $\geq$ 25 kg/m^2) increased by about 40% (from 47 to 65%) and

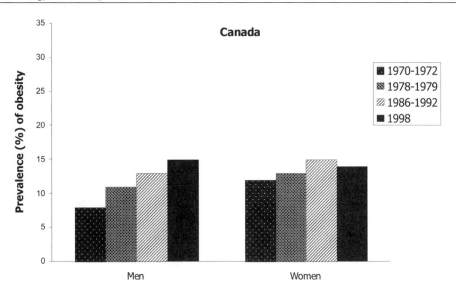

Fig. 2. Time trends in prevalence (%) of obesity (body mass index ≥ 30.0 kg/m^2) in adults (ages 20–64 yr) in Canada, 1970–1998. The data are from Nutrition Canada Survey (1970–1972), Canada Health Survey (1978–1979), Canada Heart Health Surveys (1986–1992), and National Population Health Survey (1998) *(5)*.

the prevalence of obesity (BMI ≥ 30 kg/m^2) rose by 100% (from 15 to 30%). Regarding extreme obesity (BMI ≥ 40 kg/m^2), the prevalence rose from 3% in 1988–1994 to 5% in 1999–2002. The increases in overweight and obesity have occurred in all age and racial/ethnic groups. In 1999–2002, the highest prevalence of overweight and obesity was found among non-Hispanic black women (77%).

The prevalence of obesity in Canada is lower than in the United States, but it appears to increase over time. Data from national surveys in Canada *(5)* showed that between 1970–1972 and 1998, the prevalence of obesity in adults (ages 20–64 yr) increased from about 8 to 15% in men and from 12 to 14% in women (Fig. 2).

Three national surveys were conducted in the two most populated Brazilian regions in 1975, 1989, and 1997 *(6)*. Between 1975 and 1997, the prevalence of obesity among adults over 20 yr of age increased from 2.4 to 6.9% in men and from 7.0 to 12.5% in women (Fig. 3). The most recent trend, from 1989 to 1997, indicated that the increases in obesity prevalence were more intense in men than in women, in rural than in urban settings, and in poorer than in richer families. There was a reduction in the prevalence of obesity among upper-income urban women (12.8–9.2%).

Fernald et al. *(7)* assessed the prevalence of overweight and obesity among the rural poor in Mexico in comparison with a national sample using data from two national surveys in Mexico. The first survey was conducted in 2000 in about 45,000 adults and was based on a nationally representative sample of the Mexican noninstitutionalized population. The second survey was conducted in 2003 in about 13,000 adults and was designed to be representative of the poorest rural communities in seven Mexican states. In both surveys, height and weight were measured using standardized techniques. In the nationally representative sample, the prevalence of overweight and obesity was 40.8 and 20.4%, respectively, in men. The corresponding figures in women were 36.5 and 30.2%, respectively. In the 2003 sample from low-income rural regions of Mexico, the prevalence of overweight and obesity was 38.9 and 13.6% in men, and 36.8 and 22.2% in women.

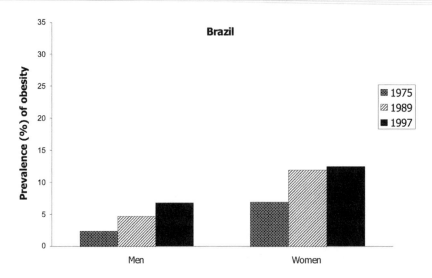

Fig. 3. Time trends in prevalence (%) of obesity (body mass index ≥ 30.0 kg/m²) in adults (ages 25–64 yr) in Brazil, 1975–1997. The data are from national household surveys in northeast and southeast Brazil *(6)*.

Europe

The Monitoring Trends and Determinants in Cardiovascular Disease (MONICA) Project includes a series of cross-sectional surveys in 26 countries, mostly in Europe *(8)*. In each survey a random sample of at least 200 persons ages 35–64 yr was selected. Standardized methods were applied for anthropometric measurements. Table 1 shows the age-standardized prevalence of obesity in the European countries included in the MONICA Project. Overall, the prevalence of obesity increased in most European populations over the 10-yr study period. In the last survey (in the early 1990s), the prevalence of obesity in the populations varied from approx 15 to 25% in men and 10 to 35% in women, with the highest prevalence in men and women from Eastern Europe. Among women, there was a significant inverse association between educational level and BMI in virtually all 26 countries; the difference in mean BMI between the highest and lowest educational tertiles ranged from –3.3 to –0.6 kg/m² in the 1990s. Among men, the association between BMI and educational level was positive in some Eastern and Central European populations and in China and also in populations with a low prevalence of obesity. By contrast, there was an inverse association between BMI and educational level in populations with a high prevalence of obesity.

Table 2 provides other national survey data from European populations. In Finland, the proportion of obese men doubled between 1972 and 1997 *(9)*, whereas the prevalence of obesity in women remained constant over the 25-yr period. The most recent data show that about 20% of men and women in Finland are obese *(9)*. Between the 1980s and 1990s, considerable increases in the prevalence of obesity have occurred in both men and women in Norway *(10)*, the Netherlands *(11)*, Sweden *(12)*, and the United Kingdom *(13)* and in men in France *(14)*.

Africa

Using data from nationally representative surveys conducted in the 1990s, the overall proportion of obese women (ages 15–49 yr) in sub-Saharan Africa was estimated to be 2.5%, ranging from 1.0% in Burkina Faso to 7.1% in Namibia *(15)*. The proportion of

Table 1
Prevalence of Obesity (BMI $\geq$ 30.0 kg/m^2)in MONICA Populations
Ages 35–64 yr in Early 1980s and Early 1990s[a]

Area	Country, center	Men (%)		Women (%)	
		1980s	1990s	1980s	1990s
Northern Europe	Denmark, Glostrup	11	13	10	12
	Finland, Kuopio Province	18	24	19	26
	Finland, North Karelia	17	23	24	24
	Finland, Turku-Loimaa	19	22	17	19
	Iceland, Iceland	11	16	11	18
	Sweden, Gothenburg	7	13	9	10
	Sweden, Northern Sweden	11	14	14	14
Western Europe	United Kingdom, Belfast	11	14	14	16
	United Kingdom, Glasgow	11	23	16	23
	Germany, Augsburg	18	17	15	21
	Germany, Augsburg, rural	20	24	22	23
	Germany, Bremen	14	16	18	21
	Belgium, Ghent	11	13	15	16
	France, Lille	14	17	19	22
	France, Strasbourg	22	22	23	19
	France, Toulouse	9	13	11	10
	Switzerland, Ticino	20	13	15	16
	Switzerland, Vaud-Fribourg	13	17	13	10
Eastern Europe	Russian Federation, Moscow	13	8	33	22
	Russian Federation, Novosibirsk	14	17	44	35
	Lithuania, Kaunas	22	20	45	32
	Poland, Warsaw	18	22	26	29
	Poland, Tarnobrzeg Voivodship	13	15	32	36
	Czech Republic, Czech Republic	21	23	32	30
Southern Europe	Spain, Catalonia	9	16	24	25
	Italy, Area Brianza	11	14	15	18
	Italy, Friuli	16	17	19	19

[a]Adapted from ref. 8.

obese women was greater in urban than in rural regions (Fig. 4). Furthermore, in general, obesity was more frequent among women with a high educational level than among women with a low educational level. This is in contrast to the Western countries with a high prevalence of obesity, where an inverse relation between educational level and BMI in women has been observed.

Asia, Western Pacific, and India

Despite an increasing prevalence of overweight and obesity in Asia, the prevalence remains low (Table 3). Based on nationwide cross-sectional surveys conducted in Japan *(16)*, the proportion of overweight and obese men increased from 14.5 and 0.8%, respectively, in the time period 1976–1980 to 20.5 and 2.0% during 1991–1995. The increasing trend was most apparent in the youngest age groups (20–29 yr) and in those from small towns. In women, the prevalence of overweight and obesity remained relatively constant over this 20-yr period, although a decreasing prevalence was noted in

Table 2
Prevalence of Obesity (BMI $\geq$ 30.0 kg/m^2) in Men
and Women in Selected European Countries

Country	Period	Age (yr)	Men (%)	Women (%)	Reference
Finland	1972	25–59	10.1	19.2	9
	1977	25–59	12.3	20.6	
	1982	25–59	14.9	18.7	
	1987	25–59	17.7	20.6	
	1992	25–59	19.9	21.3	
	1997	25–59	20.7	20.1	
France	1985–1987	35–64	10	11	14
	1995–1997	35–64	13	11	
Norway	1984–1986	$\geq$20	7.5	13.0	10
	1995–1997	$\geq$20	14.0	17.8	
The Netherlands	1976–1980	37–43	4.9	6.2	11
	1987–1991	37–43	7.4	7.6	
	1993–1997	37–43	8.5	9.3	
Sweden	1980/1981	16–84	6.6	8.8	12
	1988/1989	16–84	7.3	9.1	
	1996/1997	16–84	10.0	11.9	
United Kingdom	1987/1989	$\geq$16	7	12	13
	1993	$\geq$16	13	16	
	1994	$\geq$16	14	17	
	1995	$\geq$16	15	17	
	1996	$\geq$16	16	18	
	1997	$\geq$16	17	19	

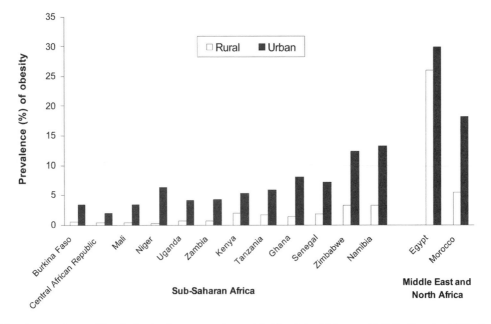

Fig. 4. Prevalence (%) of obesity in women (ages 15–49 yr) in Africa and Midle East in 1990s by rural and urban area. (From ref. *15.*)

Table 3
Prevalence of Obesity (BMI ≥ 30.0 kg/m^2) in Men and Women in Asia,
Western Pacific Regions, and India

Country	Period	Age (yr)	Men (%)	Women (%)	Reference
India					
Urban (Delhi)	1991–1995	35–64	7.1	16.4	20
Rural (Haryana)	1991–1995	35–64	0.7	2.2	
China	1989	20–45	0.4	0.2	17
	1997	20–45	0.5	1.5	
Japan, national surveys	1976–1980	≥20	0.8	2.3	16
	1981–1985	≥20	1.1	2.3	
	1986–1990	≥20	1.5	2.2	
	1991–1995	≥20	2.0	2.3	
Nepal, national surveys	1996	15–49	–	0.1	15
Australia, national surveys	1980	25–64	9.3	8.0	19
	1983	25–64	9.1	10.5	
	1989	25–64	11.5	13.2	
New Zealand, national surveys	1989	18–64	10	12	18
Papua New Guinea					
Urban coastal	1991	25–69	36	54	21
Rural coastal	1991	25–69	24	19	
Highlands	1991	25–69	5	5	
Samoa					
Urban	1978	25–69	39	59	21
	1991	25–69	58	77	
Rural	1978	25–69	18	37	
	1991	25–69	42	59	
Nauru	1987	25–69	65	70	21

younger women (ages 20–29 yr). Data from the China Health and Nutrition survey, showed that between 1989 and 1997, the prevalence of overweight almost doubled in women (from 10.3 to 19.2%) and tripled in men (from 4.6 to 13.6%) (17). Regarding obesity, the prevalence increased from 0.2 to 1.5% in women and from 0.4 to 0.5% in men over the same time period. However, there are Asian nations, such as Nepal, where the prevalence of obesity is very low (0.1% in women in 1997) (15).

In Australia and New Zealand, the prevalence of obesity was 10–13% in the late 1980s (Table 3) (18,19). Results from national surveys in Australia indicated that the proportion of obese persons increased over a 9-yr period, from about 8 to 9% in 1980 to 12 to 13% in 1989 (19). Cross-sectional surveys conducted in India in 1991–1995 (20) revealed a considerably higher prevalence of obesity in urban (7.1% in men and 16.4% in women) than in rural (0.7 in men and 2.2% in women) regions (Table 3).

Finally, there is a very high prevalence of obesity in Polynesian populations, with up to 65% of men and 80% of women being obese (21). The prevalence of obesity in Polynesian populations is higher in urban than in rural areas. Since the late 1980s, the prevalence of obesity has increased markedly in these populations (21).

Summary

The prevalence of obesity has markedly increased during the last few decades in the United States and other countries. Specifically, between the periods 1976–1980 and

Table 4
International Cutoff Points for BMI for Overweight and Obesity
by Sex Between Ages 2 and 18 yr[a]

	Overweight (kg/m^2)		Obesity (kg/m^2)	
Age (yr)	Males	Females	Males	Females
2	18.4	18.0	20.1	19.8
4	17.6	17.3	19.3	19.2
6	17.6	17.3	19.8	19.7
8	18.4	18.4	21.6	21.6
10	19.8	19.9	24.0	24.1
12	21.2	21.7	26.0	26.7
14	22.6	23.3	27.6	28.6
16	23.9	24.4	28.9	29.4
18	25.0	25.0	30.0	30.0

[a]Adapted from ref. 24.

1999–2002, the prevalence of obesity doubled among US adults, and currently about one-third of the US adult population is obese (3,4). The obesity epidemic will tremendously affect public health, because obesity is strongly associated with several chronic diseases, including cardiovascular disease, type 2 diabetes, and certain cancers. Because these conditions can be costly to treat, obesity clearly has a considerable economic impact. Obesity-related morbidity has been estimated to account for 5.5–7.8% of total health-care expenditures in the United States (22).

PREVALENCE AND TRENDS OF OBESITY IN CHILDREN AND ADOLESCENTS

Currently, there is a lack of agreement concerning the definitions for overweight and obesity in children and adolescents, which makes comparisons of prevalence across countries difficult. In the United States, the 85th and 95th percentiles of BMI for age and sex based on nationally representative survey data have been recommended as cutoff points to identify overweight and obesity (23). The European Childhood Obesity Group of the International Obesity Task Force (IOTF) (24) has proposed an international reference, age- and sex-specific BMI cutoff points, to define childhood and adolescent overweight and obesity. The IOTF reference was developed based on data from measured children and adolescents, ages 6–18 yr, across six heterogeneous nations: Brazil, Great Britain, Hong Kong, the Netherlands, Singapore, and the United States. The IOTF definitions of overweight and obesity presented in Table 4 are based on age- and sex-specific BMI cutoff points corresponding to a BMI of 25 and 30 kg/m^2, respectively, at age 18 (24).

United States and Canada

Six nationally representative examination surveys on the prevalence of overweight among children and adolescents have been conducted in the United States between the 1960s and 1999–2002: NHES 2 and 3; NHANES I, II, and III; and the continuous NHANES (4,25,26). The same standardized measurements have been used in all surveys, thus allowing a unique and comprehensive examination of the changes in overweight status. The 2000 Centers for Disease Control and Prevention growth charts for the

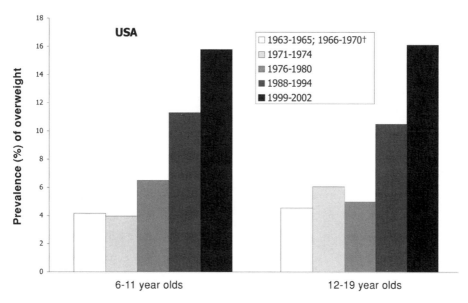

Fig. 5. Time trends in prevalence (%) of overweight (body mass index for age at 95th percentile or greater) in children and adolescents in national surveys in United States, 1963–2000. [†]Data for 1963–1965 are for children 6–11 yr of age; data for 1966–1970 are for adolescents 12–17 yr of age, not 12–19. The data are from NHES 2 (1960–1965), NHES 3 (1966–1970), and NHANES (1971–1974, 1976–1980, 1988–1994, 1999–2002) *(4,25,26).*

United States were used to define overweight and at risk for overweight among children *(23).* The BMI-for-age growth charts were developed from five of those six national surveys (NHES 2 and 3, NHANES I and II, and NHANES III for children younger than 6 yr of age). At risk for overweight was defined as a BMI at or above the 85th percentile but less than the 95th percentile of the sex-specific BMI, as defined by the growth chart. Overweight was defined as at or above the 95th percentile of the sex-specific BMI-for-age growth chart. Between the 1960s and 1999–2002, the prevalence of overweight among 6- through 11-yr-old children increased from 4.2 to 15.8% (Fig. 5). During this same period, the corresponding prevalence among 12- through 19-yr-old children increased from 4.6 to 16.1%. Among children 2 through 5 yr old, a doubling in the prevalence of overweight was noted between 1971–1974 and 1999–2002 (from 5.0 to 10.3%). The most recent data (1999–2002) further show that another 15% of children and teens ages 6–19 yr and 12% of children ages 2–5 yr are considered at risk of becoming overweight.

The prevalence of overweight in children and adolescents in Canada has also been dramatically increasing. Willms et al. *(27)* assessed the prevalence of overweight and obesity among Canadian boys and girls ages 7–13 yr. Overweight and obesity were defined according to the reference proposed by the IOTF *(24).* The results revealed that over a 15-yr period the proportion of overweight Canadian children increased almost threefold, from 11.4% in 1981 to 29.3% in 1996. The prevalence of overweight was highest in children and adolescents with low socioeconomic status.

Europe

Lissau et al. *(28)* summarized the prevalence of overweight among adolescents in 13 European countries and the United States using data from nationally (or regionally for

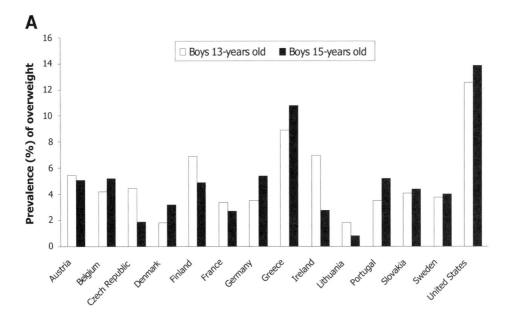

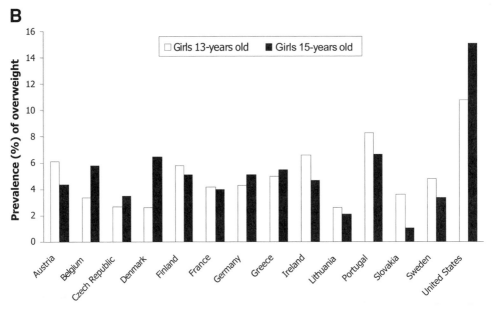

Fig. 6. Prevalence of overweight (body mass index at or above 95th percentile) in (**A**) in boys and (**B**) girls in 13 European countries and United States in 1997–1998. (From ref. *28*.)

Flemish Belgium and France) representative, cross-sectional 1997–1998 school-year surveys that used identical data collection methods. At least 1540 adolescents were included from each country. Data for BMI were based on self-reported weights and heights; these data were also used to create a reference curve (based on all 29,242 adolescents) to establish cutoff points for BMI at or above the 95th centile, defined as overweight. The prevalence of overweight was highest in the United States, Ireland, Greece, and Portugal, and lowest in Lithuania (Fig. 6).

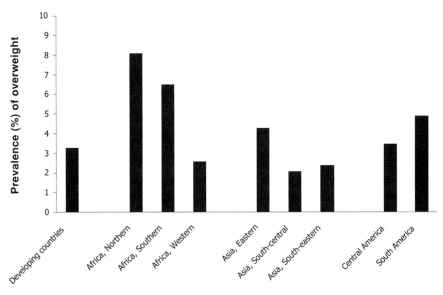

Fig. 7. Global and regional prevalence of overweight in preschool children (under 5 yr of age) in developing countries in 1995. (From ref. *29*.)

Developing Countries

de Onis and Blössner *(29)* estimated the prevalence and trends of overweight among preschool children in developing countries by using data obtained from 160 nationally representative cross-sectional surveys (in 94 countries) included in WHO's global database on child growth and malnutrition (Geneva). The data were analyzed in a standardized way to allow comparisons across countries and over time. Estimates were obtained only for regions in which the proportion of children covered by the surveys was more than 70%. Overweight was defined as a weight-for-height two standard deviations (SDs) above the international reference median value of the National Center for Health Statistics, as recommended by WHO *(30)*. Figure 7 presents the regional and global estimates of the prevalence of overweight children under 5 yr of age. The overall prevalence of overweight in children in this age group in developing countries in 1995 was estimated to be 3.3%. The highest prevalence was found in Latin America and the Caribbean (4.4%), followed by Africa (3.9%) and Asia (2.9%). The countries with the highest percentage of overweight children were in the Middle East (Quatar), North Africa (Algeria, Egypt, and Morocco), and Latin America and the Caribbean (Argentina, Chile, Bolivia, Peru, Uruguay, Costa Rica, and Jamaica). Other countries with a high prevalence of overweight were Armenia, Kiribati, Malawi, South Africa, and Uzbekistan. Of 38 countries for which trend data were available, 16 showed a rising trend, 8 showed a falling trend, and 14 showed no apparent change in the prevalence of overweight.

Other Survey Data

Wang et al. *(31)* summarized the trends of overweight in older children and adolescents ages 6–18 yr from four countries. They used nationally representative data from the United States (1971–1974 and 1988–1994), Russia (1992 and 1998), and Brazil (1975 and 1997) and nationwide survey data from China (1991 and 1997). Overweight was defined according to age- and sex-specific cutoff points recommended by IOTF *(24)*. The overweight prevalence increased during the study periods in the United States

Table 5
Time Trends in Prevalence of Overweight in Children and Adolescents in United States, Brazil, China, and Russia According to Age, Sex, and Urban or Rural Residence[a]

Overweight[b]	United States		Brazil		China		Russia	
	1971–1974	1988–1994	1974	1997	1991	1997	1992	1998
All	15.4	25.6	4.1	13.9	6.4	7.7	15.6	9.0
Children 6–9 yr	11.8	22.0	4.9	17.4	10.5	11.3	26.4	10.2
Adolescents 10–18 yr	16.8	27.3	3.7	12.6	4.5	6.2	11.5	8.5
Males	14.5	25.0	2.9	13.1	6.3	8.4	15.5	9.6
Females	16.3	26.3	5.3	14.8	6.5	7.0	15.8	8.3
Rural	16.6	26.6	3.1	8.4	5.9	6.4	17.7	11.2
Urban	14.7	24.6	4.9	18.4	7.7	12.4	14.7	8.1

[a]Adapted from ref. 31.

[b]Overweight was defined as the combined prevalence of overweight and obesity. It was calculated using IOTF standards, which were age- and sex-specific BMI cutoff points corresponding to a BMI of 25 at age 25 yr (24).

(from 15.4 to 25.6%), Brazil (from 4.1 to 13.9%), and China (from 6.4 to 7.7%), but decreased in Russia (from 15.6 to 9.0%) (Table 5). The annual rates of increase in the prevalence of overweight were 0.6% in the United States, 0.5% in Brazil, and 0.2% in China. In Russia, the overweight prevalence decreased annually by 1.1%. The proportion of overweight children and adolescents in Brazil and China was higher in urban than in rural areas (Table 4).

Summary

The past three decades have seen an explosive increase in the number of overweight children in most countries of the world. Overweight and obesity in adolescence are strong determinants of obesity and related morbidity and mortality in adulthood, with 50–80% of obese adolescents becoming obese as adults (32,33). Therefore, from a public health perspective, it is of great importance to reach children and adolescents through preventive programs addressing issues of physical inactivity and dietary practices.

PREVALENCE AND TRENDS OF TYPE 2 DIABETES IN ADULTS

United States

In the United States, the most complete information on the prevalence of type 2 diabetes has been obtained from NHANES II, NHANES III, and continuous NHANES. These surveys have provided estimates of the prevalence and time trends for both diagnosed and undiagnosed diabetes, impaired fasting glucose, and impaired glucose tolerance from representative samples of the US population. According to American Diabetes Association diagnostic criteria (34), the prevalence of diagnosed and undiagnosed diabetes in US adults ages 40–74 yr increased by 38% between 1976–1980 and 1988–1994 (from 8.9 to 12.3%) (35). During the same period, the prevalence of impaired fasting glucose increased by 49% (from 6.5 to 9.7%). Based on the most recent data from NHANES, the estimated age- and sex-adjusted prevalence of diabetes (diagnosed and undiagnosed) in the total population of adults ages 20 yr and over was

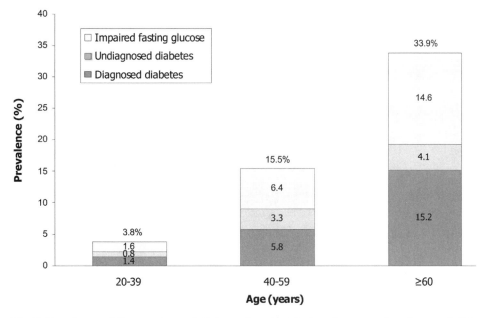

Fig. 8. Prevalence of diagnosed type 2 diabetes, impaired fasting glucose, and undiagnosed diabetes in adults ages 20 yr or over in the United States, 1999–2000. The data are from NHANES 1999–2000 *(36)*.

8.6% in 1999–2000 *(36)*. An additional 6.1% of adults had impaired fasting glucose, increasing to 14.6% for adults ages 60 yr and older. Overall, in 1999–2000, an estimated 14.5% of US adults 20 yr and over and 33.9% of those 60 yr and over had either diabetes or impaired fasting glucose (Fig. 8). The prevalence of diabetes and impaired fasting glucose was higher among non-Hispanic blacks (21.1% among those 20 yr and over) and Mexican Americans (18.8%) than among non-Hispanic whites (13.1%). The NHANES surveys observed that the proportion of undiagnosed diabetes represented approximately one-third of total diabetes and that this fraction has changed little over time.

Globally

Wild et al. *(1)* estimated the global prevalence of diabetes and the number of adults (ages 20 yr and over) with diabetes for the years 2000 and 2030. Estimates for the prevalence of diabetes by age and sex were derived from a limited number of countries and extrapolated to all 191 WHO member states and applied to United Nations population estimates for 2000 and 2030. Because most data sources did not distinguish between type 1 and type 2 diabetes, the total prevalence of diabetes was estimated. It was estimated that the prevalence of diabetes worldwide will increase by 39%, from 4.6% in 2000 to 6.4% in 2030 (Fig. 9). The prevalence is higher in developed countries than in developing countries, but the greatest relative increase in the prevalence of diabetes will occur in the developing countries in which the prevalence of diabetes is estimated to rise by 46% (from 4.1 to 6.0%). In developed countries, the prevalence is estimated to increase by 33% (from 6.3 to 8.4%). The total number of adults ages 20 yr and over with diabetes is projected to approximately double between 2000 and 2030 (from 171 million to 366 million). Overall, the prevalence of diabetes is higher in men than in women. However, more women than men have diabetes, which is most likely explained by the combined effect of a higher number of elderly women than men in

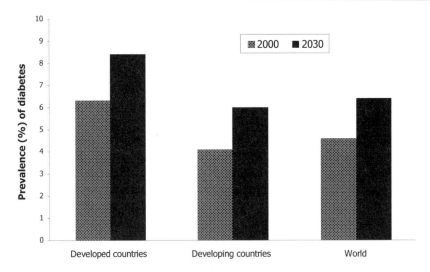

Fig. 9. Estimated prevalence (%) of type 2 diabetes in adults ages 20 yr or over in developed and developing countries and globally in years 2000 and 2030. (From ref. *1*.)

Table 6
**Top 10 Countries Globally With Highest Estimated Number
of Adults Ages 20 yr and Over With Diabetes in 2000 and 2030**[a]

		2000				*Prediction for 2030*	
Rank	*Country*	*Adults with diabetes (millions)*	*Adults with diabetes (%)*	*Rank*	*Country*	*Adults with diabetes (millions)*	*Adults with diabetes (%)*
1	India	31.6	5.5	1	India	79.3	8.0
2	China	20.7	2.4	2	China	42.2	3.7
3	United States	17.6	8.8	3	United States	30.2	11.2
4	Indonesia	8.4	6.7	4	Indonesia	21.2	10.6
5	Japan	6.8	6.7	8	Japan	8.9	8.8
6	Pakistan	5.2	7.7	5	Pakistan	13.8	8.7
7	Russian Federation	4.6	4.2	9	Philippines	7.8	10.2
8	Brazil	4.5	4.3	6	Brazil	11.3	7.0
9	Italy	4.2	9.2	10	Egypt	6.7	9.7
10	Bangladesh	3.2	4.6	7	Bangladesh	11.1	7.7

[a]Adapted from ref. *1*.

most populations and the increasing prevalence of diabetes with age. In developing countries, most adults with diabetes are in the age range of 45–65 yr, whereas in developed countries, most adults with diabetes are 65 years and above. For both 2000 and 2030, the country with the highest estimated number of adults with diabetes is India, followed by China, the United States, and Indonesia (Table 6).

Summary

The number of persons with diabetes is reaching epidemic proportions. From 2000 to 2030, the worldwide prevalence of diabetes in adults is projected to rise by 39%. The largest proportional and absolute increase will occur in developing countries, where the prevalence will rise from 4.1 to 6.0%. In India, China, and Indonesia, the adult diabetic population is estimated to more than double by 2030. In the United States, 14.5% of adults currently have diabetes (diagnosed or undiagnosed) or impaired fasting glucose.

PREVALENCE AND TRENDS OF TYPE 2 DIABETES IN CHILDREN AND ADOLESCENTS

Previously, type 2 diabetes was mainly a disease of the middle-aged and elderly. In recent decades, however, the age at onset of type 2 diabetes has decreased, and this type of diabetes has now been reported even in children and adolescents in many populations. Type 2 diabetes has been reported in children from a number of countries, including the United States, Canada, the United Kingdom, Australia, Japan, Taiwan, and India (37). National population data on the prevalence of type 2 diabetes remain limited and are unavailable for many countries. Therefore, the precise burden of type 2 diabetes in children is still unknown. However, given the rising prevalence of overweight in children, the problem is likely to be substantial.

The largest study on diabetes in children is from Japan, with about 7 million children studied between 1976 and 1997 (38). Over the 21-yr period, the incidence of type 2 diabetes increased 10-fold in children ages 6–12 yr (0.2 per 100,000/yr from 1976 to 1980 vs 2.0 per 100,000/yr from 1991 to 1995) and almost doubled among children 13–15 yr old (7.3 vs 13.9 per 100,000/yr). However, these figures are likely to be underestimated because the initial screening step of the study was a urine glucose, with blood testing reserved only for those with glycosuria. Currently, type 2 diabetes accounts for 80% of all childhood diabetes in Japan.

Data from the United States and Canada also indicate an increasing prevalence of diabetes in children. In Cincinnati, Ohio, the annual incidence of type 2 diabetes in children and adolescents 10–19 yr old increased 10-fold between 1982 and 1994 (0.7 per 100,000 vs 7.2 per 100,000) (39). Type 2 diabetes accounted for 16% of all new diagnoses of diabetes in children up to 19 yr of age and accounted for 33% of new cases among patients ages 10–19 yr (39). In Chicago, Illinois, the 10-yr average annual incidence of type 2 diabetes among African American and Latino children and adolescents (ages 0–17 yr) increased by 9% per year from 1985 (40). Among the Cree-Ojibway aboriginals in Canada, diabetes and impaired fasting glucose were observed in 1 and 3%, respectively, of children and adolescents ages 4–19 yr (41); impaired glucose tolerance was observed in 10% of those ages 10–19 yr (42).

LIFESTYLE-RELATED RISK FACTORS FOR DIABETES

Obesity and Weight Gain

Findings from epidemiological studies have repeatedly confirmed a strong positive association between excess adiposity and risk of developing type 2 diabetes. Few risk factor–disease relationships are stronger than the link between excess adiposity and diabetes. Based on data from the Behavioral Risk Factors Surveillance System conducted in the United States, Mokdad et al. (43) estimated that for every kilogram increment in self-reported body weight, the risk for diabetes increases by about 9%. Findings from a large cohort of US men, the Health Professionals Follow-up Study, showed a 7.3% increased risk of diabetes for every kilogram of weight gained (44). Using data

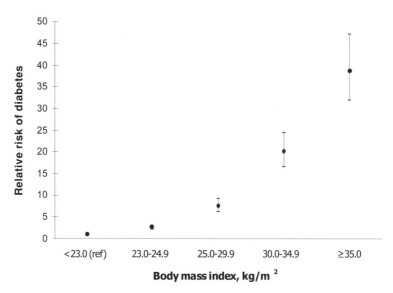

Fig. 10. Relative risk of type 2 diabetes according to body mass index in Nurses' Health Study. (From ref. *45*.)

from a large cohort of women, the Nurses' Health Study, Hu et al. *(45)* found that over-weight or obesity was the single most important determinant of diabetes, and it was estimated that approx 60% of the cases of diabetes could be attributed to overweight (BMI ≥ 25 kg/m²). Compared with women having a BMI of <23 kg/m², those with a BMI of 30–34.9 kg/m² had about a 20-fold and those with a BMI of 35 kg/m² or higher about a 40-fold increased risk of type 2 diabetes (Fig. 10) *(45)*. Results from other studies of BMI in relation to diabetes have indicated more modest associations, with approximately six- to eightfold increased risk of diabetes among those with a BMI of 30 kg/m² or higher compared with those having a BMI <23 kg/m² *(44)* or <25 kg/m² *(46,47)*. In addition to high BMI, as a measure of overall obesity, a number of studies have shown that measures of central obesity, including waist-to-hip ratio and waist cir-cumference, are important predictors of developing type 2 diabetes *(48–56)*. In some populations, central obesity has emerged as a better determinant of the development of type 2 diabetes than BMI *(50,52–55)*. For example, in a population-based cohort of Dutch men and women *(54)*, an increase of 1 SD of waist-to-thigh ratio was associated with a 42% increased risk of type 2 diabetes in men and a 92% increased risk in women, independent of BMI. After adjustment for the waist-to-thigh ratio, an increase of 1 SD of BMI was associated with a 31% increased risk of type 2 diabetes in women; BMI was not an independent determinant of risk in men *(54)*.

Weight Loss

Evidence from epidemiological studies indicates that even moderate, sustained weight loss can increase insulin sensitivity, improve insulin action, and decrease the risk of developing type 2 diabetes. In a longitudinal study of 209 Pima Indians *(57)*, a signifi-cant linear inverse relation was observed between changes in body weight and changes in insulin-stimulated glucose disposal in subjects with normal glucose tolerance and in those with impaired glucose tolerance. Improvements in insulin action after an average of 10% weight reduction were lost with weight regain but largely preserved with weight

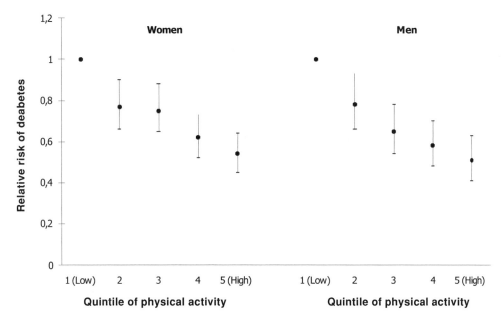

Fig. 11. Relative risk of type 2 diabetes according to total physical activity level among women in Nurses' Health Study and among men in Health Professionals Follow-up Study. (From refs. *63* and *66*.)

maintenance. In the Finnish Diabetes Prevention Study *(58)*, sustained weight reduction during a 4-yr follow-up of individuals with impaired glucose tolerance resulted in a substantial improvement in insulin sensitivity. Findings from the Framingham Study *(59)* showed that a modest amount of sustained weight loss reduced the risk of diabetes by 37% in 618 overweight individuals. The effect was even stronger for overweight (BMI $\geq$ 29 kg/m^2) individuals among whom sustained weight loss was associated with a 62% reduction in the risk of diabetes. Additionally, in the Health Professionals Follow-up Study *(44)* of 22,171 men, the risk of developing diabetes was reduced by about 50% as a result of weight loss exceeding 6 kg over a 10-yr period.

Physical Activity

A number of prospective cohort studies have indicated that physical activity is associated with a significant reduction in the risk of type 2 diabetes, whereas a sedentary lifestyle is associated with an increased risk *(45,47,60–66)*. For instance, in the Nurses' Health Study *(66)*, the risk of type 2 diabetes decreased with increasing amounts of total physical activity. Compared with women with the lowest level of total physical activity, those with the highest level had a 46% lower risk, independent of major risk factors for diabetes (Fig. 11). Moreover, the inverse dose-response relationship persisted after controlling for BMI *(66)*. In the same cohort of nurses, time spent watching television, a major sedentary behavior in the United States, was significantly positively related to the risk of diabetes *(61)*; each 2-h daily increment in watching television was associated with a 14% increase in the risk of diabetes. Similar findings were obtained from a cohort of men (the Health Professional's Follow-up Study) showing a 20% increased risk of diabetes for each 2-h daily increment in watching television *(63)*. In addition, compared with men with the lowest level of total physical activity, those with the highest level had a 49% lower risk of diabetes (Fig. 11).

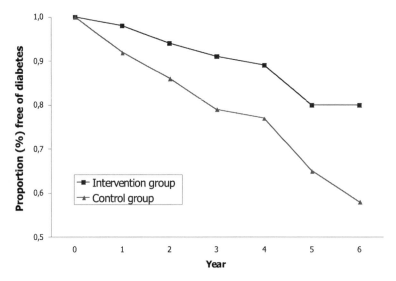

Fig. 12. Proportion of subjects remaining free of diabetes during study period in Finnish Diabetes Prevention Study. (Adapted from ref. *67*.)

Lifestyle Modification and Risk of Type 2 Diabetes

Randomized controlled trials in Finland and the United States have demonstrated the feasibility and efficiency of lifestyle intervention programs in the prevention of diabetes in individuals with impaired glucose tolerance. The lifestyle intervention program in the Finnish trial *(67)* aimed to achieve a reduction in weight of 5% or more; moderate exercise for at least 30 min/d; an intake of total and saturated fat of <30 and <10%, respectively; and an increase in fiber intake to at least 15 g/1000 kcal. Subjects in the intervention group were also recommended to consume frequently whole-grain foods, vegetables, fruits, low-fat milk and low-fat meat products, soft margarines, and vegetable oils rich in monounsaturated fatty acids. The lifestyle program was associated with a 58% reduction in risk of developing diabetes, and the 4-yr cumulative incidence of diabetes was 11% in the intervention group in comparison with 23% in the control group (Fig. 12). The US Diabetes Prevention Project *(68)* aimed to achieve and maintain a weight reduction of at least 7% through a healthy low-calorie, low-fat diet and to engage in moderate physical activity for at least 150 min/wk. This trial showed that over 3-yr, the lifestyle intervention reduced the risk of progressing from impaired glucose tolerance to diabetes by 58%, whereas the oral hypoglycemic drug metformin reduced the risk by 31%; the 3-yr cumulative incidence of diabetes was 14% in the intervention group and 29% in the control group. The results of these two trials are also similar to those from the Da Qing Impaired Glucose Tolerance and Diabetes Study in China *(69)*, showing that modification of diet and/or exercise level can significantly decrease the risk of diabetes in individuals with impaired glucose tolerance.

Summary

Besides genetic predisposition, there is ample evidence that such modifiable lifestyle factors as obesity and physical inactivity are important determinants of the development of type 2 diabetes. Furthermore, it has been demonstrated that lifestyle modifications, including changes in exercise and dietary practices, the primary factors in determining weight loss, can effectively delay or prevent the development of diabetes in high-risk groups.

CONCLUSIONS

The prevalence of obesity in adults, children, and adolescents has increased dramatically globally over the last few decades and there is no sign of it abating. About half of the adult population in the United States and other Western countries is currently estimated to be overweight or obese. Urban areas of some developing countries are approaching similar proportions.

As for obesity, the number of persons with diabetes is reaching epidemic proportions *(70)*, and it has been projected that the prevalence will grow substantially over the next several decades *(1)*. The increasing prevalence of type 2 diabetes is indicative of the effects of globalization and industrialization, which affects all nations, with obesity, sedentary lifestyle, and inappropriate diet the predominant factors involved.

Because obesity and diabetes are major causes of morbidity and mortality, reversing the obesity and diabetes epidemics is of utmost importance. The trend of increasing prevalence of obesity and diabetes all over the world has already imposed an enormous burden on health-care systems, and this will continue to increase in the future. Thus, prevention of these two diseases in adults, and especially in children and adolescents, should be an essential component of future public health intervention programs.

REFERENCES

1. Wild S, Roglic G, Green A, Sicree R, King H. Global prevalence of diabetes: estimates for the year 2000 and projections for 2030. Diabetes Care 2004;27:1047–1053.
2. WHO Consultation on Obesity. Obesity: Preventing and Managing the Global Epidemic. WHO Technical Report Series 894. World Health Organization, Geneva, Switzerland, 2000.
3. Flegal KM, Carroll MD, Ogden CL, Johnson CL. Prevalence and trends in obesity among US adults, 1999–2000. JAMA 2002;288:1723–1727.
4. Hedley AA, Ogden CL, Johnson CL, Carroll MD, Curtin LR, Flegal KM. Prevalence of overweight and obesity among US children, adolescents, and adults, 1999–2002. JAMA 2004;291:2847–2850.
5. Katzmarzyk PT. The Canadian obesity epidemic: an historical perspective. Obes Res 2002;10: 666–674.
6. Monteiro CA, D'A Benicio MH, Conde WL, Popkin BM. Shifting obesity trends in Brazil. Eur J Clin Nutr 2000;54:342–346.
7. Fernald LC, Gutierrez JP, Neufeld LM, et al. High prevalence of obesity among the poor in Mexico. JAMA 2004;291:2544, 2545.
8. Molarius A, Seidell JC, Sans S, Tuomilehto J, Kuulasmaa K. Educational level, relative body weight, and changes in their association over 10 years: an international perspective from the WHO MONICA Project. Am J Public Health 2000;90:1260–1268.
9. Lahti-Koski M, Jousilahti P, Pietinen P. Secular trends in body mass index by birth cohort in eastern Finland from 1972 to 1997. Int J Obes Relat Metab Disord 2001;25:727–734.
10. Midthjell K, Kruger O, Holmen J, et al. Rapid changes in the prevalence of obesity and known diabetes in an adult Norwegian population. The Nord-Trondelag Health Surveys: 1984–1986 and 1995–1997. Diabetes Care 1999;22:1813–1820.
11. Visscher TL, Kromhout D, Seidell JC. Long-term and recent time trends in the prevalence of obesity among Dutch men and women. Int J Obes Relat Metab Disord 2002;26:1218–1224.
12. Lissner L, Johansson SE, Qvist J, Rossner S, Wolk A. Social mapping of the obesity epidemic in Sweden. Int J Obes Relat Metab Disord 2000;24:801–805.
13. Seidell JC. The epidemiology of obesity. In: Björntorp P, ed. International Textbook of Obesity. John Wiley, Chichester, UK, 2001, pp. 23–29.
14. Marques-Vidal P, Ruidavets JB, Cambou JP, Ferrieres J. Trends in overweight and obesity in middle-aged subjects from southwestern France, 1985–1997. Int J Obes Relat Metab Disord 2002;26:732–734.
15. Martorell R, Khan LK, Hughes ML, Grummer-Strawn LM. Obesity in women from developing countries. Eur J Clin Nutr 2000;54:247–252.
16. Yoshiike N, Seino F, Tajima S, et al. Twenty-year changes in the prevalence of overweight in Japanese adults: the National Nutrition Survey 1976–1995. Obes Rev 2002;3:183–190.

17. Bell AC, Ge K, Popkin BM. Weight gain and its predictors in Chinese adults. Int J Obes Relat Metab Disord 2001;25:1079–1086.

18. Ball MJ, Wilson BD, Robertson IK, Wilson N, Russell DG. Obesity and body fat distribution in New Zealanders: a pattern of coronary heart disease risk. N Z Med J 1993;106:69–72.

19. Bennett SA, Magnus P. Trends in cardiovascular risk factors in Australia: results from the National Heart Foundation's Risk Factor Prevalence Study, 1980–1989. Med J Aust 1994;161:519–527.

20. Reddy KS, Prabhakaran D, Shah P, Shah B. Differences in body mass index and waist: hip ratios in North Indian rural and urban populations. Obes Rev 2002;3:197–202.

21. Hodge AM, Dowse GK, Zimmet PZ, Collins VR. Prevalence and secular trends in obesity in Pacific and Indian Ocean island populations. Obes Res 1995;3(Suppl 2):77s–87s.

22. Kortt MA, Langley PC, Cox ER. A review of cost-of-illness studies on obesity. Clin Ther 1998;20:772–779.

23. Kuczmarski RJ, Ogden CL, Guo SS, et al. 2000 CDC growth charts for the United States: methods and development. Vital Health Stat 11 2002;246:1–190.

24. Cole TJ, Bellizzi MC, Flegal KM, Dietz WH. Establishing a standard definition for child overweight and obesity worldwide: international survey. BMJ 2000;320:1240–1243.

25. Ogden CL, Flegal KM, Carroll MD, Johnson CL. Prevalence and trends in overweight among US children and adolescents, 1999–2000. JAMA 2002;288:1728–1732.

26. Prevalence of Overweight Among Children and Adolescents: United States, 1999. National Center for Health Statistics. Accessed June 8, 2004, at www.cdc.gov/nchs/products/pubs/pubd/hestats/overwght99.htm.

27. Willms JD, Tremblay MS, Katzmarzyk PT. Geographic and demographic variation in the prevalence of overweight Canadian children. Obes Res 2003;11:668–673.

28. Lissau I, Overpeck MD, Ruan WJ, Due P, Holstein BE, Hediger ML. Body mass index and overweight in adolescents in 13 European countries, Israel, and the United States. Arch Pediatr Adolesc Med 2004;158:27–33.

29. de Onis M, Blössner M. Prevalence and trends of overweight among preschool children in developing countries. Am J Clin Nutr 2000;72:1032–1039.

30. World Health Organization. Physical Status: The Use and Interpretation of Anthropometry. Report of a WHO Expert Committee. World Health Organ Tech Rep Ser. World Health Organization, Geneva, Switzerland, 1995: 854.

31. Wang Y, Monteiro C, Popkin BM. Trends of obesity and underweight in older children and adolescents in the United States, Brazil, China, and Russia. Am J Clin Nutr 2002;75:971–977.

32. Must A, Strauss RS. Risks and consequences of childhood and adolescent obesity. Int J Obes Relat Metab Disord 1999;23(Suppl 2):S2–S11.

33. Guo SS, Chumlea WC. Tracking of body mass index in children in relation to overweight in adulthood. Am J Clin Nutr 1999;70:145S–148S.

34. Report of the expert committee on the diagnosis and classification of diabetes mellitus. Diabetes Care 1997;20:1183–1197.

35. Harris MI, Flegal KM, Cowie CC, et al. Prevalence of diabetes, impaired fasting glucose, and impaired glucose tolerance in US adults: the Third National Health and Nutrition Examination Survey, 1988–1994. Diabetes Care 1998;21:518–524.

36. Prevalence of diabetes and impaired fasting glucose in adults—United States, 1999–2000. MMWR Morb Mortal Wkly Rep 2003;52:833–837.

37. Alberti G, Zimmet P, Shaw J, Bloomgarden Z, Kaufman F, Silink M. Type 2 diabetes in the young: the evolving epidemic: the international diabetes federation consensus workshop. Diabetes Care 2004;27:1798–1811.

38. Kitagawa T, Owada M, Urakami T, Yamauchi K. Increased incidence of non-insulin dependent diabetes mellitus among Japanese schoolchildren correlates with an increased intake of animal protein and fat. Clin Pediatr (Phila) 1998;37:111–115.

39. Pinhas-Hamiel O, Dolan LM, Daniels SR, Standiford D, Khoury PR, Zeitler P. Increased incidence of non-insulin-dependent diabetes mellitus among adolescents. J Pediatr 1996;128:608–615.

40. Lipton R, Keenan H, Onyemere KU, Freels S. Incidence and onset features of diabetes in African-American and Latino children in Chicago, 1985–1994. Diabetes Metab Res Rev 2002;18: 135–142.

41. Dean HJ, Young TK, Flett B, Wood-Steiman P. Screening for type-2 diabetes in aboriginal children in northern Canada. Lancet 1998;352:1523, 1524.

42. Harris SB, Gittelsohn J, Hanley A, et al. The prevalence of NIDDM and associated risk factors in native Canadians. Diabetes Care 1997;20:185–187.

43. Mokdad AH, Ford ES, Bowman BA, et al. Diabetes trends in the U.S.: 1990–1998. Diabetes Care 2000;23:1278–1283.

44. Koh-Banerjee P, Wang Y, Hu FB, Spiegelman D, Willett WC, Rimm EB. Changes in body weight and body fat distribution as risk factors for clinical diabetes in US men. Am J Epidemiol 2004;159:1150–1159.

45. Hu FB, Manson JE, Stampfer MJ, et al. Diet, lifestyle, and the risk of type 2 diabetes mellitus in women. N Engl J Med 2001;345:790–797.

46. Mokdad AH, Ford ES, Bowman BA, et al. Prevalence of obesity, diabetes, and obesity-related health risk factors, 2001. JAMA 2003;289:76–79.

47. Hu G, Lindstrom J, Valle TT, et al. Physical activity, body mass index, and risk of type 2 diabetes in patients with normal or impaired glucose regulation. Arch Intern Med 2004;164:892–896.

48. Chan JM, Rimm EB, Colditz GA, Stampfer MJ, Willett WC. Obesity, fat distribution, and weight gain as risk factors for clinical diabetes in men. Diabetes Care 1994;17:961–969.

49. Carey VJ, Walters EE, Colditz GA, et al. Body fat distribution and risk of non-insulin-dependent diabetes mellitus in women: the Nurses' Health Study. Am J Epidemiol 1997;145:614–619.

50. Wei M, Gaskill SP, Haffner SM, Stern MP. Waist circumference as the best predictor of noninsulin dependent diabetes mellitus (NIDDM) compared to body mass index, waist/hip ratio and other anthropometric measurements in Mexican Americans—a 7-year prospective study. Obes Res 1997;5:16–23.

51. Edelstein SL, Knowler WC, Bain RP, et al. Predictors of progression from impaired glucose tolerance to NIDDM: an analysis of six prospective studies. Diabetes 1997;46:701–710.

52. de Vegt F, Dekker JM, Jager A, et al. Relation of impaired fasting and postload glucose with incident type 2 diabetes in a Dutch population: the Hoorn Study. JAMA 2001;285:2109–2113.

53. Warne DK, Charles MA, Hanson RL, et al. Comparison of body size measurements as predictors of NIDDM in Pima Indians. Diabetes Care 1995;18:435–439.

54. Snijder MB, Dekker JM, Visser M, et al. Associations of hip and thigh circumferences independent of waist circumference with the incidence of type 2 diabetes: the Hoorn Study. Am J Clin Nutr 2003;77:1192–1197.

55. Han TS, Feskens EJ, Lean ME, Seidell JC. Associations of body composition with type 2 diabetes mellitus. Diabet Med 1998;15:129–135.

56. Okosun IS, Cooper RS, Rotimi CN, Osotimehin B, Forrester T. Association of waist circumference with risk of hypertension and type 2 diabetes in Nigerians, Jamaicans, and African-Americans. Diabetes Care 1998;21:1836–1842.

57. Weyer C, Hanson K, Bogardus C, Pratley RE. Long-term changes in insulin action and insulin secretion associated with gain, loss, regain and maintenance of body weight. Diabetologia 2000;43:36–46.

58. Uusitupa M, Lindi V, Louheranta A, Salopuro T, Lindstrom J, Tuomilehto J. Long-term improvement in insulin sensitivity by changing lifestyles of people with impaired glucose tolerance: 4-year results from the Finnish Diabetes Prevention Study. Diabetes 2003;52:2532–2538.

59. Moore LL, Visioni AJ, Wilson PW, D'Agostino RB, Finkle WD, Ellison RC. Can sustained weight loss in overweight individuals reduce the risk of diabetes mellitus? Epidemiology 2000;11:269–273.

60. Burchfiel CM, Sharp DS, Curb JD, et al. Physical activity and incidence of diabetes: the Honolulu Heart Program. Am J Epidemiol 1995;141:360–368.

61. Hu FB, Li TY, Colditz GA, Willett WC, Manson JE. Television watching and other sedentary behaviors in relation to risk of obesity and type 2 diabetes mellitus in women. JAMA 2003;289:1785–1791.

62. Helmrich SP, Ragland DR, Leung RW, Paffenbarger RS Jr. Physical activity and reduced occurrence of non-insulin-dependent diabetes mellitus. N Engl J Med 1991;325:147–152.

63. Hu FB, Leitzmann MF, Stampfer MJ, Colditz GA, Willett WC, Rimm EB. Physical activity and television watching in relation to risk for type 2 diabetes mellitus in men. Arch Intern Med 2001;161:1542–1548.

64. Lynch J, Helmrich SP, Lakka TA, et al. Moderately intense physical activities and high levels of cardiorespiratory fitness reduce the risk of non-insulin-dependent diabetes mellitus in middle-aged men. Arch Intern Med 1996;156:1307–1314.

65. Wannamethee SG, Shaper AG, Alberti KG. Physical activity, metabolic factors, and the incidence of coronary heart disease and type 2 diabetes. Arch Intern Med 2000;160:2108–2116.

66. Hu FB, Sigal RJ, Rich-Edwards JW, et al. Walking compared with vigorous physical activity and risk of type 2 diabetes in women: a prospective study. JAMA 1999;282:1433–1439.

67. Tuomilehto J, Lindstrom J, Eriksson JG, et al. Prevention of type 2 diabetes mellitus by changes in lifestyle among subjects with impaired glucose tolerance. N Engl J Med 2001;344:1343–1350.
68. Knowler WC, Barrett-Connor E, Fowler SE, et al. Reduction in the incidence of type 2 diabetes with lifestyle intervention or metformin. N Engl J Med 2002;346:393–403.
69. Pan XR, Li GW, Hu YH, et al. Effects of diet and exercise in preventing NIDDM in people with impaired glucose tolerance: the Da Qing IGT and Diabetes Study. Diabetes Care 1997;20:537–544.
70. Zimmet P. Globalization, coca-colonization and the chronic disease epidemic: can the Doomsday scenario be averted? J Intern Med 2000;247:301–310.

II GENETICS AND PATHOPHYSIOLOGY

3

Genetics of Obesity and Diabetes

Despina Sanoudou, PhD, FACMG, Cbiol, MIbiol
and Christos S. Mantzoros, MD, DSc

CONTENTS

INTRODUCTION

Obesity and diabetes mellitus are two disease states with significant morbidity and mortality, the prevalence of which is reaching the point of an international epidemic, with continuously increasing numbers of affected individuals *(1)*. Full elucidation of the pathogenesis of obesity and diabetes mellitus and, thus, the development of preventative and therapeutic approaches require delineation of the genetic defects associated with these disease states and clarification of the molecular mechanisms that lead from genotype to phenotype. This chapter focuses on recent advances in the field and, by presenting data from several large-scale human studies and a wide range of animal models, outlines researchers' current knowledge on the genetics of obesity and diabetes (with an emphasis on type 2 diabetes). A good understanding of the mutations and molecular pathways involved in the development of disease could allow presymptomatic diagnosis and more accurate prognosis and could eventually reveal better therapeutic targets.

OBESITY

Obesity is a complex trait with multifactorial etiology, including behavioral, environmental, and genetic factors. The genetic contribution to obesity in humans has been established from a series of family, twin, and adoption studies, and the estimated heritability of body mass index (BMI) seems to range between 50 and 90% *(2)*. It is, however, difficult to reconcile the genetic etiology of common human obesity with the markedly variable prevalence of the disease in individuals of different socioeconomic backgrounds and demographic origins *(3)* (see www.who.int). One of the hypotheses

From: *Contemporary Diabetes: Obesity and Diabetes*
Edited by: C. S. Mantzoros © Humana Press Inc., Totowa, NJ

based on mouse studies proposes that susceptibility to obesity is determined largely by genetic factors, but that the environment determines phenotypic expression *(4)*.

Extensive studies mainly involving the "candidate gene" and the "genome-scanning" approaches have been performed to date, in an effort to identify genes contributing to or responsible for obesity. In the majority of cases, obesity is believed to result from interactions of multiple "susceptibility" genes, and only a few rare cases have been attributed to single gene mutations *(see* "Human Monogenetic Studies" section). Significant variability has also been observed in the genetic predisposition for obesity in different ethnic groups, and different genes have been proposed to lead to obesity at different ages *(5)*. A forum entitled the "Human Obesity Gene Map" has been established that includes the findings of all genetic studies conducted to decipher the genetics of obesity (http://obesitygene.pbrc.edu/).

Animal Studies

MONOGENIC STUDIES

Genetic studies of animal models have contributed significantly to the current understanding of obesity. Approximately 10 mouse models with naturally occurring single gene mutations are available and have been extensively studied *(6)* (for an up-to-date list, visit the web site http://obesitygene.pbrc.edu/). The obese (ob) mouse model is regarded as the classic animal model of obesity, caused by a mutation in the leptin *(Lep)* gene that prevents leptin secretion from the adipose tissue *(7)*. This mouse model has been instrumental in the dissection of the leptin signaling pathway. Other single gene mutation mouse models of obesity include the agouti yellow (A^y) *(8)*, tubby (tub) *(9)*, diabetic (db) *(10)*, fat (fat) *(11)*, and mahogany (mg) *(12)* mutant mouse strains, with mutations in the nonagouti *(a)*, tubby candidate *(Tub)*, leptin receptor *(Lepr)*, carboxypeptidase E *(Cpe)*, and attractin *(Atrn)* genes, respectively. All naturally occurring single gene mutations are recessive with the exception of the agouti yellow, which is dominant. A comprehensive list of these mouse models and references on their phenotype can be found at http://obesitygene.pbrc.edu/natural.htm. Interestingly, the majority of naturally occurring mutations affect genes of the leptin-melanocortin pathway (Fig. 1).

A large number of knockout (KO) and transgenic mouse obesity models have been generated, on the background of either wild-type (WT) mouse strains or different obese mouse strains *(13)*. Examples of the mutated genes include members of the leptin-melanocortin pathway such as pro-piomelanocortin *(POMC) (14)* and melanocortin-4 receptor *(MC4R) (15)*, as well as promelanin-concentrating hormone *(PMCH)*, perilipin *(PLIN)*, and nitric oxide synthase 2 (inducible, macrophage) *(NOS2)*, which are involved in the regulation of energy expenditure (EE) and insulin resistance, respectively *(16–18)*.

β-Adrenergic receptor (βAR) *(ADRB)*-deficient mice have also been generated, establishing the role of βArs in the body's defense against diet-induced obesity *(19)*. Chemical mutagenesis recently generated the SMA1 mouse that carries a growth hormone *(GH)* mutation, reducing/eliminating its expression, which presents with excessive amounts of visceral fat *(20–23)*.

POLYGENIC STUDIES

Numerous polygenic mouse models of obesity have been generated. Some are inbred mouse lines, whereas others result from repeated selections of noninbred mice. Multiple

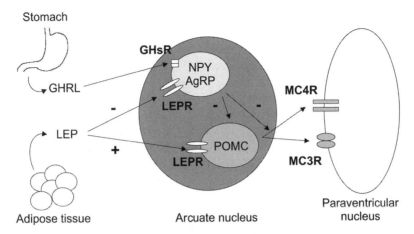

Fig. 1. The leptin-melanocortin pathway involves leptin (LEP) secretion from adipocytes into the circulation, binding to its receptor (LEPR) in the central nervous system (CNS), resulting in altered production of pro-piomelanocortin (POMC), neuropeptide Y (NPY) and agouti-related protein (AgRP). Cleavage of POMC by proprotein convertase subtilisin/kexin type 1 (PCSK1) to give α-melanocyte-stimulating hormone (α-MSH) and adrenocorticotropin (adrenocorticotropic hormone) α-MSH can, in turn, bind and activate melanocortin-3 receptor (MC3R) and MC4Rs, which inhibit food intake and alter energy homeostasis. Ghrelin (GHRL) is secreted by the stomach, acts on growth hormone secretagogue receptors (GHsR), and signals hunger.

crosses, particularly between mouse strains with extremely different phenotypes, enable the identification of >130 quantitative trait loci (QTL) associated with obesity (http://obesitygene.pbrc.edu/). It is noteworthy that different QTL have been associated with the age of onset and gender in obesity (e.g., *see* refs. *24–26*). Certain loci only contribute to obesity by interaction with other loci, whereas pairs of loci can have a coordinate effect on correlated traits such as body and muscle weight and leptin concentration *(27)*.

A number of other species, including rat *(Rattus norvegicus)*, wild pig *(Sus scrofa)*, and cow *(Bos bovis)* (e.g., *see* refs. *28–30*), have served as experimental models for obesity, and additional ones, such as baboon, are emerging as future targets *(31)*. Animal models of obesity, particularly of species genetically closer to humans, may prove to be invaluable in pharmaceutical research, especially in identifying therapeutic targets and evaluating the efficiency and side effects of drug candidates.

Human Studies

POLYGENIC STUDIES

The "Human Obesity Gene Map" includes an extensive list of susceptibility genes that can lead to obesity independently and/or by interacting with other genes and/or environmental factors.

Genomewide scans for obesity susceptibility genes have been performed in hundreds of families mostly of North American and European origin, but also African American, Asian, Mexican American, Pima Indian, and others. The two main approaches involved linkage analysis and association studies. By these approaches more than 200 obesity susceptibility loci have been identified, localizing on almost all human chromosomes, except chromosome 21 and Y. Examples of strong linkage include chromosomes 2, 5, 10, 11, and 20 *(32)*.

More than 60 candidate genes have been proved to have some role in obesity susceptibility (http://obesitygene.pbrc.edu/). One example is the β3AR *(ADRB3)* on 8p12-p11, which is involved in the regulation of lipid metabolism, leptin production, and thermogenesis. Its Trp64Arg variant has been frequently, but not always, found to correlate with increased abdominal/visceral adipocity, lower EE, and greater resistance to weight loss in various populations *(33–36)*. Variants of the adipocyte-secreted hormone adiponectin, as well as variants of the transcription factor peroxisome proliferator-activated receptor γ (PPARγ) (such as Pro12Ala, Pro115Gln, and C1431T) have also been associated with BMI *(37–41)*. The Pro12Ala variant of PPARγ2, in particular, is also thought to interact with diet *(42)*, to induce obesity and insulin resistance.

Extensive linkage studies have given rise to multiple positional gene candidates, such as insulin receptor substrate 1 *(IRS1)* and calpain 10 *(CAPN10)* on 2q34-q37; tubby-like protein 4 *(TULP4)*, acetyl-CoenzymeA acetyltransferase 2 *(ACAT2)*, and tumor necrosis factor-α-induced protein 3 *(TNFAIP3)* on 6q23-q27; glucokinase *(GK)* and neuropeptide Y *(NPY)* on 7p15-p14; and apolipoprotein A-IV *(APOA4)* and dopamine receptor 2 *(DRD2)* on 11q22-q24.

Other genes without a direct association to obesity may play a modifying role in certain aspects of obesity. For example, a polymorphism in the ghrelin *(GHRL)* gene seems to be associated with childhood-onset obesity *(43)*. A polymorphism in the hormone-sensitive lipase gene *(LIPE)* contributes to baseline body composition in a gender-, age-, and insulin-dependent manner *(44)*.

Finally, some genes have been implicated in gene–environment interactions. For example, lipoprotein lipase *(LPL)* and β2AR *(ADRB2)* gene polymorphisms have been associated with gene–exercise interactions *(45–47)*. Furthermore, a gene–gene interaction has been described for *LPL* and *ADRB2*, with combinations of certain variants having various effects on BMI *(48)*.

MONOGENIC STUDIES

Genes. A limited number of monogenic obesity cases affecting different parts of the leptin-melanocortin pathway have been identified (Fig. 1). Because only a few obese subjects have been reported to have *LEP* mutations, elevated leptin levels probably reflecting leptin resistance are the most common characteristics of human obesity and suggest that defects downstream of leptin are responsible for obesity in the vast majority of human subjects *(49–52)*. Mutations, albeit rare, have also been found in *LEPR, PCSK1*, and *POMC (14,53,54)*. The most common are mutations in the *MC4R* gene, which regulates feeding behavior and is responsible for up to 7% of pediatric obesity in several studies *(55–57)*. Other single gene mutations leading to obesity involve *PPARG*, single-minded homolog 1 *(SIM1)*, and melanocortin receptor-3 *(MC3R) (39,58–60)*. Details on the mutations and the resulting phenotype can be found at http://obesity-gene.pbrc.edu/cgi-bin/ace/sgd_table.cgi.

Syndromes. A number of genetic syndromes present with obesity as one of their clinical features, although in some of them it is more frequent than in others. In summary, there are approx 18 autosomal dominant, 15 autosomal recessive, 10 X-linked, and 1 digenic syndromes. Examples include the syndromes Prader-Willi (hypotonia, cognitive impairment, morbid obesity), Bardet-Biedl 1-7 (Table 1), WAGR (Wilms tumor, aniridia, genital anomalies, retardation), Alstrom (Table 1), Wilson-Turner (mental retardation, gynecomastia), Cohen (psychomotor retardation, hypotonia, joint laxity, progressive retinochoroidal dystrophy), and achondroplasia (abnormal bone growth).

Table 1
Monogenic Disorders Associated With Diabetes Mellitus and Obesity[a]

Condition	Gene	Gene symbol	Type of diabetes	Obesity	Additional clinical features	Mode of inheritance
Aceruloplasminemia	Ceruloplasmin	CP	1		Progressive dementia, extrapyramidal disorders, cerebellar ataxia, and diabetes mellitus	Autosomal recessive
Autoimmune Polyendocrine Syndrome type I (APS-1 or APECED)	Autoimmune regulator E	AIRE	1		Autoimmune polyendocrinopathy, candidiasis, ectodermal dystrophy	Autosomal recessive or dominant
Cystic fibrosis	Cystic fibrosis transmembrane conductance regulator	CFTR	1		Chronic sinopulmonary disease, gastrointestinal/nutritional abnormalities, obstructive azoospermia, salt loss syndromes	Autosomal recessive
Immune dysregulation, Polyendocrinopathy, Enteropahty, X-linked syndrome (IPEX or XPID)	Forkhead box P3	FOXP3	1		Immune dysregulation, polyendocrino-pathy, enteropathy	X-linked
Wolfram syndrome	Wolframin	WFS1	1		Diabetes insipidus, optic atrophy, deafness	Autosomal recessive
Bardet-Biedl syndrome (BBS)	Bardet-Biedl syndrome 1,2,4, 6–8	BBS1,2, 4,6–8	1	Yes	Mental retardation, dysphormic extremities, retinal dystrophy or pigmentary retinopathy	Autosomal recessive (triallelic inheritance)
Cystinosis, nephropathic (CTNS)	Cystinosin	CTNS	1			Under study
Multiple epiphyseal dysplasia, with early-onset diabetes mellitus (or Wolcott-Rallison syndrome)	Translation initiation factor 2-α kinase-3	EIF2AK3	1		Demineralization of bone with multiple fractures, tooth discoloration, skin abnormalities	Under study

(Continued)

43

Table 1 *(Continued)*

Condition	Gene	Gene symbol	Type of diabetes	Obesity	Additional clinical features	Mode of inheritance
Bloom syndrome (BLM)	RecQ protein-like-3	RECQL3	1 or 2		Proportionate pre- and postnatal growth deficiency; sun-sensitive, telangiectatic, hypo- and hyperpigmented skin; predisposition to malignancy; chromosomal instability	Autosomal recessive
Friedreich's ataxia	Frataxin	FRDA	1 or 2		Cerebellar degeneration, cardiomyopathy	Autosomal recessive
Alstrom syndrome	Alstrom syndrome 1	ALMS1	2	Yes	Deafness, retinal degeneration	Autosomal recessive
Berardinelli-Seip congenital lipodystrophy	Seipin; 1-acylglrlycerol-3-phosphate O-acyltransferase 2	BSCL2; AGPAT2	2	Yes	Congenital lipodystrophy, insulin resistance, hypertriglyceridemia	Autosomal recessive
Cockayne syndrome, type 1 (CKN1)	Cockayne syndrome 1 gene	CKN1	2		Dwarfism, pigmentary retinal degeneration, optic atrophy, deafness, marble epiphyses in some digits, photosensitivity, mental retardation	Autosomal recessive
Congenital disorder of glycosylation type Ia (or carbohydrate-deficient glycoprotein syndrome)	Phosphomannomutase-2	PMM2	2			Autosomal recessive
Dunnigan-type familial partial lipodystrophy (FPLD)	Lamin A/C	LMNA	2	Yes		Autosomal dominant
Hemochromatosis	Hemochromatosis gene	HFE	2		Cirrhosis, hypogonadism, hyperpigmentation	Autosomal recessive
Hyperproinsulinemia	Insulin	INS	2		Fasting hyperglycemia, impaired glucose tolerance	Autosomal dominant

Disease	Protein	Gene			Features	Inheritance
Late onset familial partial lipodystrophy (FPLD)	Peroxisome proliferator-activated receptor-γ	*PPARG*	2	Yes		Autosomal dominant
Leprechaunism (Donohue syndrome)	Insulin receptor	*IR*	2			Autosomal recessive
Mandibuloacral dysplasia (MAD)	Lamin A/C	*LMNA*	2			Autosomal recessive
Maternally Inherited Diabetes and Deafness (MIDD)	Mitochondrial leucyl tRNA 1	*MTTL1*	2		Deafness	Maternal
Maturity-Onset Diabetes of the Young 1 (MODY1)	Hepatocyte nuclear factor 4a	*HNF4A*	2		Microvascular complications	Autosomal dominant
Maturity-Onset Diabetes of the Young 2 (MODY2)	Glucokinase	*GCK*	2		Impaired fasting glucose, impaired glucose tolerance	Autosomal dominant
Maturity-Onset Diabetes of the Young 3 (MODY3)	Hepatocyte nuclear factor 1a	*HNF1A or TCF1*	2		Microvascular complications, increased sensitivity to sulfonylureas	Autosomal dominant
Maturity-Onset Diabetes of the Young 4 (MODY4)	Insulin promoter factor 1	*IPF1*	2		Pancreatic agenesis (when homozygote)	Autosomal dominant
Maturity-Onset Diabetes of the Young 5 (MODY5)	Hepatocyte nuclear factor 1b	*HNF1B or TCF2*	2		Renal cysts, urogenital malformations	Autosomal dominant
Maturity-Onset Diabetes of the Young 6 (MODY6)	Neurogenic differentiation 1	*NEUROD1*	2			Autosomal dominant

(*Continued*)

Table 1 (*Continued*)

Condition	Gene	Gene symbol	Type of diabetes	Obesity	Additional clinical features	Mode of inheritance
Myotonic dystrophy			2			Autosomal dominant
Pineal hyperplasia, insulin-resistant diabetes mellitus, and somatic abnormalities (or Rabson-Mendenhall syndrome)	Insulin receptor	IR	2	Yes	Dental and skin abnormalities, abdominal distension, phallic enlargement	Autosomal recessive
Polycystic ovarian syndrome (PCOS1 or Stein-Leventhal syndrome)	Cytochrome P450, subfamily XIA	CYP11A	2	Yes	Hirsutism, amenorrhea, hyperinsulinism	Autosomal dominant
Thiamin-responsive megaloblastic anemia syndrome (TRMA or Rogers syndrome)	Solute carrier family 19 (thiamine transporter), member 2	SLC19A2	2		Thiamine-responsive anemia, deafness	Autosomal recessive
Type A insulin resistance	Insulin receptor	IR	2		Acanthosis nigricans, hyperandrogenism	
Werner syndrome	RecQ protein-like-2	RECQL2	2		Scleroderma-like skin changes, cataract, SC calcification, premature arteriosclerosis	Autosomal recessive
Ataxia telangiectasia (AT)	Ataxia-telangiectasia mutated	ATM	2		Immune defects, predisposition to malignancy	Autosomal recessive

[a]Examples of genetic disorders associated with type 1 and/or 2 diabetes mellitus and obesity are presented.

The causative or strong candidate genes are known for the majority of these syndromes. A detailed review of obesity-related genetic syndromes is beyond the scope of this chapter. More information is available at http://obesitygene.pbrc.edu/.

DIABETES

Type 1 Diabetes

Type 1 diabetes is a heterogeneous and multifactorial autoimmune disease currently thought to result from a combination of genetic and environmental factors. The incidence of the disease is variable in different populations, ranging from approx 20 cases yearly per 100,000 individuals among Northern European populations to only 0.4–1.1 cases yearly per 100,000 individuals among Asians. This may be related to different frequencies of susceptibility genes in each population *(61)*.

ANIMAL STUDIES

Animal models with specific genetic alterations are powerful tools in the understanding of complex polygenic diseases because interindividual variation is minimized, environmental parameters can be carefully controlled, large sample numbers are easy to obtain, and all tissues can be easily accessed at any age. Therefore, the downstream effects of naturally occurring or experimentally introduced mutations can be effectively studied. A number of animal models have been used to elucidate the molecular mechanisms underlying type 1 diabetes. Spontaneous mutations in several inbred rodent lines, such as the nonobese diabetic mouse (NOD), the Bio-Breeding Diabetes-Prone rat, and the Komeda Diabetes-Prone subline of the Long-Evans Tokushima Lean rat, led to sublines that succumb to type 1 diabetes with varying incidence *(62–64)*. The NOD mouse has been used most extensively to date, with transgenic and gene-targeted models generated for a long series of different genes including major histocompatibility complex (MHC) molecules (e.g., D57, HLA-DRα, HLA-DQ6), cytokines (interleukin-2 [IL-2], tumor neurosis factor-α [TNF-α], transforming growth factor-β1), autoantigens (proinsulin, HSP60, GAD), costimulatory molecules (CD152, CD80), and T-cell receptors (BDC2.5, BOC8.3) (reviewed in ref. *65*). When defective, particularly in β-cells, some of these genes can accelerate or inhibit the development of diabetes. Despite the large number of diabetogenes, two checkpoints have been clearly defined, the first regulating the onset of insulitis at about 3 wk of age and the second controlling the transition to overt disease at about 8–12 wk *(66)*. Interestingly, it appears that IL-12 plays a crucial role in the regulation of the former *(67)*.

More recently, human genes associated with type 1 diabetes, such as MHC molecules, have also been transgenically expressed in mice *(68)* and are expected to offer important new information.

HUMAN STUDIES

The contribution of genetics to the pathogenesis of type 1 diabetes is supported by several lines of evidence demonstrating (1) that the lifetime risk of 1:300 in the general Caucasian population is in sharp contrast to the 1:6 risk in the case of affected first-degree relatives, and to 1:3 in monozygotic twins *(69)*; and (2) that the estimated monozygotic twin concordance rate range of 21–70% is significantly higher than the 0–13% range for dizygotic twins *(70)*.

Polygenic Factors. Population studies have revealed that more than 20 genetic loci, designated as insulin-dependent diabetes mellitus (IDDM) loci, are significantly linked

Table 2
Loci Linked to Type 1 Diabetes[d]

Locus	Location	Marker (candidate genes)	Reference
IDDM1	6p21	HLA (human leukocyte antigen)	[a,b,c]
IDDM2	11p15	INS VNTR (insulin)	(Bell et al. 1984)[a,b,c]
IDDM3	15q26	D15S107	(Field et al. 1996)[a,b]
IDDM4	11q13	FGF3 (fibroblast growth factor 3) (LRP5 [low-density lipoprotein receptor–related protein 5] candidate)	(Hashimoto et al. 1994)[a,b]
IDDM5	6q25.1	ESR1 (estrogen receptor 1)	(Davies et al. 1994)[a,b,c]
IDDM6	18q21	D18S487	(Merriman et al. 1997)[a,b]
IDDM7	2q31	D2S152 (NEUROD [neurogenic differentiation], G6PC2 [glucose-6-phosphatase, catalytic, 2] candidates)	(Copeman et al. 1995)[a,b,c]
IDDM8	6q27	D6S264	(Luo et al. 1995)[a,b,c]
IDDM9	3q21	D3S1576	(Mein et al. 1998)[a,b]
IDDM10	10p11	D10S193	(Davies et al. 1994)[a,b,c]
IDDM11	14q24.3	D14S67	(Field et al. 1996)[a,b]
IDDM12	2q33	CTLA4 (cytotoxic T-lymphocyte–associated protein 4)	(Nistico et al. 1996)[a,b,c]
IDDM13	2q35	D2S164	(Morahan et al. 1996)[a,b,c]
IDDM15	6q21	D6S283	(Delepine et al. 1997)[a]
IDDM16	14q32.3	D14S542 (within IGH region)	(Field et al. 2002)
IDDM17	10q25	D10S554	(Verge et al. 1998)
IDDM18	5q33	IL12B (interleukin-12B)	(Morahan et al. 2001)
Unnamed	1q42	D1S1617	(Cox et al. 2001)[a,c]
Unnamed	14q13.1	D14S70	(Mein et al. 1998)[b,c]
Unnamed	16q23.1	D16S515	(Mein et al. 1998)[b,c]
Unnamed	19q13	D19S247-D19S225	(Mein et al. 1998)[b,c]

Footnotes: These loci also included in the study of:
[a]Concannon et al. 1998
[b]Mein et al. 1998
[c]Cox et al. 2001
[d]The locus number, the chromosomal location, the marker (candidate gene), and representative references are presented. Most of the evidence is based on studies of US and UK populations, although some of the findings have also been confirmed in other populations.

to type 1 diabetes. Although the number of genes with potential association to type 1 diabetes is continuously increasing, the majority of type 1 diabetes-associated genes remain to be determined (Table 2). We discuss the most important of these genes next.

Human Leukocyte Antigen Genes. The human leukocyte antigen (HLA) genes, part of the MHC, were the first to be linked to susceptibility for the disease IDDM1 and still remain the major contributors, accounting for >42% of familial type 1 diabetes cases *(71,72)*. Complex and strong associations with type 1 diabetes have been shown for class II genes (gene groups: HLA-DR, -DQ, and -DP), and a weaker association for class I genes (gene groups: HLA-A, -B, -C), whereas associations with class III genes have been inconsistent. Class I genes encode antigens that are an integral part of the plasma membrane of nucleated cells; class II molecules are expressed primarily on B-lymphocytes, macrophages, and activated T-lymphocytes. The class II DQB1 and DRB1 alleles are the major IDDM1 contributors to type 1 diabetes, and other HLA loci can further modify the final disease risk *(73–75)*. Moreover, DQ genes are the common denominators to type 1 diabetes susceptibility across various ethnic groups. Interestingly, a number of HLA alleles confer protection against the disease and can even override the effect of strong susceptibility alleles *(76,77)*. The HLA-DQ molecules associated with protection from type 1 diabetes give more stable dimers, particularly at neutral pH, than those conferring susceptibility *(78)*.

Insulin Gene. In general, class I alleles of the 14-bp variable number tandem repeat (26–63 repeats) polymorphic region, upstream of the insulin gene translational start site, predispose to type 1 diabetes, and class III alleles (140–210 repeats) confer a dominant protective effect *(79–81)*.

Other IDDM Loci and Candidate Genes. Preliminary evidence suggests a potential association of several other genes to type 1 diabetes. For example, the vitamin D receptor gene polymorphism and the MHC class I chain-related gene-A *(MIC-A)* have been associated with type 1 diabetes *(82,83)*, and polymorphisms in the IL receptor 4 *(IL4R)* gene, as well as specific combinations of genotypes at the IL-4R and the IL-4 *(IL4)* and IL-13 *(IL13)* loci are now being reported to increase the risk of type 1 diabetes *(84)*. Other examples include the T-cell-specific factor 7 *(TCF7)* and the IL-10 *(IL10) (85,86)*. Elucidating the mechanisms underlying the relationship between these polymorphisms and type 1 diabetes as well as any potential interactions could enable future presymptomatic diagnosis and early use of preventative measures.

Monogenic Factors. Monogenic forms of type 1 diabetes are extremely rare (Table 1), but their study has been instrumental in understanding the molecular pathways leading to diabetes, because they allow the identification of disease-causative gene mutations and, consequently, point to disease-related molecular pathways. Two characteristic forms are the autoimmune polyendocrine syndrome type I (APS-I) or autoimmune polyendocrinopathy, candidiasis, and ectodermal dystrophy, and the immune dysregulation, polyendocrinopathy, enteropathy, X-linked syndrome (IPEX) or X-linked polyendocrinopathy, immune dysfunction, and diarrhea. APS-I is an autosomal recessive autoimmune polyglandular syndrome with type 1 diabetes as one of its potential manifestations, caused by mutations in the *AIRE* gene, which is involved in the induction of tolerance to self-antigens *(87)*. IPEX is associated with overwhelming neonatal autoimmunity and is usually lethal in infancy. It is caused by mutations in the *FOXP3* gene, which codes for a transcription factor expressed in $CD4^+$ lymphocytes *(88)*.

Type 2 Diabetes

Type 2 diabetes is a heterogeneous metabolic disorder, characterized by defects in both insulin secretion and insulin action, and its current prevalence of 5 to 6% is projected to rise by approx 50% by the year 2010 *(89)*, bringing the total of affected individuals worldwide close to 215 million. Type 2 diabetes is generally attributed to a combination of environmental and genetic factors acting on a number of intermediate traits of relevance to the diabetic phenotype, including β-cell mass, insulin secretion, insulin action, fat distribution, and obesity, but the specific contribution of genetic and environmental factors may vary in different type 2 diabetes subtypes, with highly genetic forms at one end of the spectrum, and genetic susceptibility strongly associated with environmental factors at the other end.

Evidence to support the genetic aspect of type 2 diabetes arises from twin (43% concordance between Danish dizygotic twins and 63% in monozygotic twins) and family studies (20–30% increased risk for siblings), as well as the marked differences in disease prevalence among various racial groups *(90–94)*. Although several rare monogenic forms of type 2 diabetes have been described, it is currently believed that type 2 diabetes is primarily a polygenic disorder.

Similarly to other complex disorders with multifactorial inheritance, the approaches employed for the genetic study of type 2 diabetes have mainly included animal studies, the "candidate gene," and "genomewide-scanning" approaches.

ANIMAL STUDIES

Monogenic Studies

Insulin Signaling. The understanding of type 2 diabetes has been significantly enriched by the study of a range of KO and transgenic mouse models (summarized in Table 3) targeting specific pathways of insulin action and insulin signaling.

Regarding insulin action, the crucial role of the insulin receptor (IR) (Fig. 2) was confirmed in homozygous $IR^{-/-}$ mice, which develop a severe form of diabetes and die within the first week of life from diabetic ketoacidosis *(95,96)*. Heterozygote $IR^{+/-}$ mice, however, do not present with any metabolic abnormalities, suggesting that a decrease in IR number does not necessarily lead to insulin resistance. *IR* tissue–specific KOs in muscle (MIRKO) exhibited features of the metabolic syndrome with normal blood glucose, serum insulin, and glucose tolerance but severely impaired skeletal muscle glucose uptake and obesity *(97,98)*. On the contrary, liver-specific *IR* KOs (LIRKO) had severe insulin resistance and increased β-cell mass, and β-cell-specific knockouts (βIRKO) developed glucose intolerance with aging *(99,100)*. Finally, neuron-specific *IR* KOs (NIRKO) presented not only with insulin resistance, but also diet-induced obesity *(101)*. Mouse KO models of the insulin receptor substrates (IRSs) 1–4, the major substrates of IR (Fig. 2), have shown that $IRS1^{-/-}$ mice do not develop frank diabetes, but β-cell hyperplasia and mild insulin resistance, which is mainly localized in skeletal muscle, a phenotype similar to the human syndrome X *(102,103)*, whereas $IRS2^{-/-}$ mice develop overt type 2 diabetes early on in life, with severe liver insulin resistance and lack of β-cell hyperplasia *(104,105)*, and $IRS3^{-/-}$ mice present with only mild glucose intolerance *(106)*.

Regarding insulin signaling, KO models of molecules downstream of IRS in the insulin-signaling cascade (see Fig. 2) such as p85α (or p85β or p85α/p55α/p50α) and AKT2 result in quite different phenotypes with increased insulin sensitivity in the former and insulin resistance at the level of skeletal muscle and liver leading to type 2 diabetes in the latter *(107–111)*. $GLUT4^{-/-}$ mice present with only moderate insulin resistance, whereas male $GLUT4^{+/-}$ mice develop type 2 diabetes *(112,113)*. Muscle (MG4KO)– and liver (FG4KO)–specific KOs for *GLUT4* present with insulin resistance *(114,115)*, which is seen in both the muscles and the liver of the latter mouse model.

B-Cell Dysfunction. In addition to insulin resistance, dysfunction of β-cells, which are responsible for the secretion of insulin, and impaired insulin secretion is another major cause of type 2 diabetes. The study of transgenic mice overexpressing the human insulin gene led to the conclusion that chronic hyperinsulinemia can lead to insulin resistance in the fasting state *(116)*. Single homogeneous insulin gene KO mice $INS1^{-/-}$or $INS2^{-/-}$ did not develop insulin deficiency, however, and the pancreatic insulin content was similar to WT levels, partly owing to the increase in the β-cell population

Table 3

Genetically Engineered Mouse Models of Insulin Pathways

Monogenic—all tissues/ref.	Monogenic—tissue specific/ref.	Phenotype[a]
IGF1$^{-/-}$ (210)		Growth deficiency; liver-specific insulin insensitivity in muscle
IGF2$^{-/-}$ (212)		Growth deficiency
IGF2 overexpression (213)		Increased fetal size, abnormal shape of β-cells
IR$^{-/-}$ (95,96)	Muscle (98); liver (99); β-cells (100); neurons (101)	Diabetic ketoacidosis, early postnatal death, decreased brown and adipose tissue, triglycerides and FFA levels raised, reduced hepatic glycogen content; muscle specific—elevated fat mass, serum triglycerides, and FFA; liver specific—glucose intolerant
IR$^{+/-}$ (95,96)	IR-dominant negative in muscle (215)	Normal by glucose tolerance tests
	IR-dominant negative in muscle/fat (214)	Glycogen reduced, glucose and insulin increased
IRS-1$^{-/-}$ (107)		"Prodromal" features of type 2 diabetes without becoming diabetic
IRS-2$^{-/-}$ (105)		Growth retardation, insulin resistance, normal–mild glucose intolerance Disturbed peripheral insulin signaling and glucose homeostasis, reduced β-cell mass, early diabetes
IRS-3$^{-/-}$ (106)		Normal growth, glucose, insulin
IGF1R$^{-/-}$ (210)	β-Cells (216)	Developmental delay in ossification, abnormal CNS, epidermis; β-cell-specific age-dependent impairment of glucose tolerance
p85α$^{-/-}$ (110)		Hypoglycemia, increased insulin sensitivity
pik3r1$^{-/-}$ (108)		Perinatal lethality, hepatocyte necrosis, enlarged skeletal muscle fibers, brown fat necrosis, calcification of cardiac tissue
pik3r1$^{+/-}$ (109)		Improved glucose homeostasis
pik3r2$^{+/-}$ (111)		Significantly increased insulin sensitivity
AKT2$^{-/-}$ (107)		Increased glucose
GK$^{-/-}$ (121)	Liver (122); β-cells (119)	Severe hyperglycemia, perinatal death; liver specific—mild hyperglycemia, profound glycogen synthesis deficiency
GK$^{+/-}$ (217)	β-Cells (119)	Increased fasting glucose, decreased glucose tolerance, abnormal liver glucose metabolism, mild diabetes

(Continued)

51

Table 3 (Continued)

Monogenic—all tissues/ref.	Monogenic—tissue specific/ref.	Phenotype[a]
GLUT4−/− (113)	Muscle (115); fat (114)	Growth retarded, cardiac hypertrophy, severely reduced adipose tissue deposits, postprandial hyperinsulinemia, hypoglycemia only in male; muscle specific—severe insulin resistance and glucose intolerance; fat specific—glucose intolerance, insulin resistance
GLUT4+/− (112)		Insulin resistance, increased glucose and insulin, reduced muscle glucose uptake, hypertension, no obesity
GLUT2−/− (120)		Diabetes, glucose intolerance, hyperglycemic, hypoinsulinemic, increased FFA and glucagon, abnormal glucose tolerance, early death
Kir6.2−/− (124)		Mild impairment of glucose tolerance
SUR−/− (123)		Mild glucose intolerance, neonatal hyperinsulinemic hypoglycemia
RPS6KB1−/− (218)		Hypoinsulinemic, glucose intolerant

Polygenic—all tissues/ref.	Polygenic—tissue specific/ref.	Phenotype
INS1−/−/INS2−/− (118)		Diabetes, ketoacidosis, liver steatosis, death within 48 h
IR+/−/IRS-1+/− (126)		Diabetes in 50% adult mice, severe insulin resistance in muscle and liver, β-cell hyperplasia
IR+/−/IRS-2+/− (125)		Diabetes in adults, severe insulin resistance in liver, limited β-cell hyperplasia
IRS-1+/−/IRS-2+/− (219)		Mild glucose intolerance, hyperinsulinemia
IR+/−/IRS-1+/−/IRS-2+/− (125)		Early diabetes, severe insulin resistance in muscle and liver, marked β-cell hyperplasia
IRS-1−/−/IRS-3−/− (220)		Early severe lipoatrophy, hyperglycemia, hyperinsulinemia, insulin resistance
IRS-1−/−/IRS-4−/− (220)		Similar to IRS-1−/− phenotype
IRS-1−/−/GK+/− (127)	β-Cells GK+/− (127)	Diabetes in adults, insulin resistance, β-cell hyperplasia
IR+/−/IRS-1+/−/p85α+/− (109)		Protection from diabetes
IGF1−/−/IGF1R−/− (210)		Organ hypoplasia, developmental delay in ossification, abnormal CNS, epidermis
IGF2−/−/IGF1R−/− (210)		30% normal height, organ hypoplasia, developmental delay in ossification, abnormal CNS, epidermis
IGF1−/−/IGF2−/− (210)		30% normal height, organ hypoplasia, developmental delay in ossification, abnormal CNS, epidermis
IR−/−/IGFR1−/− (221)	IGF1R/IR-dominant negative muscle (222)	90% decrease in exocrine pancreas size; Diabetes, insulin resistance
IGFR1+/−/IRS-2+/− (219)		Glucose tolerance, mild hyperinsulinemia, reduced β-cell mass

[a]FFA, free fatty acid.

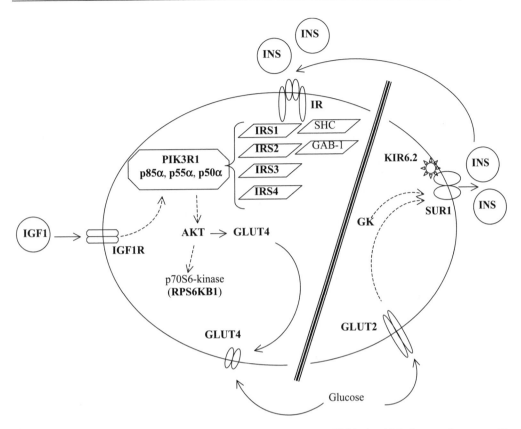

Fig. 2. Insulin (INS) binds to insulin receptor (IR) and activates IRS1–4, which, in turn, interact with the p85α, p55α, and p50α subunits of the phosphoinositide-3-kinase, regulatory subunit, polypeptide 1 (PIK3R1) and activate it. INS and IR have very similar structures to insulin-like growth factor (IGF) and IGF receptor (IGFR). On binding of IGF to its receptor, a cascade is triggered that leads to PIK3R1 activation. This, in turn, stimulates a series of molecular interactions, one of which leads to AKT activation. AKT stimulates the translocation of glucose transporter 4 (GLUT4) to the cell membrane. GLUT4 is the main glucose transporter in certain tissues such as muscle. In addition to GLUT4, GLUT2, a glucose transporter mainly expressed in the β-cells of the pancreas, functions as a glucose sensor. Together with glucokinase (GK), β-cell K^+ATP channel subunits SUR1 and KIR6.2 are responsible for glucose-regulated insulin secretion. GLUT4 is predominantly found in muscle and fat cells, and GLUT2 in liver and β-cells. Genes for which KO or transgenic mouse models are available are indicated in bold (see art).

(117,118). Homozygous KO mice of either one of two key sensors of ambient glucose levels and, thus, regulators of the β-cell glucose-stimulated insulin secretion (i.e., glucose transporter 2 [*GLUT2*] and *GK*) develop type 2 diabetes, which leads to early death (Fig. 2) *(119–121)*. *GK* tissue–specific KOs have been generated for both β-cells and liver, with a more severe phenotype in the former *(119,121,122)*. Finally, homozygous KOs have been generated for the potassium inwardly rectifying channel, subfamily J, member 11 (*KCNJ11* or *KIR6.2*), and for the adenosine triphosphate (ATP)-binding cassette, subfamily C (CFTR/MRP), member 8 (*ABCC8* or *SUR1*), which make up the β-cell K_{ATP} channels and are responsible for glucose and sulfonylurea-regulated insulin secretion (Fig. 2) *(123,124)*. The respective mouse phenotypes involve mild glucose intolerance and impaired response to glucose blood levels.

Polygenic Studies. Building on combinations of monogenic mouse models, a number of polygenic models have also been developed in an effort to understand the interactions between different molecular pathways involved in type 2 diabetes and, ultimately, its polygenic etiology. For example, double heterozygous mice for *IR* and *IRS1*, as well as triple heterozygous mutations for *IR*, *IRS1*, and *IRS2*, develop severe insulin resistance in both muscle and liver, whereas the IR$^{+/-}$/IRS2$^{+/-}$ mice show insulin resistance only in liver *(125,126)*. IR$^{-/-}$/GK$^{+/-}$ mice have moderate insulin resistance *(127)*. All of these mouse models result in different degrees of β-cell hyperplasia. Diabetes developed the earliest and was most severe in the triple heterozygous mice. Double homozygous mice Ins1$^{-/-}$/Ins2$^{-/-}$ are growth retarded, develop severe diabetic ketoacidosis, and die soon after birth *(118)*. However, an improvement in insulin sensitivity has also been achieved in IR$^{+/-}$/IRS1$^{+/-}$/p85$^{+/-}$ mice, revealing the complex interactions between different diabetogenes predisposing to insulin resistance and sensitivity, respectively *(109)*.

Conclusion. Significant novel insights into the pathophysiology of type 2 diabetes have been derived from studies in genetically engineered mice. For example, phosphatidylinositol-3-kinase was directly shown, for the first time, to participate in glucose homeostasis *(110)*, and varying levels of GLUT4 were suggested to alter whole-body glucose disposal *(128)*. Direct evidence showed, for the first time, that GK serves as a glucose sensor for insulin secretion with a pivotal role in glucose homeostasis particularly in β-cells *(119,122)*. The role of the liver in glucose homeostasis proved to be much greater than previously thought, with liver-confined insulin resistance leading to glucose intolerance and muscle-confined insulin resistance associated with altered fat metabolism but not diabetes *(98,99)*. Moreover, it became apparent that both IRS-dependent and IRS-independent pathways of insulin and IGF signal transduction are present *(102)*. Tyrosine-phosphorylated IRS2 and IRS3 were found to assume a compensatory role in the absence of IRS1 in liver and muscle, respectively *(129–131)*, and IRS2$^{-/-}$ was the first single gene deficiency to cause both peripheral insulin resistance and β-cell deficiency in a type 2 diabetes animal model *(104,105)*. Studies of polygenic mouse models revealed the complexity of gene interactions leading to diabetes, with combinations of diabetic-gene mutations almost reversing the increased diabetes risk, and combinations of nondiabetic genes acting additively and leading to diabetes *(109,127)*. In general, it appears that compensatory mechanisms can lead to milder than expected phenotypes, while an intimate communication exists between pancreatic β-cells and insulin-target tissues.

Although animal models are critical in dissecting the molecular pathways involved in type 2 diabetes, they have a number of differences from humans that are important to bear in mind when interpreting the data. For example, mice are probably more sensitive to insulin than humans, as demonstrated by the observations that, unlike in humans, *IRS1* mutations do not lead to a diabetic phenotype in mice, and *IRS2* mutations, which lead to typical type 2 diabetes in homozygous KO mice, have not been found in humans to date *(132)*.

HUMAN STUDIES

The vast majority of type 2 diabetes cases are polygenic. Multiple loci have demonstrated associations or linkage to type 2 diabetes. Genomewide scans have identified very few chromosomal regions with significant or consistent correlation to type 2 diabetes. Loci with significant linkage to type 2 diabetes (LOD [log of odds] scores >3.6 and supporting evidence of linkage by more than two studies) were 1q21-q24, 1q25.3,

2q37.3, 3p24.1, 3q28, 10q26.13, 12q24.31, and 18p11.22 *(133–139)*; reviewed in ref. *140*. The locus 2q37.3 has received a great deal of attention since it was first associated with type 2 diabetes in Mexican Americans, and it has been named NIDDM1 *(133)*. NIDDM1 was later shown to host the gene *CAPN10*, a member of the calpain (calcium-activated neutral proteases) family of nonlysosomal cysteine proteases that catalyze the endoproteolytic cleavage of specific substrates involved in a number of cellular functions, including intracellular signaling *(141,142)*. Associations of certain *CAPN10* polymorphisms and type 2 diabetes have been reported in some populations; however, they have not been reproduced by other studies, and the precise genotype–phenotype correlation remains unclear *(143–146)*.

A wide range of candidate genes have been assessed for association to type 2 diabetes. More than 200 candidate genes have been tested and more than 40 different gene associations have been described. However, very few have been reproduced by multiple studies *(147)*. The main problems with these studies include inadequate statistical power, multiple hypothesis testing, population stratification, publication bias, and phenotypic differences. Larger studies and meta-analysis using thousands rather than hundreds of subjects are the most favorable solutions *(148–151)*.

The strongest and most reproducible association for type 2 diabetes to date has been described for the transcription factor PPARγ, a target for the insulin-sensitizing drugs thiazolidinediones, which plays a central role in adipocyte development. A common amino acid substitution (Pro12Ala) in PPARγ has been associated with a higher BMI, insulin resistance, and an increased risk of type 2 diabetes *(152,153)*. Although the effect of Pro12Ala for an individual carrier may be weak, the high frequency of this allele leads to a high population risk of about 25% *(154)*. Interestingly, dominant negative mutations in PPARG can also act as a monogenic cause of type 2 diabetes, as seen in two families to date *(58)*.

Significant associations with type 2 diabetes have also been found for *SUR1*; *KIR6.2*; glucagon receptor *(GCGR)*; glucokinase *(GCK)*; and solute carrier family 2 (facilitated glucose transporter), member 1 *(SLC2A1* or *GLUT1)* after meta-analyses *(140)*.

Other Specific Types of Diabetes

The monogenic forms make up approx 5% of type 2 diabetes cases. They often present in childhood or early adulthood, and according to the 1997 American Diabetes Association guidelines, they are classified as "other specific types of diabetes" *(155)*. Certain monogenic forms of type 2 diabetes such as maturity-onset diabetes of the young (MODY), mitochondrial diabetes syndromes, and hyperproinsulinemia are associated with defective insulin secretion. The most common among them is the MODY. MODY is genetically, metabolically, and clinically heterogeneous, encompassing monogenic forms of diabetes of β-cell origin. MODY displays autosomal dominant inheritance and is the result of mutations identified in six different genes, each one associated with a different form of MODY (Table 1). Mitochondrial diabetes syndromes involve mutations in mitochondrial genes (such as rRNA and tRNA genes or NADH dehydrogenase) and, thus, they are strictly maternally inherited. Some patients with mitochondrial diabetes syndromes may display an acute-onset insulin-dependent form of diabetes, although in most individual patients, the monogenic forms are clinically indistinguishable from other type 2 diabetes cases. Hyperproinsulinemia, caused by mutations in the insulin gene that lead to structurally abnormal, functionally inactive insulin, can also lead to type 2 diabetes *(156)*.

A number of other monogenic forms of type 2 diabetes are associated with insulin resistance. Examples include leprechaunism (or Donahue syndrome) *(157)*, Rabson-Mendenhall syndrome *(158)*, and Type A insulin resistance *(159,160)* (Table 1). However, a wide range of additional monogenic syndromes display type 2 diabetes as one of their symptoms. Some are primary lipoatrophy syndromes such as Berardinelli-Seip congenital lipodystrophy *(161,162)*, Dunnigan-type familial partial lipodystrophy (FPLD) *(163)*, and late-onset FPLD *(164)*, whereas others are complex syndromes associated with lipoatrophy such as mandibuloacral dysplasia *(165)*, Werner syndrome *(166)*, and Cockayne syndrome *(167)*. The specific manifestations of these syndromes are briefly presented in Table 1; a more detailed description is beyond the scope of this chapter and can be found elsewhere *(168)*.

Gene Polymorphisms in Complications of Type 1 and 2 Diabetes

Both type 1 and 2 diabetes are associated with a series of complications, such as nephropathy, retinopathy, and cardiovascular disease, which seriously compromise the quality of life and longevity of patients with diabetes. In addition to a genetic predisposition to developing diabetes, accumulating evidence suggests a genetic component for developing these complications as well. Although a wide range of genes have been assessed for their association with increased risk of such complications *(169–172)*, only a few studies have revealed significant and consistent results in both type 1 and 2 diabetes *(173)*, including the nephropathy-associated angiotensin-converting enzyme (ACE), and the microvascular disease-associated aldose reductase (AR) *(174–178)*. Thus, more work is required to elucidate the genetics of complications of diabetes.

OBESITY AND DIABETES: A DIRECT LINK?

There is considerable evidence supporting the link among a high-fat diet, obesity, and diabetes; however, the mechanisms behind these associations are only beginning to emerge (*see* Chapter 7). Although it is obesity that is traditionally thought to result in insulin resistance, it is currently believed that this association is bidirectional. Insulin signaling is considered critical for the development of obesity *(179)*. In addition, adipose tissue plays a key role in the development of insulin resistance by expressing and secreting proteins with multiple endocrine functions *(180)*. Leptin is an adipocyte-derived hormone that regulates energy homeostasis and neuroendocrine function. Leptin deficiency leads to insulin resistance and diabetes, which may be corrected by the administration ofr-metHuLeptin *(181)*. Leptin secretion is also influenced by several factors such as TNF-α, a cytokine, the levels of which increase with obesity and induce insulin resistance *(182–185)*. A TNF-α-related increase in plasminogen activator inhibitor 1 levels has also been associated with obesity and insulin resistance *(186)*. By contrast, the expression of the adipoise tissue–derived endogenous insulin sensitizer adiponectin is decreased in obesity. Administration of adiponectin improves insulin resistance, and combined administration of adiponectin and leptin can completely reverse insulin resistance in lipoatrophy and obesity *(187)*. The adipose tissue-secreted proteins IL-6, macrophages and monocyte chemoattractant protein 1, adipsin, acylation-stimulating protein, and resistin, as well as proteins of the renin angiotensin system present additional links between obesity and insulin resistance, which are covered in detail in other chapters of this textbook *(188–193)*. The transcription factor PPARγ plays a key role in high-fat-diet-induced obesity and insulin resistance at least in part by altering leptin and adiponectin expression *(194)*. Spontaneous or engineered animal models of leptin, its receptor, adiponectin, and TNF-α deficiency have been extensively studied and shown to develop insulin resistance *(7,195–197)*, in contrast to resistin KO mice, which do not develop insulin resistance, only hyperglycemia *(198)*. Finally, several single nucleotide polymorphisms (SNPs) of these molecules have been linked to the development of insulin resistance and diabetes *(199–202)*. In summary, there is considerable evidence to support the link between diabetes and obesity, but extensive work is still required to decipher the complex molecular pathways behind it.

FUTURE DIRECTIONS

Although many chromosomal loci and genes have been associated with diabetes and obesity, and the rate of progress is increasing, the search for their genetic causes is far from complete. The completion of the Human Genome Project and the expanding knowledge on SNPs combined with findings from genomewide scans, as well as advances in genomic technologies and data analysis, hold considerable promise *(203–206)*. The rapid progress in genomics and proteomics, e.g., could enable the accelerated transition from mutations to transcriptional changes to protein changes and hence, a better understanding of the molecular pathways involved in the development of disease. Large-scale screens based on chemical mutagenesis of whole animals and transposon insertions in embryonic stem cells are also likely to play a key role in the pace of future developments *(207,208)*. The identification of disease-causing mutations, particularly in the context of gene–gene and gene–environment interactions of low- or moderate-penetrance genes, may eventually enable presymptomatic genetic testing and early use of preventative measures and/or medications. Characterization of the molecular pathways involved in the development and progression of disease promises to reveal new therapeutic targets, and the availability of a wide range of animal models will expedite the testing phase of the various drug candidates. Meantime, progress in pharmacogenomics could ultimately permit the selection of "individualized" drugs, which will take into consideration potential interactions of the individual's genome with the drug, thus minimizing potential drug side effects. Finally, in-depth genetic studies are expected to help clarify the complex interpopulation differences. It is hoped that researchers will eventually achieve the incorporation of appropriate tests, preventative measures, and medications in a better suited, individualized preventative and therapeutic regimen.

Glossary

Term	Definition
Allele	Alternative form of a genetic locus; a single allele for each locus is inherited from each parent
Association studies	Genetic association studies do not focus on families where a praticular disease is segregating, instead samples of affected and unaffected individuals are drawn from the population, and the frequency with which certain alleles are present in each of these groups is tested for association with a disease
Candidate gene approach	It involves analysis of genes that are a priori suspected to be involved in the disease, either due to previous knowledge from animal models or due to their physiological role. For example, the main criteria for consideration as a type II diabetes candidate

(Continued)

Term	Definition
	genes include 1. known or presumed biological role in glucose or energy metabolism in humans (e.g., insulin secretion or insulin-signaling pathways); 2. involved in other subtypes of diabetes (e.g., MODY) or diseases that display diabetes mellitus as one of their symptoms (e.g., Wolfram syndrome); 3. association with diabetes or related symptoms in animal models; 4. differential expression in diabetic and normal tissues. The candidate gene approach evaluates statistically the co-occurrence of alleles or phenotypes. In this approach, an LOD score of 3 is usually taken as strong evidence of linkage and corresponds to a *p*-value of 0.0001, suggesting that linkage of that gene to the disease is 1000 times more likely than the alternative of no linkage (*see* LOD score below).
Chemical mutagenesis	Method in which a chemical agent such as ethylmethanesulphonate (EMS) or *N*-ethyl-*N*-nitrosourea (ENU) is used to induce point mutations in DNA, leading to a variety of genetic lesions that may result in complete loss of function, reduced function, increased function or altered function.
Genome wide scan	The entire genome is evaluated for chromosomal regions carrying polymorphisms that are associated with the disease, by association studies or linkage analysis (for example, ~350 to ~370 polymorphic markers are tested, with an average spacing of 10cM). It investigates the possibility of a specific genetic relationship between chromosomal loci. For this approach, more stringent LOD score criteria have been proposed than for the "candidate gene approach" (strong evidence requires LOD score > 3.3), owing to the large number of linkage tests that are performed in order to scan the entire genome *(209)*.
Genomics	The study of genes and their function.
Haplotype	The combination of alleles (for different genes) which are located closely together on the same chromosome and tend to be inherited together.
HLA genes	The human leukocyte antigen genes are the most polymorphic genes known in humans, with some of them having hundreds of different alleles. The HLA alleles on a given chromosome are so closely linked that they are transmitted together as a haplotype.
Linkage analysis	Analysis that searches for an increased sharing of genotypes between affected family members above the levels expected from the family relationships alone. It normally creates associations within families, but not among unrelated people. The traditional, statistical measure for linkage is the LOD score (logarithm of the likelihood ration for linkage). Where the family and the population merge, then linkage and association merge.
Locus	The position on a chromosome of a gene or other chromosome marker; also, the DNA at that position. The use of locus is sometimes restricted to mean expressed DNA regions.
LOD score	Logarithm of the odd score; a measure of the likelihood of two loci being within a measurable distance of each other.
Meta-analysis	The combination of data from several studies to produce a single estimate using multifactorial methods.

(Continued)

Glossary *(Continued)*

Term	*Definition*
Pharmacogenomics	The study of the interaction of an individual's genetic makeup and response to a drug.
Polymorphism	A polymorphism is a difference in DNA sequence that occurs in a population with a frequency higher than 1%.
Proteomics	The study of the full set of proteins encoded by a genome.
QTL	Quantitative trait locus; a polymorphic locus that contains alleles that differentially affect the expression of a continuously distributed phenotypic trait.
SNPs	Single nucleotide polymorphisms; DNA sequence variations that occur when a single nucleotide (A, T, C, or G) in the genome sequence is altered.
Translational start site	The sequence determining where the translation of mRNA into protein will start from.
VNTR	Variable number tandem repeats; any gene whose alleles contain different numbers of tandemly repeated oligonucleotide sequences.
Gene expression studies	The study of which genes are "activated" or "switched on" to make protein.

REFERENCES

1. Wild S, Roglic G, Green A, Sicree R, King H. Global prevalence of diabetes: estimates for the year 2000 and projections for 2030. Diabetes Care 2004;27:1047–1053.
2. Maes HH, Neale MC, Eaves LJ. Genetic and environmental factors in relative body weight and human adiposity. Behav Genet 1997;27:325–351.
3. Hill JO, Peters JC. Environmental contributions to the obesity epidemic. Science 1998;280:1371–1374.
4. West DB, Waguespack J, McCollister S. Dietary obesity in the mouse: interaction of strain with diet composition. Am J Physiol 1995;268:R658–R665.
5. Rice T, Sjostrom CD, Perusse L, Rao DC, Sjostrom L, Bouchard C. Segregation analysis of body mass index in a large sample selected for obesity: the Swedish Obese Subjects study. Obes Res 1999;7:246–255.
6. Tschop M, Heiman ML. Rodent obesity models: an overview. Exp Clin Endocrinol Diabetes 2001;109:307–319.
7. Zhang Y, Proenca R, Maffei M, Barone M, Leopold L, Friedman JM. Positional cloning of the mouse obese gene and its human homologue. Nature 1994;372:425–432.
8. Miller MW, Duhl DM, Vrieling H, et al. Cloning of the mouse agouti gene predicts a secreted protein ubiquitously expressed in mice carrying the lethal yellow mutation. Genes Dev 1993;7:454–467.
9. Kleyn PW, Fan W, Kovats SG, et al. Identification and characterization of the mouse obesity gene tubby: a member of a novel gene family. Cell 1996;85:281–290.
10. Tartaglia LA, Dembski M, Weng X, et al. Identification and expression cloning of a leptin receptor, OB-R. Cell 1995;83:1263–1271.
11. Naggert JK, Fricker LD, Varlamov O, et al. Hyperproinsulinaemia in obese fat/fat mice associated with a carboxypeptidase E mutation which reduces enzyme activity. Nat Genet 1995;10:135–142.
12. Gunn TM, Miller KA, He L, et al. The mouse mahogany locus encodes a transmembrane form of human attractin. Nature 1999;398:152–156.
13. Butler AA, Cone RD. Knockout models resulting in the development of obesity. Trends Genet 2001;17:S50–S54.
14. Krude H, Biebermann H, Luck W, Horn R, Brabant G, Gruters A. Severe early-onset obesity, adrenal insufficiency and red hair pigmentation caused by POMC mutations in humans. Nat Genet 1998;19:155–157.
15. Huszar D, Lynch CA, Fairchild-Huntress V, et al. Targeted disruption of the melanocortin-4 receptor results in obesity in mice. Cell 1997;88:131–141.

16. Marsh DJ, Weingarth DT, Novi DE, et al. Melanin-concentrating hormone 1 receptor-deficient mice are lean, hyperactive, and hyperphagic and have altered metabolism. Proc Natl Acad Sci USA 2002;99:3240–3245.

17. Martinez-Botas J, Anderson JB, Tessier D, et al. Absence of perilipin results in leanness and reverses obesity in Lepr(db/db) mice. Nat Genet 2000;26:474–479.

18. Perreault M, Marette A. Targeted disruption of inducible nitric oxide synthase protects against obesity-linked insulin resistance in muscle. Nat Med 2001;7:1138–1143.

19. Bachman ES, Dhillon H, Zhang CY, et al. betaAR signaling required for diet-induced thermogenesis and obesity resistance. Science 2002;297:843–845.

20. Hrabe de Angelis MH, Flaswinkel H, Fuchs H, et al. Genome-wide, large-scale production of mutant mice by ENU mutagenesis. Nat Genet 2000;25:444–447.

21. Nolan PM, Peters J, Strivens M, et al. A systematic, genome-wide, phenotype-driven mutagenesis programme for gene function studies in the mouse. Nat Genet 2000;25:440–443.

22. Justice MJ. Capitalizing on large-scale mouse mutagenesis screens. Nat Rev Genet 2000;1:109–115.

23. Meyer CW, Korthaus D, Jagla W, et al. A novel missense mutation in the mouse growth hormone gene causes semidominant dwarfism, hyperghrelinemia, and obesity. Endocrinology 2004;145: 2531–2541.

24. Morris KH, Ishikawa A, Keightley PD. Quantitative trait loci for growth traits in C57BL/6J x DBA/2J mice. Mamm Genome 1999;10:225–228.

25. Rance KA, Heath SC, Keightley PD. Mapping quantitative trait loci for body weight on the X chromosome in mice. II. Analysis of congenic backcrosses. Genet Res 1997;70:125–133.

26. Taylor BA, Tarantino LM, Phillips SJ. Gender-influenced obesity QTLs identified in a cross involving the KK type II diabetes-prone mouse strain. Mamm Genome 1999;10:963–968.

27. Brockmann GA, Kratzsch J, Haley CS, Renne U, Schwerin M, Karle S. Single QTL effects, epistasis, and pleiotropy account for two-thirds of the phenotypic F(2) variance of growth and obesity in DU6i x DBA/2 mice. Genome Res 2000;10:1941–1957.

28. Kloting I, Kovacs P, van den Brandt J. Quantitative trait loci for body weight, blood pressure, blood glucose, and serum lipids: linkage analysis with wild rats (Rattus norvegicus). Biochem Biophys Res Commun 2001;284:1126–1133.

29. Andersson L, Haley CS, Ellegren H, et al. Genetic mapping of quantitative trait loci for growth and fatness in pigs. Science 1994;263:1771–1774.

30. MacNeil MD, Grosz MD. Genome-wide scans for QTL affecting carcass traits in Hereford x composite double backcross populations. J Anim Sci 2002;80:2316–2324.

31. Comuzzie AG, Cole SA, Martin L, et al. The baboon as a nonhuman primate model for the study of the genetics of obesity. Obes Res 2003;11:75–80.

32. Clement K, Boutin P, Froguel P. Genetics of obesity. Am J Pharmacogenomics 2002;2:177–187.

33. Shuldiner AR, Sabra M. Trp64Arg beta3-adrenoceptor: when does a candidate gene become a disease-susceptibility gene? Obes Res 2001;9:806–809.

34. Sakane N, Yoshida T, Umekawa T, Kogure A, Takakura Y, Kondo M. Effects of Trp64Arg mutation in the beta 3-adrenergic receptor gene on weight loss, body fat distribution, glycemic control, and insulin resistance in obese type 2 diabetic patients. Diabetes Care 1997;20:1887–1890.

35. Kim-Motoyama H, Yasuda K, Yamaguchi T, et al. A mutation of the beta 3-adrenergic receptor is associated with visceral obesity but decreased serum triglyceride. Diabetologia 1997;40:469–472.

36. Walston J, Andersen RE, Seibert M, et al. Arg64 beta3-adrenoceptor variant and the components of energy expenditure. Obes Res 2003;11:509–511.

37. Pihlajamaki J, Vanhala M, Vanhala P, Laakso M. The Pro12Ala polymorphism of the PPAR gamma 2 gene regulates weight from birth to adulthood. Obes Res 2004;12:187–190.

38. Stumvoll M, Tschritter O, Fritsche A, et al. Association of the T-G polymorphism in adiponectin (exon 2) with obesity and insulin sensitivity: interaction with family history of type 2 diabetes. Diabetes 2002;51:37–41.

39. Ristow M, Muller-Wieland D, Pfeiffer A, Krone W, Kahn CR. Obesity associated with a mutation in a genetic regulator of adipocyte differentiation. N Engl J Med 1998;339:953–959.

40. Menzaghi C, Ercolino T, Di Paola R, et al. A haplotype at the adiponectin locus is associated with obesity and other features of the insulin resistance syndrome. Diabetes 2001;51:2306–2312.

41. Doney A, Fischer B, Frew D, et al. Haplotype analysis of the PPARgamma Pro12Ala and C1431T variants reveals opposing associations with body weight. BMC Genet 2002;3:21.

42. Luan J, Browne PO, Harding AH, et al. Evidence for gene-nutrient interaction at the PPARgamma locus. Diabetes 2001;50:686–689.

43. Miraglia del Giudice E, Santoro N, Cirillo G, et al. Molecular screening of the ghrelin gene in Italian obese children: the Leu72Met variant is associated with an earlier onset of obesity. Int J Obes Relat Metab Disord 2004;28:447–450.

44. Garenc C, Perusse L, Chagnon YC, et al. The hormone-sensitive lipase gene and body composition: the HERITAGE Family Study. Int J Obes Relat Metab Disord 2002;26:220–227.

45. Meirhaeghe A, Helbecque N, Cottel D, Amouyel P. Beta2-adrenoceptor gene polymorphism, body weight, and physical activity. Lancet 1999;353:896.

46. Meirhaeghe A, Helbecque N, Cottel D, Amouyel P. Impact of polymorphisms of the human beta2-adrenoceptor gene on obesity in a French population. Int J Obes Relat Metab Disord 2000; 24:382–387.

47. Meirhaeghe A, Luan J, Selberg-Franks P, et al. The effect of the Gly16Arg polymorphism of the beta(2)-adrenergic receptor gene on plasma free fatty acid levels is modulated by physical activity. J Clin Endocrinol Metab 2001;86:5881–5887.

48. Corella D, Guillen M, Portoles O, et al. Gender specific associations of the Trp64Arg mutation in the beta3-adrenergic receptor gene with obesity-related phenotypes in a Mediterranean population: interaction with a common lipoprotein lipase gene variation. J Intern Med 2001;250:348–360.

49. Montague CT, Farooqi IS, Whitehead JP, et al. Congenital leptin deficiency is associated with severe early-onset obesity in humans. Nature 1997;387:903–908.

50. Strobel A, Issad T, Camoin L, Ozata M, Strosberg AD. A leptin missense mutation associated with hypogonadism and morbid obesity. Nat Genet 1998;18:213–215.

51. Ozata M, Ozdemir IC, Licinio J. Human leptin deficiency caused by a missense mutation: multiple endocrine defects, decreased sympathetic tone, and immune system dysfunction indicate new targets for leptin action, greater central than peripheral resistance to the effects of leptin, and spontaneous correction of leptin-mediated defects. J Clin Endocrinol Metab 1999;84:3686–3695.

52. Considine RV, Sinha MK, Heiman ML, et al. Serum immunoreactive-leptin concentrations in normal-weight and obese humans. N Engl J Med 1996;334:292–295.

53. Clement K, Vaisse C, Lahlou N, et al. A mutation in the human leptin receptor gene causes obesity and pituitary dysfunction. Nature 1998;392:398–401.

54. Jackson RS, Creemers JW, Ohagi S, et al. Obesity and impaired prohormone processing associated with mutations in the human prohormone convertase 1 gene. Nat Genet 1997;16:303–306.

55. Vaisse C, Clement K, Durand E, Hercberg S, Guy-Grand B, Froguel P. Melanocortin-4 receptor mutations are a frequent and heterogeneous cause of morbid obesity. J Clin Invest 2000;106: 253–262.

56. Farooqi IS, Keogh JM, Yeo GS, Lank EJ, Cheetham T, O'Rahilly S. Clinical spectrum of obesity and mutations in the melanocortin 4 receptor gene. N Engl J Med 2003;348:1085–1095.

57. Branson R, Potoczna N, Kral JG, Lentes KU, Hoehe MR, Horber FF. Binge eating as a major phenotype of melanocortin 4 receptor gene mutations. N Engl J Med 2003;348:1096–1103.

58. Barroso I, Gurnell M, Crowley VE, et al. Dominant negative mutations in human PPARgamma associated with severe insulin resistance, diabetes mellitus and hypertension. Nature 1999;402:880–883.

59. Holder JL Jr, Butte NF, Zinn AR. Profound obesity associated with a balanced translocation that disrupts the SIM1 gene. Hum Mol Genet 2000;9:101–108.

60. Lee YS, Poh LK, Loke KY. A novel melanocortin 3 receptor gene (MC3R) mutation associated with severe obesity. J Clin Endocrinol Metab 2002;87:1423–1426.

61. Park Y, Eisenbarth GS. Genetic susceptibility factors of Type 1 diabetes in Asians. Diabetes Metab Res Rev 2001;17:2–11.

62. Kawano K, Hirashima T, Mori S, Natori T. OLETF (Otsuka Long-Evans Tokushima Fatty) rat: a new NIDDM rat strain. Diabetes Res Clin Pract 1994;24(Suppl):S317–S320.

63. Nakhooda AF, Like AA, Chappel CI, Murray FT, Marliss EB. The spontaneously diabetic Wistar rat: metabolic and morphologic studies. Diabetes 1977;26:100–112.

64. Delovitch TL, Sing B. The nonobese diabetic mouse as a model of autoimmune diabetes: immune dysregulation gets the NOD. Immunity 1997;7:727–738.

65. Adorini L, Gregori S, Harrison LC. Understanding autoimmune diabetes: insights from mouse models. Trends Mol Med 2002;8:31–38.

66. Andre I, Gonzalez A, Wang B, Katz J, Benoist C, Mathis D. Checkpoints in the progression of autoimmune disease: lessons from diabetes models. Proc Natl Acad Sci USA 1996;93:2260–2263.

67. Katz J, Benoist C, Mathis D. Major histocompatibility complex class I molecules are required for the development of insulitis in non-obese diabetic mice. Eur J Immunol 1993;23:3358–3360.

68. Fugger L. Human autoimmunity genes in mice. Curr Opin Immunol 2000;12:698–703.

69. Harper PS. Endocrine and reproductive disorders. In: Practical Genetic Counselling. Butterworth Heinemann, Oxford, UK, 268–270.

70. Redondo MJ, Fain PR, Eisenbarth GS. Genetics of type 1A diabetes. Recent Prog Horm Res 2001;56:69–89.

71. Singal DP, Blajchman MA. Histocompatibility (HL-A) antigens, lymphocytotoxic antibodies and tissue antibodies in patients with diabetes mellitus. Diabetes 1973;22:429–432.

72. Davies JL, Kawaguchi Y, Bennett ST, et al. A genome-wide search for human type 1 diabetes susceptibility genes. Nature 1994;371:130–136.

73. Herr M, Dudbridge F, Zavattari P, et al. Evaluation of fine mapping strategies for a multifactorial disease locus: systematic linkage and association analysis of IDDM1 in the HLA region on chromosome 6p21. Hum Mol Genet 2000;9:1291–1301.

74. Nejentsev S, Reijonen H, Adojaan B, et al. The effect of HLA-B allele on the IDDM risk defined by DRB1*04 subtypes and DQB1*0302. Diabetes 1997;46:1888–1892.

75. Noble JA, Valdes AM, Thomson G, Erlich HA. The HLA class II locus DPB1 can influence susceptibility to type 1 diabetes. Diabetes 2000;49:121–125.

76. Undlien DE, Friede T, Rammensee HG, et al. HLA-encoded genetic predisposition in IDDM: DR4 subtypes may be associated with different degrees of protection. Diabetes 1997;46:143–149.

77. Van der Auwera B, Van Waeyenberge C, Schuit F, et al. DRB1*0403 protects against IDDM in Caucasians with the high-risk heterozygous DQA1*0301-DQB1*0302/DQA1*0501-DQB1*0201 genotype: Belgian Diabetes Registry. Diabetes 1995;44:527–530.

78. Ettinger RA, Liu AW, Nepom GT, Kwok WW. Exceptional stability of the HLA-DQA1*0102/DQB1*0602 alpha beta protein dimer, the class II MHC molecule associated with protection from insulin-dependent diabetes mellitus. J Immunol 1998;161:6439–6445.

79. Bennett ST, Lucassen AM, Gough SC, et al. Susceptibility to human type 1 diabetes at IDDM2 is determined by tandem repeat variation at the insulin gene minisatellite locus. Nat Genet 1995;9:284–292.

80. Bennett ST, Wilson AJ, Esposito L, et al. Insulin VNTR allele-specific effect in type 1 diabetes depends on identity of untransmitted paternal allele: the IMDIAB Group. Nat Genet 1997;17:350–352.

81. Vafiadis P, Ounissi-Benkalha H, Palumbo M, et al. Class III alleles of the variable number of tandem repeat insulin polymorphism associated with silencing of thymic insulin predispose to type 1 diabetes. J Clin Endocrinol Metab 2001;86:3705–3710.

82. Gambelunghe G, Ghaderi M, Cosentino A, Falorni A, Brunetti P, Sanjeevi CB. Association of MHC Class I chain-related A (MIC-A) gene polymorphism with Type I diabetes. Diabetologia 2000;43:507–514.

83. Motohashi Y, Yamada S, Yanagawa T, et al. Vitamin D receptor gene polymorphism affects onset pattern of type 1 diabetes. J Clin Endocrinol Metab 2003;88:3137–3140.

84. Bugawan TL, Mirel DB, Valde AM, Panelo A, Pozzilli P, Erlich HA. Association and interaction of the IL4R, IL4, and IL13 loci with type 1 diabetes among Filipinos. Am J Hum Genet 2003;72:1505–1514.

85. Noble JA, White AM, Lazzeroni LC, et al. A polymorphism in the TCF7 gene, C883A, is associated with type 1 diabetes. Diabetes 2003;52:1579–1582.

86. Ide A, Kawasaki E, Abiru N, et al. Genetic association between interleukin-10 gene promoter region polymorphisms and type 1 diabetes age-at-onset. Hum Immunol 2002;63:690–695.

87. Anderson MS, Venanzi ES, Klein L, et al. Projection of an immunological self shadow within the thymus by the aire protein. Science 2002;298:1395–1401.

88. Bennett CL, Christie J, Ramsdell F, et al. The immune dysregulation, polyendocrinopathy, enteropathy, X-linked syndrome (IPEX) is caused by mutations of FOXP3. Nat Genet 2001;27:20, 21.

89. Amos AF, McCarty DJ, Zimmet P. The rising global burden of diabetes and its complications: estimates and projections to the year 2010. Diabet Med 2001;14(Suppl 5):S1–S85.

90. Poulsen P, Kyvik KO, Vaag A, Beck-Nielsen H. Heritability of type II (non-insulin-dependent) diabetes mellitus and abnormal glucose tolerance—a population-based twin study. Diabetologia 1999;42:139–145.

91. Knowler WC, Pettitt DJ, Saad MF, Bennett PH. Diabetes mellitus in the Pima Indians: incidence, risk factors and pathogenesis. Diabetes Metab Rev 1990;6:1–27.

92. Zimmet P, Taylor R, Ram P, et al. Prevalence of diabetes and impaired glucose tolerance in the biracial (Melanesian and Indian) population of Fiji: a rural-urban comparison. Am J Epidemiol 1983;118:673–688.

93. Newman B, Selby JV, King MC, Slemenda C, Fabsitz R, Friedman GD. Concordance for type 2 (non-insulin-dependent) diabetes mellitus in male twins. Diabetologia 1987;30:763–768.

94. Barnett AH, Eff C, Leslie RD, Pyke DA. Diabetes in identical twins: a study of 200 pairs. Diabetologia 1981;20:87–93.

95. Joshi RL, Lamothe B, Cordonnier N, et al. Targeted disruption of the insulin receptor gene in the mouse results in neonatal lethality. Embo J 1996;15:1542–1547.

96. Accili D, Drago J, Lee EJ, et al. Early neonatal death in mice homozygous for a null allele of the insulin receptor gene. Nat Genet 1996;12:106–109.

97. Kim JK, Michael MD, Previs SF, et al. Redistribution of substrates to adipose tissue promotes obesity in mice with selective insulin resistance in muscle. J Clin Invest 2000;105:1791–1797.

98. Bruning JC, Michael MD, Winnay JN, et al. A muscle-specific insulin receptor knockout exhibits features of the metabolic syndrome of NIDDM without altering glucose tolerance. Mol Cell 1998;2:559–569.

99. Michael MD, Kulkarni RN, Postic C, et al. Loss of insulin signaling in hepatocytes leads to severe insulin resistance and progressive hepatic dysfunction. Mol Cell 2000;6:87–97.

100. Kulkarni RN, Bruning JC, Winnay JN, Postic C, Magnuson MA, Kahn CR. Tissue-specific knockout of the insulin receptor in pancreatic beta cells creates an insulin secretory defect similar to that in type 2 diabetes. Cell 1999;96:329–339.

101. Bruning JC, Gautam D, Burks DJ, et al. Role of brain insulin receptor in control of body weight and reproduction. Science 2000;289:2122–2125.

102. Tamemoto H, Kadowaki T, Tobe K, et al. Insulin resistance and growth retardation in mice lacking insulin receptor substrate-1. Nature 1994;372:182–186.

103. Araki E, Haag BL 3rd, Kahn CR. Cloning of the mouse insulin receptor substrate-1 (IRS-1) gene and complete sequence of mouse IRS-1. Biochim Biophys Acta 1994;1221:353–356.

104. Kubota N, Tobe K, Terauchi Y, et al. Disruption of insulin receptor substrate 2 causes type 2 diabetes because of liver insulin resistance and lack of compensatory beta-cell hyperplasia. Diabetes 2000;49:1880–1889.

105. Withers DJ, Gutierrez JS, Towery H, et al. Disruption of IRS-2 causes type 2 diabetes in mice. Nature 1998;391:900–904.

106. Liu SC, Wang Q, Lienhard GE, Keller SR. Insulin receptor substrate 3 is not essential for growth or glucose homeostasis. J Biol Chem 1999;274:18,093–18,099.

107. Cho H, Mu J, Kim JK, et al. Insulin resistance and a diabetes mellitus-like syndrome in mice lacking the protein kinase Akt2 (PKB beta). Science 2001;292:1728–1731.

108. Fruman DA, Mauvais-Jarvis F, Pollard DA, et al. Hypoglycaemia, liver necrosis and perinatal death in mice lacking all isoforms of phosphoinositide 3-kinase p85 alpha. Nat Genet 2000;26:379–382.

109. Mauvais-Jarvis F, Ueki K, Fruman DA, et al. Reduced expression of the murine p85alpha subunit of phosphoinositide 3-kinase improves insulin signaling and ameliorates diabetes. J Clin Invest 2002;109:141–149.

110. Terauchi Y, Tsuji Y, Satoh S, et al. Increased insulin sensitivity and hypoglycaemia in mice lacking the p85 alpha subunit of phosphoinositide 3-kinase. Nat Genet 1999;21:230–235.

111. Ueki K, Yballe CM, Brachmann SM, et al. Increased insulin sensitivity in mice lacking p85beta subunit of phosphoinositide 3-kinase. Proc Natl Acad Sci USA 2002;99:419–424.

112. Stenbit AE, Tsao TS, Li J, et al. GLUT4 heterozygous knockout mice develop muscle insulin resistance and diabetes. Nat Med 1997;3:1096–1101.

113. Katz EB, Stenbit AE, Hatton K, DePinho R, Charron MJ. Cardiac and adipose tissue abnormalities but not diabetes in mice deficient in GLUT4. Nature 1995;377:151–155.

114. Abel ED, Peroni O, Kim JK, et al. Adipose-selective targeting of the GLUT4 gene impairs insulin action in muscle and liver. Nature 2001;409:729–733.

115. Zisman A, Peroni OD, Abel ED, et al. Targeted disruption of the glucose transporter 4 selectively in muscle causes insulin resistance and glucose intolerance. Nat Med 2000;6:924–928.

116. Marban SL, DeLoia JA, Gearhart JD. Hyperinsulinemia in transgenic mice carrying multiple copies of the human insulin gene. Dev Genet 1989;10:356–364.

117. Leroux L, Desbois P, Lamotte L, et al. Compensatory responses in mice carrying a null mutation for Ins1 or Ins2. Diabetes 2001;50(Suppl 1):S150–S153.

118. Duvillie B, Cordonnier N, Deltour L, et al. Phenotypic alterations in insulin-deficient mutant mice. Proc Natl Acad Sci USA 1997;94:5137–5140.

119. Terauchi Y, Sakura H, Yasuda K, et al. Pancreatic beta-cell-specific targeted disruption of glucokinase gene: diabetes mellitus due to defective insulin secretion to glucose. J Biol Chem 1995; 270:30,253–30,256.

120. Guillam MT, Hummler E, Schaerer E, et al. Early diabetes and abnormal postnatal pancreatic islet development in mice lacking Glut-2. Nat Genet 1997;17:327–330.
121. Grupe A, Hultgren B, Ryan A, Ma YH, Bauer M, Stewart TA. Transgenic knockouts reveal a critical requirement for pancreatic beta cell glucokinase in maintaining glucose homeostasis. Cell 1995;83:69–78.
122. Postic C, Shiota M, Niswender KD, et al. Dual roles for glucokinase in glucose homeostasis as determined by liver and pancreatic beta cell–specific gene knock-outs using Cre recombinase. J Biol Chem 1999;274:305–315.
123. Seghers V, Nakazaki M, DeMayo F, Aguilar-Bryan L, Bryan J. Sur1 knockout mice: a model for K(ATP) channel-independent regulation of insulin secretion. J Biol Chem 2000;275:9270–9277.
124. Miki T, Nagashima K, Tashiro F, et al. Defective insulin secretion and enhanced insulin action in KATP channel-deficient mice. Proc Natl Acad Sci USA 1998;95:10,402–10,406.
125. Kido Y, Burks DJ, Withers D, et al. Tissue-specific insulin resistance in mice with mutations in the insulin receptor, IRS-1, and IRS-2. J Clin Invest 2000;105:199–205.
126. Bruning JC, Winnay J, Bonner-Weir S, Taylor SI, Accili D, Kahn CR. Development of a novel polygenic model of NIDDM in mice heterozygous for IR and IRS-1 null alleles. Cell 1997;88:561–572.
127. Terauchi Y, Iwamoto K, Tamemoto H, et al. Development of non-insulin-dependent diabetes mellitus in the double knockout mice with disruption of insulin receptor substrate-1 and beta cell glucokinase genes: genetic reconstitution of diabetes as a polygenic disease. J Clin Invest 1997;99:861–866.
128. Rossetti L, Stenbit AE, Chen W, et al. Peripheral but not hepatic insulin resistance in mice with one disrupted allele of the glucose transporter type 4 (GLUT4) gene. J Clin Invest 1997;100:1831–1839.
129. Bruning JC, Winnay J, Cheatham B, Kahn CR. Differential signaling by insulin receptor substrate 1 (IRS-1) and IRS-2 in IRS-1-deficient cells. Mol Cell Biol 1997;17:1513–1521.
130. Kaburagi Y, Satoh S, Tamemoto H, et al. Role of insulin receptor substrate-1 and pp60 in the regulation of insulin-induced glucose transport and GLUT4 translocation in primary adipocytes. J Biol Chem 1997;272:25,839–25,844.
131. Yamauchi T, Tobe K, Tamemoto H, et al. Insulin signalling and insulin actions in the muscles and livers of insulin-resistant, insulin receptor substrate 1-deficient mice. Mol Cell Biol 1996;16:3074–3084.
132. Kalidas K, Wasson J, Glaser B, et al. Mapping of the human insulin receptor substrate-2 gene, identification of a linked polymorphic marker and linkage analysis in families with Type II diabetes: no evidence for a major susceptibility role. Diabetologia 1998;41:1389–1391.
133. Hanis CL, Boerwinkle E, Chakraborty R, et al. A genome-wide search for human non-insulin-dependent (type 2) diabetes genes reveals a major susceptibility locus on chromosome 2. Nat Genet 1996;13:161–166.
134. Hanson RL, Ehm MG, Pettitt DJ, et al. An autosomal genomic scan for loci linked to type II diabetes mellitus and body-mass index in Pima Indians. Am J Hum Genet 1998;63:1130–1138.
135. Ehm MG, Karnoub MC, Sakul H, et al. Genomewide search for type 2 diabetes susceptibility genes in four American populations. Am J Hum Genet 2000;66:1871–1881.
136. Duggirala R, Blangero J, Almasy L, et al. Linkage of type 2 diabetes mellitus and of age at onset to a genetic location on chromosome 10q in Mexican Americans. Am J Hum Genet 1999;64:1127–1140.
137. Parker A, Meyer J, Lewitzky S, et al. A gene conferring susceptibility to type 2 diabetes in conjunction with obesity is located on chromosome 18p11. Diabetes 2001;50:675–680.
138. Vionnet N, Hani El H, Dupont S, et al. Genomewide search for type 2 diabetes-susceptibility genes in French whites: evidence for a novel susceptibility locus for early-onset diabetes on chromosome 3q27-qter and independent replication of a type 2-diabetes locus on chromosome 1q21-q24. Am J Hum Genet 2000;67:1470–1480.
139. Das SK, Hasstedt SJ, Zhang Z, Elbein SC. Linkage and association mapping of a chromosome 1q21-q24 type 2 diabetes susceptibility locus in northern European Caucasians. Diabetes 2004;53:492–499.
140. Florez JC, Hirschhorn J, Altshuler D. The inherited basis of diabetes mellitus: implications for the genetic analysis of complex traits. Annu Rev Genomics Hum Genet 2003;4:257–291.
141. Sreenan SK, Zhou YP, Otani K, et al. Calpains play a role in insulin secretion and action. Diabetes 2001;50:2013–2020.
142. Horikawa Y, Oda N, Cox NJ, et al. Genetic variation in the gene encoding calpain-10 is associated with type 2 diabetes mellitus. Nat Genet 2000;26:163–175.
143. Tsai HJ, Sun G, Weeks DE, et al. Type 2 diabetes and three calpain-10 gene polymorphisms in Samoans: no evidence of association. Am J Hum Genet 2001;69:1236–1244.
144. Rasmussen SK, Urhammer SA, Berglund L, et al. Variants within the calpain-10 gene on chromosome 2q37 (NIDDM1) and relationships to type 2 diabetes, insulin resistance, and impaired acute insulin secretion among Scandinavian Caucasians. Diabetes 2002;51:3561–3567.

145. Fingerlin TE, Erdos MR, Watanabe RM, et al. Variation in three single nucleotide polymorphisms in the calpain-10 gene not associated with type 2 diabetes in a large Finnish cohort. Diabetes 2002;51:1644–1648.

146. Daimon M, Oizumi T, Saitoh T, et al. Calpain 10 gene polymorphisms are related, not to type 2 diabetes, but to increased serum cholesterol in Japanese. Diabetes Res Clin Pract 2002;56:147–152.

147. Hirschhorn JN, Lohmueller K, Byrne E, Hirschhorn K. A comprehensive review of genetic association studies. Genet Med 2002;4:45–61.

148. Dahlman I, Eaves IA, Kosoy R, et al. Parameters for reliable results in genetic association studies in common disease. Nat Genet 2002;30:149, 150.

149. Demenais F, Kanninen T, Lindgren CM, et al. A meta-analysis of four European genome screens (GIFT Consortium) shows evidence for a novel region on chromosome 17p11.2-q22 linked to type 2 diabetes. Hum Mol Genet 2003;12:1865–1873.

150. Ioannidis JP, Ntzani EE, Trikalinos TA, Contopoulos-Ioannidis DG. Replication validity of genetic association studies. Nat Genet 2001;29:306–309.

151. Lohmueller KE, Pearce CL, Pike M, Lander ES, Hirschhorn JN. Meta-analysis of genetic association studies supports a contribution of common variants to susceptibility to common disease. Nat Genet 2003;33:177–182.

152. Deeb SS, Fajas L, Nemoto M, et al. A Pro12Ala substitution in PPARgamma2 associated with decreased receptor activity, lower body mass index and improved insulin sensitivity. Nat Genet 1998;20:284–287.

153. Yen CJ, Beamer BA, Negri C, et al. Molecular scanning of the human peroxisome proliferator activated receptor gamma (hPPAR gamma) gene in diabetic Caucasians: identification of a Pro12Ala PPAR gamma 2 missense mutation. Biochem Biophys Res Commun 1997;241:270–274.

154. Altshuler D, Hirschhorn JN, Klannemark M, et al. The common PPARgamma Pro12Ala polymorphism is associated with decreased risk of type 2 diabetes. Nat Genet 2000;26:76–80.

155. Report of the expert committee on the diagnosis and classification of diabetes mellitus. Diabetes Care 1997;20:1183–1197.

156. Haneda M, Polonsky KS, Bergenstal RM, et al. Familial hyperinsulinemia due to a structurally abnormal insulin: definition of an emerging new clinical syndrome. N Engl J Med 1984;310:1288–1294.

157. Psiachou H, Mitton S, Alaghband-Zadeh J, Hone J, Taylor SI, Sinclair L. Leprechaunism and homozygous nonsense mutation in the insulin receptor gene. Lancet 1993;342:924.

158. Accili D, Frapier C, Mosthaf L, et al. A mutation in the insulin receptor gene that impairs transport of the receptor to the plasma membrane and causes insulin-resistant diabetes. EMBO J 1989;8:2509–2517.

159. Kahn CR, Flier JS, Bar RS, et al. The syndromes of insulin resistance and acanthosis nigricans: insulin-receptor disorders in man. N Engl J Med 1976;294:739–745.

160. Moller DE, Cohen O, Yamaguchi Y, et al. Prevalence of mutations in the insulin receptor gene in subjects with features of the type A syndrome of insulin resistance. Diabetes 1994;43:247–255.

161. Agarwal AK, Arioglu E, De Almeida S, et al. AGPAT2 is mutated in congenital generalized lipodystrophy linked to chromosome 9q34. Nat Genet 2002;31:21–23.

162. Magre J, Delepine M, Khallouf E, et al. Identification of the gene altered in Berardinelli-Seip congenital lipodystrophy on chromosome 11q13. Nat Genet 2001;28:365–370.

163. Cao H, Hegele RA. Nuclear lamin A/C R482Q mutation in canadian kindreds with Dunnigan-type familial partial lipodystrophy. Hum Mol Genet 2000;9:109–112.

164. Agarwal AK, Garg A. A novel heterozygous mutation in peroxisome proliferator-activated receptor-gamma gene in a patient with familial partial lipodystrophy. J Clin Endocrinol Metab 2002;87:408–411.

165. Novelli G, Muchir A, Sangiuolo F, et al. Mandibuloacral dysplasia is caused by a mutation in LMNA-encoding lamin A/C. Am J Hum Genet 2002;71:426–431.

166. Yu CE, Oshima J, Fu YH, et al. Positional cloning of the Werner's syndrome gene. Science 1996;272:258–262.

167. Henning KA, Li L, Iyer N, et al. The Cockayne syndrome group A gene encodes a WD repeat protein that interacts with CSB protein and a subunit of RNA polymerase II TFIIH. Cell 1995;82:555–564.

168. Flier JS, Mantzoros C. Syndromes of severe insulin resistance. In: De Groot L ed. Endocrinology Saunders, Philadelphia, PA, pp. 799–810.

169. Wagenknecht LE, Bowden DW, Carr JJ, Langefeld CD, Freedman BI, Rich SS. Familial aggregation of coronary artery calcium in families with type 2 diabetes. Diabetes 2001;50:861–866.

170. Pettitt DJ, Saad MF, Bennett PH, Nelson RG, Knowler WC. Familial predisposition to renal disease in two generations of Pima Indians with type 2 (non-insulin-dependent) diabetes mellitus. Diabetologia 1990;33:438–443.

171. Freedman BI, Tuttle AB, Spray BJ. Familial predisposition to nephropathy in African-Americans with non-insulin-dependent diabetes mellitus. Am J Kidney Dis 1995;25:710–713.

172. O'Dea DF, Murphy SW, Hefferton D, Parfrey PS. Higher risk for renal failure in first-degree relatives of white patients with end-stage renal disease: a population-based study. Am J Kidney Dis 1998;32:794–801.

173. Bowden DW. Genetics of diabetes complications. Curr Diabetes Rep 2002;2:191–200.

174. Yamamoto T, Sato T, Hosoi M, et al. Aldose reductase gene polymorphism is associated with progression of diabetic nephropathy in Japanese patients with type 1 diabetes mellitus. Diabetes Obes Metab 2003;5:51–57.

175. Jacobsen P, Tarnow L, Carstensen B, Hovind P, Poirier O, Parving HH. Genetic variation in the Renin-Angiotensin system and progression of diabetic nephropathy. J Am Soc Nephrol 2003; 14:2843–2850.

176. Fujisawa T, Ikegami H, Kawaguchi Y, et al. Meta-analysis of association of insertion/deletion polymorphism of angiotensin I-converting enzyme gene with diabetic nephropathy and retinopathy. Diabetologia 1998;41:47–53.

177. Kunz R, Bork JP, Fritsche L, Ringel J, Sharma AM. Association between the angiotensin-converting enzyme-insertion/deletion polymorphism and diabetic nephropathy: a methodologic appraisal and systematic review. J Am Soc Nephrol 1998;9:1653–1663.

178. Demaine AG. Polymorphisms of the aldose reductase gene and susceptibility to diabetic microvascular complications. Curr Med Chem 2003;10:1389–1398.

179. Bluher M, Michael MD, Peroni OD, et al. Adipose tissue selective insulin receptor knockout protects against obesity and obesity-related glucose intolerance. Dev Cell 2002;3:25–38.

180. Kershaw EE, Flier JS. Adipose tissue as an endocrine organ. J Clin Endocrinol Metab 2004; 89:2548–2556.

181. Masuzaki H, Ogawa Y, Aizawa-Abe M, et al. Glucose metabolism and insulin sensitivity in transgenic mice overexpressing leptin with lethal yellow agouti mutation: usefulness of leptin for the treatment of obesity-associated diabetes. Diabetes 1999;48:1615–1622.

182. Bjorbaek C, Kahn BB. Leptin signaling in the central nervous system and the periphery. Recent Prog Horm Res 2004;59:305–331.

183. Hotamisligil GS, Shargill NS, Spiegelman BM. Adipose expression of tumor necrosis factor-alpha: direct role in obesity-linked insulin resistance. Science 1993;259:87–91.

184. Hotamisligil GS. Inflammatory pathways and insulin action. Int J Obes Relat Metab Disord 2003;27 (Suppl 3):S53–S55.

185. Ruan H, Lodish HF. Insulin resistance in adipose tissue: direct and indirect effects of tumor necrosis factor-alpha. Cytokine Growth Factor Rev 2003;14:447–455.

186. Juhan-Vague I, Alessi MC, Mavri A, Morange PE. Plasminogen activator inhibitor-1, inflammation, obesity, insulin resistance and vascular risk. J Thromb Haemost 2003;1:1575–1579.

187. Yamauchi T, Kamon J, Waki H, et al. The fat-derived hormone adiponectin reverses insulin resistance associated with both lipoatrophy and obesity. Nat Med 2001;7:941–946.

188. Fernandez-Real JM, Ricart W. Insulin resistance and chronic cardiovascular inflammatory syndrome. Endocr Rev 2003;24:278–301.

189. Sartipy P, Loskutoff DJ. Monocyte chemoattractant protein 1 in obesity and insulin resistance. Proc Natl Acad Sci USA 2003;100:7265–7270.

190. Cianflone K, Xia Z, Chen LY. Critical review of acylation-stimulating protein physiology in humans and rodents. Biochim Biophys Acta 2003;1609:127–143.

191. Banerjee RR, Lazar MA. Resistin: molecular history and prognosis. J Mol Med 2003;81:218–226.

192. Engeli S, Schling P, Gorzelniak K, et al. The adipose-tissue renin-angiotensin-aldosterone system: role in the metabolic syndrome? Int J Biochem Cell Biol 2003;35:807–825.

193. Goossens GH, Blaak EE, van Baak MA. Possible involvement of the adipose tissue renin-angiotensin system in the pathophysiology of obesity and obesity-related disorders. Obes Rev 2003;4:43–55.

194. Kadowaki T, Hara K, Yamauchi T, Terauchi Y, Tobe K, Nagai R. Molecular mechanism of insulin resistance and obesity. Exp Biol Med (Maywood) 2003;228:1111–1117.

195. Reue K, Peterfy M. Mouse models of lipodystrophy. Curr Atheroscler Rep 2000;2:390–396.

196. Halaas JL, Gajiwala KS, Maffei M, et al. Weight-reducing effects of the plasma protein encoded by the obese gene. Science 1995;269:543–546.

197. Uysal KT, Wiesbrock SM, Marino MW, Hotamisligil GS. Protection from obesity-induced insulin resistance in mice lacking TNF-alpha function. Nature 1997;389:610–614.

198. Banerjee RR, Rangwala SM, Shapiro JS, et al. Regulation of fasted blood glucose by resistin. Science 2004;303:1195–1198.

199. Liu YJ, Rocha-Sanchez SM, Liu PY, et al. Tests of linkage and/or association of the LEPR gene polymorphisms with obesity phenotypes in Caucasian nuclear families. Physiol Genomics 2004;17:101–106.

200. Gonzalez Sanchez JL, Serrano Rios M, Fernandez Perez C, Laakso M, Martinez Larrad MT. Effect of the Pro12Ala polymorphism of the peroxisome proliferator-activated receptor gamma-2 gene on adiposity, insulin sensitivity and lipid profile in the Spanish population. Eur J Endocrinol 2002; 147:495–501.

201. Hu FB, Doria A, Li T, et al. Genetic variation at the adiponectin locus and risk of type 2 diabetes in women. Diabetes 2004;53:209–213.

202. Yiannakouris N, Yannakoulia M, Melistas L, Chan JL, Klimis-Zacas D, Mantzoros CS. The Q223R polymorphism of the leptin receptor gene is significantly associated with obesity and predicts a small percentage of body weight and body composition variability. J Clin Endocrinol Metab 2001; 86:4434–4439.

203. Risch N, Merikangas K. The future of genetic studies of complex human diseases. Science 1996;273:1516–1517.

204. Allison DB, Neale MC, Zannolli R, Schork NJ, Amos CI, Blangero J. Testing the robustness of the likelihood-ratio test in a variance-component quantitative-trait loci-mapping procedure. Am J Hum Genet 1999;65:531–544.

205. Allison DB, Schork NJ. Selected methodological issues in meiotic mapping of obesity genes in humans: issues of power and efficiency. Behav Genet 1997;27:401–421.

206. Marth GT, Korf I, Yandell MD, et al. A general approach to single-nucleotide polymorphism discovery. Nat Genet 1999;23:452–456.

207. Hrabe de Angelis M, Balling R. Large scale ENU screens in the mouse: genetics meets genomics. Mutat Res 1998;400:25–32.

208. Brown SD, Nolan PM. Mouse mutagenesis-systematic studies of mammalian gene function. Hum Mol Genet 1998;7:1627–1633.

209. Lander E, Kruglyak L. Genetic dissection of complex traits: guidelines for interpreting and reporting linkage results. Nat Genet 1995;11:241–247.

210. Liu JP, Baker J, Perkins AS, Robertson EJ, Efstratiadis A. Mice carrying null mutations of the genes encoding insulin-like growth factor I (Igf-1) and type 1 IGF receptor (Igf1r). Cell 1993;75:59–72.

211. Yakar S, Liu JL, Fernandez AM, et al. Liver-specific igf-1 gene deletion leads to muscle insulin insensitivity. Diabetes 2001;50:1110–1118.

212. Filson AJ, Louvi A, Efstratiadis A, Robertson EJ. Rescue of the T-associated maternal effect in mice carrying null mutations in Igf-2 and Igf2r, two reciprocally imprinted genes. Development 1993;118:731–736.

213. Petrik J, Pell JM, Arany E, et al. Overexpression of insulin-like growth factor-II in transgenic mice is associated with pancreatic islet cell hyperplasia. Endocrinology 1999;140:2353–2363.

214. Lauro D, Kido Y, Castle AL, et al. Impaired glucose tolerance in mice with a targeted impairment of insulin action in muscle and adipose tissue. Nat Genet 1998;20:294–298.

215. Chang PY, Benecke H, Le Marchand-Brustel Y, Lawitts J, Moller DE. Expression of a dominant-negative mutant human insulin receptor in the muscle of transgenic mice. J Biol Chem 1994; 269: 16,034–16,040.

216. Xuan S, Kitamura T, Nakae J, et al. Defective insulin secretion in pancreatic beta cells lacking type 1 IGF receptor. J Clin Invest 2002;110:1011–1019.

217. Bali D, Svetlanov A, Lee HW, et al. Animal model for maturity-onset diabetes of the young generated by disruption of the mouse glucokinase gene. J Biol Chem 1995;270:21,464–21,467.

218. Pende M, Kozma SC, Jaquet M, et al. Hypoinsulinaemia, glucose intolerance and diminished beta-cell size in S6K1-deficient mice. Nature 2000;408:994–997.

219. Withers DJ, Burks DJ, Towery HH, Altamuro SL, Flint CL, White MF. Irs-2 coordinates Igf-1 receptor-mediated beta-cell development and peripheral insulin signalling. Nat Genet 1999;23:32–40.

220. Laustsen PG, Michael MD, Crute BE, et al. Lipoatrophic diabetes in Irs1(–/–)/Irs3(–/–) double knockout mice. Genes Dev 2002;16:3213–3222.

221. Kido Y, Nakae J, Hribal ML, Xuan S, Efstratiadis A, Accili D. Effects of mutations in the insulin-like growth factor signaling system on embryonic pancreas development and beta-cell compensation to insulin resistance. J Biol Chem 2002;277:36,740–36,747.

222. Fernandez AM, Kim JK, Yakar S, et al. Functional inactivation of the IGF-I and insulin receptors in skeletal muscle causes type 2 diabetes. Genes Dev 2001;15:1926–1934.

4

Nutrients and Peripherally Secreted Molecules in Regulation of Energy Homeostasis

Greeshma K. Shetty, MD, Diana Barb, MD and Christos S. Mantzoros, MD, DSc

CONTENTS

INTRODUCTION

Obesity, a growing epidemic with a current prevalence of 30.9% in the United States *(1)*, is directly responsible for the rapidly increasing morbidity and mortality from insulin resistance and the metabolic syndrome, diabetes, cardiovascular disease, cancer, respiratory ailments, arthritis, reproductive challenges, and psychosocial problems *(2)*. Obesity is responsible for approx 300,000 deaths in the United States every year and was thus recently declared the major public health problem in this country, superceding smoking *(3)*. Moreover, the recent rapid increase in the incidence of obesity in children has resulted in nearly half of all children with newly diagnosed diabetes now having type 2 diabetes *(4)*, which, in turn, is expected to result in increasing morbidity and mortality at relatively younger ages in the future, a fact with enormous public health consequences.

The recent exponential increase in the morbidity and mortality related to obesity has led to the intensification of research efforts aimed at elucidating its etiology and treatment. Although Kennedy *(5)* proposed a biological basis for body fat regulation about 50 yr ago, the nature of the first endocrine feedback loop regulating body weight remained elusive until the discovery of the adipocyte-secreted hormone leptin in 1994 *(6)*. This discovery led to a transformation of researchers' conception of adipose tissue from that of an inert reservoir of stored energy to an active organ producing and secreting many molecules that regulate energy homeostasis. Moreover, it has only recently become

From: *Contemporary Diabetes: Obesity and Diabetes*
Edited by: C. S. Mantzoros © Humana Press Inc., Totowa, NJ

Table 1
Adipocyte-Expressed and/or -Secreted Molecules

Category	*Molecules[a]*
Hormones	Leptin, resistin, adiponectin, estrogens, AGT
Cytokines	IL-6, TNF-α
Other immune-related proteins	MCP-1
Extracellular matrix proteins	Type I, II, IV, VI collagen; fibronectin; osteonectin; laminin; entactin; matrix metalloproteinases 2 and 9
Complement factors	Adipsin (complement factor D), complement C3, complement factor B, ASP
Enzymes	Cytochrome P450-dependent aromatase, 17β-HSD, 11β-HSD1, LPL, CETP
Proteins of RAS	Renin, AGT, AT1, AT2, ACE
Acute-phase response proteins	α1-Acid glycoprotein, haptoglobin
Proteins involved in fibrinolytic system	PAI-1, tissue factor
Other	Apolipoprotein E, prostacyclin, FFAs, PPARγ

[a]LPL, lipoprotein lipase; CETP, cholesterol ester transfer protein.

apparent that other peripheral organs such as the pancreas and the gastrointestinal (GI) tract secrete several molecules, which also signal information on energy intake and balance. Signals from both adipose tissue and other peripheral organs not only are integrated centrally in the brain to alter energy homeostasis, but may also influence other physiological functions, such as the neuroendocrine and reproductive hormone systems (*see* Chapter 5).

In this chapter, we review molecules expressed in the periphery, which affect substrate utilization and/or energy partitioning. We then present the role of nutrients and hormonal signals secreted by the adipose tissue, the pancreas, and the GI system in response to acute or chronic changes in energy homeostasis. The integration of all these peripheral signals in the central nervous system (CNS) and hypothalamus is discussed in Chapter 5.

ADIPOSE TISSUE

Adipocytes are not only energy depots that store triglycerides during feeding and release fatty acids during fasting, but cells that also secrete numerous proteins and bioactive peptides known as adipokines, which, in turn, act at both the local (paracrine/autocrine) and systemic (endocrine) level. Therefore, today adipose tissue is considered a true endocrine organ *(7)* (see Table 1 and Fig. 1). Although several adipose tissue-generated molecules have been recently discovered and proposed to play an important role in energy homeostasis, those best understood as the most important ones are leptin, interleukin-6 (IL-6), and tumor necrosis factor-α (TNF-α), whereas adiponectin recently emerged as a potentially very important molecule.

Leptin

Leptin (from the Greek word *leptos*, meaning thin) is a 167 amino acid protein, which was discovered in 1994 by positional cloning of the *obese* (*ob*) gene *(6)*. Mutations in the *ob* gene (leptin gene), as well as the diabetes (*db*) gene (leptin receptor gene), result in

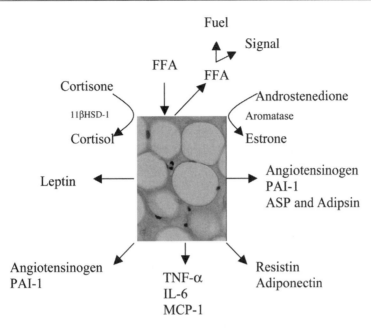

Fig. 1. Adipocyte as an endocrine cell.

morbid obesity and diabetes in rodents and humans *(6,8,9)*. Leptin is thought to act as a lipostat: as the amount of fat stored in adipocytes rises, leptin is released into the blood and signals to the brain adequacy of energy stores. Leptin levels decrease in response to caloric restriction and weight loss *(10)*, and leptin levels increase in response to overfeeding and increasing adipose tissue mass. Leptin secretion is also increased by insulin, glucocorticoids, TNF-α, and estrogens and is decreased in response to starvation, β3 adrenergic activity, androgens, free fatty acids (FFAs), growth hormone (GH), and peroxisome proliferator-activated receptor γ (PPARγ) agonists *(7)*. However, the effect of the latter on circulating leptin levels in humans is null, because these molecules also increase the subject's overall fat mass.

Administration of leptin to leptin-deficient (*ob/ob*) and healthy rodents results in significant weight loss, demonstrating that leptin is directly involved in the regulation of food intake, energy expenditure (EE), and neuroendocrine function by signaling body fat depot size to the brain *(6,11–13)*. However, administration of leptin to diet-induced obese mice, a model of human obesity, results in only minimal weight loss *(14)*, demonstrating that these hyperleptinemic mice are leptin resistant, probably owing to receptor or postreceptor defects *(15)*.

Leptin circulates in the bloodstream in a free and a bound form and mediates its metabolic effects by binding to and activating the long isoform of a specific leptin/class 1 cytokine receptor (also known as ObRb), which signals via the Janus kinase (JAK)-signal transducer and activators of transcription (STAT) system *(16)*. Signaling pathways downstream of leptin include the JAK-STAT pathway, mitogen-activated protein kinase (MAPK), and phosphatidylinositol-3-kinase (PI-3K). These pathways can be activated by leptin in vitro and in vivo *(17)*. Leptin receptors are mainly, but not exclusively, found centrally in hypothalamic nuclei (arcuate hypothalamus [ARC] and paraventricular nucleus) and brain stem. Activation of the centrally expressed leptin receptors triggers appetite-inhibiting circuits (mainly through upregulation of α-melanocyte-stimulating

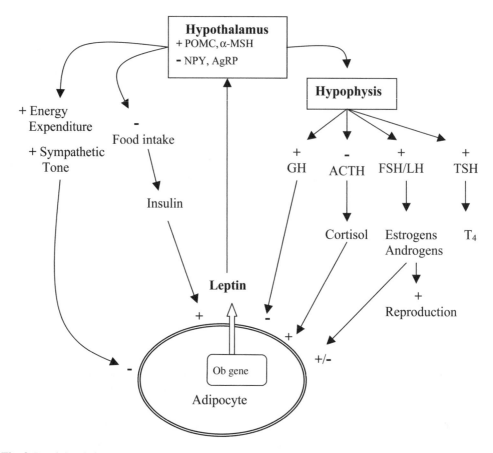

Fig. 2. Leptin's role in energy homeostasis and reproduction: regulation of leptin secretion by overfeeding, insulin, cortisol, and sex hormones. ACTH, adrenocorticotropic hormone; FSH/LH, follicle-stimulating hormone/luteinizing hormone; TSH, thyroid-stimulating hormone; T_4, thyroxine.

hormone [α-MSH] [proopiomelanocortin, POMC]) and inhibits appetite stimulatory circuits (mainly by suppressing neuropeptide Y [NPY] and agouti-related peptide [AgRP] expression in hypothalamic nuclei) *(18)*. Activation of leptin receptors in the ventromedial hypothalamus (VMN) and ARC results in modulation of autonomic nervous system (ANS) activity. Indeed, some studies have shown that acute leptin injections (intravenously, intracerebroventricularly, or intrahypothalamically into the VMN) increase sympathetic nerve activity *(19–21)*. Through activation of sympathetic nerves, leptin stimulates FFA oxidation and thermogenesis in brown adipose tissue (BAT). Leptin also increases glucose uptake in several tissues, including muscle and BAT, and thus seems to play a role in modulating peripheral insulin sensitivity. The latter is likely to involve activation of central melanocortin neurons as well. Finally, it is not only leptin, but also other peripherally secreted molecules (e.g., insulin, adiponectin, gut peptides) that interact with the hypothalamus–ANS axis and modulate glucose homeostasis, energy expenditure, thermogenesis, and lipid metabolism (lipolysis and fatty acids oxidation) *(22)*. Other endocrine effects (via direct action on peripheral tissue including muscle and pancreatic β-cells) include regulation of immune function; hematopoiesis; angiogenesis *(23)*; and, finally, bone metabolism, which is affected by both direct and indirect mechanisms of leptin action *(7)*. Figure 2 summarizes the complex role of leptin.

In humans, leptin is mainly expressed in adipose tissue, but has also been found in the hypothalamus, pituitary, placenta, skeletal muscle, and gastric epithelium (24). Studies in humans have demonstrated that only a distinct minority of morbidly obese subjects have either congenital leptin deficiency (25) or inactivating mutations of the leptin receptor gene (14). Leptin and/or leptin receptor mutations result in extreme obesity, hypogonadotropic hypogonadism, growth delay, and secondary hypothyroidism (26), suggesting that the leptin pathway plays a significant role in the central regulation of energy balance and hypothalamic endocrine functions. In the vast majority of obese subjects, however, serum leptin levels are directly proportional to their adiposity (27) and are secreted in greater amounts from sc than visceral adipose tissue (7), indicating that common human obesity is characterized by elevated leptin levels owing to leptin insensitivity or resistance. Molecular mechanisms proposed to underlie leptin resistance are (1) defects in leptin transport across the blood–brain barrier into the CNS; and (2) reduced hypothalamic leptin signaling, in part owing to upregulation of specific inhibitors of leptin signaling (18). More specifically, besides its primary role in regulating energy homeostasis (mediated via hypothalamic pathways), leptin may act as a critical link between the adipose tissue and the reproductive system by directly influencing the hypothalamic–gonadal axis. Leptin-deficient mice and humans have markedly increased appetite, develop obesity, and fail to go through puberty. All these abnormalities are corrected by therapy with recombinant leptin (17). Moreover, extremely thin women with hypothalamic amenorrhea and/or anorexia nervosa have low leptin levels (28,29). Because exogenous administration of leptin to normalize falling leptin levels in response to starvation restores neuroendocrine function in healthy men (30), and leptin treatment of strenuously exercising women normalizes neuroendocrine and reproductive function, as well as bone markers in women with relative hypoleptinemia (31), it has been proposed that leptin's main role in humans is to signal to the brain information on energy deficiency or sufficiency (7), rather than energy excess.

IL-6 and TNF-α

IL-6 and TNF-α are two cytokines mainly produced by immune cells, but also expressed in adipose tissue. Adipocytes also express both TNF-α and IL-6 receptors. In contrast to TNF-α, which is expressed mainly locally, and circulates in low levels, suggesting that it has mainly paracrine rather than endocrine functions, IL-6 circulates at high levels in the bloodstream. Adipose tissue generates up to 25–30% of circulating IL-6. IL-6 tissue expression and serum levels increase with increasing adiposity and decrease in response to diet-induced weight loss (32). Moreover, IL-6-deficient rodents develop obesity, mainly owing to lack of central IL-6 action, whereas intracerebroventricular administration of IL-6 decreases body fat (33). More importantly, IL-6 levels in the CNS correlate inversely with sc and total body fat in overweight and obese humans, suggesting a relative deficiency of IL-6 centrally in obesity (34). Thus, increased production of IL-6 by the adipose tissue of obese subjects may represent a compensatory mechanism attempting to limit obesity, but increased expression of this cytokine in adipose tissue, especially visceral adipose tissue (35), leads to insulin-signaling defects and thus insulin resistance (35,36). Therefore, plasma IL-6 concentrations predict the development of type 2 diabetes and cardiovascular disease (CVD) (7).

Similar to IL-6, TNF-α causes lipolysis and inhibits adipogenesis (37). Initially suspected to play a role in cachexia (because it has been shown to be identical to cachexin, a factor secreted by macrophages in vitro), TNF-α is now implicated in the pathogenesis of obesity and insulin resistance by impairing insulin signaling. This effect is mediated directly by activation of a serine kinase that increases serine phosphorylation of insulin receptor substrate-1 (IRS-1) and insulin receptor substrate-2 (IRS-2), thus making them poor substrates for insulin receptor kinases and increasing their degradation. TNF-α also acts indirectly by increasing serum FFAs, which induce insulin resistance *per se* in multiple tissues *(7)*. Increased TNF-α expression in obese humans and animals has been proposed to reflect a defective compensatory autocrine/paracrine mechanism to limit obesity *(37)*, because increased TNF-α expression also leads to insulin resistance *(37)*. Thus, both cytokines play a role in inflammation and obesity-mediated insulin resistance, and we have recently shown that soluble TNF-α receptor levels, a marker of activation of the TNF-α system, also predict cardiovascular disease in patients with diabetes (unpublished observations) *(38)*.

Macrophages and Monocyte Chemoattractant Protein-1

Monocyte chemoattractant protein-1 (MCP-1) is a chemokine that recruits monocytes to the site of inflammation and is expressed in adipocytes and stromavascular cells in the adipose tissue. MCP-1 may contribute to insulin resistance, either directly by decreasing insulin-stimulated glucose uptake and insulin-induced insulin receptor phosphorylation, or indirectly through inflammatory factors secreted by the activated macrophages (TNF-α and IL-6) *(7)*.

Adiponectin

Adiponectin, a 247 amino acid protein produced exclusively by adipocytes, circulates in tightly associated trimers and higher-order oligomers *(39–42)*. Eight adiponectin isoforms, each having a variable potency *(42)*, bind and activate at least two adiponectin receptors, which, in turn, alter the phosphorylation state of 5 adenosine monophosphate-(AMP) kinase *(42,43)*. Adiponectin receptor 1 (AdipoR1), which is expressed ubiquitously, but most abundantly in skeletal muscle, has a high affinity for globular adiponectin and a very low affinity for full-length adiponectin, whereas adiponectin receptor 2 (AdipoR2), which is found predominantly in the liver, has an intermediate affinity for both forms *(44)*.

Adiponectin decreases with increasing overall and central adiposity *(40,45)*, and increases with long-term weight reduction *(46)*. Studies in rodents have revealed that peripheral administration of adiponectin increases FFA oxidation and glucose uptake and regulates EE, thus reducing body weight and visceral adiposity without affecting food intake *(47,48)*. In addition, accumulating evidence indicates that adiponectin regulates insulin sensitivity *(44,49–52)*. Adiponectin levels are low in states of insulin resistance and, conversely, levels are higher in a state of improved insulin sensitivity, such as after weight reduction or treatment with insulin-sensitizing drugs, such as thiazolidindiones *(42)*. In addition to its insulin-sensitizing effects, adiponectin exerts potent antiinflammatory *(53)* and atheroprotective effects *(54,55)*. Within the vascular wall, adiponectin inhibits monocyte adhesion and macrophage transformation to foam cells, and it also increases nitric oxide (NO) production in endothelial cells, thus promoting vasodilatation and stimulating angiogenesis *(7,23)*. AdipoR1, which has a higher affinity for globular adiponectin, is more abundant in endothelial cells. One of the major signaling effects of adiponectin in the endothelial cells is activation of the AMP kinase, which, in turn, activates endothelial NO synthase (eNOS) and enhances NO production. eNOS activation is also dependent on signaling through Akt kinase (Akt) and its upstream mediator PI-3K.

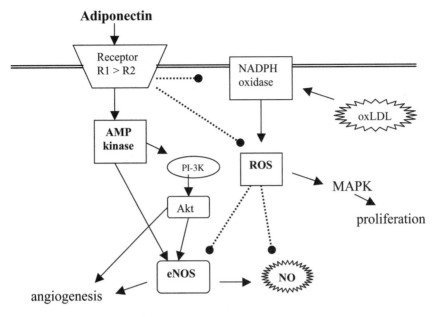

Fig. 3. Multiple potential signaling pathways for adiponectin.

Both eNOS and Akt activation contribute to the effects of adiponectin on angiogenesis. Another potential mechanism is inhibition from adiponectin of oxidized low-density lipoprotein (oxLDL)-induced superoxide production (ROS), possibly through inhibition of cellular nicotinamide adenine dinucleotide phosphate (NADPH) oxidase activity. Consequently, reduced ROS generation may enhance NO production (by ameliorating the suppression of eNOS activity by ROS) and diminish cell proliferation (by blocking oxLDL-induced MAPK activation) *(23)* (Fig. 3).

Resistin

Resistin, a recently identified 114 amino acid protein with a 20 amino acid signal sequence, is almost exclusively expressed in white adipose tissue, and especially in visceral vs sc adipose tissue. Resistin is secreted as a 94 amino acid polypeptide with 11 cysteine residues *(56)* and circulates as a dimer *(18)*. Initial animal and in vitro studies demonstrated that administration of recombinant resistin impairs glucose and lipid metabolism *(56,57)*, but these initial findings were challenged by subsequent observations in mice *(58,59)*, and a null association between circulating resistin and insulin resistance in humans *(60,61)*. More recent data indicate that resistin may act to negate leptin's and adiponectin's effect to induce MAPK phosphorylation and regulate metabolism in obese mice *(62)*, but these data have not been independently confirmed. Our data in mice reveal no evidence of an association between resistin and insulin resistance *(60,63)*. Whether resistin influences obesity either directly or by altering glucose and insulin levels, and/or whether resistin plays a direct or indirect role in inflammation associated with obesity *(64,65)* warrants further investigation.

Plasminogen Activator Inhibitor-1

Plasminogen activor inhibitor-1 (PAI-1), a primary inhibitor of fibrinolysis, is also secreted by adipocytes, and its secretion is greater by the visceral than by sc adipose tissue. Plasma PAI-1 levels are elevated in obesity and the insulin resistance syndrome and predict future risk for type 2 diabetes and CVD (7).

Acylation-Stimulating Protein

Acylation-stimulating protein (ASP), a complement protein, is a 76 amino acid protein composed of three components: complement factor C, factor B, and adipsin (complement factor D). Some studies in humans indicate that ASP positively correlates with fat mass, insulin resistance, dyslipidemia, and CVD (66). ASP affects both lipid and glucose metabolism (1) by promoting fatty acid uptake in the adipose tissue and triglyceride synthesis by increasing the activity of diacylglycerol (DAG) acyltransferase, (2) by decreasing lypolysis and the release of FFAs from adipocytes, and (3) by increasing glucose transport into adipocytes (7). Thus, some studies suggest that fasting ASP level may be predictive of postprandial triglyceride and FFA clearance in humans (67). Further studies are needed, however, to elucidate fully the understanding of the production, regulation, and physiological role of ASP in humans.

Proteins of Renin Angiotensin System

Proteins of the renin angiotensin system (RAS), which include renin, angiotensinogen (AGT), AGT I, AGT II, AGT receptor type 1 (AT1) and type 2 (AT2), and angiotensin-converting enzyme (ACE), are expressed in the adipose tissue as well, with their expression directly correlated with adipose mass and are higher in the visceral compared to sc compartment. Adipose tissue AGT expression is decreased by fasting and increased by refeeding, a fact reflected also in corresponding changes in blood pressure. The effects of the activation of RAS (increase in vascular tone, aldosterone secretion, and, consequently, sodium and water retention) indicate that the adipose tissue RAS could be a potential link between obesity and hypertension (7).

Enzymes Involved in Metabolism of Steroid Hormones

Intracellular levels of glucocorticoids may also regulate fat metabolism and the metabolic syndrome. 11β-hydroxysteroid dehydrogenase type 1 (11β-HSD1) is an enzyme expressed in adipose tissue, liver, and pancreas that catalyzes the activation of cortisone into cortisol in humans and 11-dehydrocorticosterone into corticosterone, the active metabolite in mice. Mice overexpressing 11β-HSD1 have increased levels of corticosterone, visceral obesity, insulin resistance, and hyperlipidemia (68). By contrast, 11β-HSD1-deficient mice have decreased gluconeogenesis during stress and on exposure to high-fat diets and have a diabetes-resistant phenotype (69). In human idiopathic obesity, 11β-HSD1 expression and activity are increased in adipose tissue and are correlated with total and regional adiposity. In addition, 11β-HSD1 inhibitors (such as carbenoxolone) improve insulin sensitivity and glycemic control, as well as decrease visceral adiposity and overall obesity in humans, suggesting a potential therapeutic role of these agents (70).

Adipose tissue expresses aromatase, an important enzyme for transforming androstenedione into estrone and testosterone into estradiol. Consequently, adipose tissue is the most important source of estrogens in postmenopausal women. The rate of conversion of androstenedione into estrone increases with age and body mass index and also affects body fat distribution. Aromatase-deficient mice have increased visceral adiposity, insulin resistance, dyslipidemia, and hepatic steatosis (71).

Peroxisome Proliferator-Activated Receptor γ

PPARγ, a nuclear receptor involved in the regulation of adipocyte differentiation, has recently become a target in the treatment of type 2 diabetes, hyperlipidemia, inflammation, and malignancy *(72)*. Administration of high-affinity PPARγ ligands, such as thiazolidine-diones, increases fat mass, whereas specific single-nucleotide polymorphisms of PPARγ have been associated with protection from obesity and insulin resistance on exposure to high-fat diets, as well as decreased triglyceride content throughout the body *(72)*.

ENDOCRINE PANCREAS

The most important hormone regulating energy homeostasis is insulin. Insulin, a 51 amino acid hormone composed of two peptide chains linked together by two disulfide bonds, is secreted from pancreatic β-cells and acts by binding to and activating a het-erotetrameric glycoprotein insulin receptor expressed on the plasma membrane of almost all cells. Insulin binding results in tyrosine phosphorylation of the insulin receptor and initiation of intracellular signaling via subsequent phosphorylation and activation of IRSs and other molecules that regulate key cellular activities, including gene expression; glucose uptake and oxidation; and synthesis of glycogen, triglyc-erides, and protein *(73)*.

Insulin-binding sites have been identified in key areas of food intake control, such as the arcuate nucleus (ARC) in the hypothalamus *(74)*, and intracerebroventricular infusion of insulin dramatically decreases food intake and body weight in animals *(75)*. By contrast, neuron-specific insulin receptor knockout (KO) mice demonstrate increased food intake, body weight, and adiposity, suggesting that insulin, similar to leptin, plays a key role in regulating energy balance *(76,77)*. Animal models of diet-induced obesity and leptin resistance are also characterized by insulin resistance and reduced insulin transport into the brain, suggesting that in addition to defective leptin transport and lep-tin resistance, weight gain and increased food intake may be owing to decreased central insulin levels *(78)*. Moreover, changes in nutrient availability and body weight induce adaptive responses in feeding behavior and in metabolic processes and promote weight gain and insulin resistance *(79)*. Thus, insulin resistance is also regarded as a maladap-tive response to increased nutrient availability *(see* Nutrients section).

Insulin, similar to leptin, circulates in levels proportional to the degree of adiposity *(80)*, which may serve to increase central insulin levels and/or to overcome impaired insulin-mediated intracellular signaling *(73)*. Finally, negative regulators of both leptin and insulin signal transduction, such as inhibitors of protein tyrosine phosphatase 1B, may provide opportunities for the treatment of both obesity and insulin resistance *(81)*.

GASTROINTESTINAL SIGNALS

Gut signals also regulate energy balance. Of the many GI tract-generated molecules, we focus herein on those newly discovered and considered to be the most important, ghrelin, peptide YY (PYY), glucagon-like peptide 1 (GLP1) and oxyntomodulin, bombesin like peptides, cholecystokinin (CCK), and gastric inhibitory peptide (GIP).

Ghrelin

Ghrelin, a 28 amino acid peptide with a labile octanoyl fatty acid side chain at the serine residue three, is mainly expressed in enterochromaffin cells in the mucosa of the stomach fundus *(82)*. In addition to being a potent GH secretagogue *(82)*, ghrelin increases food intake and decreases fat utilization *(83–85)*. Ghrelin is unique because it is the only gut hormone that stimulates food intake. In healthy humans, ghrelin levels rise before meals *(83)* and in response to diet-induced weight loss *(86)* and fall acutely after feeding. This fall is absent or blunted in obese humans *(87)*, a fact that has been proposed to contribute to the development of their obesity. By contrast, obese patients who undergo gastric bypass surgery have decreased ghrelin levels, which could contribute to maintaining decreased weight after bypass surgery *(86)*. Furthermore, recent data on humans have demonstrated an inverse and independent-of-adiposity correlation between ghrelin and leptin, but no regulation of ghrelin by administration of leptin over a short-term period of a few hours to a few days *(88)*. Whether ghrelin, alone or in concert with leptin, plays an important role in regulating energy homeostasis in humans remains to be shown by interventional studies.

Peptide YY

Peptide YY (PYY) is a 36 amino acid peptide with a tyrosine residue at both C- and N-terminals *(89)*, that is secreted from the L-cells of the small and large bowel *(90)*. PYY has structural homology with and belongs to the same peptide family as pancreatic polypeptide and neuropeptide Y (NPY), a potent central orexigenic peptide *(91)*. Unlike ghrelin, which signals energy insufficiency and stimulates food intake, PYY inhibits food intake through a gut–hypothalamic pathway that involves inhibition of NPY via Y2 receptors in the ARC and the dorsal motor nucleus of the vagus nerve *(92)*. PYY levels decrease with fasting and increase rapidly after a meal *(93)*, and peripheral injections of PYY to achieve normal postprandial levels decrease food intake and reduce body weight in rodents *(94)*. PYY reduces appetite and food intake when administered to obese or normal weight subjects, and endogenous levels of PYY may be lower in obese subjects, suggesting that a relative PYY deficiency may contribute to the development of obesity *(95)*. We have recently found that PYY levels are higher in obese patients after gastric bypass surgery (unpublished observation), a fact that may underlie the increased efficacy of this procedure in decreasing body weight. Thus, ongoing clinical trials involving the administration of PYY are awaited with great anticipation.

GLP1/Oxyntomodulin

GLP1, a 30 amino acid hormone *(96)* with a 50% amino acid homology with pancreatic glucagon, and oxyntomodulin, a 37 amino acid peptide, are both secreted by the enteroendocrine L-cells of the small and large intestines in a nutrient-dependent manner *(97)*. Although initial interest in GLP1 was fueled by its ability to lower blood glucose levels *(97)* and stimulate islet cell proliferation and neogenesis *(98)*, exogenous GLP1 was also found to decrease body weight and adipose tissue mass in rodents *(99,100)*. Moreover, mice deficient in dipeptidyl peptidase IV, an inhibitor of GLP1 degradation, are resistant to diet-induced obesity and insulin resistance. In contrast, immunoblockade of central GLP1 with antibodies resulted in increased energy intake. Although GLP1 is presumed to produce its anorectic effect by acting centrally, the exact mechanism of its action and its potential efficacy in humans have yet to be fully elucidated *(97)*.

Bombesin-Like Peptides

Bombesin-like peptides include gastrin-releasing peptide (GRP), which is processed into the smaller peptides GRP_{1-27} and GRP_{18-27}, and neuromedin B (NMB), which is processed into NMB_{1-32} and NMB_{23-32}. These peptides are released from the GI tract in response to food intake, and result in decreased food intake *(101)* and duration of feeding *(102,103)* by binding to a G protein-coupled receptor *(104)* that signals information on energy intake to the brain *(101,105)*. These receptors are widely expressed both in the GI tract and centrally, and bombesin receptor 3 KO mice display hyperphagia, mild obesity, diabetes, and hypertension.

Cholecystokinin

CCK is a peptide with several isoforms ranging in size from 4 to 83 amino acids, that is released by the duodenum and jejunum in response to food ingestion *(106)* and stimulates pancreatic enzyme secretion, gallbladder contraction, intestinal motility *(107)*, as well as gastric distension and slowing of gastric emptying, which, in turn, results in reduced food intake *(107,108)*. CCK acts via specific receptors to cause termination of an individual meal *(109–111)*. CCK receptor antagonists increase food intake in rodents *(112)*, and peripheral administration of CCK reduces food intake acutely in animals and humans *(107)*, but may also lead to a compensatory increase in daily meal number and thus results in little weight loss.

Gastric Inhibitory Peptide

GIP, a peptide secreted by the duodenal K-cells on absorption of fat or glucose, is a potent insulin incretin and is oversecreted in the diet-induced mouse model of obesity. Mice lacking the GIP receptor are protected from obesity and insulin resistance *(113)*, indicating that GIP is implicated in a peripheral, possibly leptin-independent, decrease in EE and fat oxidation, rather than an alteration in energy intake.

NUTRIENTS

Circulating nutrients (glucose, fatty acids, amino acids) are derived from two main sources: exogenous (from food intake) and endogenous (from tissue production such as glucose and lipid production by the liver). Fasting and weight loss are associated with decreased EE, whereas excess nutrients lead to thermogenic responses. Thus, the availability of nutrients can regulate EE. The availability of nutrients can be sensed at central sites (hypothalamus), as well as directly in peripheral tissues (such as muscle and fat) through nutrient-sensing pathways. The hypothalamus is where these signals are integrated and feeding behavior and metabolism are modulated. A prolonged period of excess food intake activates nutrient-sensing pathways, which, in turn, leads to weight gain and insulin resistance. It also stimulates secretion of insulin and leptin, which act to counterregulate weight gain and insulin resistance via their hypothalamic receptors by decreasing food intake and production of endogenous nutrients and by increasing EE. The hypothalamus can also directly sense nutrients via neural nutrient-sensing pathways and trigger counterregulatory neural responses to reverse weight gain and insulin resistance, functioning as a true negative feedback system. Thus, alteration in the balance in the nutrient-sensing pathways/nutrient-activated mechanisms could lead finally to the development of obesity and type 2 diabetes *(79)*.

Proposed cellular fuel sensors or nutrient-sensing pathways are now better understood and are briefly discussed next.

Malonyl-CoA Sensor

The malonyl-CoA sensor is implicated in the switch of oxidation from fatty acids to glucose; this molecule is an inhibitor of carnityl-palmitoyl transferase (CPT1), the rate-limiting enzyme implicated in long-chain fatty acid (LCFA) oxidation. In the presence of high concentrations of glucose and insulin, the accumulation of malonyl-CoA inhibits CPT1 and reduces lipid oxidation, favoring lipid storage into triglycerides, thus causing insulin resistance in pheripheral tissues. Hypothalamic neurons can also directly sense LCFA-CoA. In the hypothalamus, activation of malonyl-CoA triggers counterregulatory responses to decrease food intake and glucose production *(79)*.

Hexosamine Biosynthesis Pathway

The hexosamine biosynthesis pathway (HBP) is activated by increased glucose fluxes. Only 1–3% of incoming glucose enters the HBP after conversion into fructose-6-phosphate (Fru-6P) by the enzyme glutamine-fructose-6-phosphate aminotransferase (6FAT), which also regulates the flux to this pathway. The final step is production of uridine diphosphate (UDP)-*N*-acetylglucosamine (GlucNAc), the main substrate for protein glycosylation. Glycosylation of the proteins implicated in the multiple sites of insulin-signaling cascade induces insulin resistance by decreasing tyrosine phosphorylation of the IRS proteins. This, in turn, decreases insulin action on glucose transport, metabolism, and gene expression. Not only glucose but also FFAs can influence the activation of HBP. FFAs can inhibit the entry of Fru-6P into the glycolytic pathway and therefore cause a shunt of Fru-6P toward the HBP. Short-term overfeeding with a high-fat diet induces increased fluxes into the HBP and increases the levels of UDP-GlucNAc in skeletal muscle. Activation of HBP decreases EE and leptin expression, suggesting a role for this pathway in the regulation of energy balance.

Protein Kinase C

An Increase in plasma FFAs elevates the cytosolic concentration of LCFA-CoA and increases triglycerides and DAG synthesis. DAG activates protein kinase C, in both muscle and liver, which induces serine phosphorylation and reduces tyrosine phosphorylation of the IRS-1 and inhibits activation of PI-3k, thus promoting insulin resistance *(114)*.

Mammalian Target of Rapamycine Kinase

Mammalian target of rapamycine (mTOR) kinase is an evolutionary very well-conserved kinase that integrates signals from nutrients (amino acids and energy) and growth factors to regulate both cell growth and cell-cycle progression. The bacterially derived drug rapamycin (sirolimus), a Food and Drug Administration-approved immunosuppressive and cardiology drug, specifically inhibits TOR, resulting in reduced cell growth, reduced rate of cell-cycle progression, and reduced rate of proliferation *(115)*. The main downstream effector of the mTOR kinase, the ribosomal protein S6 kinase 1 (S6K1), is also activated by amino acids and growth factors. Mice with genetically ablated S6K1 are protected against age- and high-fat diet-induced obesity while enhancing insulin sensitivity *(116)*. EE is increased in these mice, by increasing thermogenesis, lipolysis, and oxygen consumption. At a molecular level, mitochondrial density is increased in muscle and adipose tissue, as is the expression of genes critical for mitochondrial function, fatty acid oxidation, and enhanced insulin signaling at both receptor and postreceptor levels. Conversely, enhanced S6K1 activity, under the condition of nutrient excess, is linked to insulin resistance by negatively regulating insulin signaling *(116,117)*.

AMP-Activated Protein Kinase

AMP-activated protein kinase (AMPK) is an important energy and nutrient sensor, activated by leptin, adiponectin, and exercise, that has beneficial effects on insulin resistance. It decreases the activation of mTOR and S6K1 and modulates expression of proliferator-activated receptor coactivator 1 (PGC-1) *(117)*. AMPK functions also as an energy and nutrient sensor in the hypothalamus. Via central actions, and probably by inhibiting AMPK, glucose can modulate food intake as well as peripheral insulin sensitivity *(22)*.

Modulation of Gene Expression

Direct modulation of gene expression by nutrients is also a potential mechanism.

All these pathways converge finally to decrease expression of PGC-1 α and β, key coactivators of PPARα, PPARγ, and PPARδ, leading to mitochondrial dysfunction and reduced EE, all of which enhance the risk for obesity and insulin resistance *(117)*.

CONCLUSIONS

Recent developments in basic research are elucidating the mechanisms responsible for energy homeostasis and are expected to lead to the development of new treatment options for obesity and related disorders, thus offering tangible benefits to the increasing percentage of the population striving to control their body weight and prevent comorbidities.

REFERENCES

1. Flegal KM, Troiano RP. Changes in the distribution of body mass index of adults and children in the US population. Int J Obes Relat Metab Disord 2000;24(7):807–818.
2. Overweight, obesity, and health risk: National Task Force on the Prevention and Treatment of Obesity. Arch Intern Med 2000;160(7):898–904.
3. Manson JE, Skerrett PJ, Greenland P, VanItallie TB. The escalating pandemics of obesity and sedentary lifestyle: a call to action for clinicians. Arch Intern Med 2004;164(3):249–258.
4. Fagot-Campagna A, Pettitt DJ, Engelgau MM, et al. Type 2 diabetes among North American children and adolescents: an epidemiologic review and a public health perspective. J Pediatr 2000; 136(5):664–672.
5. Kennedy GC. The role of depot fat in the hypothalamic control of food intake in the rat. Proc R Soc Lond 1953;140:579–592.
6. Zhang Y, Proenca R, Maffei M, Barone M, Leopold L, Friedman JM. Positional cloning of the mouse obese gene and its human homologue. Nature 1994;372(6505):425–432.
7. Kershaw EE, Flier JS. Adipose tissue as an endocrine organ. J Clin Endocrinol Metab 2004;89(6): 2548–2556.
8. Coleman DL. Obese and diabetes: two mutant genes causing diabetes-obesity syndromes in mice. Diabetologia 1978;14(3):141–148.
9. Friedman JM, Leibel RL. Tackling a weighty problem. Cell 1992;69(2):217–220.
10. Mantzoros CS, Flier JS. Editorial: leptin as a therapeutic agent—trials and tribulations. J Clin Endocrinol Metab 2000;85(11):4000–4002.
11. McMinn JE, Sindelar DK, Havel PJ, Schwartz MW. Leptin deficiency induced by fasting impairs the satiety response to cholecystokinin. Endocrinology 2000;141(12):4442–4448.
12. Doring H, Schwarzer K, Nuesslein-Hildesheim B, Schmidt I. Leptin selectively increases energy expenditure of food-restricted lean mice. Int J Obes Relat Metab Disord 1998;22(2):83–88.
13. Ahima RS, Saper CB, Flier JS, Elmquist JK. Leptin regulation of neuroendocrine systems. Front Neuroendocrinol 2000;21(3):263–307.

14. Halaas JL, Boozer C, Blair-West J, Fidahusein N, Denton DA, Friedman JM. Physiological response to long-term peripheral and central leptin infusion in lean and obese mice. Proc Natl Acad Sci USA 1997;94(16):8878–8883.
15. Mantzoros CS. The role of leptin in human obesity and disease: a review of current evidence. Ann Intern Med 1999;130(8):671–680.
16. Auwerx J, Staels B. Leptin. Lancet 1998;351(9104):737–742.
17. Flier JS. Obesity wars: molecular progress confronts an expanding epidemic. Cell 2004;116(2): 337–350.
18. Gale SM, Castracane VD, Mantzoros CS. Energy homeostasis, obesity and eating disorders: recent advances in endocrinology. J Nutr 2004;134(2):295–298.
19. Kamohara S, Burcelin R, Halaas JL, Friedman JM, Charron MJ. Acute stimulation of glucose metabolism in mice by leptin treatment. Nature 1997;389(6649):374–377.
20. Haque MS, Minokoshi Y, Hamai M, Iwai M, Horiuchi M, Shimazu T. Role of the sympathetic nervous system and insulin in enhancing glucose uptake in peripheral tissues after intrahypothalamic injection of leptin in rats. Diabetes 1999;48(9):1706–1712.
21. Minokoshi Y, Haque MS, Shimazu T. Microinjection of leptin into the ventromedial hypothalamus increases glucose uptake in peripheral tissues in rats. Diabetes 1999;48(2):287–291.
22. Alquier T, Kahn BB. Peripheral signals set the tone for central regulation of metabolism. Endocrinology 2004;145(9):4022–4024.
23. Goldstein BJ, Scalia R. Adiponectin: a novel adipokine linking adipocytes and vascular function. J Clin Endocrinol Metab 2004;89(6):2563–2568.
24. Moschos S, Chan JL, Mantzoros CS. Leptin and reproduction: a review. Fertil Steril 2002;77(3): 433–444.
25. Farooqi IS, Keogh JM, Yeo GS, Lank EJ, Cheetham T, O'Rahilly S. Clinical spectrum of obesity and mutations in the melanocortin 4 receptor gene. N Engl J Med 2003;348(12):1085–1095.
26. Clement K, Vaisse C, Lahlou N, et al. A mutation in the human leptin receptor gene causes obesity and pituitary dysfunction. Nature 1998;392(6674):398–401.
27. Considine RV, Sinha MK, Heiman ML, et al. Serum immunoreactive-leptin concentrations in normal-weight and obese humans. N Engl J Med 1996;334(5):292–295.
28. Miller KK, Parulekar MS, Schoenfeld E, et al. Decreased leptin levels in normal weight women with hypothalamic amenorrhea: the effects of body composition and nutritional intake. J Clin Endocrinol Metab 1998;83(7):2309–2312.
29. Laughlin GA, Yen SS. Hypoleptinemia in women athletes: absence of a diurnal rhythm with amenorrhea. J Clin Endocrinol Metab 1997;82(1):318–321.
30. Chan JL, Heist K, DePaoli AM, Veldhuis JD, Mantzoros CS. The role of falling leptin levels in the neuroendocrine and metabolic adaptation to short-term starvation in healthy men. J Clin Invest 2003;111(9):1409–1421.
31. Welt CK, Chan JL, Bullen J, et al. Recombinant human leptin in women with hypothalamic amenorrhea. N Engl J Med 2004;351(10):987–997.
32. Bastard JP, Jardel C, Bruckert E, et al. Elevated levels of interleukin 6 are reduced in serum and subcutaneous adipose tissue of obese women after weight loss. J Clin Endocrinol Metab 2000;85(9): 3338–3342.
33. Wallenius K, Wallenius V, Sunter D, Dickson SL, Jansson JO. Intracerebroventricular interleukin-6 treatment decreases body fat in rats. Biochem Biophys Res Commun 2002;293(1):560–565.
34. Stenlof K, Wernstedt I, Fjallman T, Wallenius V, Wallenius K, Jansson JO. Interleukin-6 levels in the central nervous system are negatively correlated with fat mass in overweight/obese subjects. J Clin Endocrinol Metab 2003;88(9):4379–4383.
35. Fried SK, Bunkin DA, Greenberg AS. Omental and subcutaneous adipose tissues of obese subjects release interleukin-6: depot difference and regulation by glucocorticoid. J Clin Endocrinol Metab 1998;83(3):847–850.
36. Hotamisligil GS, Arner P, Caro JF, Atkinson RL, Spiegelman BM. Increased adipose tissue expression of tumor necrosis factor-alpha in human obesity and insulin resistance. J Clin Invest 1995;95(5):2409–2415.
37. Warne JP. Tumour necrosis factor alpha: a key regulator of adipose tissue mass. J Endocrinol 2003;177(3):351–355.
38. Harris MI, Hadden WC, Knowler WC, Bennett PH. Prevalence of diabetes and impaired glucose tolerance and plasma glucose levels in U.S. population aged 20–74 yr. Diabetes 1987;36(4): 523–534.

39. Scherer PE, Williams S, Fogliano M, Baldini G, Lodish HF. A novel serum protein similar to C1q, produced exclusively in adipocytes. J Biol Chem 1995;270(45):26,746–26,749.

40. Arita Y, Kihara S, Ouchi N, et al. Paradoxical decrease of an adipose-specific protein, adiponectin, in obesity. Biochem Biophys Res Commun 1999;257(1):79–83.

41. Wang Y, Xu A, Knight C, Xu LY, Cooper GJ. Hydroxylation and glycosylation of the four conserved lysine residues in the collagenous domain of adiponectin: potential role in the modulation of its insulin-sensitizing activity. J Biol Chem 2002;277(22):19,521–19,529.

42. Chandran M, Phillips SA, Ciaraldi T, Henry RR. Adiponectin: more than just another fat cell hormone? Diabetes Care 2003;26(8):2442–2450.

43. Yamauchi T, Kamon J, Ito Y, et al. Cloning of adiponectin receptors that mediate antidiabetic metabolic effects. Nature 2003;423(6941):762–769.

44. Kubota N, Terauchi Y, Yamauchi T, et al. Disruption of adiponectin causes insulin resistance and neointimal formation. J Biol Chem 2002;277(29):25,863–25,866.

45. Gavrila A, Chan JL, Yiannakouris N, et al. Serum adiponectin levels are inversely associated with overall and central fat distribution but are not directly regulated by acute fasting or leptin administration in humans: cross-sectional and interventional studies. J Clin Endocrinol Metab 2003;88(10): 4823–4831.

46. Yang WS, Lee WJ, Funahashi T, et al. Weight reduction increases plasma levels of an adipose-derived anti-inflammatory protein, adiponectin. J Clin Endocrinol Metab 2001;86(8):3815–3819.

47. Masaki T, Chiba S, Yasuda T, et al. Peripheral, but not central, administration of adiponectin reduces visceral adiposity and upregulates the expression of uncoupling protein in agouti yellow (Ay/a) obese mice. Diabetes 2003;52(9):2266–2273.

48. Fruebis J, Tsao TS, Javorschi S, et al. Proteolytic cleavage product of 30-kDa adipocyte complement-related protein increases fatty acid oxidation in muscle and causes weight loss in mice. Proc Natl Acad Sci USA 2001;98(4):2005–2010.

49. Yamauchi T, Kamon J, Waki H, et al. The fat-derived hormone adiponectin reverses insulin resistance associated with both lipoatrophy and obesity. Nat Med 2001;7(8):941–946.

50. Bluher M, Michael MD, Peroni OD, et al. Adipose tissue selective insulin receptor knockout protects against obesity and obesity-related glucose intolerance. Dev Cell 2002;3(1):25–38.

51. Stefan N, Vozarova B, Funahashi T, et al. Plasma adiponectin concentration is associated with skeletal muscle insulin receptor tyrosine phosphorylation, and low plasma concentration precedes a decrease in whole-body insulin sensitivity in humans. Diabetes 2002;51(6):1884–1888.

52. Lindsay RS, Funahashi T, Hanson RL, et al. Adiponectin and development of type 2 diabetes in the Pima Indian population. Lancet 2002;360(9326):57, 58.

53. Yokota T, Oritani K, Takahashi I, et al. Adiponectin, a new member of the family of soluble defense collagens, negatively regulates the growth of myelomonocytic progenitors and the functions of macrophages. Blood 2000;96(5):1723–1732.

54. Ouchi N, Kihara S, Arita Y, et al. Novel modulator for endothelial adhesion molecules: adipocyte-derived plasma protein adiponectin. Circulation 1999;100(25):2473–2476.

55. Ouchi N, Kihara S, Arita Y, et al. Adipocyte-derived plasma protein, adiponectin, suppresses lipid accumulation and class A scavenger receptor expression in human monocyte-derived macrophages. Circulation 2001;103(8):1057–1063.

56. Steppan CM, Bailey ST, Bhat S, et al. The hormone resistin links obesity to diabetes. Nature 2001;409(6818):307–312.

57. McTernan PG, Fisher FM, Valsamakis G, et al. Resistin and type 2 diabetes: regulation of resistin expression by insulin and rosiglitazone and the effects of recombinant resistin on lipid and glucose metabolism in human differentiated adipocytes. J Clin Endocrinol Metab 2003;88(12):6098–6106.

58. Steppan CM, Lazar MA. Resistin and obesity-associated insulin resistance. Trends Endocrinol Metab 2002;13(1):18–23.

59. Way JM, Gorgun CZ, Tong Q, et al. Adipose tissue resistin expression is severely suppressed in obesity and stimulated by peroxisome proliferator-activated receptor gamma agonists. J Biol Chem 2001;276(28):25,651–25,653.

60. Lee JH, Chan JL, Yiannakouris N, et al. Circulating resistin levels are not associated with obesity or insulin resistance in humans and are not regulated by fasting or leptin administration: cross-sectional and interventional studies in normal, insulin-resistant, and diabetic subjects. J Clin Endocrinol Metab 2003;88(10):4848–4856.

61. Silha JV, Krsek M, Hana V, et al. Perturbations in adiponectin, leptin and resistin levels in acromegaly: lack of correlation with insulin resistance. Clin Endocrinol (Oxf) 2003;58(6):736–742.

62. Banerjee RR, Rangwala SM, Shapiro JS, et al. Regulation of fasted blood glucose by resistin. Science 2004;303(5661):1195–1198.

63. Lee JH, Bullen JW Jr, Stoyneva VL, Mantzoros CS. Circulating resistin in lean, obese and insulin-resistant mouse models: lack of association with insulinemia and glycemia. Am J Physiol Endocrinol Metab 2005;288:E625–E632.

64. Holcomb IN, Kabakoff RC, Chan B, et al. FIZZ1, a novel cysteine-rich secreted protein associated with pulmonary inflammation, defines a new gene family. EMBO J 2000;19(15):4046–4055.

65. Shetty GK, Economides PA, Horton ES, Mantzoros CS, Veves A. Circulating adiponectin and resistin levels in relation to metabolic factors, inflammatory markers, and vascular reactivity in diabetic patients and subjects at risk for diabetes. Diabetes Care 2004;27(10):2450–2457.

66. Cianflone K, Xia Z, Chen LY. Critical review of acylation-stimulating protein physiology in humans and rodents. Biochim Biophys Acta 2003;1609(2):127–143.

67. Cianflone K, Zakarian R, Couillard C, Delplanque B, Despres JP, Sniderman A. Fasting acylation-stimulating protein is predictive of postprandial triglyceride clearance. J Lipid Res 2004;45(1):124–131.

68. Masuzaki H, Paterson J, Shinyama H, et al. A transgenic model of visceral obesity and the metabolic syndrome. Science 2001;294(5549):2166–2170.

69. Kotelevtsev Y, Holmes MC, Burchell A, et al. 11beta-hydroxysteroid dehydrogenase type 1 knock-out mice show attenuated glucocorticoid-inducible responses and resist hyperglycemia on obesity or stress. Proc Natl Acad Sci USA 1997;94(26):14,924–14,929.

70. Masuzaki H, Flier JS. Tissue-specific glucocorticoid reactivating enzyme, 11 beta-hydroxysteroid dehydrogenase type 1 (11 beta-HSD1)—a promising drug target for the treatment of metabolic syndrome. Curr Drug Targets Immune Endocr Metab Disord 2003;3(4):255–262.

71. Takeda K, Toda K, Saibara T, et al. Progressive development of insulin resistance phenotype in male mice with complete aromatase (CYP19) deficiency. J Endocrinol 2003;176(2):237–246.

72. Gurnell M. PPARgamma and metabolism: insights from the study of human genetic variants. Clin Endocrinol (Oxf) 2003;59(3):267–277.

73. Niswender KD, Schwartz MW. Insulin and leptin revisited: adiposity signals with overlapping physiological and intracellular signaling capabilities. Front Neuroendocrinol 2003;24(1):1–10.

74. Marks JL, Porte D Jr, Stahl WL, Baskin DG. Localization of insulin receptor mRNA in rat brain by in situ hybridization. Endocrinology 1990;127(6):3234–3236.

75. Woods SC, Lotter EC, McKay LD, Porte D Jr. Chronic intracerebroventricular infusion of insulin reduces food intake and body weight of baboons. Nature 1979;282(5738):503–505.

76. Bruning JC, Gautam D, Burks DJ, et al. Role of brain insulin receptor in control of body weight and reproduction. Science 2000;289(5487):2122–2125.

77. Cohen P, Zhao C, Cai X, et al. Selective deletion of leptin receptor in neurons leads to obesity. J Clin Invest 2001;108(8):1113–1121.

78. Kaiyala KJ, Prigeon RL, Kahn SE, Woods SC, Schwartz MW. Obesity induced by a high-fat diet is associated with reduced brain insulin transport in dogs. Diabetes 2000;49(9):1525–1533.

79. Obici S, Rossetti L. Minireview: nutrient sensing and the regulation of insulin action and energy balance. Endocrinology 2003; 144(12):5172-5178.

80. Bagdade JD, Bierman EL, Porte D Jr. The significance of basal insulin levels in the evaluation of the insulin response to glucose in diabetic and nondiabetic subjects. J Clin Invest 1967;46(10):1549–1557.

81. Dadke S, Chernoff J. Protein-tyrosine phosphatase 1B as a potential drug target for obesity. Curr Drug Targets Immune Endocr Metab Disord 2003;3(4):299–304.

82. Kojima M, Hosoda H, Date Y, Nakazato M, Matsuo H, Kangawa K. Ghrelin is a growth-hormone-releasing acylated peptide from stomach. Nature 1999;402(6762):656–660.

83. Cummings DE, Purnell JQ, Frayo RS, Schmidova K, Wisse BE, Weigle DS. A preprandial rise in plasma ghrelin levels suggests a role in meal initiation in humans. Diabetes 2001;50(8):1714–1719.

84. Wren AM, Small CJ, Ward HL, et al. The novel hypothalamic peptide ghrelin stimulates food intake and growth hormone secretion. Endocrinology 2000;141(11):4325–4328.

85. Tschop M, Smiley DL, Heiman ML. Ghrelin induces adiposity in rodents. Nature 2000;407(6806):908–913.

86. Cummings DE, Weigle DS, Frayo RS, et al. Plasma ghrelin levels after diet-induced weight loss or gastric bypass surgery. N Engl J Med 2002;346(21):1623–1630.

87. English PJ, Ghatei MA, Malik IA, Bloom SR, Wilding JP. Food fails to suppress ghrelin levels in obese humans. J Clin Endocrinol Metab 2002;87(6):2984–2987.

88. Chan JL, Bullen J, Lee JH, Yiannakouris N, Mantzoros CS. Ghrelin levels are not regulated by recombinant leptin administration and/or three days of fasting in healthy subjects. J Clin Endocrinol Metab 2004;89(1):335–343.

89. Tatemoto K, Mutt V. Isolation of two novel candidate hormones using a chemical method for finding naturally occurring polypeptides. Nature 1980;285(5764):417, 418.

90. Adrian TE, Ferri GL, Bacarese-Hamilton AJ, Fuessl HS, Polak JM, Bloom SR. Human distribution and release of a putative new gut hormone, peptide YY. Gastroenterology 1985;89(5): 1070–1077.

91. Tatemoto K, Carlquist M, Mutt V. Neuropeptide Y—a novel brain peptide with structural similarities to peptide YY and pancreatic polypeptide. Nature 1982;296(5858):659–660.

92. Korner J, Leibel RL. To eat or not to eat—how the gut talks to the brain. N Engl J Med 2003;349(10): 926–928.

93. Anini Y, Fu-Cheng X, Cuber JC, Kervran A, Chariot J, Roz C. Comparison of the postprandial release of peptide YY and proglucagon-derived peptides in the rat. Pflügers Arch 1999;438(3): 299–306.

94. Batterham RL, Cowley MA, Small CJ, et al. Gut hormone PYY(3-36) physiologically inhibits food intake. Nature 2002;418(6898):650–654.

95. Batterham RL, Cohen MA, Ellis SM, et al. Inhibition of food intake in obese subjects by peptide YY3-36. N Engl J Med 2003;349(10):941–948.

96. Kieffer TJ, Habener JF. The glucagon-like peptides. Endocr Rev 1999;20(6):876–913.

97. Drucker DJ, Philippe J, Mojsov S, Chick WL, Habener JF. Glucagon-like peptide I stimulates insulin gene expression and increases cyclic AMP levels in a rat islet cell line. Proc Natl Acad Sci USA 1987;84(10):3434–3438.

98. Xu G, Stoffers DA, Habener JF, Bonner-Weir S. Exendin-4 stimulates both beta-cell replication and neogenesis, resulting in increased beta-cell mass and improved glucose tolerance in diabetic rats. Diabetes 1999;48(12):2270–2276.

99. Greig NH, Holloway HW, De Ore KA, et al. Once daily injection of exendin-4 to diabetic mice achieves long-term beneficial effects on blood glucose concentrations. Diabetologia 1999;42(1):45–50.

100. Szayna M, Doyle ME, Betkey JA, et al. Exendin-4 decelerates food intake, weight gain, and fat deposition in Zucker rats. Endocrinology 2000;141(6):1936–1941.

101. Merali Z, McIntosh J, Anisman H. Role of bombesin-related peptides in the control of food intake. Neuropeptides 1999;33(5):376–386.

102. Flynn FW. Fourth ventricular injection of selective bombesin receptor antagonists facilitates feeding in rats. Am J Physiol 1993;264(1 Pt 2):R218–R221.

103. Gutzwiller JP, Drewe J, Hildebrand P, Rossi L, Lauper JZ, Beglinger C. Effect of intravenous human gastrin-releasing peptide on food intake in humans. Gastroenterology 1994;106(5):1168–1173.

104. Battey JF, Way JM, Corjay MH, et al. Molecular cloning of the bombesin/gastrin-releasing peptide receptor from Swiss 3T3 cells. Proc Natl Acad Sci USA 1991;88(2):395–399.

105. Gibbs J, Kulkosky PJ, Smith GP. Effects of peripheral and central bombesin on feeding behavior of rats. Peptides 1981;2(Suppl 2):179–183.

106. Go VLW. The physiology of cholecystokinin. In: Gut Hormones. Bloom SR, ed. Churchill Livingstone, Edinburgh, 1978, pp. 203–207.

107. Kissileff HR, Carretta JC, Geliebter A, Pi-Sunyer FX. Cholecystokinin and stomach distension combine to reduce food intake in humans. Am J Physiol Regul Integr Comp Physiol 2003;285(5):R992–R998.

108. Moran TH, McHugh PR. Cholecystokinin suppresses food intake by inhibiting gastric emptying. Am J Physiol 1982;242(5):R491–R497.

109. Bi S, Moran TH. Actions of CCK in the controls of food intake and body weight: lessons from the CCK-A receptor deficient OLETF rat. Neuropeptides 2002;36(2–3):171–181.

110. Moran TH, Robinson PH, Goldrich MS, McHugh PR. Two brain cholecystokinin receptors: implications for behavioral actions. Brain Res 1986;362(1):175–179.

111. Wank SA, Harkins R, Jensen RT, Shapira H, de Weerth A, Slattery T. Purification, molecular cloning, and functional expression of the cholecystokinin receptor from rat pancreas. Proc Natl Acad Sci USA 1992;89(7):3125–3129.

112. Corp ES, Curcio M, Gibbs J, Smith GP. The effect of centrally administered CCK-receptor antagonists on food intake in rats. Physiol Behav 1997;61(6):823–827.

113. Miyawaki K, Yamada Y, Ban N, et al. Inhibition of gastric inhibitory polypeptide signaling prevents obesity. Nat Med 2002;8(7):738–742.

114. Boden G, Carnell LH. Nutritional effects of fat on carbohydrate metabolism. Best Pract Res Clin Endocrinol Metab 2003;17(3):399–410.
115. Fingar DC, Blenis J. Target of rapamycin (TOR): an integrator of nutrient and growth factor signals and coordinator of cell growth and cell cycle progression. Oncogene 2004;23(18): 3151–3171.
116. Um SH, Frigerio F, Watanabe M, et al. Absence of S6K1 protects against age- and diet-induced obesity while enhancing insulin sensitivity. Nature 2004;431(7005):200–205.
117. Patti ME, Kahn BB. Nutrient sensor links obesity with diabetes risk. Nat Med 2004;10(10): 1049, 1050.

5

Central Integration of Peripheral Signals in Regulation of Energy Homeostasis

Greeshma K. Shetty, MD,
George Karanastasis, MD,
and Christos S. Mantzoros, MD, DSc

CONTENTS

INTRODUCTION
AFFERENT CNS SIGNALS CONVEYING NUTRITIONAL STATUS
NEUROANATOMIC STRUCTURES MEDIATING ENERGY HOMEOSTASIS
CENTRAL NEUROPEPTIDES REGULATING ENERGY BALANCE
CONCLUSIONS
REFERENCES

INTRODUCTION

The growing epidemic of obesity, a disease state emerging from an imbalance between energy intake and energy expenditure (EE), has recently attracted the attention of many researchers, leading to efforts to investigate and characterize the mechanisms underlying energy homeostasis. As a result, there has been an explosion of research in the area and the discovery of an ever-increasing number of molecules, that play an active role in normal physiology and pathophysiology.

Friedman's discovery of leptin in 1994 conceptualized a model of communication between peripheral endocrine organs and the central nervous system (CNS) in the control of energy homeostasis. The investigation of leptin signaling, along with the study of other recently discovered hormones such as ghrelin and PYY-(36), has led to the identification and study of a distinct group of centrally expressed neuropeptides, that integrate several signals from the periphery in response to changing nutritional states (Fig. 1).

The purpose of this chapter is to summarize the current understanding of the central pathways regulating energy homeostasis. Its focus lies mainly on central neuropeptides and their regulation by peripheral hormones and dietary nutrients, the latter discussed only sparingly in the context of integration and subsequent regulation of energy balance.

From: *Contemporary Diabetes: Obesity and Diabetes*
Edited by: C. S. Mantzoros © Humana Press Inc., Totowa, NJ

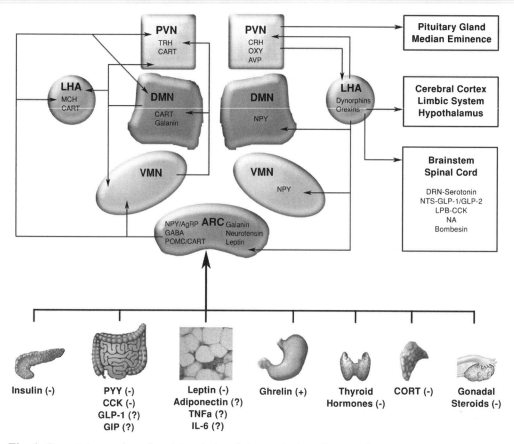

Fig. 1. Central integration of peripheral signals in regulation of energy homeostasis: ARC, arcuate nucleus; VMN, ventromedial nucleus; DMN, dorsomedial nucleus; PVN, paraventricular nucleus; LHA, lateral hypothalamus; LPB, lateral parabrachial nucleus; DRN, dorsal reticular nucleus; TRH, thyrotropin-releasing hormone; OXY, oxytocin; AVP, vasopressin; NTS, nucleus tractus solitarius; GLP-1/2, glucagon-like peptide 1/2; GIP, gastric inhibitory peptide; TNFa, tumor necrosis factor alpha; IL-6, interleukin 6; NA, noradrenaline; (+), orexigenic effect; (–), anorexigenic effect; (?), unknown effect. (Adapted from ref. *1*.)

AFFERENT CNS SIGNALS CONVEYING NUTRITIONAL STATUS

The afferent signals to the brain conveying information regarding nutrient availability, or lack thereof, can be classified into three distinct types: endocrine, metabolic, and neural. Hormones are released from peripheral endocrine organs, such as the pancreas (insulin), intestine (cholecystokinin [CCK]), white adipose tissue (leptin), and stomach (ghrelin), and their levels in the bloodstream fluctuate in response to changing levels of energy availability. These hormones convey information on the energy status of the organism to the CNS by binding to receptors specific to each hormone strategically located throughout widespread neuronal subpopulations, principally within the hypothalamic nuclei. These receptor–ligand interactions are followed by the downstream stimulation or inhibition of discrete neural centers, which ultimately modulate the energy balance in response to the initiating signal. As discussed subsequently, the central effectors of peripheral signaling have been divided into orexigenic (energy intake promoting) and anorexigenic (energy intake restricting). In addition to peripheral regulation, these centers exert stimulatory and/or inhibitory effects on each other through numerous redundant interconnections.

The metabolic influence on central energy homeostasis is similar to that of the endocrine factors just discussed. Hypothalamic neurons express surface enzymes *(1)* and ion channels *(2,3)* that also act as direct sensors of nutrient availability and further activate intracellular second-messenger pathways to appropriate a response. The most extensively studied nutrients are carbohydrates and lipids, and research on carbohydrate metabolism has revealed that declining blood glucose levels activate the orexigenic group of neurons, whereas elevated postprandial glucose levels activate the anorexigenic group. A detailed discussion of the role of nutrients in energy homeostasis is presented in Chapter 4.

Neural afferent signals from the periphery travel mainly via the vagus nerve, which densely innervates the gastrointestinal tract. During the process of food ingestion, these neurons are activated by a combination of mechanical factors (e.g., luminal distention) *(4)* and peripheral hormones (e.g., CCK) *(5)*. Afferents relay information to the nucleus tractus solitarius, located centrally in the medulla oblongata, and carry out the short-term regulation of feeding.

NEUROANATOMIC STRUCTURES MEDIATING
ENERGY HOMEOSTASIS

The current understanding of the energy homeostasis model ascribes a central role to the hypothalamus in the integration of peripheral signals *(6)*. Within the hypothalamus, the arcuate nucleus (ARC) is a major site of energy signal integration; it is considered to be the key sensor of peripheral energy input and has been described as the "*primum movens* of metabolism regulation" *(7)*. This theory of central importance, although under considerable debate, is based on the anterior location of the ARC in relation to the other hypothalamic nuclei, which makes the ARC the area first encountered and activated by circulating signals *(7)*; the immediate surroundings of the ARC not being shielded by the blood–brain barrier and allowing unrestricted access to afferent inputs *(7)*; and, finally, the two subpopulations of neurons colocated in this nucleus with opposing actions on energy homeostasis *(7)* (discussed below).

The paraventricular nucleus (PVN), the lateral hypothalamus–perifornical area, and the ventromedial and dorsomedial nuclei are the other main hypothalamic areas identified as effectors of peripheral information *(8,9)*. These structures are divided into two categories. The lateral hypothalamus–perifornical area constitutes the orexigenic limb, whereas the ventromedial, dorsomedial, and paraventricular nuclei comprise the anorexigenic division of the hypothalamus. The connections between these two areas are not only abundant, but are highly redundant as well. During a positive energy balance, neurochemical signaling inhibits orexigenic centers and activates anorexigenic centers, whereas during negative energy states the opposite occurs. In accordance with this agonist–antagonist model and the redundant regulation, it is important to note that the entire mechanism underlying energy homeostasis is redundantly and reciprocally controlled at several levels of execution, and not solely in the CNS.

In addition to the hypothalamus, the brain stem appears to have an important role in the signal integration of energy availability *(10)*. Several sensors of nutrient intake and expenditure, as well as receptors of peripheral hormones, including leptin and insulin, have been identified throughout the caudal brain stem *(7)*. These findings, coupled with the presence of energy-modulating neuropeptides in brain stem neurons, highlight this structure's role in the regulation of energy homeostasis *(7)*.

CENTRAL NEUROPEPTIDES REGULATING ENERGY BALANCE

As discussed, the CNS structures responsible for regulating energy homeostasis mediate their effects through the release of specific neuropeptides. For the sake of clarity, we have grouped these peptides into orexigenic and anorexigenic subcategories and presented then separately. However, it must be mentioned that they act in a combined manner, either synergistically or antagonistically.

Orexigenic Pathways

Several orexigenic neuropeptides have been identified, the most important being neuropeptide Y (NPY), agouti-related protein (AgRP), melanin-concentrating hormone (MCH), orexin, and galanin (GAL). These neuropeptides are expressed centrally and integrate peripheral signals to reduce EE and/or increase energy intake.

NEUROPEPTIDE Y

NPY is a 36 amino acid peptide expressed throughout the CNS, but especially in hypothalamic nuclei and the locus ceruleus of the brain stem *(11)*. NPY, considered to be one of the most potent orexigenic signals, is colocalized with AgRP in the ARC *(12,13)* and mediates its effects via six known NPY receptors, but regulation of feeding is mainly attributed to NPY1 and NPY5 receptors found in the PVN *(14)*.

A state of negative energy balance results in increased levels of NPY *(15)*. Conversely, a positive energy balance, associated with increased leptin and insulin levels, results in decreased NPY levels *(16)*. Similarly, peptide YY (PYY) inhibits NPY expression in the ARC via the Y2 receptor *(17)*, whereas ghrelin increases the expression of NPY and AgRP in the ARC *(18)*. Furthermore, regulation of NPY by peripheral hormones has been demonstrated with the administration of corticosterone (CORT), a glucoregulatory adrenal steroid released in energy-deficient states, which binds to surface glucocorticoid type II receptors, increasing NPY gene expression and, thus, NPY-induced feeding *(19–22)*.

In addition to hormonal regulation, dietary nutrients, most notably glucose, may also exert a regulatory effect on NPY. The increase in NPY expression observed in rats during states of hypoglycemia with normal circulating triglyceride and leptin levels demonstrates the potential regulation of NPY by glucose *(23–25)*. Furthermore, it establishes the role of NPY in initiating spontaneous feeding when preprandial glucose levels drop *(26,27)*.

Central administration of NPY increases food intake and lipogenesis as well as decreases energy expenditure and sympathetic outflow to brown adipose tissue *(12,28)*. Interestingly, NPY knockout (KO) mice have a normal phenotype and feeding behavior *(29)*, with the exception of an attenuated feeding response to fasting *(30)*, indicating that the system responsible for energy homeostasis is not dependent on any single hormone but, rather, has built-in redundancy.

AGOUTI-RELATED PROTEIN

AgRP is a 132 amino acid peptide primarily coexpressed with NPY in the ARC *(12,31,32)*. Together, these two peptides constitute the orexigenic limb of the central melanocortin system. AgRP mediates its effects mainly by blocking α-melanocyte-stimulating harmone (α-MSH) (a potent anorexigenic peptide; discussed later) from binding to MC4R and MC3R in the brain *(12)*. Central administration of AgRP in rodents increases feeding and body weight *(33,34)*. AgRP also affects energy expenditure and thermogenesis via the thyrotropin-releasing hormone system, such that exogenous

AgRP in rats results in a decreased thyroid-stimulating hormone and total levorotatory thyroxine simulating the hypothyroid state present during fasting (35). The hormonal and dietary regulation of AgRP closely parallels that of NPY. Rising leptin and insulin levels decrease AgRP expression, whereas the reverse is observed with increased ghrelin and CORT levels (36–38). Similar to NPY, declining carbohydrate stores and hypoglycemia result in increased expression of AgRP (39).

AgRP and NPY potentiate each other's effect on feeding behavior (40). Together, these neuropeptides comprise a redundant system of energy homeostasis aimed at replenishing and maintaining adequate nutrient stores in a negative energy balance. This redundancy could explain the minor alterations in feeding behavior observed in AgRP-deficient mice (29). Furthermore, it is suggested that these neuropeptides are not tonically active, because NPY and AgRP double KO mice do not become obese when nutrients are administered in a controlled fashion (41).

MELANIN-CONCENTRATING HORMONE

MCH is a cyclic 19 amino acid peptide produced in the lateral hypothalamus (LHA) and the zona incerta. MCH mediates its effects via G protein-coupled receptors (GPCRs) called the melanin-concentrating hormone receptor 1 (MCH1-R) and MCH2-R (12,42). Similar to the peptides of the ARC, MCH levels increase during fasting and decrease with rising leptin levels. However, in contrast to the former peptides, insulin is a stimulator of MCH (43) whereas ghrelin does not influence its expression to a significant extent (44). Additionally, it is declining fatty acid levels, rather than glucose, that result in increased expression of MCH (45,46).

Central administration of MCH causes hyperphagia (47), whereas MCH KO mice and mice with bilateral lesions of the LHA have reduced weight and are lean owing to hypophagia (12), and possibly increased EE (42). Mice with targeted disruption of MCH1-R display excessive feeding, hyperactivity, increased metabolic rate, and resistance to diet-induced obesity (48). This resistance to weight gain in the setting of hyperphagia suggests that MCH may promote a positive energy balance mainly by decreasing activity and EE, rather than by increasing nutrient intake.

OREXINS

The orexins (also known as hypocretins) are neuropeptides found in the lateral hypothalamus and perifornical area and are processed into orexin A, a 33 amino acid peptide, and orexin B, a 28 amino acid peptide (12). Similar to NPY and AgRP, orexins are stimulated by a negative energy balance and by rising levels of glucocorticoids and ghrelin (40,49–54). However, in contrast to the former, insulin also exerts a stimulatory effect on the expression of orexin mRNA (55,56). Furthermore, leptin does not significantly regulate orexin levels, with obesity and hyperphagia (hyperleptinemic states) actually being associated with increased levels of these neuropeptides (49,57–60). The considerable rise in orexin mRNA observed in response to declining blood sugar and the subsequent stimulating effects of orexins on locomotor activity and searching behavior suggest a role in hypothalamic arousal (49,55,61–63).

GALANIN

GAL is a 29 amino acid peptide expressed in the hypothalamus, primarily in the paraventricular and ARC nuclei, as well as the LHA and perifornical area (64). Two receptors (GALR1, GALR2) mediating the effects of this peptide have been identified throughout the hypothalamus (64–67). The regulation of GAL from peripheral endocrine signals markedly differs from that of NPY and AgRP *(22,68–72)*. Similarly, declining glucose levels fail to elicit changes in GAL mRNA expression *(73)*. However, GAL levels have been found to increase in the PVN in response to high-fat diets *(74–77)*. Exogenous administration of GAL stimulates feeding behavior, as well as decreases energy expenditure and sympathetic nervous system (SNS) activity *(78)*. Interestingly, this response is blunted significantly when fats are eliminated from the diet *(22,74,75,79,80)*. These observations suggest that GAL has a role in regulating carbohydrate metabolism in the setting of a high-fat diet *(81)*, but further research into the pathophysiological role of this peptide is needed.

Anorexigenic Pathways

Signals of a positive energy balance are integrated centrally via anorexigenc neuropeptides, including α-MSH, cocaine- and amphetamine-regulated transcript (CART), GAL-like peptide (GALP), the corticotropin-releasing hormone (CRH) family of peptides, serotonin, β-adrenergic receptors (β-ARs) and dopamine (DA).

MELANOCORTINS

Melanocortins, the main central signal of energy abundance, are peptides cleaved from proopiomelanocortin ([POMC]; the anorexigenic limb of the central melanocortin system) and subsequently processed to yield the 13 amino acid peptide α-MSH and the 12 amino acid peptide γ-MSH *(82)*. Melanocortins mediate their effects via five GPCRs (MCR) expressed throughout the body. MC3R, expressed in many areas of the CNS and in several peripheral sites, and MC4R, expressed mostly in the CNS *(83)*, are the receptors most relevant to energy regulation. Peripheral signals of energy abundance, such as insulin and leptin *(84,85)*, act mainly in the ARC of the hypothalamus to increase the expression of POMC and, thus, the secretion of α-MSH *(86,87)*, which, in turn, activates MC3R and MC4R to decrease energy intake and increase EE *(88)*. In contrast to the orexigenic peptides, dietary nutrients exert no regulatory control over POMC expression *(89–91)*.

MC4R KO mice are obese and MC4R antagonists administered centrally decrease food intake dramatically *(82)*. MC3R KO mice have reduced lean body mass and increased fat mass, despite hypophagia and normal metabolic rates *(92)*. Furthermore, several MC4R mutations have been identified in obese humans *(93,94)*, accounting for approx 5% of morbid obesity in children *(95,96)*, usually presenting with severe obesity, increased height, fat mass, and hyperinsulinemia; but normal lipid and gonadotropin levels *(95)*. Melanocortin agonists reduce both food intake and body weight in several mouse models of obesity *(88,97)*, and their role in humans is being evaluated in ongoing trials.

COCAINE- AND AMPHETAMINE-REGULATED TRANSCRIPT

CART is a 116 amino acid anorexigenic neuropeptide mainly expressed in the ARC, LHA, and paraventricular nuclei *(98)*. CART expression increases in response to elevated levels of leptin, insulin, and glucocorticoids *(99)*. Irrespective of leptin levels, high-fat diets also exert a stimulatory effect on CART mRNA expression.

Direct intracerebroventricular administration of CART decreases nocturnal, as well as fasting-induced food intake in rodents *(12)*. Although no specific receptor has been identified to date, there is evidence that neurons synthesizing CART are indirectly responsible for the effects of leptin through the innervation of preganglionic sympathetic neurons in the thoracic spinal cord and, thus, SNS activation *(100)*. CART may also act as a modulator of the rebound thermogenic effect taking place in states of hypothermia *(101,102)*.

GALANIN-LIKE PEPTIDE

GALP is a 60 amino acid peptide structurally related to GAL expressed mainly in the ARC *(103)*. GALP is a selective agonist of GALR2 *(103)*. In contrast to GAL, GALP mRNA levels increase in response to leptin and food restriction *(104)*. Although further studies must be conducted to determine the dietary control of this peptide, administration of glucose has been shown to increase GALP entry into the brain *(105)*. Central injection of this hormone results in decreased feeding and body weight *(106)*. Additionally, a thermogenic response has been observed following acute administration of GALP *(107)*.

CRH FAMILY OF PEPTIDES

The CRH family of peptides comprises corticotropin-releasing factor (CRF) and the endogenous CRF receptor ligands, the urocortins *(108)*. CRF, a 41 amino acid peptide primarily expressed in the PVN, is responsible for adrenocorticotropic hormone release from the anterior pituitary and subsequent release of CORT from the adrenal glands *(109,110)*. CRF mRNA expression is tightly controlled by CORT levels *(111,112)*, which are also an important regulator of glucose metabolism. Interventional studies have demonstrated that central administration of CRF results in hypophagia, increased EE and blood glucose, and decreased insulin secretion *(109,113–117)*. The effects of urocortin administration are similar to those of CRF in nature, but are of higher potency and longer duration *(118–121)*. These findings indicate that the CRH family of peptides plays an important role in preserving glycemic balance, while counteracting the anorexigenic hormones in a positive energy state. In short, they promote a negative energy balance while maintaining tight glycemic control through the effects of adrenal steroids.

SEROTONIN (5-HT)

Serotonin (5-HT) has an important anorexigenic role by mediating leptin's weight-reducing effect *(86)* and by stimulating POMC neurons to release α-MSH *(122)*. 5-HT$_{2C}$ receptor KO mice have decreased oxygen consumption and increased food intake and body weight *(86)*. Several antiobesity drugs act by increasing 5-HT receptor signaling.

β-ADRENERGIC RECEPTORS

Stimulation of central α1- or β2-adrenergic receptors reduces food intake. β-ARs are considered the most important receptors in the adrenergic family for regulation of energy expenditure in response to dietary excess. Ablation of all three β-ARs (β-less) in mice results in obesity, largely due to lower EE, and this effect is enhanced when mice are challenged with caloric excess *(123)*. Thus, β-less mice are mildly obese on a regular diet, but become massively obese on a high-fat diet. These data are further supported by the fact that mutations of β-ARs are clearly associated with human obesity.

DOPAMINE

DA also plays a central role in energy intake, as seen in the abnormal feeding associated with pharmacological depletion and/or genetic disruption of DA synthesis *(86)*. Striatal extracellular DA increases with food intake in normal-weight subjects *(124)*, but in obese subjects there is reduced brain DA activity, which may predispose them to excessive food intake *(124)*. Further studies are needed to define the specific DA receptor isoforms (D_1–D_5) that will have the most significant weight-reducing effects, while avoiding behavioral side effects or addiction.

CONCLUSIONS

Peripherally generated signals are integrated in the brain by anorexigenic and orexigenic pathways to regulate energy balance. Notably, almost all peripheral signals activate both pathways in opposing directions to generate a complex system of signal integration. The mapping of this complex and redundant system has improved the understanding of energy homeostasis in normal and diseased states. It is hoped that these new insights will lead to effective therapeutics in the near future.

REFERENCES

1. Lynch RM, Tompkins LS, Brooks HL, et al. Localization of glucokinase gene expression in the rat brain. Diabetes 2000;49(5):693–700.
2. Akabayashi A, Zaia CT, Silva I, et al. Neuropeptide Y in the arcuate nucleus is modulated by alterations in glucose utilization. Brain Res 1993;621(2):343–348.
3. Muroya S, Yada T, Shioda S, Takigawa M. Glucose-sensitive neurons in the rat arcuate nucleus contain neuropeptide Y. Neurosci Lett 1999;264(1–3):113–116.
4. Burdyga G, Spiller D, Morris R, et al. Expression of the leptin receptor in rat and human nodose ganglion neurones. Neuroscience 2002;109(2):339–347.
5. Moriarty P, Dimaline R, Thompson DG, Dockray GJ. Characterization of cholecystokininA and cholecystokininB receptors expressed by vagal afferent neurons. Neuroscience 1997;79(3):905–913.
6. Barsh GS, Schwartz MW. Genetic approaches to studying energy balance: perception and integration. Nat Rev Genet 2002;3(8):589–600.
7. Horvath TL, Diano S, Tschop M. Brain circuits regulating energy homeostasis. Neuroscientist 2004;10(3):235–246.
8. Kalra SP, Dube MG, Pu S, et al. Interacting appetite-regulating pathways in the hypothalamic regulation of body weight. Endocr Rev 1999;20(1):68–100.
9. Saper CB, Chou TC, Elmquist JK. The need to feed: homeostatic and hedonic control of eating. Neuron 2002;36(2):199–211.
10. Berthoud HR. Multiple neural systems controlling food intake and body weight. Neurosci Biobehav Rev 2002;26(4):393–428.
11. Allen YS, Adrian TE, Allen JM, et al. Neuropeptide Y distribution in the rat brain. Science 1983;221(4613):877–879.
12. Hillebrand JJ, de Wied D, Adan RA. Neuropeptides, food intake and body weight regulation: a hypothalamic focus. Peptides 2002;23(12):2283–2306.
13. Sawchenko PE, Pfeiffer SW. Ultrastructural localization of neuropeptide Y and galanin immunoreactivity in the paraventricular nucleus of the hypothalamus in the rat. Brain Res 1988;474(2):231–245.
14. Hu Y, Bloomquist BT, Cornfield LJ, et al. Identification of a novel hypothalamic neuropeptide Y receptor associated with feeding behavior. J Biol Chem 1996;271(42):26,315–26,319.
15. Shiraishi T, Oomura Y, Sasaki K, Wayner MJ. Effects of leptin and orexin-A on food intake and feeding related hypothalamic neurons. Physiol Behav 2000;71(3–4):251–261.
16. Krysiak R, Obuchowicz E, Herman ZS. Interactions between the neuropeptide Y system and the hypothalamic-pituitary-adrenal axis. Eur J Endocrinol 1999;140(2):130–136.
17. Batterham RL, Cowley MA, Small CJ, et al. Gut hormone PYY(3-36) physiologically inhibits food intake. Nature 2002;418(6898):650–654.
18. Nakazato M, Murakami N, Date Y, et al. A role for ghrelin in the central regulation of feeding. Nature 2001;409(6817):194–198.
19. Akabayashi A, Watanabe Y, Wahlestedt C, et al. Hypothalamic neuropeptide Y, its gene expression and receptor activity: relation to circulating corticosterone in adrenalectomized rats. Brain Res 1994;665(2):201–212.
20. McKibbin PE, Cotton SJ, McCarthy HD, Williams G. The effect of dexamethasone on neuropeptide Y concentrations in specific hypothalamic regions. Life Sci 1992;51(16):1301–1307.

21. Stanley BG, Lanthier D, Chin AS, Leibowitz SF. Suppression of neuropeptide Y-elicited eating by adrenalectomy or hypophysectomy: reversal with corticosterone. Brain Res 1989;501(1):32–36.

22. Tempel DL, Leibowitz SF. Adrenal steroid receptors: interactions with brain neuropeptide systems in relation to nutrient intake and metabolism. J Neuroendocrinol 1994;6(5):479–501.

23. Giraudo SQ, Kotz CM, Grace MK, et al. Rat hypothalamic NPY mRNA and brown fat uncoupling protein mRNA after high-carbohydrate or high-fat diets. Am J Physiol 1994;266(5 Pt 2): R1578–R1583.

24. Wang J, Akabayashi A, Dourmashkin J, et al. Neuropeptide Y in relation to carbohydrate intake, corticosterone and dietary obesity. Brain Res 1998;802(1–2):75–88.

25. Welch CC, Kim EM, Grace MK, et al. Palatability-induced hyperphagia increases hypothalamic Dynorphin peptide and mRNA levels. Brain Res 1996;721(1–2):126–131.

26. Campfield LA, Smith FJ. Blood glucose dynamics and control of meal initiation: a pattern detection and recognition theory. Physiol Rev 2003;83(1):25–58.

27. Campfield LA, Smith FJ, Rosenbaum M, Hirsch J. Human eating: evidence for a physiological basis using a modified paradigm. Neurosci Biobehav Rev 1996;20(1):133–137.

28. Billington CJ, Briggs JE, Grace M, Levine AS. Effects of intracerebroventricular injection of neuropeptide Y on energy metabolism. Am J Physiol 1991;260(2 Pt 2):R321–R327.

29. Erickson JC, Clegg KE, Palmiter RD. Sensitivity to leptin and susceptibility to seizures of mice lacking neuropeptide Y. Nature 1996;381(6581):415–421.

30. Bannon AW, Seda J, Carmouche M, et al. Behavioral characterization of neuropeptide Y knockout mice. Brain Res 2000;868(1):79–87.

31. Baskin DG, Hahn TM, Schwartz MW. Leptin sensitive neurons in the hypothalamus. Horm Metab Res 1999;31(5):345–350.

32. Broberger C, Johansen J, Johansson C, et al. The neuropeptide Y/agouti gene-related protein (AGRP) brain circuitry in normal, anorectic, and monosodium glutamate-treated mice. Proc Natl Acad Sci USA 1998;95(25):15,043–15,048.

33. Small CJ, Kim MS, Stanley SA, et al. Effects of chronic central nervous system administration of agouti-related protein in pair-fed animals. Diabetes 2001;50(2):248–254.

34. Ghilardi N, Ziegler S, Wiestner A, et al. Defective STAT signaling by the leptin receptor in diabetic mice. Proc Natl Acad Sci USA 1996;93(13):6231–6235.

35. Kim MS, Small CJ, Stanley SA, et al. The central melanocortin system affects the hypothalamo-pituitary thyroid axis and may mediate the effect of leptin. J Clin Invest 2000;105(7):1005–1011.

36. Chen P, Li C, Haskell-Luevano C, et al. Altered expression of agouti-related protein and its colocalization with neuropeptide Y in the arcuate nucleus of the hypothalamus during lactation. Endocrinology 1999;140(6):2645–2650.

37. Hahn TM, Breininger JF, Baskin DG, Schwartz MW. Coexpression of Agrp and NPY in fasting-activated hypothalamic neurons. Nat Neurosci 1998;1(4):271, 272.

38. Mizuno TM, Mobbs CV. Hypothalamic agouti-related protein messenger ribonucleic acid is inhibited by leptin and stimulated by fasting. Endocrinology 1999;140(2):814–817.

39. Karatayv O, Chang GQ, Davydova Z, Wang J, Leibowitz SF. Circulating glucose and relation to hypothalamic peptides involved in eating and body weight. Paper presented at the SFN 33rd Annual Meeting, New Orleans, November 8–12, 2003.

40. Wirth MM, Giraudo SQ. Agouti-related protein in the hypothalamic paraventricular nucleus: effect on feeding. Peptides 2000;21(9):1369–1375.

41. Qian S, Chen H, Weingarth D, et al. Neither agouti-related protein nor neuropeptide Y is critically required for the regulation of energy homeostasis in mice. Mol Cell Biol 2002;22(14):5027–5035.

42. Tritos NA, Maratos-Flier E. Two important systems in energy homeostasis: melanocortins and melanin-concentrating hormone. Neuropeptides 1999;33(5):339–349.

43. Bahjaoui-Bouhaddi M, Fellmann D, Griffond B, Bugnon C. Insulin treatment stimulates the rat melanin-concentrating hormone-producing neurons. Neuropeptides 1994;27(4):251–258.

44. Toshinai K, Mondal MS, Nakazato M, et al. Upregulation of Ghrelin expression in the stomach upon fasting, insulin-induced hypoglycemia, and leptin administration. Biochem Biophys Res Commun 2001;281(5):1220–1225.

45. Sergeev VG, Akmaev IG. Effects of blockers of carbohydrate and lipid metabolism on expression of mRNA of some hypothalamic neuropeptides. Bull Exp Biol Med 2000;130(8):766–768.

46. Sergeyev V, Broberger C, Gorbatyuk O, Hokfelt T. Effect of 2-mercaptoacetate and 2-deoxy-D-glucose administration on the expression of NPY, AGRP, POMC, MCH and hypocretin/orexin in the rat hypothalamus. Neuroreport 2000;11(1):117–121.

47. Qu D, Ludwig DS, Gammeltoft S, et al. A role for melanin-concentrating hormone in the central regulation of feeding behaviour. Nature 1996;380(6571):243–247.

48. Shimada M, Tritos NA, Lowell BB, et al. Mice lacking melanin-concentrating hormone are hypophagic and lean. Nature 1998;396(6712):670–674.

49. Cai XJ, Widdowson PS, Harrold J, et al. Hypothalamic orexin expression: modulation by blood glucose and feeding. Diabetes 1999;48(11):2132–2137.

50. Mondal MS, Nakazato M, Date Y, et al. Widespread distribution of orexin in rat brain and its regulation upon fasting. Biochem Biophys Res Commun 1999;256(3):495–499.

51. Sakurai T, Amemiya A, Ishii M, et al. Orexins and orexin receptors: a family of hypothalamic neuropeptides and G protein-coupled receptors that regulate feeding behavior. Cell 1998;92(5):696,697.

52. Stricker-Krongrad A, Beck B. Modulation of hypothalamic hypocretin/orexin mRNA expression by glucocorticoids. Biochem Biophys Res Commun 2002;296(1):129–133.

53. Lawrence CB, Snape AC, Baudoin FM, Luckman SM. Acute central ghrelin and GH secretagogues induce feeding and activate brain appetite centers. Endocrinology 2002;143(1):155–162.

54. Olszewski PK, Li D, Grace MK, et al. Neural basis of orexigenic effects of ghrelin acting within lateral hypothalamus. Peptides 2003;24(4):597–602.

55. Griffond B, Risold PY, Jacquemard C, et al. Insulin-induced hypoglycemia increases preprohypocretin (orexin) mRNA in the rat lateral hypothalamic area. Neurosci Lett 1999;262(2):77–80.

56. Moriguchi T, Sakurai T, Nambu T, et al. Neurons containing orexin in the lateral hypothalamic area of the adult rat brain are activated by insulin-induced acute hypoglycemia. Neurosci Lett 1999;264(1–3):101–104.

57. Beck B, Richy S. Hypothalamic hypocretin/orexin and neuropeptide Y: divergent interaction with energy depletion and leptin. Biochem Biophys Res Commun 1999;258(1):119–122.

58. Taheri S, Mahmoodi M, Opacka-Juffry J, et al. Distribution and quantification of immunoreactive orexin A in rat tissues. FEBS Lett 1999;457(1):157–161.

59. Wortley KE, Chang GQ, Davydova Z, Leibowitz SF. Peptides that regulate food intake: orexin gene expression is increased during states of hypertriglyceridemia. Am J Physiol Regul Integr Comp Physiol 2003;284(6):R1454–R1465.

60. Yamamoto Y, Ueta Y, Date Y, et al. Down regulation of the prepro-orexin gene expression in genetically obese mice. Brain Res Mol Brain Res 1999;65(1):14–22.

61. Briski KP, Sylvester PW. Hypothalamic orexin-A-immunpositive neurons express Fos in response to central glucopenia. Neuroreport 2001;12(3):531–534.

62. Cai XJ, Evans ML, Lister CA, et al. Hypoglycemia activates orexin neurons and selectively increases hypothalamic orexin-B levels: responses inhibited by feeding and possibly mediated by the nucleus of the solitary tract. Diabetes 2001;50(1):105–112.

63. Yamanaka A, Beuckmann CT, Willie JT, et al. Hypothalamic orexin neurons regulate arousal according to energy balance in mice. Neuron 2003;38(5):701–713.

64. Gundlach AL, Burazin TC, Larm JA. Distribution, regulation and role of hypothalamic galanin systems: renewed interest in a pleiotropic peptide family. Clin Exp Pharmacol Physiol 2001;28(1–2):100–105.

65. Leibowitz SF. Brain peptides and obesity: pharmacologic treatment. Obes Res 1995;3(Suppl 4):573S–589S.

66. Tempel DL, Leibowitz SF. Diurnal variations in the feeding responses to norepinephrine, neuropeptide Y and galanin in the PVN. Brain Res Bull 1990;25(6):821–825.

67. Wynick D, Bacon A. Targeted disruption of galanin: new insights from knock-out studies. Neuropeptides 2002;36(2–3):132–144.

68. Bergonzelli GE, Pralong FP, Glauser M, et al. Interplay between galanin and leptin in the hypothalamic control of feeding via corticotropin-releasing hormone and neuropeptide Y. Diabetes 2001;50(12):2666–2672.

69. Cheung CC, Hohmann JG, Clifton DK, Steiner RA. Distribution of galanin messenger RNA-expressing cells in murine brain and their regulation by leptin in regions of the hypothalamus. Neuroscience 2001;103(2):423–432.

70. Seth A, Stanley S, Jethwa P, et al. Galanin-like peptide stimulates the release of gonadotropin-releasing hormone in vitro and may mediate the effects of leptin on the hypothalamo-pituitary-gonadal axis. Endocrinology 2004;145(2):743–750.

71. Akabayashi A, Watanabe Y, Gabriel SM, et al. Hypothalamic galanin-like immunoreactivity and its gene expression in relation to circulating corticosterone. Brain Res Mol Brain Res 1994;25(3–4):305–312.

72. Hedlund PB, Koenig JI, Fuxe K. Adrenalectomy alters discrete galanin mRNA levels in the hypothalamus and mesencephalon of the rat. Neurosci Lett 1994;170(1):77–82.

73. Wang J, Akabayashi A, Yu HJ, et al. Hypothalamic galanin: control by signals of fat metabolism. Brain Res 1998;804(1):7–20.

74. Akabayashi A, Koenig JI, Watanabe Y, et al. Galanin-containing neurons in the paraventricular nucleus: a neurochemical marker for fat ingestion and body weight gain. Proc Natl Acad Sci USA 1994;91(22):10,375–10,379.

75. Leibowitz SF. Hypothalamic galanin, dietary fat, and body fat. In: Bray GA, Ryan DH, eds. Nutrition, Genetics, and Obesity. Louisiana State University Press, Baton Rouge, 1999, pp. 338–381.

76. Leibowitz SF, Akabayashi A, Wang J. Obesity on a high-fat diet: role of hypothalamic galanin in neurons of the anterior paraventricular nucleus projecting to the median eminence. J Neurosci 1998;18(7):2709–2719.

77. Odorizzi M, Max JP, Tankosic P, et al. Dietary preferences of Brattleboro rats correlated with an overexpression of galanin in the hypothalamus. Eur J Neurosci 1999;11(9):3005–3014.

78. Kyrkouli SE, Stanley BG, Leibowitz SF. Galanin: stimulation of feeding induced by medial hypothalamic injection of this novel peptide. Eur J Pharmacol 1986;122(1):159–160.

79. Barton C, Lin L, York DA, Bray GA. Differential effects of enterostatin, galanin and opioids on high-fat diet consumption. Brain Res 1995;702(1–2):55–60.

80. Nagase H, Nakajima A, Sekihara H, et al. Regulation of feeding behavior, gastric emptying, and sympathetic nerve activity to interscapular brown adipose tissue by galanin and enterostatin: the involvement of vagal-central nervous system interactions. J Gastroenterol 2002;37(Suppl 14):118–127.

81. Nemeth PM, Rosser BW, Choksi RM, et al. Metabolic response to a high-fat diet in neonatal and adult rat muscle. Am J Physiol 1992;262(2 Pt 1):C282–C286.

82. MacNeil DJ, Howard AD, Guan X, et al. The role of melanocortins in body weight regulation: opportunities for the treatment of obesity. Eur J Pharmacol 2002;450(1):93–109.

83. Gantz I, Fong TM. The melanocortin system. Am J Physiol Endocrinol Metab 2003;284(3): E468–E474.

84. Cowley MA, Smart JL, Rubinstein M, et al. Leptin activates anorexigenic POMC neurons through a neural network in the arcuate nucleus. Nature 2001;411(6836):480–484.

85. Kieffer TJ, Habener JF. The adipoinsular axis: effects of leptin on pancreatic beta-cells. Am J Physiol Endocrinol Metab 2000;278(1):E1–E14.

86. Schwartz MW, Woods SC, Porte D Jr, et al. Central nervous system control of food intake. Nature 2000;404(6778):661–671.

87. Spiegelman BM, Flier JS. Obesity and the regulation of energy balance. Cell 2001;104(4):531–543.

88. Pierroz DD, Ziotopoulou M, Ungsunan L, et al. Effects of acute and chronic administration of the melanocortin agonist MTII in mice with diet-induced obesity. Diabetes 2002;51(5):1337–1345.

89. Clegg DJ, Benoit SC, Air EL, et al. Increased dietary fat attenuates the anorexic effects of intracerebroventricular injections of MTII. Endocrinology 2003;144(7):2941–2946.

90. Harrold JA, Williams G, Widdowson PS. Changes in hypothalamic agouti-related protein (AGRP), but not alpha-MSH or pro-opiomelanocortin concentrations in dietary-obese and food-restricted rats. Biochem Biophys Res Commun 1999;258(3):574–577.

91. Torri C, Pedrazzi P, Leo G, et al. Diet-induced changes in hypothalamic pro-opio-melanocortin mRNA in the rat hypothalamus. Peptides 2002;23(6):1063–1068.

92. Chen AS, Marsh DJ, Trumbauer ME, et al. Inactivation of the mouse melanocortin-3 receptor results in increased fat mass and reduced lean body mass. Nat Genet 2000;26(1):97–102.

93. Yeo GS, Farooqi IS, Aminian S, et al. A frameshift mutation in MC4R associated with dominantly inherited human obesity. Nat Genet 1998;20(2):111, 112.

94. Vaisse C, Clement K, Guy-Grand B, Froguel P. A frameshift mutation in human MC4R is associated with a dominant form of obesity. Nat Genet 1998;20(2):113, 114.

95. Farooqi IS, Keogh JM, Yeo GS, et al. Clinical spectrum of obesity and mutations in the melanocortin 4 receptor gene. N Engl J Med 2003;348(12):1085–1095.

96. O'Rahilly S, Farooqi IS, Yeo GS, Challis BG. Minireview: human obesity-lessons from monogenic disorders. Endocrinology 2003;144(9):3757–3764.

97. Bluher S, Ziotopoulou M, Bullen JW Jr, et al. Responsiveness to peripherally administered melanocortins in lean and obese mice. Diabetes 2004;53(1):82–90.

98. Hurd YL, Fagergren P. Human cocaine- and amphetamine-regulated transcript (CART) mRNA is highly expressed in limbic- and sensory-related brain regions. J Comp Neurol 2000;425(4): 583–598.

99. Kristensen P, Judge ME, Thim L, et al. Hypothalamic CART is a new anorectic peptide regulated by leptin. Nature 1998;393(6680):72–76.

100. Elias CF, Lee C, Kelly J, et al. Leptin activates hypothalamic CART neurons projecting to the spinal cord. Neuron 1998;21(6):1375–1385.

101. Savontaus E, Conwell IM, Wardlaw SL. Effects of adrenalectomy on AGRP, POMC, NPY and CART gene expression in the basal hypothalamus of fed and fasted rats. Brain Res 2002;958(1): 130–138.

102. Vrang N, Larsen PJ, Tang-Christensen M, et al. Hypothalamic cocaine-amphetamine regulated transcript (CART) is regulated by glucocorticoids. Brain Res 2003;965(1–2):45–50.

103. Larm JA, Gundlach AL. Galanin-like peptide (GALP) mRNA expression is restricted to arcuate nucleus of hypothalamus in adult male rat brain. Neuroendocrinology 2000;72(2):67–71.

104. Jureus A, Cunningham MJ, McClain ME, et al. Galanin-like peptide (GALP) is a target for regulation by leptin in the hypothalamus of the rat. Endocrinology 2000;141(7):2703–2706.

105. Kastin AJ, Akerstrom V, Hackler L. Food deprivation decreases blood galanin-like peptide and its rapid entry into the brain. Neuroendocrinology 2001;74(6):423–432.

106. Krasnow SM, Fraley GS, Schuh SM, et al. A role for galanin-like peptide in the integration of feeding, body weight regulation, and reproduction in the mouse. Endocrinology 2003;144(3):813–822.

107. Lawrence CB, Baudoin FM, Luckman SM. Centrally administered galanin-like peptide modifies food intake in the rat: a comparison with galanin. J Neuroendocrinol 2002;14(11):853–860.

108. Richard D, Lin Q, Timofeeva E. The corticotropin-releasing factor family of peptides and CRF receptors: their roles in the regulation of energy balance. Eur J Pharmacol 2002;440(2–3):189–197.

109. Richard D, Huang Q, Timofeeva E. The corticotropin-releasing hormone system in the regulation of energy balance in obesity. Int J Obes Relat Metab Disord 2000;24(Suppl 2):S36–S39.

110. Whitnall MH. Regulation of the hypothalamic corticotropin-releasing hormone neurosecretory system. Prog Neurobiol 1993;40(5):573–629.

111. Cai A, Wise PM. Age-related changes in the diurnal rhythm of CRH gene expression in the paraventricular nuclei. Am J Physiol 1996;270(2 Pt 1):E238–E243.

112. Moldow RL, Fischman AJ. Circadian rhythm of corticotropin releasing factor-like immunoreactivity in rat hypothalamus. Peptides 1984;5(6):1213–1215.

113. Arase K, York DA, Shimizu H, et al. Effects of corticotropin-releasing factor on food intake and brown adipose tissue thermogenesis in rats. Am J Physiol 1988;255(3 Pt 1):E255–E259.

114. Egawa M, Yoshimatsu H, Bray GA. Effect of corticotropin releasing hormone and neuropeptide Y on electrophysiological activity of sympathetic nerves to interscapular brown adipose tissue. Neuroscience 1990;34(3):771–775.

115. Glowa JR, Barrett JE, Russell J, Gold PW. Effects of corticotropin releasing hormone on appetitive behaviors. Peptides 1992;13(3):609–621.

116. Inui A. Transgenic approach to the study of body weight regulation. Pharmacol Rev 2000;52(1):35–61.

117. Rothwell NJ. Central effects of CRF on metabolism and energy balance. Neurosci Biobehav Rev 1990;14(3):263–271.

118. Currie PJ, Coscina DV, Bishop C, et al. Hypothalamic paraventricular nucleus injections of urocortin alter food intake and respiratory quotient. Brain Res 2001;916(1–2):222–228.

119. Krahn DD, Gosnell BA, Levine AS, Morley JE. Behavioral effects of corticotropin-releasing factor: localization and characterization of central effects. Brain Res 1988;443(1–2):63–69.

120. Spina M, Merlo-Pich E, Chan RK, et al. Appetite-suppressing effects of urocortin, a CRF-related neuropeptide. Science 1996;273(5281):1561–1564.

121. Wang C, Mullet MA, Glass MJ, et al. Feeding inhibition by urocortin in the rat hypothalamic paraventricular nucleus. Am J Physiol Regul Integr Comp Physiol 2001;280(2):R473–R480.

122. Heisler LK, Cowley MA, Kishi T, et al. Central serotonin and melanocortin pathways regulating energy homeostasis. Ann N Y Acad Sci 2003;994:169–174.

123. Bachman ES, Dhillon H, Zhang CY, et al. betaAR signaling required for diet-induced thermogenesis and obesity resistance. Science 2002;297(5582):843–845.

124. Wang GJ, Volkow ND, Fowler JS. The role of dopamine in motivation for food in humans: implications for obesity. Expert Opin Ther Targets 2002;6(5):601–609.

6

Role of Energy Expenditure in Regulation of Energy Homeostasis

Eric S. Bachman, MD, PhD

INTRODUCTION

Obesity has emerged as a major threat to human health. Numerous morbidities are associated with obesity, including type 2 diabetes mellitus, which now affects adolescents in alarming numbers *(1)*. Understanding the pathogenic mechanisms that lead to obesity, therefore, represents one of the great challenges to medicine today. Obesity is defined arbitrarily as an increase in body fat stores compared to lean body mass and can be estimated clinically as a body mass index (BMI) of more than 30 kg/m². According to the first law of thermodynamics, the total energy of a system plus the surroundings is constant. Obesity can result, therefore, from a relative increase in energy intake (food) compared to energy expenditure (EE) (metabolic rate and digestion). Whereas many of the central pathways that regulate food intake are being elucidated, much less is known about the regulation of EE and its role in body weight homeostasis. Discovery of the fat hormone leptin as part of an "adipostatic" endocrine system of body weight regulation has revolutionized our understanding of body weight homeostasis *(2)*. Figure 1 presents a proposed wiring diagram for the control of EE.

COMPONENTS OF EE

Models that categorize EE into obligatory (basal) and adaptive (facultative) thermogenesis are useful for discussion but are not mechanistically exclusive. Obligatory EE includes all processes that are involved in the maintenance of basic metabolic and

From: *Contemporary Diabetes: Obesity and Diabetes*
Edited by: C. S. Mantzoros © Humana Press Inc., Totowa, NJ

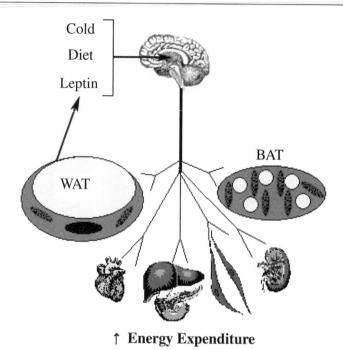

↑ **Energy Expenditure**

Fig. 1. Model for adaptive thermogenesis. Leptin, cold, and diet are sensed by hypothalamic nuclei in the brain, which activate descending pathways from the sympathetic nervous system (SNS), and these innervate potential thermogenic target tissues, including from left to right white adipose tissue (WAT), heart, liver, skeletal muscle, kidney, and brown adipose tissue (BAT). Lipid droplets are depicted by white spaces, and mitochondria by black ovals.

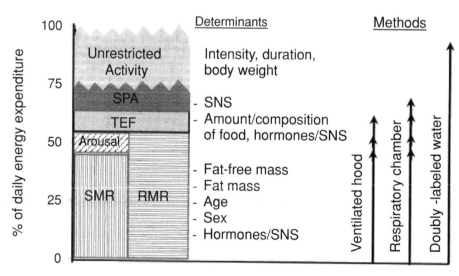

Fig. 2. Components of EE. The physiological determinants and methods for measurement are given. TEF, thermic effect of food; SPA, spontaneous physical activity. *(7)*

physiological processes, including the maintenance of ion gradients, muscle tone, digestion, and blood flow (standard metabolic rate [SMR]; Fig. 2). Adaptive thermogenesis includes cold-induced thermogenesis and diet-induced thermogenesis (DIT). As an example of the mechanistic overlap between obligatory and adaptive thermogenesis,

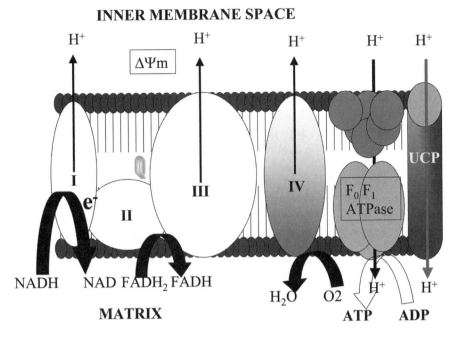

Fig. 3. Mitochondrial respiration. Reducing equivalents (NADH, FADH$_2$) from glucose and fatty acid metabolism donate protons to the electron transport chain in the inner mitochondrial membrane, resulting in proton (H) transport and a proton-motive, electrochemical gradient ($\Delta\psi$m). The energy from the proton gradient can result in ATP synthesis via F$_0$F$_1$ ATPase, or protons can reenter the mitochondrial matrix via specific uncoupling proteins (UCP) or nonspecific pathways, thereby generating heat. I, II, III, IV: electron transport complexes; Q: coenzyme Q.

thyroid hormone (TH) is required for up to 30% of SMR, adaptive increases in TH are required for normal cold-induced thermogenesis *(3,4)*. Furthermore, physical activity can have long-lasting effects on resting metabolic rate (RMR) *(5)*. Finally, physical activity is often considered a separate category, although increased physical activity may also elicit stimuli that activate adaptive thermogenesis, such as caloric excess *(6)*. Approximate contributions for the various EE components are RMR (70%), physical activity (20%), and facultative (10%), with physical activity representing the most variable component *(7)*. At the cellular level, the majority (approx 90%) of EE in mammals derives form oxidative phosphorylation of substrates in mitochondria *(8)*.

Mitochondrial Metabolism

Mitochondria are the major source of cellular adenosine triphosphate (ATP). Approximately (90%) of cellular metabolism occurs in mitochondria, whereas the other 10% of mammalian EE is nonmitochondrial, or owing to other oxidases *(8)*. The most active mitochondria are characterized by densely packed membrane cristae, and these contain abundant membrane proteins involved in oxidative phosphorylation (Fig. 3). Metabolic fuels are converted into reducing equivalents (NADH, FADH$_2$), which donate electrons to the electron transport chain (Fig. 3). The transfer of electrons through the electron transport chain in mitochondria is coupled to proton translocation across the inner mitochondrial membrane, mediated by complexes I, III, and IV, and creation of an electrochemical proton gradient ($\Delta\psi$m). The energy derived from protons reentering the matrix can be captured by complex V (adenosine triphosphatase [ATPase]), which catalyzes the phosphorylation of adenosine $5'$-diphosphate from inorganic phosphate, forming ATP and water (9). In summary, oxidative phosphorylation is a tightly coupled series of reactions that allow cells to efficiently synthesize ATP from metabolic fuels.

The transfer of energy through the electron transport chain in mitochondria presents many opportunities for the control of EE. Proton leak across the mitochondrial membrane, e.g., is a major pathway that regulates EE and has received enormous attention for its potential role in regulating EE and body weight. The electrochemical gradient across the inner mitochondrial membrane ($\Delta\psi$m; Fig. 3) allows protons to reenter mitochondria through ATPase, as already described, or in a manner that is not coupled (uncoupled) to ATP synthesis (10). This can occur via either specific uncoupling proteins (UCPs) or nonspecific membrane leak. Species differences in EE across a wide spectrum of body masses have been shown to relate to differences in proton leak and composition of mitochondrial phospholipids (11). The finding that certain tissues, especially BAT, possess a unique, inducible UCP that lowers the mitochondrial membrane potential has led to great excitement among researchers that such a mechanism regulates EE and body weight specifically in mammals ([12]; see discussion under Brown Adipose Tissue). Altered EE then could theoretically be controlled in numerous ways in mitochondria, including changes in UCP levels, changes in UCP activity, or via wholesale changes in mitochondrial protein levels, biogenesis, and electron transport (13). Defective mitochondrial biogenesis, e.g., has recently been shown to affect EE and body weight regulation (14). A high level of respiratory control must be maintained in mitochondria, however, in order to preserve ATP levels in the face of greatly varying metabolic rates.

Measuring Metabolism

Numerous techniques are available to measure EE (Fig. 2). The most accurate method is direct calorimetry, which can be performed either by water immersion or closed chamber heat convection. Doubly labeled water ingestion, in which EE can be interpolated from the amount of $^2H_2{}^{18}O$ ingested and the amount of ^2H and ^{18}O released as water and CO_2, has been shown to be accurate to within 5% of indirect calorimetry (15). As stated, >90% of oxygen consumption arises from mitochondrial metabolism (8). Given this fact, and the ease of measuring EE indirectly via O_2 consumption, indirect calorimetry methods have been widely used. Many indirect calorimeters calculate an approximate mass-independent EE by incorporating oxygen consumption (VO_2), CO_2 production (VCO_2), respiratory exchange ratio (RER = VCO_2/VO_2), and protein catabolism according to Weir, whereas other investigators normalize EE to relative tissue contributions (16,17):

Weir's Equation (18)

Energy expenditure (kcal/min) = $3.941 \times VO_2 + 1.106 \times VCO_2 - 2.17 \times$ g urinary nitrogen

Finally, Kleiber has proposed a predictive model to estimate EE across species and among organisms of different mass (19):

Kleiber's Equation (Modified After ref. 20)

$$B \sim M^{0.75}\, e^{-E_i}/kT$$

in which B = metabolic rate, M = body mass, E_i = activation energy, k = Boltzmann's constant, and T = temperature. The predictive accuracy of these models argue that metabolic rate, or EE, represents a similar set of basic biological processes across all living organisms.

ABNORMAL REGULATION OF EE IN OBESITY

Small differences in the ratio of energy intake to EE could result in significant adipose gain. For example, the current epidemic of obesity could be stabilized by lowering food intake by 100 kcal/d, according to one estimate (1). The notoriously high failure rate of calorie-restricted diets has led to the concept that powerful homeostatic mechanisms exist in mammals, which maintain body weight via changes in food intake and EE. Whereas there is abundant evidence that increased food intake causes obesity, there has been less evidence that decreased EE specifically leads to obesity. For example, compared to lean subjects, obese patients have increased EE (7). Thus, only relative differences in EE might account for predisposition to obesity. Evidence exists both to support and refute an important role for defective EE in human obesity.

Evidence in Support of a Role for Abnormal EE in Obesity

Numerous studies support a pathogenic role for reduced EE in the development of obesity. Early studies demonstrating large, inferred differences in EE based on self-reported food intake compared to body weight gain were later cast into doubt by the doubly labeled water technique, proving that patients consistently underestimate food intake (15,21,22). Nonetheless, evidence has emerged that lower EE is genetically determined and predisposes to obesity. For example, RMR is highly heritable and is independent of fat-free mass, age, and sex as a predictor of EE (23). Overfeeding studies in monozygotic twins show a high degree of similarity in weight gain between but not among twins, arguing strongly that genetic factors play a major role in controlling EE (24). In adition, the environment in which twins are raised has little influence over eventual BMI in identical twins (25). Finally, direct and indirect measurements of EE and respiratory quotient have shown small but measurable differences between obese and lean patients, particularly in certain ethnic groups such as Pima Indians (26,27). Longitudinal studies have confirmed that differences in EE are associated with a tendency to develop obesity over a period of years (28).

Evidence Against a Role for Abnormal EE in Obesity

Other reports have failed to support the hypothesis that abnormal regulation of EE leads to obesity. For example, EE increases linearly with increasing BMI, and, thus, increased EE at higher body weight would function to resist further change in body weight (7). Indeed, longitudinal follow-up of nondiabetic Pima Indians reveals that increased EE accompanies increases in body weight (Fig. 4), even when adjusted for body composition (29). Similarly, 5- to 10-yr old children with varying, known susceptibility to obesity have similar increases in RMR (30). Furthermore, a large number of studies have failed to find obesity-promoting mechanisms to explain differences between lean and obese subjects, including SNS nerve activity (31), catecholamine turnover (32), lipolysis (33), thermic effect of food (7), and THs (34). Finally, rare cases of obesity in humans, including Prader-Willi syndrome (35), as well as those caused by monogenic mutations in leptin, leptin receptor, and melanocortin receptor deficiency are not characterized by noticeable differences in EE (36–38). In summary, the hypothesis that relatively low EE contributes to the development of obesity has been supported by some but not all studies. It remains unclear whether stimulation of EE in humans will be an effective approach for the treatment of obesity.

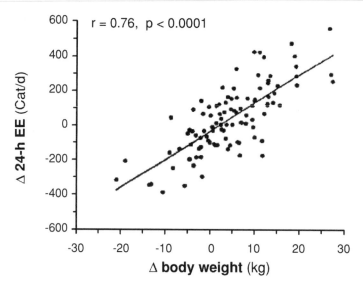

Fig. 4. Adjusted changes in EE with increases in body weight among Pima Indians. EE increases linearly with increasing body weight within individuals. (After ref. *30.*)

MECHANISMS THAT MAINTAIN BODY WEIGHT AT A SET POINT

The very existence of antiobesity mechanisms in mammals has been questioned because of the following observations: (1) mammals are more likely to have had to adapt evolutionarily to caloric deficit rather than surfeit; (2) almost all obese mammals show resistance to high levels of leptin; and (3) numerous, redundant mechanisms exist that stimulate food intake *(39)*. The "thrifty gene" hypothesis states that humans are predisposed to storing rather than expending calories *(40,41)*. This hypothesis is supported by the presence of hyperleptinemia in most obese humans and rodent models, in which, despite high leptin levels, obesity develops in a state of leptin resistance. The actions of leptin for most humans are thus more likely to be most important in the lower physiological range of leptin, as seen in starvation. In fact, leptin has potent effects on metabolism in its lower physiological range, which provides the basis for the argument that the role of leptin is to signal declining, not increasing, adipose stores *(42–46)*.

EE and Body Weight Set-Point Alterations

Energy balance in most humans is regulated with fine precision over a lifetime *(47)*, arguing that powerful physiological mechanisms maintain body weight within a narrow "set point." One theory proposes that specific thermogenic mechanisms (such as DIT) have evolved in mammals to allow consumption of large quantities of low-quality diets, e.g., and dissipation of excess EE *(48,49)*. High net consumption of nutrient-poor food, e.g., would then allow sufficient amino acids to be obtained. The phenomenon of DIT has indeed been demonstrated in BAT *(50)*. Recently, DIT in rodents was shown to be a critically important antiobesity mechanism, especially in response to caloric excess *(51)*. Likewise, studies in humans support the existence of mechanisms that increase EE in response to overfeeding and obesity *(24,25,52)*. Some thermogenic mechanisms are now known, including leptin-induced increases in EE that regulate adipose tissue selectively *(37,53)*. Other mechanisms that defend human body weight set point are demonstrated in under-and overfeeding studies (Fig. 5) *(54)*. Thus,

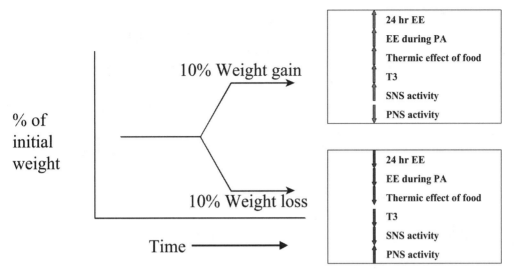

Fig. 5. Physiological changes that accompany weight gain and loss in mammals. PA, physical activity. (Adapted from ref. *55*.)

overfeeding human subjects results in increased SNS activity, decreased parasympathetic nervous system (PNS) activity, and an inferred form of physical activity known as nonexercise activity thermogenesis (NEAT) *(55)*. The significance of thermogenic, antiobesity mechanisms in humans, in contrast to well-established mechanisms in rodents, remains a critical area of question that will greatly influence approaches to treating obesity *(51)*.

REGULATION OF EE

Physical Activity

Physical activity is the most variable component of daily EE, ranging from less than 100 kcal/d in sedentary adults to thousands of kcal/d in endurance athletes. Physical activity has effects on EE both acutely, with large increases in maximal oxygen consumption, and chronically, via increased mitochondrial proliferation *(56)*. Thus, physical activity represents an ideal mechanism to resist obesity in the setting of increased food intake. Studies in 5-to 10-yr-old Pima Indians have indeed shown an inverse relationship between physical activity and eventual obesity *(30,57)*. Only 10% of the variability in human body weight is estimated to be owing to differences in physical activity, however *(58)*, and other studies have shown decreased physical activity but no change in overall EE between lean and obese adolescents *(59)*. In humans, sustained weight loss is most successful with a combination of decreased food intake and physical activity *(60)*. Coordinated physical activity is a complex behavior, however, and is likely to be regulated by numerous mechanisms in the central nervous system (CNS) that are at present poorly understood. Recently, evidence that physical activity is, in fact, a specific, regulated component of the "adipostatic" system of body weight regulation has emerged. For example, mice lacking melanocortin receptor 4, which lies downstream of leptin signaling, fail to engage in running-wheel behavior in response to increasing adiposity *(6)*. Further investigation into the regulation of physical activity as a specific mechanism to control body fat stores will clearly be of great importance in the field of obesity.

A separate category of physical activity that is related to adiposity is called NEAT. Studies of careful overfeeding in lean humans showed that the majority of increased EE in response to caloric excess occurs not via increases in thermic effect of food, RMR, or coordinated physical activity but, rather, most likely in increased NEAT *(55)*. While formally a subclass of physical activity, NEAT includes all tasks of daily living, including posture, fidgeting, and even chewing gum *(61)*. NEAT can be accurately measured by sensors in humans and rodents *(62)*. At least a portion of increased EE in hyperthyroidism is attributable to an increase in NEAT *(63)*. Insight into the role and regulation of NEAT in human obesity will therefore be critical for the understanding of body weight regulation.

Thyroid Hormone

The critical role that TH (including levorotatory thyroxine [T_4] and trilodothyronine [T_3]) plays in EE is well documented, although, overall, TH is not believed to play a specific role in regulating adiposity. Briefly, T_4 is converted into its more active congener, T_3, by deiodinases in tissues. T_3 binds to TH receptors in the nucleus, which then alter transcription of numerous genes *(64)*. Approximately 30% of basal thermogenesis is TH mediated, and in mammals, the main function of TH is to maintain temperature homeostasis *(4)*. Numerous, diverse pathways, anabolic and catabolic, are stimulated in response to TH (reviewed in ref. *4*). In addition, increased ATP turnover and heat production are probably derived from baseline increases in metabolic flux through many cellular pathways, such as the maintenance of ion gradients, ion cycling, and uncoupling, the sum of which is to increase EE *(65)*.

The effects of TH on body weight regulation are small, however, when one notes that the effects of varying TH doses over a wide range results in a 15% difference in EE but little effect on body weight *(66)*. Additional evidence against a specific role for TH in adipose-specific EE includes the following: First, a deficiency of TH results in only mild obesity and lipid accumulation *(67)*. Second, thyroid dysfunction is not associated with many models of obesity that are characterized by low EE. Third, TH receptors (TRα and TRβ) are not required for normal body weight regulation *(68)*. Finally, THs are normal or elevated in human obesity *(34,68)*. As shown in Fig. 6, low TH levels are associated with reduced EE during weight loss and act to resist body weight change in obesity *(69)*. In this way, decreased TH in response to dietary restriction limits the clinical effectiveness of such a lifestyle change.

Tissue-specific regulation of TH represents a potential mechanism for manipulation of EE. It is well known that systemic hyperthyroidism causes increased EE, often resulting in reduced body weight *(64)*, albeit from both adipose and protein tissue depletion *(70)*. The mechanisms that mediate body weight loss in response to TH are not fully described, however, and may involve multiple pathways including those that are independent of β-adrenergic stimulation *(71)*. BAT is a major thermogenic tissue in rodents and has the capacity to increase thermogenesis via expression of type 2 deiodinase (D2), which converts T_4 into T_3 *(72)*. This conversion is under SNS control, results in increased T_3 in BAT, and is required for cold-induced adaptive thermogenesis (Fig. 6) *(3,73,74)*. Failure to induce D2 activity in response to cold is observed in obesity-prone, β-adrenergic receptor (βAR)-less mice *(51)*. Thus, thermogenesis via uncoupling mechanisms in BAT, and in humans in skeletal muscle, represents a potentially important mechanism for increasing EE *(65)*. Loss of function of D2 via gene disruption has no demonstrable effect on body weight in mice, however *(75)*. Additionally,

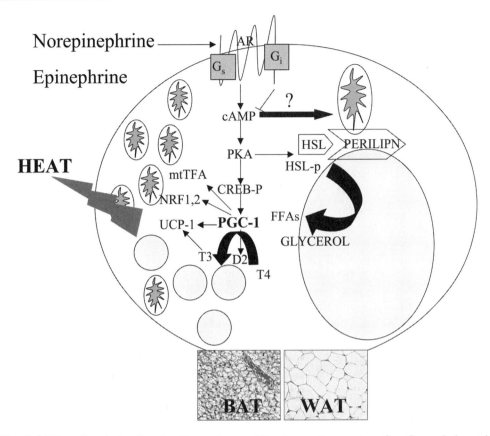

Fig. 6. βAR-mediated signaling in adipose tissues. AR, adrenergic receptors; $G_{i,s}$, G-coupled protein receptors; PKA, protein kinase A; CREB-P, phosphorylated cyclic adenosine monophosphate cAMP-responsive transcription factor; NRF, nuclear respiratory factors; mtTFA, mitochondrial transcription factor A.

lack of TH does not affect body weight, DIT, or biochemical evidence of BAT activation in response to high-fat feeding *(76)*. Nonetheless, stimulation of TH receptor-specific agonists, possibly in a tissue-specific manner, with ensuing increased EE, represents a potential approach for the treatment of obesity.

SNS and Adrenergic Receptors

The SNS has a rich history in the scientific literature as a critical regulator of EE *(77)*. The origins of the SNS have been mapped to CNS nuclei in the hypothalamus, midbrain, and brain stem *(78)*. First-order, leptin-responsive neurons innervate thoracolumbar sympathetic ganglia, which then synapse in target organs. Postganglionic neurons release either norepinephrine (NE) (sympathetic) or acetylcholine (parasympathetic) from terminals (Figs. 1 and 6) (reviewed in ref. *77*). NE and epinephrine stimulate adrenergic receptors of two classes, α (αARs) and β (βARs), based on molecular and pharmacological similarity. βARs are the most important receptors in the adrenergic family for regulation of EE in response to dietary excess *(79)*. A popular model for increased EE in response to caloric excess, and resistance to obesity, is shown in Fig. 1. This is supported by numerous studies. For example, low SNS activity can be associated with a propensity for future weight gain *(77,80)*. Low SNS activity is also seen in most rodent models of obesity, and activation of this pathway by βAR agonists is effective in reducing obesity *(81,82)*. Numerous attempts to perturb SNS function (surgical, chemical, immunological, genetic) failed to affect body weight, however, and the importance of SNS-mediated DIT therefore lacked support *(83–86)*. Ablation of all three βARs (β-less) in mice, however, results in obesity that is entirely owing to lower EE, and this deficit is magnified when challenged with caloric excess *(51)*. Thus, β-less mice are mildly obese on a regular diet but become massively obese when challenged with a high-fat diet. These results are supported by numerous genetic studies in humans, as already discussed, which describe mutations in βARs that are associated with human obesity. The relative contribution of individual tissues to DIT in mammals is not known at this time *(71,79)*.

Futile Cycles

Futile cycles represent a potential mechanism for the regulation of EE in mammals. The earliest work on thermogenic futile cycles came from studies in bumblebees, in which simultaneous activity of phosphofructokinase and fructose bisphosphatase, creating no net progression through glycolysis, increases muscle temperature at the expense of ATP *(87)*. Calcium cycling can also be thermogenic, as seen in tuna and billfish, which use a modified extraocular muscle that can provide heat by ATP-dependent calcium cycling between the sarcoplasmic reticulum (SR) and cytosol *(88)*. This process involves the α ryanodine receptor, which has been reported to cause malignant hyperthermia in humans *(89,90)*. Futile cycles have not yet been shown to play a significant role in mammalian body weight regulation *(91)*, although lipogenic/lipolytic futile cycles are stimulated in WAT in response to peroxisome proliferator-activated receptor γ (PPARγ) agonists *(92)*. Potentially important futile cycles that regulate body weight via increased EE in mammals include calcium, sodium, and proton cycles in cells. Recently, the molecular cloning and demonstration of a partially uncoupling, SR calcium ATPase (SERCA I) in mouse BAT raises the interesting possibility that calcium cycling contributes to adaptive thermogenesis *(93)*.

Intermediary Metabolism Genes That Regulate EE and Body Weight

The roles of leptin and melanocortin-stimulated EE for normal body weight regulation in humans are not as clear as their role in food intake, possibly owing to the difficulty in comparing and "normalizing" EE in humans who differ markedly in body mass and composition. Increasing evidence is emerging, however, that EE in mammals is controlled at numerous rate-limiting and in some cases leptin-mediated steps in glucose and fatty acid metabolism (Fig. 7). For example, loss of function of key synthetic enzymatic steps in fatty acid synthesis results in increased EE, reduced body weight, and obesity resistance in many rodent models *(94–97)*. In humans, polymorphisms in the rate-limiting enzyme for triglyceride synthesis are associated with lean kindreds *(98)*. An emerging, central mediator of these critical steps in fatty acid metabolism is adenosine monophosphate kinase (AMPK). This enzyme is regulated by leptin, and AMPK regulates fatty acid synthesis and β-oxidation of fatty acids via acetyl CoA carboxylase (ACCoA) in muscle and the brain, thereby affecting appetite and EE *(99,100)*. The role of the leptin–AMPK–fatty acid metabolism pathway in humans remains to be confirmed *(101)*.

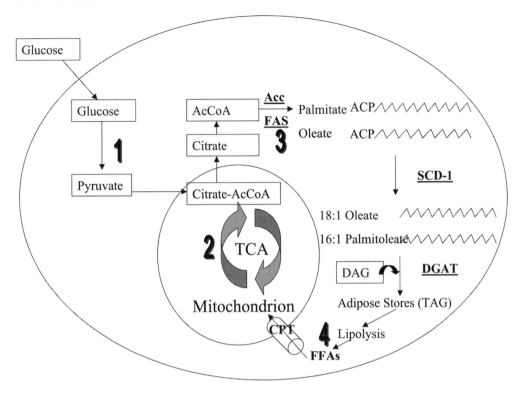

Fig. 7. Metabolic control of EE. Cellular metabolism with respect to glucose and fatty acid oxidation is shown. Steps that are required for normal EE and body weight dysregulation, as demonstrated by gene disruption studies in rodents, are underlined. Major metabolic processes are denoted by numbers: 1 (glycolysis), 2 (Krebs cycle), 3 (fatty acid synthesis), 4 (lipolysis). ACC, acetyl CoA carboxylase; ACP, acyl carrier protein; CPT, carnitine palmitoyl transferases; DAG, diacylglycerol; FFA, fatty acids; FAS, fatty acid synthase; TCA, tricarboxylic acid cycle.

THERMOGENIC TISSUES

Many tissues have the metabolic potential to mediate thermogenesis as a specific response to increased body weight and adipose stores.

Brown Adipose Tissue

The sine qua non of tissue thermogenesis, BAT, plays a critical role in thermogenesis and body weight regulation in rodents *(102)* but might not represent an attractive target for antiobesity treatment owing to its apparent absence in adult humans *(103)*. Originally described as a thermogenic organ in hibernating animals *(104)*, BAT is recognized as a specialized form of adipose tissue that is highly thermogenic (Fig. 6). Numerous depots of BAT can be found in mice, and this specialized adipose tissue is characterized by multilocular lipid droplets, densely packed mitochondria and vascularity, and the capacity to generate heat when stimulated by catecholamines (Fig. 6) *(105)*. Stimulation of βARs by catecholamines or synthetic β-agonists markedly stimulates EE, primarily in BAT *(48)*. High-fat feeding results in marked BAT hypertrophy and increased EE, suggesting that BAT plays a role in resisting obesity *(48,50)*. Subsequent isolation and cloning of a 32-kDa protein, then-called thermogenin, spawned a decade-long search for the function of such proteins (UCPs) that uncouple oxidative phosphorylation and thus have the capacity to produce heat *(12)*. The molecular pathway that leads to increased EE in BAT is diagrammed in Fig. 6.

Nonetheless, subsequent studies showed that whereas UCP-1 is required for cold-induced thermogenesis *(106)* and NE-induced thermogenesis in BAT *(107)*, UCP-1 is not required for normal body weight regulation *(106,108)* or NE-induced thermogenesis in WAT *(109)*. Furthermore, there is no evidence that close relatives of UCP-1, UCP-2 and UCP-3, are involved in thermogenesis or body weight regulation *(110–113)*. The findings of some studies support a role for UCPs in more specialized forms of thermogenesis. For example, overexpression of UCP-1 in WAT results in the appearance of brown adipocytes in WAT depots and obesity resistance *(114)*. In addition, overexpression of UCP-3 in mouse skeletal muscle results in hyperphagic, lean mice. However, these results have been criticized as being owing to overexpression artifacts *(115)*. Thus, a paradox emerges: BAT is necessary for normal body weight regulation, but the major thermogenic protein, UCP-1, is not required. This paradox may be solved by finding another thermogenic mediator in BAT, or investigating other tissues as potential mediators of DIT.

White Adipose Tissue

Since the identification of leptin as the afferent limb of an adipostatic feedback loop, the understanding of WAT as a critical mediator of mammalian physiology has emerged. Via regulation of glucose uptake, lipolysis, response to β- and α- adrenergic stimulation, and release of numerous cytokines (leptin, acylation-stimulating protein, adiponectin, resistin) *(116)*, WAT clearly participates actively in many metabolic processes (Fig. 6) *(117)*. Furthermore, the metabolic rate of WAT is often cited as negligible, despite strong support that significant EE derives from WAT *(109,118)*. This can be seen diagrammatically in Fig. 6, with lipolysis and increased free fatty acid (FFA) activation of UCP-1 in BAT representing two mechanisms for increased EE. Moreover, WAT has a unique physiological capacity for nearly unlimited expansion; a review of secreted WAT-specific cytokines, including leptin, adiponectin, resistin, and other substances, is provided in ref. *117*. WAT can therefore be viewed not only as a storage depot, but as an important endocrine organ that integrates afferent metabolic information and responds with efferent, secretory products that profoundly affect EE and body weight.

Although there has been only limited evidence in humans that primary defects in WAT function contribute to obesity *(119,120)*, WAT represents an important potential antiobesity target via increased EE. The process of lipolysis, as shown diagrammatically in Fig. 7, causes significant increases in EE *(105,109)*. Stimulation of βARs on WAT activates signal transduction pathways that result in PKA-induced phosphorylation of hormone-sensitive lipase (HSL), translocation of HSL to lipid droplets, and lipolysis *(105)*. Stimulation of this pathway indeed has demonstrated that WAT has the capacity to develop BAT morphology and function, and that this process accompanies resistance to obesity *(121)*. The origin of BAT cells within WAT depots is not known. Cloning of the predominant β3AR in WAT led to an ardent search for highly selective agonists that would be effective in humans *(121)*. Despite intense effort and proof of concept for βAR-mediated weight loss in primates, β-agonists have not been effective in treating humans with obesity, probably because of the low abundance of β3AR in human tissues, lack of specificity for the human β3AR, and intolerable side effects. These considerations have made the use of β-agonists for human obesity uncertain *(122)*.

LEPTIN

The discovery of an adipostatic system for body weight regulation, mediated by leptin, has revolutionized the understanding of body weight regulation. Studies on leptin-deficient *ob/ob* mice revealed that lack of this circulating hormone leads to hyperphagia, reduced EE, and massive obesity *(123)*. Successful cloning of the gene whose defect leads to this phenotype was a major advance in the field of obesity research *(2)*. Leptin, from the Greek word *leptos,* meaning thin, is released from adipocytes and acts on the brain to reduce food intake and increase EE. Leptin treatment depletes body fat specifically *(53)*, and most obese humans and almost all mouse models of obesity (except *ob/ob*) have elevated levels of leptin in serum consistent with leptin resistance *(124)*. Nonetheless, the few leptin-deficient human subjects described recapitulate the response to treatment seen in *ob/ob* mice, albeit mostly via reduced food intake *(125)*. Experimental evidence points to both acute and chronic effects of leptin to increase EE, both via activation of BAT and increases in SNS firing *per se (126,127)*. Indeed, acute effects of leptin include increased catecholamine turnover in BAT *(126)*, increased SNS firing in numerous thermogenic tissues *(127)*, and lipolysis *(128)*. The overall magnitude of these effects is small, however, given that the effects of leptin treatment on EE and body weight are identical to those in acutely pair-fed animals. The acute effects of leptin may be important for body weight regulation because leptin prevents the decrease in EE that normally accompanies decreased food intake *(53)*.

Muscle

Skeletal muscle comprises approx 40% of the body mass in mammals and has the capacity for 10-fold increases in EE in response to physical activity. This fact, in addition to very close correlations between overall EE and fat-free mass *(129)*, suggests that muscle may play an important role in body weight regulation by regulating EE in response to caloric excess *(130)*. Indeed, careful measurements of oxygen extraction in muscle tissues correlate closely with overall resting EE *(130)*, and a large fraction (40%) of epinephrine-induced increases in EE occurs in muscle *(131)*. As in BAT, PPARγ, coactivator-1 (PGC-1) *(132)* plays a major role in cold-activated changes in EE by coactivating numerous factors that result in mitochondrial biogenesis *(133)* (Fig. 6). Surprisingly, transgenic overexpression of PGC-1 does not result in obesity resistance despite an increase in mitochondria and oxidative muscle fibers, and improved muscle performance *(134)*. Potential mediators of increased EE in skeletal muscle include leptin, which stimulates the SNS (αARs); AMPK; and inhibition of acetyl ACCoA, leading to increased fat oxidation *(99,101)*. Finally, muscle may be an important thermogenic tissue via other pathways, such as catecholamine-mediated stimulation of βARs *(79)*.

Liver

The liver plays a major role in the metabolism of glucose and fatty acids and, thus, has the potential to regulate EE. ACC1 and ACC2 are enzymes that generate malonyl CoA, which is a substrate for subsequent fatty acid synthesis and also inhibits entry of fatty acids into mitochondria via carnitine palmitoyl transferases. ACC1 and ACC-2 are found abundantly in liver and muscle, and lack of this enzyme results in significant increases in EE and obesity resistance *(97)*. The liver also expresses the rate-limiting enzyme for the synthesis of monounsaturated fatty acids, stearoyl CoA desaturase (SCD). Cohen et al. *(135)* found this enzyme in a carefully designed screen for genes that are altered by leptin treatment and subsequently discovered that suppression of SCD and reduced body weight are associated with increased AMPK activity, reduced ACC activity, and increased oxidation of fat in liver *(135,136)*. Thus, the pathway shown in Fig. 7 plays an important role in EE and body weight regulation *(137)*.

APPROACHES TO TREAT OBESITY VIA MANIPULATION OF EE

The major antiobesity pathways that have been targeted for manipulation of EE include mitochondrial uncoupling, activation of the SNS, and TH. With the possible exception of the medicines discussed in "Sympathomimetics", none of these has been successful in treating human obesity owing to either intolerable side effects or lack of efficacy. Efficacy is judged by prevention of further weight gain, 5–10% loss of weight, metabolic improvement, and long-term maintenance *(138)*.

Uncoupling Oxidative Phosphorylation

Compounds that short-circuit the mitochondrial membrane potential, called uncouplers, preceded the isolation and characterization of endogenous UCPs. These compounds (2,4-dinitrophenol), which are effective treatments for obesity via their ability to increase oxygen consumption, nonetheless fell out of favor owing to a narrow therapeutic window and intolerable side effects *(139)*. Although loss-of-function studies in mice do not demonstrate an important role for uncoupling in general for body weight regulation and EE, gain-of-function approaches to increasing uncoupling processes in specific tissues remain a viable area for investigation.

Hormones

LEPTIN

Leptin is an adipocyte-derived cytokine that stimulates numerous pathways in the CNS including weight loss. Exogenous leptin results in a decreased food intake and, presumably via the SNS, a modest increase in EE and fat mobilization. The majority of obese human patients have elevated leptin levels in serum, however, indicating that there is resistance to leptin. The mechanism of leptin resistance has not been established, but possibilities include low free leptin levels in serum, decreased transport across the blood–brain barrier and lower levels in the hypothalamus, or cellular resistance to leptin-receptor-mediated signaling. The effects of exogenous leptin on body weight loss in humans are variable across a wide patient population, most likely owing to already high leptin levels in obese patients and resistance to its effects *(140)*. The changes in EE owing to exogenous leptin are modest, however, and may represent an effect of leptin as just described to prevent the lower EE that accompanies caloric restriction. Leptin-deficient patients respond dramatically to leptin treatment, although these patients are rare *(125,141)*. Rare patients with partial leptin deficiency may respond to exogenous leptin treatment *(142)*. Larger prospective double-blind and placebo-controlled clinical trials in obese patients have shown only modest, dose-dependent weight loss in patients along with a high degree of variability in response *(143)*.

THYROID HORMONE

Activation of TH receptor β (TRβ) increases metabolic rate and causes weight loss in mice and may become a drug target for obesity *(144)*. Subtype-specific compounds that are selective for a single TRβ isoform are potential approaches to making antiobesity compounds *(145)*. The mechanisms for these effects are unclear but may include membrane effects, uncoupling of oxidative phosphorylation, and induction of ion cycling *(65)*.

Sympathomimetics

Sibutramine is a nonselective NE/serotonin reuptake inhibitor that acts as both an appetite suppressant *(146)* and an activator of SNS activity via the β3AR *(147)*. Sibutramine is currently indicated for the treatment of obesity in the absence of known cardiovascular disease and is effective at reducing body weight by 5–10% *(148)*. Dose-limiting toxicity and potential side effects include increased heart rate and blood pressure. Patients should be screened for evidence of underlying atherosclerotic heart disease and followed periodically while taking sibutramine.

Ephedrine is a sympathomimetic agent that increases numerous SNS activity responses including heart rate, blood pressure, and basal metabolic rate. The mechanism of action of ephedrine is direct activation of adrenergic receptors. Its efficacy is limited by cardiovascular side effects and relatively low efficacy in the treatment of obesity, although in combination with caffeine shows greater weight loss than placebo *(149)*. Ma huang (*Ephedra sinica*) is an over-the-counter source of ephedrine that has been linked to serious adverse cardiovascular consequences owing to unrestricted use *(146)*.

Nicotine stimulates NE release from sympathetic nerve terminals, resulting in modest (5%) thermogenesis *(150)*. Smoking cessation may have contributed to the increase in the prevalence of obesity owing to withdrawal of nicotine, which acts as both an appetite suppressant and a stimulator of thermogenesis *(151,152)*.

Caffeine stimulates thermogenesis by inhibiting of adenosine receptors on tissues, resulting in increased intracellular cAMP and lipolysis *(153)*. Caffeine may be useful to a small extent as a treatment for obesity, especially in combination with other compounds such as ephedrine or nicotine *(150,153)*.

A discussion of sympathomimetics would not be complete without mentioning the major efforts by numerous groups to synthesize compounds that selectively activate βARs, increase EE, and effect weight loss. The ability of βAR agonists to reverse obesity in rodent models led to great hope that these would become effective treatments in humans *(82)*. β3 agonists, in particular, would seem to be ideal targets, because their expression is restricted to adipose tissue and they effectively reduce body weight in rodents *(105)*. The potential mechanisms of action of β-gonists are multiple, including increased mitochondrial function and abundance, differentiation of BAT in WAT depots, lipolysis, and increased fatty acid oxidation. As already discussed, however, the limited expression of β3AR in human tissues, difficulty in synthesizing full agonists for the human β3AR, combined with intolerable side effects in humans renders the future of β-agonists as effective antiobesity treatments unclear *(154,155)*.

PROSPECTS

Numerous pathways that regulate body weight via changes in EE have been elucidated. Many of these are centrally mediated pathways that alter EE via the SNS and via unknown mechanisms in peripheral tissues. Prime candidates for antiobesity drug targets include fat oxidation in adipose tissue, muscle, and liver via AMPK-mediated mechanisms. In addition, increased mitochondrial respiration, selective uncoupling, and futile cycles remain fertile areas for future investigation into the mechanisms that control body weight via EE.

REFERENCES

1. Hill JO, Wyatt HR, Reed GW, Peters JC. Science 2003;299:853–855.
2. Zhang Y, Proenca R, Maffei M, Barone M, Leopold L, Friedman JM. Nature 1994;372:425–432.
3. de Jesus LA, Carvalho SD, Ribeiro MO, et al. J Clin Invest 2001;108:1379–1385.
4. Silva JE. Ann Intern Med 2003;139:205–213.
5. Speakman JR, Selman C. Proc Nutr Soc 2003;62:621–634.
6. Butler AA, Marks DL, Fan W, Kuhn CM, Bartolome M, Cone RD. Nat Neurosci 2001;4:605–611.
7. Ravussin E, Swinburn BA. Lancet 1992;340:404–408.
8. Rolfe DF, Brown GC. Physiol Rev 1997;77:731–758.
9. Mitchell P, Moyle J. Nature 1967;213:137–139.
10. Rousset S, Alves-Guerra MC, Mozo J, et al. Diabetes 2004;53(Suppl 1):S130–S135.
11. Porter RK, Hulbert AJ, Brand MD. Am J Physiol 1996;271:R1550–R1560.
12. Nicholls DG. Biochem Soc Trans 2001;29:751–755.
13. Spiegelman BM, Flier JS. Cell 2001;104:531–543.
14. Nisoli E, Clementi E, Paolucci C, et al. Science 2003;299:896–899.
15. Ravussin E, Harper IT, Rising R, Bogardus C. Am J Physiol 1991;261:E402–E409.
16. Wang Z, O'Connor TP, Heshka S, Heymsfield SB. J Nutr 2001;131:2967–2970.
17. Bosy-Westphal A, Eichhorn C, Kutzner D, Illner K, Heller M, Muller MJ. J Nutr 2003;133:2356–2362.
18. Weir JB. Nutrition 1990;6:213–221.
19. Kleiber M. J Theor Biol 1975;53:199–204.
20. Gillooly JF, Brown JH, West GB, Savage VM, Charnov EL. Science 2001;293:2248–2251.
21. Livingstone MB. Br J Biomed Sci 1995;52:58–67.
22. Champagne CM, Baker NB, DeLany JP, Harsha DW, Bray GA. J Am Diet Assoc 1998;98:426–433.
23. Bogardus C, Lillioja S, Ravussin E, et al. N Engl J Med 1986;315:96–100.
24. Bouchard C, Tremblay A, Despres JP, et al. N Engl J Med 1990;322:1477–1482.
25. Stunkard AJ, Harris JR, Pedersen NL, McClearn GE. N Engl J Med 1990;322:1483–1487.
26. Zurlo F, Lillioja S, Esposito-Del Puente A, et al. Am J Physiol 1990;259:E650–E657.
27. Tataranni PA, Harper IT, Snitker S, et al. Int J Obes Relat Metab Disord 2003;27:1578–1583.
28. Ravussin E, Lillioja S, Knowler WC, et al. N Engl J Med 1988;318:467–472.
29. Weyer C, Pratley RE, Salbe AD, Bogardus C, Ravussin E, Tataranni PA. J Clin Endocrinol Metab 2000;85:1087–1094.
30. Salbe AD, Weyer C, Harper I, Lindsay RS, Ravussin E, Tataranni PA. Pediatrics 2002;110:307–314.
31. Scherrer U, Randin D, Tappy L, Vollenweider P, Jequier E, Nicod P. Circulation 1994;89:2634–2640.
32. Rumantir MS, Vaz M, Jennings GL, et al. J Hypertens 1999;17:1125–1133.
33. Jansson PA, Larsson A, Smith U, Lonnroth P. J Clin Invest 1992;89:1610–1617.
34. Kokkoris P, Pi-Sunyer FX. Endocrinol Metab Clin North Am 2003;32:895–914.
35. Goldstone AP, Brynes AE, Thomas EL, et al. Am J Clin Nutr 2002;75:468–475.
36. Clement K, Vaisse C, Lahlou N, et al. Nature 1998;392:398–401.
37. O'Rahilly S, Farooqi IS, Yeo GS, Challis BG. Endocrinology 2003;144:3757–3764.
38. Branson R, Potoczna N, Kral JG, Lentes KU, Hoehe MR, Horber FF. N Engl J Med 2003;348: 1096–1103.
39. Schwartz MW, Woods SC, Seeley RJ, Barsh GS, Baskin DG, Leibel RL. Diabetes 2003;52:232–238.
40. Ravussin E, Bogardus C. Infusionstherapie 1990;17:108–112.
41. Neel JV. Nutr Rev 1999;57:S2–S9.
42. Ahima RS, Kelly J, Elmquist JK, Flier JS. Endocrinology 1999;140:4923–4931.
43. Cusin I, Rouru J, Visser T, Burger AG, Rohner-Jeanrenaud F. Diabetes 2000;49:1101–1105.
44. Ahima RS, Prabakaran D, Mantzoros C, et al. Nature 1996;382:250–252.
45. Chan JL, Heist K, DePaoli AM, Veldhuis JD, Mantzoros CS. J Clin Invest 2003;111:1409–1421.
46. Welt CK, Chan JL, Bullen J, et al. N Engl J Med 2004;351:987–997.
47. Friedman JM. Science 2003;299:856–858.
48. Rothwell NJ, Stock MJ. Nature 1979;281:31–35.
49. Stock MJ. Int J Obes Relat Metab Disord 1999;23:1105–1117.
50. Glick Z, Teague RJ, Bray GA. Science 1981;213:1125–1127.
51. Bachman ES, Dhillon H, Zhang CY, et al. Science 2002;297:843–845.
51. Saad MF, Alger SA, Zurlo F, Young JB, Bogardus C, Ravussin E. Am J Physiol 1991;261:E789–E794.
53. Halaas JL, Boozer C, Blair-West J, Fidahusein N, Denton DA, Friedman JM. Proc Natl Acad Sci USA 1997;94:8878–8883.

54. Rosenbaum M, Leibel RL, Hirsch J. N Engl J Med 1997;337:396–407.
55. Levine JA, Eberhardt NL, Jensen MD. Science 1999;283:212–214.
56. Irrcher I, Adhihetty PJ, Joseph AM, Ljubicic V, Hood DA. Sports Med 2003;33:783–793.
57. Salbe AD, Weyer C, Harper I, Lindsay RS, Ravussin E, Tataranni PA. Am J Clin Nutr 2003; 78,193, 194; author reply 194, 195.
58. Ravussin E, Bogardus C. Br J Nutr 2000;83(Suppl 1):S17–S20.
59. Ekelund U, Aman J, Yngve A, Renman C, Westerterp K, Sjostrom M. Am J Clin Nutr 2002;76:935–941.
60. Jakicic JM. Endocrinol Metab Clin North Am 2003;32:967–980.
61. Levine J, Baukol P, Pavlidis I. N Engl J Med 1999;341, 2100.
62. Levine J, Melanson EL, Westerterp KR, Hill JO. Am J Physiol Endocrinol Metab 2001;281:E670–E675.
63. Levine JA, Nygren J, Short KR, Nair KS. J Appl Physiol 2003;94:165–170.
64. Brent GA. N Engl J Med 1994;331:847–853.
65. Lebon V, Dufour S, Petersen KF, et al. J Clin Invest 2001;108:733–737.
66. al-Adsani H, Hoffer LJ, Silva JE. J Clin Endocrinol Metab 1997;82:1118–1125.
67. Larsen PR, Davies TF. In: Larsen PR, Kronenberg HM, Melmed S, Polonsky K, eds. Williams Textbook of Endocrinology,10th ed. Saunders, Philadelphia, 2003; pp. 423–457.
68. Gauthier K, Chassande O, Plateroti M, et al. Embo J 1999;18:623–631.
69. Rosenbaum M, Hirsch J, Murphy E, Leibel RL. Am J Clin Nutr 2000;71:1421–1432.
70. Larsen PR, Davies TF. In: Larsen PR, Kronenberg HM, Melmed S, Polonsky, K, eds. Williams Textbook of Endocrinology,10th ed. Saunders, Philadelphia, pp. 374–421.
71. Bachman ES, Hampton TG, Dhillon H, et al. Endocrinology 2004;145:2767–2774.
72. Leonard JL, Mellen SA, Larsen PR. Endocrinology 1983;112:1153–1155.
73. Silva JE, Larsen PR. Nature 1983;305:712, 713.
74. Ribeiro MO, Carvalho SD, Schultz JJ, et al. J Clin Invest 2001;108:97–105.
75. Schneider MJ, Fiering SN, Pallud SE, Parlow AF, St Germain DL, Galton VA. Mol Endocrinol 2001;15:2137–2148.
76. Curcio C, Lopes AM, Ribeiro MO, et al. Endocrinology 1999;140:3438–3443.
77. Snitker S, Macdonald I, Ravussin E, Astrup A. Obes Rev 2000;1:5–15.
78. Elmquist JK. Physiol Behav 2001;74:703–708.
79. Lowell BB, Bachman ES. J Biol Chem 2003;278:29,385–29,388.
80. Tataranni PA, Young JB, Bogardus C, Ravussin E. Obes Res 1997;5:341–347.
81. Arch JR, Ainsworth AT, Cawthorne MA, et al. Nature 1984;309:163–165.
82. Himms-Hagen J, Cui J, Danforth E Jr, et al. Am J Physiol 1994;266:R1371–R1382.
83. Levin BE, Triscari J, Marquet E, Sullivan AC. Am J Physiol 1984;247:R979–R987.
84. Rohrer DK, Chruscinski A, Schauble EH, Bernstein D, Kobilka BK. J Biol Chem 1999;274: 16,701–16,708.
85. Thomas SA, Palmiter RD. Nature 1997;387:94–97.
86. Susulic VS, Frederich RC, Lawitts J, et al. J Biol Chem 1995;270:29,483–29,492.
87. Leite A, Neto JA, Leyton JF, Crivellaro O, el-Dorry HA. J Biol Chem 1988;263:17,527–17,533.
88. Block BA, O'Brien J, Meissner G. J Cell Biol 1994;127:1275–1287.
89. Denborough M. Lancet 1998;352:1131–1136.
90. Ducreux S, Zorzato F, Muller CR, et al. J Biol Chem 2004;42:43,838–43,846.
91. Wolfe RR. In: Kinney JM, Tucker HN, eds. Energy Metabolism: Tissue Determinants and Cellular Corollaries. Raven, New York, pp. 495–523.
92. Guan HP, Li Y, Jensen MV, Newgard CB, Steppan CM, Lazar MA. Nat Med 2002;8:1122–1128.
93. de Meis L. J Biol Chem 2003;278:41,856–41,861.
94. Ntambi JM, Miyazaki M, Stoehr JP, et al. Proc Natl Acad Sci USA 2002;99:11,482–11,486.
95. Smith SJ, Cases S, Jensen DR, et al. Nat Genet 2000;25:87–90.
96. Stone SJ, Myers HM, Watkins SM, et al. J Biol Chem 2004;279:11,767–11,776.
97. Abu-Elheiga L, Matzuk MM, Abo-Hashema KA, Wakil SJ. Science 2001;291:2613–2616.
98. Ludwig EH, Mahley RW, Palaoglu E, et al. Clin Genet 2002;62:68–73.
99. Minokoshi Y, Kim YB, Peroni OD, et al. Nature 2002; 415:339–343.
100. Minokoshi Y, Alquier T, Furukawa N, et al. Nature 2004;428:569–574.
101. Unger RH. Cell 2004;117:145, 146.
102. Lowell BB, VSS, Hamann A, et al. Nature 1993;366:740–742.
103. Heaton JM. J Anat 1972;112:35–39.
104. Horwitz BA, Smith RE, Pengelley ET. Am J Physiol 1967;241:115–121.
105. Robidoux J, Martin TL, Collins S. Annu Rev Pharmacol Toxicol 2004;44:297–323.

106. Enerback S, Jacobsson A, Simpson EM, et al. Nature 1997;387:90–94.
107. Matthias A, Ohlson KB, Fredriksson JM, Jacobsson A, Nedergaard J, Cannon B. J Biol Chem 2000; 275:25,073–25,081.
108. Liu X, Rossmeisl M, McClaine J, Riachi M, Harper ME, Kozak LP. J Clin Invest 2003;111:399–407.
109. Granneman JG, Burnazi M, Zhu Z, Schwamb LA. Am J Physiol Endocrinol Metab 2003; 285:E1230–E1236.
110. Vidal-Puig AJ, Grujic D, Zhang CY, et al. J Biol Chem 2000;275:16,258–16,266.
111. Zhang CY, Baffy G, Perret P, et al. Cell 2001;105:745–755.
112. Gong DW, Monemdjou S, Gavrilova O, et al. J Biol Chem 2000;275:16,251–16,257.
113. Arsenijevic D, Onuma H, Pecqueur C, et al. Nat Genet 2000;26:435–439.
114. Kopecky J, Clarke G, Enerback S, Spiegelman B, Kozak LP. J Clin Invest 1995;96:2914–2923.
115. Clapham JC, Arch JR, Chapman H, et al. Nature 2000;406:415–418.
116. Klaus S. Curr Drug Targets 2004;5:241–250.
117. Havel PJ. Diabetes 2004;53(Suppl 1):S143–S151.
118. Goran MI, Kaskoun M, Johnson R. J Pediatr 1994;125:362–367.
119. Clement K, Vaisse C, Manning BS, et al. N Engl J Med 1995;333:352–354.
120. Snitker S, Hellmer J, Boschmann M, et al. J Clin Endocrinol Metab 1998;83:4054–4058.
121. Emorine LJ, Marullo S, Briend-Sutren MM, et al. Science 1989;245:1118–1121.
122. Weyer C, Gautier JF, Danforth E Jr. Diabetes Metab 1999;25:11–21.
123. Coleman DL. Diabetologia 1982;22:205–211.
124. Mantzoros CS. Ann Intern Med 1999;130:671–680.
125. Farooqi IS, Jebb SA, Langmack G, et al. N Engl J Med 1999;341:879–884.
126. Collins S, Kuhn CM, Petro AE, Swick AG, Chrunyk BA, Surwit RS. Nature 1996;380,677.
127. Haynes WG, Morgan DA, Walsh SA, Mark AL, Sivitz WI. J Clin Invest 1997;100:270–278.
128. Hucking K, Hamilton-Wessler M, Ellmerer M, Bergman RN. J Clin Invest 2003;111:257–264.
129. Ravussin E, Lillioja S, Anderson TE, Christin L, Bogardus C. J Clin Invest 1986;78:1568–1578.
130. Zurlo F, Larson K, Bogardus C, Ravussin E. J Clin Invest 1990;86:1423–1427.
131. Simonsen L, Bulow J, Madsen J, Christensen NJ. Am J Physiol 1992;263:E850–E855.
132. Puigserver P, Wu Z, Park CW, Graves R, Wright M, Spiegelman BM. Cell 1998;92:829–839.
133. Wu Z, Puigserver P, Andersson U, et al. Cell 1999;98:115–124.
134. Lin J, Wu H, Tarr PT, et al. Nature 2002;418:797–801.
135. Cohen P, Miyazaki M, Socci ND, et al. Science 2002;297:240–243.
136. Dobrzyn P, Dobrzyn A, Miyazaki M, et al. Proc Natl Acad Sci USA 2004;101:6409–6414.
137. Ntambi JM, Miyazaki M, Stoehr JP, et al. Proc Natl Acad Sci USA 2002;99:11,482–11,486.
138. Campfield LA, Smith FJ, Burn P. Science 1998;280:1383–1387.
139. Harper JA, Dickinson K, Brand MD. Obes Rev 2001;2:255–265.
140. Gura T. Science 2003;299:849–852.
141. O'Rahilly S. Nutr Rev 2002;60:S30–S34; discussion S68–S84, 85–87.
142. Farooqi IS, Keogh JM, Kamath S, et al. Nature 2001;414:34–35.
143. Heymsfield SB, Greenberg AS, Fujioka K, et al. JAMA 1999;282:1568–1575.
144. Grover GJ, Mellstrom K, Ye L, et al. Proc Natl Acad Sci USA 2003;100:10,067–10,072.
145. Wagner RL, Huber BR, Shiau AK, et al. Mol Endocrinol 2001;15:398–410.
146. Yanovski SZ, Yanovski JA. N Engl J Med 2002;346:591–602.
147. Connoley IP, Liu YL, Frost I, Reckless IP, Heal DJ, Stock MJ. Br J Pharmacol 1999;126:1487–1495.
148. Thearle M, Aronne LJ. Endocrinol Metab Clin North Am 2003;32:1005–1024.
149. Daly PA, Krieger DR, Dulloo AG, Young JB, Landsberg L. Int J Obes Relat Metab Disord 1993; 17(Suppl 1), S73–S78.
150. Jessen AB, Toubro S, Astrup A. Am J Clin Nutr 2003;77:1442–1447.
151. Hofstetter A, Schutz Y, Jequier E, Wahren J. N Engl J Med 1986;314:79–82.
152. Flegal KM, Troiano RP, Pamuk ER, Kuczmarski RJ, Campbell SM. N Engl J Med 1995; 333:1165–1170.
153. Astrup A, Toubro S, Christensen NJ, Quaade F. Am J Clin Nutr 1992;55:246S–248S.
154. Arch JR. Eur J Pharmacol 2002;440:99–107.
155. Hu B, Jennings LL. Prog Med Chem 2003;41:167–194.

7 Pathophysiology of Diabetes in Obesity

Geetha R. Soodini, MD
and Osama Hamdy, MD, PhD

INTRODUCTION

Obesity is diagnosed when the percentage of body fat is high in relation to the lean body mass or when the body mass index (BMI) is 30 kg/m^2 or more, and individuals with a BMI between 25 and 29.9 kg/m^2 are considered overweight. According to the Department of Health and Human Services, 60% of the US population in 2001 was either overweight or obese. Such prevalence is much higher among patients with type 2 diabetes, 80% of whom are either overweight or obese *(1,2)*. The situation is almost equally dismal around the globe, including many developing countries, where the adverse health consequences of overweight and obesity have begun to replace undernutrition and infection as the main causes of early death and disability *(3)*.

ASSOCIATION BETWEEN OBESITY AND TYPE 2 DIABETES

It has been quite clear that the prevalence of type 2 diabetes increases with the increasing prevalence of overweight and obesity among different racial and ethnic groups *(4)*. Follow-up of middle-aged women in the Nurses' Health Study and of men in the Health Professionals Follow-up Study for 10 yr has clearly shown that the risk of developing type 2 diabetes is rising in parallel with increasing severity of overweight and obesity *(5)*. Interestingly, the risk of developing diabetes starts to increase even with modest weight gain *(6,7)*. It has thus been reported that a period of gradual weight gain usually precedes the onset of type 2 diabetes. This observation is evident, e.g., in the Pima Indian population, which has a high prevalence of type 2 diabetes. Body

From: *Contemporary Diabetes: Obesity and Diabetes*
Edited by: C. S. Mantzoros © Humana Press Inc., Totowa, NJ

weight of Pima Indians has been noted to increase by an average of 30 kg above their ideal body weight in the years immediately preceding the diagnosis of diabetes *(8)*. By contrast, weight reduction is associated with decreased incidence of type 2 diabetes. In the Nurses Health Study, a weight loss of 5 kg or more reduced the risk of developing type 2 diabetes by approx 50% *(6)*. This observation was later documented in the Diabetes Prevention Program, in which an approximate 7% of weight reduction maintained for an average duration of 2.8 yr was associated with a 58% reduction in the risk of developing type 2 diabetes in prediabetic individuals with impaired glucose tolerance (IGT) *(9)*. Weight reduction through increased physical activity or bariatric surgery also leads to similar results *(10,11)*. Dixon and O'Brien *(12)* found that an average weight reduction of 27 kg 1 yr after laparoscopic adjustable gastric band surgery in a group of severely obese patients with type 2 diabetes resulted in remission of diabetes in 64% of them and major improvement in glucose control in another 26%.

Insulin resistance and hyperinsulinemia are often seen in overweight and obese individuals and are by far the best predictors of type 2 diabetes. Both conditions are currently considered an outcome of the interaction between increased body weight and underlying genetic factors. It has also been reported that although the degree of insulin sensitivity may be quite similar between the nondiabetic offspring of parents with type 2 diabetes and the offspring of nondiabetic parents whose body weight is close to the ideal weight, insulin sensitivity declines more rapidly with increasing body weight in those with a family history of diabetes *(13)*.

The development of type 2 diabetes in overweight and obese individuals is characterized by progressive deterioration of glucose tolerance over several years. Cross-sectional and prospective data suggested that weight gain and abnormal or deficient insulin secretion and insulin action together with increased endogenous hepatic glucose production underlie this deterioration *(14–17)*. It has also been observed that these abnormalities are sequential, with impairments of insulin action and insulin secretion occurring earlier during the transition from normal glucose tolerance to IGT and worsening as an individual moves toward diabetes; the increased endogenous hepatic glucose production starts only during the late transition from IGT to diabetes *(18)*. These findings suggest that intervention(s) to prevent diabetes in high-risk individuals with overweight or obesity should start very early, especially in subjects with a positive family history of diabetes among first-degree relatives.

PATHOGENESIS OF TYPE 2 DIABETES IN OBESITY

The mechanism through which obesity increases insulin resistance is currently thought to be related to the increased circulating free fatty acids (FFAs), altered levels of adipocytokines, altered body fat distribution, or a combination of the three. Serum FFA levels are frequently high in obese subjects. It has been reported that elevated levels of FFAs could potentially be the major contributor to peripheral insulin resistance in patients with type 2 diabetes mellitus *(19,20)*. Chronically elevated serum FFA levels stimulate gluconeogenesis, induce hepatic and muscle insulin resistance, and impair insulin secretion in genetically predisposed individuals *(21)*. FFAs also tend to increase the accumulation of triglycerides in both liver and skeletal muscle, which correlates with the degree of insulin resistance in these tissues *(22,23)*. In addition, since triglycerides are in a state of constant turnover, their metabolites, such as acyl coenzymes A, ceramides, and diacylglycerol, contribute toward both impaired hepatic and peripheral insulin action. This sequence of events is frequently called lipotoxicity *(24)*. Accumulating evidence suggests that such lipotoxicity may also be an important contributor to the pancreatic β-cell dysfunction seen in patients with type 2 diabetes *(25)*.

ROLE OF ADIPOCYTOKINES

Adipose tissue recently has been recognized as an endocrine organ capable of secreting a large number of adipocytokines *(26)*. Some of these cytokines are expressed almost exclusively in adipose tissue (e.g., leptin, adiponectin, and resistin), whereas others are produced by both the adipose tissue and adipose tissue–resident macrophages as well as possibly other organs or systems (e.g., tumor necrosis factor-α [TNF-α], interleukin-6 [IL-6], plasminogen activator inhibitor-1 [PAI-1], monocyte chemoattractant protein-1). With the exception of adiponectin, which is decreased, all other adipokines are increased in overweight and obese individuals. Adiponectin increases tissue sensitivity to insulin. Animal studies have shown that a deficiency of adiponectin is important in the pathogenesis of insulin resistance *(27–30)*, and adiponectin levels have been shown to correlate positively with insulin sensitivity *(31,32)* in both animals and humans. In humans, plasma adiponectin levels are decreased in both obesity and type 2 diabetes *(33,34)*. Conversely, it has been shown that a 7% reduction in body weight, by a combination of caloric reduction and increased physical activity for 6 mo, resulted in a significant increase in plasma adiponectin level in obese type 2 diabetic patients with insulin resistance *(35)*. Similar observations have been reported in patients after weight reduction by bariatric surgery *(36)*. Recently, it has been assumed that increased adiponectin levels may protect against later development of type 2 diabetes *(37)*, whereas decreased adiponectin levels may predispose to diabetes independent of obesity *(37)*. Finally, adiponectin has anti-inflammatory properties and may also protect against development or progression of atherosclerosis *(38,39)*.

In contrast to adiponectin, TNF-α is a potent proinflammatory cytokine *(40)* implicated in the development of atherosclerosis and possibly insulin resistance and type 2 diabetes. Circulating TNF-α levels are increased both in obese individuals without diabetes *(41)* and in type 2 diabetes *(42)*, but the correlation between insulin resistance and plasma levels of TNF-α is weak in both groups *(43)*. It has been postulated that tissue insulin resistance may be more strongly related to the local tissue TNF-α concentration than to its plasma levels and that the circulating levels of TNF receptors may reflect more accurately the status of activation of the TNF-α system. Studies in genetically obese animals suggest that increased release of TNF-α from adipocytes may play a major and direct role in the impairment of insulin action *(44,45)*. TNF-α influences insulin signaling through serine phosphorylation of the insulin and insulin receptor substrate-1, thus inhibiting insulin action at the organ level through autocrine and paracrine mechanisms *(46)*.

IL-6 is another important systemic proinflammatory citokine. It regulates hepatic production of C-reactive protein (CRP) and other acute-phase proteins. In animal studies, IL-6 has been implicated in the development of insulin resistance in the muscle as well as in β-cell apoptosis *(25,47)*. In humans with type 2 diabetes, IL-6 levels have been found to be increased, and to correlate with severity of inflammation, as indicated by the serum levels of CRP, as well as glucose intolerance *(48,49)*. The interrelationship between the two proinflammatory cytokines TNF-α and IL-6 is complex, because not only does TNF-α stimulate IL-6 production and consequently CRP production, but IL-6 also exerts a feedback inhibitory effect on TNF-α production *(50)*. Interventions that mainly increase IL-6, such as exercise, may have an anti-inflammatory effect through suppression of TNF-α, which is one of the major inducers of inflammation *(51)*.

Leptin is exclusively expressed in adipose tissue, especially sc fat. It may exert a direct effect in metabolically important tissues and/or indirect effects by activating specific centers in the hypothalamus to decrease food intake and increase energy expenditure, thus influencing glucose and fat metabolism (52). Food intake is reduced by systemic administration of leptin in normal-weight animals, but the response is decreased in obese animals (53). It has also been found that leptin mRNA content of adipocytes and thus leptin production are twice as high in obese vs normal-weight subjects (54). These observations suggest that obese persons are insensitive to endogenous leptin production. In addition, animal studies have shown that the administration of leptin has an insulin-sensitizing effect in muscle cells and adipocytes (55–57). In humans, mutations of the leptin gene have been associated with severe obesity, glucose intolerance, and insulin resistance, which are reversed by the administration of leptin (58–60). Whether leptin also plays an important role in the inflammation associated with type 2 diabetes and atherosclerosis by acting directly on macrophages to augment their phagocytic activity and to increase their production of other inflammatory cytokines (61,62) remains to be fully elucidated.

PAI-1 is another cytokine that may link obesity to type 2 diabetes and cardiovascular disease. This serine protease inhibits the fibrinolytic cascade. Elevated PAI-1 levels cause an imbalance between the thrombotic and fibrinolytic systems, favoring the formation of microthrombi and accelerating the atherosclerotic process (63). Adipose tissue is one of the major sources of PAI-1. Obese subjects and those with type 2 diabetes have elevated levels of PAI-1 (64,65). It has also been noted that hyperinsulinemia, which usually accompanies insulin-resistant states, is a potent stimulus for PAI-1 production by adipose tissue (66,67).

Resistin is another adipokine that has recently been reported to correlate closely with hepatic insulin resistance (68). Recent studies have demonstrated that circulating resistin leves and resistin expression in fat cells are increased in type 2 diabetes and obesity (69,70), but it is not yet clear whether high levels of circulating resistin contribute to insulin resistance, are the result of insulin resistance, or are an innocent bystander (71,72).

ROLE OF BODY FAT DISTRIBUTION IN PATHOGENESIS OF TYPE 2 DIABETES

In addition to total body fat content, the pattern of body fat distribution is an important predictor of insulin sensitivity. So far, it is still controversial whether all adipose tissue has exactly the same endocrine role or whether its endocrine function is solely dependent on its anatomic location. Individuals with upper-body fat accumulation or higher visceral fat mass are more insulin resistant than those with a predominantly lower-body fat accumulation and more sc fat (73–75). Accurate quantification of body fat compartments requires imaging techniques such as magnetic resonance imaging or computed tomography, which are too expensive to be routinely used in clinical practice. Waist circumference or waist-to-hip ratio (WHR) has been shown to correlate significantly with the visceral fat volume, however. The association between visceral fat accumulation and insulin resistance has been attributed to the increased sensitivity of visceral fat to lipolytic stimuli. This increases the flux of FFA into the portal and systemic circulations (76). In contrast to sc fat, visceral fat cells produce excessive amounts of proinflammatory adipocytokines such as TNF-α, IL-6, and PAI-1 and decreased amounts of insulin-sensitizing adipocytokines such as adiponectin (77–79).

As with total body fat, the distribution of body fat between visceral and sc compartments has a significant genetic basis *(80)*. Recent evidence indicates that there may be several loci determining the propensity to store fat in the abdominal region *(81)*. Differences in gene expression of visceral fat compared with sc fat may account for the differences in metabolic risk between the two fat depots. Of the 1660 genes that are expressed in adipose tissue, 297 (17.9%) have shown a twofold or higher difference in their expression between the visceral fat and sc fat. Many of these genes are involved in glucose homeostasis and insulin action (peroxisomei proliferator-activated receptor γ, insulin-like growth factor binding protein-3, insulin-like growth factor-1, GLUT1), or in lipid metabolism (HMG-CoA synthase, hormone-sensitive lipase). Gonadal steroids may also play a major role in the distribution of body fat. At the onset of puberty, men become more muscular and have less fat, whereas women start to have a higher percentage of body fat in relation to their muscle mass. These differences persist throughout life and are reflected in the typical male and female fat distribution. With advancing age, both gonadal steroid and growth hormone (GH) secretion decline, resulting in increased accumulation of visceral fat, particularly in men. In women, higher serum testosterone concentrations are usually associated with increased visceral fat. Thus, the decline in GH and the loss of estrogen at the time of menopause may explain the relatively rapid increase in visceral fat in postmenopausal women.

Organ-specific deposition of fat is a predictor of insulin resistance. Increased intramyocellular triglyceride content correlates closely with muscle insulin resistance and is a better predictor of impaired insulin action than visceral adiposity *(82,83)*. Intrahepatic fat accumulation is also associated with hepatic insulin resistance *(84,85)*. Inherited forms of lipodystrophy in humans are characterized by selective loss of sc and visceral fat and are associated with metabolic abnormalities such as hyperglycemia, insulin resistance, and dyslipidemia. Insufficient adipose tissue mass leads to excessive storage of ingested fat in skeletal muscle and liver and the development of severe insulin resistance in these organs *(86)*. Replacement therapy with leptin mobilizes fat out of the liver and muscle, leading to dramatic improvements in hepatic and muscle sensitivity to insulin as well as improved glycemic control *(87)*. Surgical transplantation of adipose tissue in lipodystrophic animals resulted in mobilization of fat out of the liver and muscle. This fat mobilization was found to be associated with improvement in insulin sensitivity in these organs and normalization of glucose intolerance *(88)*. Conversely, surgical removal of adipose tissue in normal glucose-tolerant hamsters resulted in fat accumulation in liver and muscle, insulin resistance, and glucose intolerance *(87)*.

Finally, differences in adipose tissue cellularity have also been suggested as a possible link between obesity and diabetes. It has been shown that obese people with a large sc abdominal adipocyte size are on average more hyperinsulinemic and glucose intolerant than those with a similar degree of adiposity but with a relatively smaller sc abdominal adipocyte size *(88)*.

REFERENCES

1. Mokdad AH, Bowman BA, Ford ES, et al. The continuing epidemics of obesity and diabetes in the United Sates. JAMA 2001;286:1195–1200.
2. Mokdad AH, Ford ES, Bowman BA, et al. Prevalence of obesity, diabetes and obesity-related health risk factors, 2001. JAMA 2003;289:76–79.
3. Caballero B. Obesity in developing countries: biological and ecological factors. J Nutr 2001; 131:866S–870S.

4. Must A, Spadano J, Coakley EH, et al. The disease burden associated with overweight and obesity. JAMA 1999;282:1523–1529.

5. Field AE, Coakley EH, Must A, et al. Impact of overweight on the risk of developing common chronic diseases during a 10-year period. Arch Intern Med 2001;161:1581–1586.

6. Colditz GA, Willet WC, Rotnitzky A, et al. Weight gain as a risk factor for clinical diabetes mellitus in women. Ann Intern Med 1995;122:481–486.

7. Chan JM, Rimm EB, Colditz GA. Obesity, fat distribution and weight gain as risk factors for clinical diabetes in men. Diabetes Care 1994;17:961–969.

8. Felber JP. From obesity to diabetes: pathophysiological considerations. Int J Obes Relat Metab Disord 1992;16:937–952.

9. Knowler WC, Barrett-Conner E, Fowler E, et al. Reduction in the incidence of type 2 diabetes with lifestyle intervention or metformin. N Engl J Med 2002;346:393–403.

10. Helmrich SP, Ragland DR, Leung RW, et al. Physical activity and reduced occurrence of non-insulin dependent diabetes mellitus. N Engl J Med 1991;325:147–152.

11. Sjostrom CD, Lissner L, Wedel H, et al. Reduction in incidence of diabetes, hypertension and lipid disturbances after intentional weight loss induced by bariatric surgery: the SOS Intervention Study. Obes Res 1999;7:477–484.

12. Dixon JB, O'Brien PE. Health outcomes of severely obese type 2 diabetic subjects 1 year after laparoscopic adjustable gastric banding. Diabetes Care 2002;25(2):358–363.

13. Bays H, DeFronzo RA, Ferranini E. Insulin resistance: a multifaceted syndrome responsible for NIDDM, obesity, hypertension, dyslipidemia and atherosclerotic cardiovascular disease. Diabetes Care 1991;14:173–194.

14. Reaven GM, Hollenbeck CB, Chen YD. Relationship between glucose tolerance, insulin secretion and insulin action in non-obese individuals with varying degrees of glucose tolerance. Diabetologia 1998;32:52–55.

15. Haffner SM, Miettinen H, Gaskill SP, et al. Decreased insulin action and insulin secretion predict the development of impaired glucose tolerance. Diabetologia 1996;39:1201–1207.

16. Martin BC, Warram JH, Krolewski AS. Role of glucose and insulin resistance in development of type 2 diabetes: results of a 25 year follow-up study. Lancet 1992;340:925–929.

17. Warram JH, Sigal RJ, Martin BC, et al. Natural history of impaired glucose tolerance: follow-up at the Joslin Clinic. Diabet Med 1996;13:S40–S45.

18. Weyer C, Bogardus C, Mott DM. The natural history of insulin secretory dysfunction and insulin resistance in the pathogenesis of type 2 diabetes mellitus. J Clin Invest 1999;104:787–794.

19. Boden G, Chen X. Effects of fat on glucose uptake and utilization in patients with non-insulin dependent diabetes. J Clin Invest 1995;96:1261–1268.

20. Paolisso G, Tataranni PA, Foley JE, et al. A high concentration of fasting plasma non-esterified fatty acids is a risk factor for the development of NIDDM. Diabetologia 1995;38:1213–1217.

21. Bays H, Mandarino L, DeFronzo RA. Role of adipocyte, free fatty acids, and ectopic fat in the pathogenesis of type 2 diabetes mellitus: peroxisomal proliferator-activated receptor agonists provide a rational therapeutic approach. J Clin Endocrinol Metab 2004;89:463–478.

22. Greco AV, Mingrone G, Giancaterini A, et al. Insulin resistance in morbid obesity: reversal with intramyocellular fat depletion. Diabetes 2002;51:144–151.

23. Seppala-Lindroos A, Vehkavaara S, Hakkinen A.-M., et al. Fat accumulation in the liver is associated with defects in insulin suppression of glucose production and serum free fatty acids independent of obesity in normal men. J Clin Endocrinol Metab 2002;87:3023–3028.

24. Unger RH. Lipotoxicity in the pathogenesis of obesity-dependent NIDDM: genetic and clinical implications. Diabetes 1996;45:273–283.

25. Shimabukuro M, Zhou YT, Leve M, Unger RH. Fatty acid induced β cell apoptosis. Proc Natl Acad Sci USA 1998;95:2498–2502.

26. Fruhbeck G, Gomez-Ambrosi J, Muruzabal FJ, Burrell MA. The adipocyte: a model for integration of endocrine and metabolic signaling in energy metabolism regulation. Am J Physiol 2001;280: E827–E847.

27. Yamauchi T, Kamon J, Waki H, et al. The fat derived hormone adiponectin reverses insulin resistance associated with both lipoatrophy and obesity. Nat Med 2001;7:941–946.

28. Nadler ST, Stoehr JP, Schueler KL, et al. The expression of adipogenic genes is decreased in obesity and diabetes mellitus. Proc Natl Acad Sci USA 2000;97:11,371–11,376.

29. Hotta K, Funahashi T, Bodkin NL, et al. Circulating concentrations of the adipocyte protein adiponectin are decreased in parallel with reduced insulin sensitivity during the progression to type 2 diabetes in rhesus monkeys. Diabetes 2001;50:1126–1133.

30. Maeda N, Shimomura I, Kishida K, et al. Diet-induced insulin resistance in mice lacking adiponectin/ACRP30. Nat Med 2002;8:731–737.
31. Weyer C, Funahashi T, Tanaka S, et al. Hypoadiponectinemia in obesity and type 2 diabetes: close association with insulin resistance and hyperinsulinemia. J Clin Endocrinol Metab 2001;86:1930–1935.
32. Abbasi F, Chu JW, Mclaughlin T, et al. Obesity versus insulin resistance in modulation of plasma adiponectin concentration. Diabetes 2002;52(Suppl 1): A81.
33. Arita Y, Kihara S, Ouchi N, et al. Paradoxical decrease of an adipose-specific protein, adiponectin, in obesity. Biochem Biophys Res Commun 1999;257:79–83.
34. Hotta K, Funahashi T, Arita Y, et al. Plasma concentration of a novel adipose-specific protein, adiponectin, in type 2 diabetic patients. Arterioscler Thromb Vasc Biol 2000;20:1595–1599.
35. Monzillo LU, Hamdy O, Horton ES, et al. Effect of lifestyle modification on adipokine levels in obese subjects with insulin resistance. Obes Res 2003;11:1048–1054.
36. Yang WS, Lee WJ, Funahashi T, et al. Weight reduction increases plasma levels of an adipose-derived anti-inflammatory protein, adiponectin. J Clin Endocrinol Metab 2001;86:3815–3819.
37. Lindsay RS, Funahashi T, Hanson RL, et al. Adiponectin and development of type 2 diabetes in the Pima Indian population. Lancet 2002;360:57, 58.
38. Yokota T, Oritani K, Takahashi I, Ishikawa J, Matsuyama A, Ouchi N. Adiponectin, a new member of the family of soluble defense collagens, negatively regulated the growth of myelmonocytic progenitors and the functions of macrophages. Blood 2000;96:1723–1732.
39. Matsuda M, Shimomura I, Sata M, et al. Role of adiponectin in preventing vascular stenosis: the missing link of adipo-vascular axis. J Biol Chem 2002;277:37,487–37,491.
40. Uzui H, Harpf A, Liu M, et al. Increased expression of membrane type 3-matrix metalloproteinase in human atherosclerotic plaque: role of activated macrophages and inflammatory cytokines. Circulation 2002;106(24):3024–3030.
41. Hotamisligil GS, Arner P, Caro JF, et al. Increased adipose tissue expression of tumor necrosis factor-alpha in human obesity and insulin resistance. J Clin Invest 1995;95:2409–2415.
42. Miyazaki Y, Pipek R, Mandarino LJ, DeFronzo RA. Tumor necrosis factor α and insulin resistance in obese type 2 diabetic patients. Int J Obes 2003;27:88–94.
43. Zinman B, Hanley AJ, Harris SB, et al. Circulating tumor necrosis factor α concentrations in a native Canadian population with high rates if type 2 diabetes mellitus. J Clin Endocrinol Metab 1999; 84:272–278.
44. Hotamisligil GS, Peraldi P, Budavari A, et al. IRS-1 mediated inhibition of insulin receptor tyrosine kinase activity in TNF-α and obesity induced insulin resistance. Science 1996;271:665–668.
45. Uysal KT, Wiesbrock SM, Marino MW, Hotamisligil GS. Protection from obesity-induced insulin resistance in mice lacking TNF-alpha function. Nature 1997;389:610–614.
46. Hofmann C, Lorenz K, Braithwaite SS, et al. Altered gene expression for tumor necrosis factor-alpha and its receptors during drug and dietary modulation of insulin resistance. Endocrinology 1994;134:264–270.
47. Sandler S, Bendtzen K, Eizirik DL, Welsh M. Interleukin-6 affects insulin secretion and glucose metabolism of rat pancreatic islets in vitro. Endocrinology 1990;126:1288–1294.
48. Pradhan AD, Manson JE, Rifai N, et al. C-reactive protein, interleukin 6 and the risk of developing type 2 diabetes. JAMA 2001;286:327–334.
49. Pickup JC, Chusney GD, Thomas SM, Burt D. Plasma interleukin 6, tumor necrosis factor and blood cytokine production in type 2 diabetes. Life Sci 2000;67:291–300.
50. Suzuki K, Nakaji S, Yamada M, et al. Systemic inflammatory response to exhaustive exercise: cytokine kinetics. Exerc Immunol Rev 2002;8:6–48.
51. Starkie R, Ostrowski SR, Jauffred S, et al. Exercise and IL-6 infusion inhibit endotoxin-induced TNF-alpha production in humans. FASEB J 2003;17:884–886.
52. Lonnqvist F, Arner P, Nordfors L, Schalling M. Overexpression of the obese (ob) gene in adipose tissue of human obese subjects. Nat Med 1995;1:950–993.
53. Van Heek M, Compton DS, France CF, et al. Diet-induced obese mice develop peripheral, but not central, resistance to leptin. J Clin Invest 1997;99:385–390.
54. Considine RV, Sinha MK, Heiman ML, et al. Serum immunoreactive-leptin concentrations in normal-weight and obese humans. N Engl J Med 1996;334:292–295.
55. Ceddia RB, William WN Jr, Curi R. Comparing effects of leptin and insulin on glucose metabolism in skeletal muscle: evidence for an effect of leptin on glucose uptake and decarboxylation. Int J Obes Rel Metab Disord 1999;23:75–82.
56. Kamohara S, Burcelin R, Halaas JL, Freidman JM. Acute stimulation of glucose metabolism in mice by leptin treatment. Nature 1997;389:374–377.

57. Muoio DM, Dohm GL. Peripheral metabolic actions of leptin. Best Pract Res Clin Endocrinol Metab 2002;16:653–666.
58. Clement K, Vaisse C, Lahlou N, et al. A mutation in the human leptin receptor gene causes obesity and pituitary dysfunction. Nature 1998;392:398–401.
59. Farooqui IS, Jebb SA, Langmack G, et al. Effects of recombinant leptin therapy in a child with congenital leptin deficiency. N Engl J Med 1999;341:879–884.
60. Mantzoros CS, Flier JS. Editorial: leptin as a therapeutic agent-trials and tribulations. J Clin Endocrinol Metab 2000;85:4000–4002.
61. Santos-Alvarez J, Goberna R, Sanchez-Margalet V: Human leptin stimulates proliferation and activation of human circulating monocytes. Cell Immunol 1999;194:6–11.
62. Giansford T, Willson TA, Metcalf D, et al. Leptin can induce proliferation, differentiation, and functional activation of hemopoietic cells. Proc Natl Acad Sci USA 1996;93:14,564–14,568.
63. Yudkin JS. Abnormalities of coagulation and fibrinolysis in insulin resistance: evidence for a common antecedent? Diabetes Care 1999;22:C25–C30.
64. Alessi MC, Bastelica D, Morange P, et al. Plasminogen activator inhibitor 1, transforming growth factor-β1 and ABMI are closely associated in human adipose tissue during morbid obesity. Diabetes 2000;49:1374–1380.
65. Alessi MC, Peiretti F, Morange P, et al. Production of plasminogen activator inhibitor1 by human adipose tissue: possible link between visceral fat accumulation and vascular disease. Diabetes 1997; 46:860–867.
66. Smith SR, Bai F, Charbonneau C, et al. A promoter genotype and oxidative stress potentially link resistin to human insulin resistance. Diabetes 2003;52:1611–1618.
67. Wang H, Chu WS, Hemphill C, Elbein SC. Human resistin gene: molecular scanning and evaluation of association with insulin sensitivity and type 2 diabetes in Caucasians. J Clin Endocrinol Metab 2002;87:2520–2524.
68. Vidal-Puig A, O'Rahilly S. Resistin: a new link between obesity and insulin resistance? Clin Endocrinol (Oxf) 2001;55:437–438.
69. Kissebah AH, Peiris AN. Biology of regional body fat distribution: relationship to non-insulin-dependent diabetes mellitus. Diabetes Metab Rev 1989;5:83–109.
70. Despres JP, Lemieux S, Lamarche B, et al. The insulin resistance-dyslipidemic syndrome: contribution of visceral obesity and therapeutic implications. Int J Obes Related Metab Disord 1995; 19(Suppl): S76–S86.
71. Lee JH, Bullen JW Jr, Stoyneva VL, Mantzoros CS. Circulating resistin in lean, obese and insulin-resistant mouse models: lack of association with insulinemia and glycemia. Am J Physiol Endocrinol Metab 2005;288:E625–E632.
72. Lee JH, Chan JL, Yiannakouris N, et al. Circulating resistin levels are not associated with obesity or insulin resistance in humans and are not regulated by fasting or leptin administration: cross-sectional and interventional studies in normal, insulin-resistant, and diabetic subjects. J Clin Endocrinol Metab 2003;88:4848–4856.
73. Albu JB, Kovera AJ, Johnson JA. Fat distribution and health in obesity. Ann NY Acad Sci 2000;904:491–501.
74. Zeirath JR, Livingston JN, Thorne J, et al. Regional difference in insulin inhibition of non-esterified fatty acid release from human adipocytes: relation to insulin receptor phosphorylation and intracellular signaling through the insulin receptor substrate-1-pathway. Diabetologia 1998;41:1343–1354.
75. Arner P. Regional differences in protein production by human adipose tissue. Biochem Soc Trans 2001;29:72–75.
76. Motoshima H, Wu X, Sinha MK, et al. Differential regulation of adiponectin secretion from cultured human omental and subcutaneous adipocytes: effects of insulin and rosiglitazone. J Clin Endocrinol Metab 2002;87:5662–5667.
77. Sewter CP, Blows F, Vidal Puig A, O'Rahilly S. Regional differences in the response of human pre-adipocytes to PPARγ and RXRα agonists. Diabetes 2002;51:7218–7223.
78. Bouchard C, Depress JP, Mauriege P. Genetics and nongenetic determinants of regional fat distribution. Endocr Rev 1993;14:72–93.
79. Perusse L, Rice T, Chagnon YC, et al. genome-wide scan for abdominal fat assessed by computed tomography in the Quebec Family Study. Diabetes 2001;50:614–621.
80. Pan DA, Lillioja S, Kriketos AD, et al. Skeletal muscle triglyceride levels are inversely related to insulin action. Diabetes 1997;46:983–988.

81. Goodpaster BH, Thaete FL, Simoneau JA, Kelley DE. Subcutaneous abdominal fat and thigh muscle composition predict insulin sensitivity independently of visceral fat. Diabetes 1997;46:1579–1585.

82. Bajaj M, Surramornkul S, Pratipanawatr T, et al. Pioglitazone reduces hepatic fat content and augments splanchnic glucose uptake in patients with type 2 diabetes mellitus. Diabetes 2003; 52:1364–1370.

83. Bajaj M, Surramonkul S, Piper P, et al. Decreased plasma adiponectin concentrations are closely related to hepatic fat content and hepatic insulin resistance in pioglitazone treated type 2 diabetic patients. J Clin Endocrinol Metab 2004;89:200–206.

84. Robbins DC, Horton ES, Tulp O, Sims EA. Familial partial lipodystrophy; complications of obesity in the non-obese? Metabolism 1982;31:445–452.

85. Oral EA, Simha V, Ruiz E, et al. Leptin replacement therapy for lipodystrophy. N Engl J Med 2002;346:57–78.

86. Gavrilova O, Marcus-Samuels B, Graham D, et al. Surgical implantation of adipose tissue reverses diabetes in lipoatrophic mice. J Clin Invest 2000;105:271–278.

87. Weber RV, Buckley MC, Fried SK, Kral JG. Subcutaneous lipectomy causes a metabolic syndrome in hamsters. Am J Physiol 2000;279: R936–R943.

88. Weyer C, Foley JE, Bogardus PA, Tataranni REP. Enlarged subcutaneous abdominal adipocyte size, but not obesity itself, predicts type 2 diabetes independent of insulin resistance. Diabetologia 2000;43:1498–1506.

III | DIAGNOSIS, CLINICAL MANIFESTATIONS, AND COMPLICATIONS

8

Diagnosing Obesity, Diabetes Mellitus, and Insulin Resistance Syndrome

Diana Barb, MD
and Christos S. Mantzoros, MD, DSc

CONTENTS

DIAGNOSING AND SCREENING FOR OBESITY

Obesity is a disease state that has reached epidemic proportions, with increasing prevalence and serious health care consequences; therefore, it is important to diagnose and evaluate it properly. In this first part of the chapter, we present criteria for the diagnosis of overweight and obesity and evaluation of the obese and overweight patient and emphasize the importance of determining the specific type of obesity and the possible presence of other risk factors in obese individuals. We also review obesity-screening recommendations and rationale.

Introduction

Obesity is a chronic disease state characterized by an excessive accumulation of fat. Obesity should be differentiated from increased body weight, because lean but very muscular individuals may be classified as overweight by arbitrary standards without actually having increased adiposity (1). Obesity is closely associated with an overlapping group of disease states including insulin resistance syndrome (IRS) and type 2 diabetes (Fig. 1). Moreover, obesity increases the risk of developing several comorbidities, including type 2 diabetes, hypertension, dyslipidemia, cardiovascular disease (CVD), arthritis, sleep apnea, and some tumors (2).

Definition and Classification

The current clinical definition of obesity, as defined by expert committees, is based on body mass index (BMI), which is simply derived by dividing weight by height squared. A BMI of 30 kg/m^2 or more is diagnostic for obesity and a BMI greater than 25 kg/m^2 is diagnostic for overweight in adults (3). However, in children, this criteria

From: *Contemporary Diabetes: Obesity and Diabetes*
Edited by: C. S. Mantzoros © Humana Press Inc., Totowa, NJ

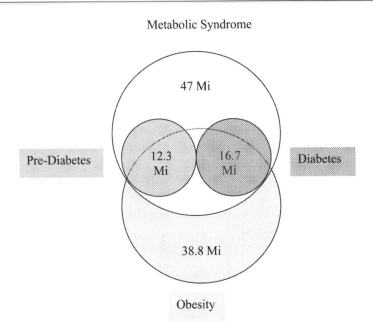

Fig. 1. Overlapping aspects of metabolic syndrome. By applying the prevalence estimates from NHANES III to the US population for the year 2000, it was found that approx 47 million (Mi) people in the United States had metabolic syndrome *(86)*, and 38.8 million American adults met the classification of obesity, defined as having a BMI ≥30 kg/m². According to NHANES III, an estimated 16.7 Mi persons age ≥20 yr had diagnosed and undiagnosed diabetes and 12.3 Mi persons age ≥20 yr had IFG (pre-diabetes) *(112)*.

cannot apply, because BMI must be adjusted for age and sex. Therefore, obesity in children is defined as a BMI greater than the 95th percentile for age and sex (Fig. 2) and/or as weight-for-height measurement greater than 120% of expected *(4)*. Criteria for defining obesity in pregnant women are currently not very clear, but guidelines of weight gain during pregnancy according to weight before pregnancy have been published *(5,6)* (Table 1). Pregnant obese women are at increased risk of pregnancy complications *(7)*, and, in addition, excessive weight gain during pregnancy is a risk factor for developing obesity later. For example, a Swedish study concluded that women who gain more than 16 kg (35 lb) during pregnancy have a higher risk of becoming overweight or obese later in life *(8)*.

There are several classification schemes for obesity (Table 2). According to the first criterion and the definition just mentioned, BMI is used not only to identify obesity classes, but also to assess the risk of morbidity and mortality. According to the second criterion, body fat distribution (i.e., android vs gynoid type of obesity) is also important, because increased central adiposity is associated with increased morbidity and mortality. Finally, a classification of obesity according to its etiology is also commonly used, as illustrated in Table 2.

Methods for Estimating Body Fat and Body Fat Distribution

IDEAL BODY WEIGHT

"Ideal body weight" (IBW) *(9)* corresponds to the weight associated with the lowest mortality rate *(10)*. According to insurance company calculations (Metropolitan Life

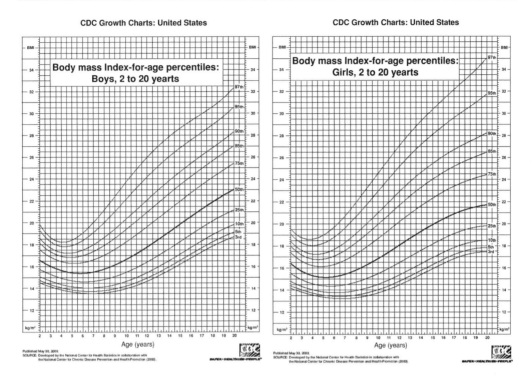

Fig. 2. Body mass index (BMI) for age and sex. The following percentile cutoff points have been established to identify overweight and obesity in children: overweight if BMI for age is ≥85th percentile to <95th percentile and obesity if BMI for age is ≥95th percentile. (CDC growth charts are available at www.cdc.gov/nchs/howto.htm.)

Table 1
Recommended Total Weight Gain in Pregnant Woman by
Prepregnancy BMI[a]

BMI (kg/m²)	Recommended total gain (kg)
<19.8	12.5–18
19.8–26.0	11.5–16
26.0–29.0	7–11.5
>29.0	≥6.0

[a]Adolescents and African-American women should strive for gains at the upper end of the recommended range. Short women (<1.57 cm) should strive for gains at the lower end of the range. (Adapted from refs. 5 and 6.)

tables available at www.metlife.com/Lifeadvice/Tools/Heightnweight), the highest life expectancy is achieved by maintaining weights at the level of the ideal Broca value minus 10% in males, and minus 15% in females.

IBW using the Broca method is calculated in kilograms by subtracting 100 from the subject's height in centimeters: Weight (in kg) = Height (in cm) – 100 ± 15% for women, and Weight (in kg) = (Height (in cm) – 100 ± 10% for men. This index has been criticized as being not specific enough and too simple. Men, short people, and older

Table 2
Classification of Obesity Using Different Criteria[a]

A. BMI (kg/m²)

BMI ranges	Classes	Health risk based on BMI	Health risk adjusted for presence of comorbid conditions
18–24.9	Normal	Minimal	Low
25.0–29.9	Overweight	Low	Moderate
30.0–34.9	Obesity class I	High	Very high
35.0–39.9	Obesity class II	Very high	Extremely high
40 or greater	Obesity class III	Extremely high	Extremely high

B. WC or W/H ratio

WC ≥ 102 cm (40 in.); W/H > 0.95 (males) WC ≥ 88 cm (35 in.); W/H > 0.85 (females)	Android/abdominal/apple-shaped obesity
WC < 102 cm (40 in.); W/H < 0.95 (males) WC < 88 cm (35 in.); W/H < 0.85 (females)	Gynoid/pelvic/pear-shaped obesity

C. Etiology

Simple obesity	Dietary
	Sedentary lifestyle
Endocrine	Cushing syndrome
	Hypothyroidism
	Insulinoma
	GH deficiency
Disorders involving the hypothalamus	Injuries, infections, tumors, infiltrative disorders
Genetic	Prader-Willi-Labhart syndrome
	Laurance-Moon-Bardet-Biedl syndrome
	Babinski-Frohlich syndrome
	Psedo-Frohlich syndrome
	Ahlstrom syndrome
	Carpenter syndrome
	Cohen syndrome
	Biemond syndrome
Drug induced	Antipsychotics
	Antidepressants
	Lithium
	Antiepileptics
	Insulin, sulfonylureas, thiazolidinediones
	Contraceptives
	Corticosteroids
	β- and α-blockers

[a]The risk of associated disease according to BMI was adapted from ref *113*.

people are evaluated too severely and women, tall people, and younger people too leniently, whereas the formula cannot be used for children at all. Another similar method commonly used to calculate the ideal weight of a patient (±10%) is by using

Table 3

**Summary of USPSTF Recommendations and Description of Classification
of USPSTF Recommendations[a]**

Grade	Summary of USPSTF recommendations
B	The USPSTF recommends that clinicians screen all adult patients for obesity and offer intensive counseling and behavioral interventions to promote sustained weight loss for obese adults.
I	The USPSTF concludes that the evidence is insufficient to recommend for or against the use of moderate- or low-intensity counseling together with behavioral interventions to promote sustained weight loss in obese adults.
I	The USPSTF concludes that the evidence is insufficient to recommend for or against the use of counseling of any intensity and behavioral interventions to promote sustained weight loss in overweight adults.

Grade	Classification of USPSTF recommendations
A	The USPSTF strongly recommends that clinicians routinely provide [the service][b] to eligible patients. The USPSTF found good evidence that [the service] improves important health outcomes and concludes that benefits substantially outweigh harms.
B	The USPSTF recommends that clinicians routinely provide [the service] to eligible patients. The USPSTF found at least fair evidence that [the service] improves important health outcomes and concludes that benefits outweigh harms.
C	The USPSTF makes no recommendation for or against routine provision of [the service]. The USPSTF found at least fair evidence that [the service] can improve health outcomes but concludes that the balance of benefits and harms is too close to justify a general recommendation.
D	The USPSTF recommmmends against routinely providing [the service] to asymptomatic patients. The USPSTF found at least fair evidence that [the service] is ineffective or that harms outweigh benefits.
I	The USPSTF concludes that the evidence is insufficient to recommend for or against routinely providing [the service]. Evidence that [the service] is effective is lacking, of poor quality, or conflicting and the balance of benefits and harms cannot be determined.

[a]Adapted from ref. *24.*

[b]In this case, [the service] refers to screening adults for obesity and providing counseling and behavioral interventions.

the Lorentz's formula: IBW = (Height in cm − 100) − (Height in cm − 150)/4 for men, and IBW = (Height in cm − 100) − (Height in cm − 150)/2.5 for women.

BODY MASS INDEX

BMI is currently the most commonly used method internationally to express weight in relation to body height for clinical purposes. It is calculated using the following formula: Body weight (kg) divided by body height squared (m) = kg/m^2 or BMI = weight $(kg)/height^2$ (m) or BMI = weight (lb) × 704/height squared (in.).

Tables for the calculation of BMI (*see* Table 3 in Chapter 26) and special nomograms that help in calculating BMI are also available (Fig. 3). In adults age 18 yr and older, BMI should range between 18.5 and 25 kg/m^2. BMI is used differently in children

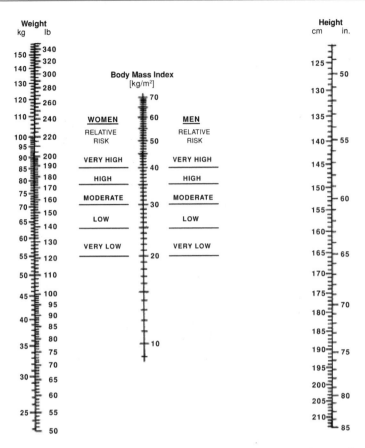

Fig. 3. Nomogram for determining BMI. To use this nomogram, place a ruler or other straight edge between the body weight (without clothes) in kilograms or pounds located on the left-hand line and the height (without shoes) in centimeters or inches located on the right-hand line. BMI is read from the middle of the scale and is in metric units. (Copyright 1978, George A. Bray, MD. Used with permission.)

than in adults. Because children's body fatness changes over the years as they grow, BMI is age, gender, and ethnicity specific in children *(11,12)*. This is why BMI for children is also referred to as BMI for age. Reference data for BMI in children have been published *(13–15),* and percentile cutoff points have been established to identify overweight and obesity in children (Fig. 2).

BMI is only an indirect correlation of the amount of body fat but, at the same time, the easiest and most practical one. Its drawbacks are that it can overestimate fat in muscular or athletic individuals and that it can underestimate fat in individuals who have lost body muscle, such as in the elderly and sedentary people.

The current practical use of BMI as an index of obesity is based on the observed associations between increasing BMI and health risks including mortality, rather than association between BMI and body composition *per se.* More specifically, large-scale epidemiological studies have established that there is a strong association between BMI and mortality *(16,17),* which is continuous and curvilinear *(18).* These curves became steeper at a cutoff value of approx 30, and this is why this BMI value is recognized internationally as a threshold for obesity in both men and women, while severe obesity is defined as a BMI greater than 40 kg/m^2. *Overweight* is a term used for individuals having a BMI between 25 and 29.9 kg/m^2. Adjusted BMI for fat distribution and other comorbid conditions (see Table 5 in Chapter 26) is a newer and probably better tool to estimate the risk of morbidity and mortality. A clinical association of comorbidities and a BMI over certain threshold values increases health risk to the next level (Table 2) (2,3).

WAIST CIRCUMFERENCE AND WAIST-TO-HIP RATIO

Waist circumference (WC) has become the most widely used measure of regional fat distribution and has largely replaced the waist-to-hip (W/H) circumference ratio because it is much easier to measure. WC is measured at the midpoint between the lower border of the rib cage and the upper border of the pelvis. A WC >102 cm (40 in.) and a W/H ratio >0.95 in men or a WC >88 cm (35 in.) and a W/H ratio >0.85 in women indicates android, central, or abdominal type of obesity, which provides a substantially increased risk of metabolic complications and other comorbidities over that of the gynoid or peripheral type (see Diagnosing IRS) (19).

SKINFOLD THICKNESS

Anthropometry and growth measurements are the most important components of the nutritional assessment in children. The triceps skinfold thickness reflects body fat and is widely used in pediatrics because it is very easy to perform. However, it is less accurate than the measurement of height and weight, and it under/overestimates body fat mass by as much as 10% (20).

OTHER APPROACHES/TECHNIQUES

If the objective is to measure fat mass directly, several methods, including densitometry, magnetic resonance imaging, computed tomography, dual energy X-ray absorptiometry, ultrasounds, and electrical impedance, can be used (21). Because of the costs and time limitations associated with their performance, these techniques are reserved only for research purposes.

Evaluation: Clinical and Laboratory

Information from the past history regarding age at onset and duration of obesity; weight gain since age 18; pregnancy history, including weight gain during pregnancy; and use of medications that could lead to and cause obesity (e.g., glucocorticoids, insulin; see Table 2) is important to obtain.

At initial clinical examination, the following data should be collected: weight, height, BMI, WC, hip circumference, W/H ratio, blood pressure (BP). Physical examination can also reveal acanthosis nigricans, which infers insulin resistance; cushingoid features; signs of hypothyroidism; growth hormone (GH) deficiency or hypogonadism; hirsutism and/or amenorrhea (suggestive of polycystic ovary syndrome [PCOS]); and other signs of potential diseases states that are to be ruled out. The work-up of an obese patient must also include serum lipid measurements; fasting plasma glucose (FPG) (and oral glucose tolerance test [OGTT] if necessary); plasma uric acid; thyroid-stimulating hormone and cortisol or other hormone measurements when the clinical condition is highly suggestive; sleep apnea studies in morbid obesity, as needed.

Evaluation of obesity class and type based on BMI, WC, and W/H ratio is the next step. Bray and colleagues (22,23) recommend that BMI be calculated and then adjusted for fat distribution and other comorbidities (e.g., dyslipidemia or hypertension) because the adjusted BMI appears to be a better index to evaluate a patient's risk of morbidity and mortality and can be used to guide treatment as well (see Tables 5 and 6 in Chapter 26).

Screening

The US Preventive Services Task Force (USPSTF) recommends that clinicians screen all adult patients for obesity and subsequently provide counseling and behavioral interventions in order to promote sustained weight loss for obese adults. This is stated as a grade B recommendation (Table 3) (24,25). BMI is the simplest and most practical method to screen for obesity, and, thus, according to USPSTF, it is also a reliable tool for risk assesment owing to overweight and obesity. It is highly reliable, and with the aforementioned caveats correlates well with an individual's percentage of body fat and subsequent risk of morbidity and mortality (26,27). Despite lack of direct evidence that behavioral interventions (diet, exercise, weight reduction) lower mortality or morbidity from obesity (see Chapter 26), weight reduction of 5–7% body weight reduces insulin resistance and BP and improves dyslipidemia and glucose metabolism (28). These changes provide indirect evidence for health benefits as concluded by USPSTF. In morbid obesity however, accumulating evidence, as revealed by a recent meta-analysis, suggests that effective weight loss after surgical treatment (bariatric surgery) has been proven to decrease obesity-induced morbidity. In this study a substantial majority of patients with diabetes, hyperlipidemia, hypertension, and obstructive sleep apnea experienced complete resolution or improvement. Diabetes was completely resolved in 76.8% of patients and resolved or improved in 86%. Hyperlipidemia was improved in 70% or more of patients. Hypertension was resolved in 61.7% of patients and resolved or improved in 78.5%. Obstructive sleep apnea was resolved in 85.7% of patients and was resolved or improved in 83.6% of patients (29).

DIAGNOSING AND SCREENING FOR DIABETES MELLITUS

Diabetes mellitus is a heterogeneous and multifactorial disorder with serious health consequences. Currently, an estimated 18 million persons in the United States and more than 150 million globally have diabetes. Because the recommendations for the classification, diagnosis, and screening of diabetes are revised every few years, reflecting new information from research and clinical practice, the goal of this part of the chapter is to discuss the available diagnostic tests and to present the current diagnostic criteria for diabetes mellitus. Screening procedures for type 2 diabetes mellitus are necessary because of the well-known association of diabetes with increased morbidity and mortality from acute and chronic complications and because as many as 50% of the diabetic population remain undiagnosed, at any given time.

Introduction

Diabetes mellitus is a metabolic disorder characterized by abnormal carbohydrate, fat, and protein metabolism, which is clinically diagnosed on the basis of hyperglycemia. The chronic hyperglycemia of diabetes is associated with long-term complications in the eyes, kidneys, nerves, and blood vessels. Depending on the etiology of diabetes mellitus, factors contributing to hyperglycemia may include reduced insulin secretion and/or insulin resistance (IR) (30).

Table 4
Etiological Classification of Diabetes Mellitus[a]

I. Type 1 diabetes
    A. Type 1A autoimmune and LADA
    B. Type 1B idiopathic
II. Type 2 diabetes
III. Other specific types of diabetes
    A. Genetic defects of β-cell function
    B. Genetic defects in insulin action
    C. Diseases of the exocrine pancreas
    D. Endocrinopathies: acromegaly, Cushing syndrome, glucagonoma, pheochromocytoma, hyperthyroidism, somatostatinoma, aldosteronoma
    E. Drug or chemical induced
    F. Infections: congenital rubella, cytomegalovirus, coxsackie
    G. Uncommon forms of immune-mediated diabetes: "stiff-man" syndrome, anti-insulin receptor antibodies
    H. Other genetic syndromes sometimes associated with diabetes: Down syndrome, Klinefelter syndrome, Turner syndrome, Wolfram syndrome, Friedreich ataxia, Huntington chorea, Laurence-Moon-Biedl syndrome, myotonic dystrophy, porphyria, Prader-Willi syndrome
IV. GDM

[a]Adapted from ref. *31*.

Terminology and Classification

Terms such as *insulin-dependent, noninsulin-dependent, juvenile- maturity-onset, and maturity-onset diabetes of the young* are not used in recent classifications and are to be eliminated *(31,32)*. The terms type 1 and type 2 diabetes, reflecting etiological differences, are recommended to be used instead of descriptions based on age at onset or treatment modality *(33)*. The category in between normality and diabetes (prediabetes or latent diabetes) is now called either impaired fasting glucose (IFG) or impaired glucose tolerance (IGT), depending on whether the plasma glucose was measured in the fasting state or after a standard OGTT *(34)*.

ETIOLOGICAL CLASSIFICATION

Based on etiology, diabetes is classified as follows:

- Type 1 diabetes results from absolute insulin deficiency. Type 1 diabetes is divided into two subtypes. Type 1A results from autoimmune destruction of pancreatic β-cells, which can be documented by the presence of autoantibodies (anti-islet cell autoantibodies, autoantibodies to glutamic acid decarboxylase (GAD), anti-insulin autoantibodies, and autoantibodies to the tyrosine phosphatases). The adult form of type 1 diabetes is known as latent autoimmune diabetes of the adult (LADA). Type 1B diabetes is also called idiopathic diabetes and is a subtype for which there is no evidence of autoimmunity, or other causes of β-cell destruction *(35)*.
- Type 2 diabetes, the most common type of diabetes, is usually associated with obesity and IR. Usually, these patients have only relative insulin deficiency and, at least initially, they do not need insulin treatment to survive.
- Other specific types of diabetes are provided in Table 4.
- Gestational diabetes mellitus (GDM) is classified as a separate entity.

Diagnostic Tests/Tests of Glycemia

RANDOM PLASMA GLUCOSE

Random, or "casual," plasma glucose measurement is inexpensive and easily accomplished but not always diagnostic. In the absence of unequivocal hyperglycemia or metabolic decompensation, a patient with a random plasma glucose level of 200 mg/dL (11.1 mmol/L) or higher should have a second confirmatory test for the diagnosis of diabetes to be established.

FASTING PLASMA GLUCOSE

FPG requires an overnight fast of at least 8 h. It is inexpensive and risk free and, thus, is the test of choice. The results of FPG are more reproducible over a short term than those of OGTT. Studies that have compared the two tests found coefficients of variation (CVs) almost two times higher in OGTT than in FPG *(36–38)*.

ORAL GLUCOSE TOLERANCE TEST

In compliance with the most recent American Diabetes Association (ADA) recommendations, OGTT is not indicated for routine use with the exception of pregnancy. One reason is the reduced overall test–retest reproducibility (some studies report only 65.6% reproducibility) *(39)*. In addition, FPG is easier to perform and more cost-effective. However, renewed emphasis of the importance of the postprandial hyperglycemia (PPG) and OGTT has been given with the recently published results of the Diabetes Prevention Program *(28)*, in which diet/exercise, as well as drug therapy (metformin and troglitazone), was shown to slow/prevent the progression of IGT to overt diabetes mellitus. It has thus been proposed that performing an OGTT could be considered in selected individuals (e.g., obese patients, or patients who share the features of metabolic syndrome) in order to identify diabetes or any degree of glucose intolerance at an early stage *(40)*.

A minimum of 150–200 g of carbohydrates/d should be included in the diet for at least 3 d preceding an OGTT in order to optimize insulin secretion. After an overnight fast, adults are given a glucose load of 75 g in 300 mL of water to be consumed within 5 min. Children are given 1.75 g of glucose/kg of ideal body weight. Recently, the test has been simplified and requires only an overnight fasting measurement (0 min) and one at 2 h (120 min) after ingestion of glucose. Samples at 30, 60, and 90 min are no longer required. Insulin levels can also be measured during the OGTT but are rarely of clinical usefulness and, thus, are reserved only for research purposes *(41)*.

Interpretation of the OGTT in nonpregnant adults (Table 5) differs from that of the OGTT in pregnancy (*see* Diagnosis of Gestational Diabetes). False-positive results may occur in severe debilitating conditions (infections, emotional stress, or in malnourished patients) and with certain drugs (diuretics, oral contraceptives, glucocorticoids, excess thyroxin, phenytoin, nicotinic acid) *(41)*.

INTRAVENOUS GLUCOSE TOLERANCE TEST

The intravenous glucose tolerance test (IVGTT) is an important dynamic test used to evaluate residual β-cell function in patients with type 1 diabetes mellitus *(42)*. It is also useful in the screening of siblings of patients with type 1 diabetes or in the evaluation of glucose tolerance in patients with malabsorbtion. However, caution must be exercised in the clinical interpretation of the results because the IVGTT bypasses normal physiology of glucose absorption *(41)*.

Table 5

Diagnostic Thresholds for Diabetes and Impaired Glucose Regulation[a]

	Test	
Category	FPG	2-h Plasma glucose
Normal	<100 mg/dL or <5.6 mmol/L[c]	<140 mg/dL or <7.8 mmol/L
IFG	100–125 mg/dL or 5.6–6.9 mmol/L	—
IGT	—	140–199 mg/dL or 7.8–11.0 mmol/L
Diabetes[b]	≥126 mg/dL or ≥7.0 mmol/L	≥200 mg/dL or ≥11.1 mmol/L

[a]Adapted from ref. 32.

[b]An FPG at or >126 is diagnostic of diabetes if confirmed in a subsequent day to be in the same diabetic range.

[c]To convert glucose level from nmol/L into mg/dL multiply by 18 or divide by 0.05551.

GLYCOSYLATED HEMOGLOBIN (HbA1c)

HbA1c, or glycated hemoglobin, glycohemoglobin, or glycosylated hemoglobin, is a term used to describe a series of stable minor hemoglobin components formed nonenzymatically from hemoglobin and glucose. The level of HbA1c in a blood sample provides a glycemic history of the previous 120 d, the average erythrocyte life span. The optimal use of HbA1c testing requires standardization of HbA1c assays. The National Glycohemoglobin Standardization Program has established standard assays for HbA1c based on the results of the Diabetes Control and Complications Trial (DCCT) (43,44).

Advantages of the test are very good reproducibility; low intraindividual CV (45,46); and very good correlation with FPG, PPG, and 2-h plasma glucose levels. HbA1c level is also a very good predictor of diabetes-specific complications (47,48) and thus provides the current basis for treatment decision in patients with diabetes (49).

Disadvantages of the test are a lack of standardization of HbgA1c assays; lack of correlation between FPG and HbA1c level (50); and limited sensitivity for very mildly elevated levels of glycemia, particularly PPG (51). The test cannot be used in situations in which erythrocyte survival is decreased (anemia or hemoglobinopathies) (52,53) and is subject to interference in the presence of associated comorbidities (alcoholism, renal failure, opiate addiction, lead poisoning, excessive use of salicylates) (54).

Some investigators have suggested that HbA1c may be a suitable screening test for diabetes (55–60), but this has not yet been translated into clinical practice, because it remains a controversial issue (45,61,62). For example, Davidson et al. (60) suggested that in patients with an FPG between 110 and 139 mg/dL, the next step should be to measure HbA1c instead of a second FPG measurement. Barr et al. (59) recommended an alternative strategy for the diagnosis of type 2 diabetes. First, casual plasma glucose is measured, and if this is ≥200 and the HbA1c is >2 standard deviations (SDs) above the mean, then diabetes is diagnosed and should be managed according to the HbA1c level. If the result of only one of these two tests is positive, an FPG should be tested to evaluate the patient for impaired fasting glucose (IFG) (refer to Table 5 or "Diagnostic Criteria") and diabetes (59). Rohlfing et al. (57) proposed that an HbA1c cutoff value of 6.1% (2 SDs above the normal mean) could identify individuals with undiagnosed diabetes who are at risk of diabetes complications. At this cutoff value, the sensitivity is 63.2% and the specificity is 97.4%, but these cutoff points may vary according to the race and/or ethnic group of the patient.

The ADA currently recommends the measurement of HbA1c only for the monitoring of glycemic control in patients with known diabetes and for documentation of the degree of glycemic control at initial assessment but not for routine screening of diabetes (31,43). The importance of HbA1c as an index of diabetes control has been reinforced by the DCCT (44) and the United Kingdom Prospective Diabetes Study (63). These studies demonstrated a direct correlation between glycemic control as assessed by HbA1c and the likelihood of developing long-term diabetes-related complications.

GLYCOSYLATED SERUM PROTEINS

The degree of glycation of serum proteins (mostly albumin and fructosamine) provides an index of glycemic status over the preceding 1 to 2 wk (the half-life of albumin is 14–20 d). This test is useful especially in a situation in which HbA1c assay is subject to interference and also in order to document relatively short-term changes in glycemic status, such as in diabetic pregnancy or after major changes in therapy (43).

Diagnostic Criteria and Screening for Diabetes Mellitus

In a 2003 ADA report, the thresholds (Table 5) of PFG were decreased and subsequently the following definitions have been changed (32):

- **Normal:** FPG < 100 mg/dL (5.6 mmol/L).
- **IFG:** FPG between 100 and 125 mg/dL (5.6–6.9 mmol/L) rather than between 110 and 125 mg/dL (6.1–6.9 mmol/L).
- **IGT:** 2-h plasma glucose after a standard OGTT between 140–199 mg/dL (7.8–11.1 mmol/L).
- **Diabetes mellitus** (criteria unchanged):
  1. Symptoms of diabetes (polyuria, polydipsia, weight loss, visual blurring) plus a random (any time of day, regardless of time interval since last meal) plasma glucose concentration ≥200 mg/dL (11.1 mmol/L).
  2. FPG ≥ 126 mg/dL (7.0 mmol/L) after an overnight fast of at least 8 h.
  3. Two-hour plasma glucose ≥200 mg/dL (11.1 mmol/L) during a standard 75-mg OGTT.

The diagnosis of diabetes can be based on any of these criteria but should be confirmed by repeat testing on a different day. The ADA diagnostic criteria strongly suggest that the diagnosis of diabetes should be made mainly on the basis of fasting glucose and, thus, do not recommend OGTT for routine use (31). The World Health Organization (WHO) agrees with the new definitions but considers continued use of the OGTT for patients with IFG (blood glucose values between 100 and 125 mg/dL or 5.6 and 6.9 mmol/L) to exclude the presence of diabetes (32,64).

The use of HbA1c for the diagnosis of diabetes is not recommended at this time because in addition to the reasons mentioned, there is no "gold standard" assay and many countries do not have ready access to the test (31).

Importantly, the cutoff value for FPG for diagnosing diabetes was lowered to 126 mg/dL (7.0 mmol/L), and a new diagnostic category, IFG, has been added to IGT in the 1997 ADA report (50). This was done to emphasize the increased risk of CVD and diabetes in these categories (IFG and/or IGT), which are also referred to as "prediabetes." Such patients are usually obese (having especially android obesity) and share the features of metabolic syndrome (which includes abdominal obesity, IR with IFG and/or IGT, dyslipidemia, and hypertension). Although both IFG and IGT are predictors of cardiovascular risk, observational studies (DECODE study *[65]*, Framingham Offspring Study *[66]*) have reported that IGT is a better predictor than IFG and is strongly associated with cardiovascular morbidity and mortality.

SCREENING FOR TYPE 2 DIABETES

Widespread use of FPG as a screening test (Fig. 4) is recommended because undiagnosed type 2 diabetes is very common (up to 50% of the affected people) *(67)* with an estimated lag of 5–7 yr between onset and diagnosis *(68)*. A large number of individuals who meet the criteria are unaware and asymptomatic, and as many as 50% of individuals with type 2 diabetes have one or more diabetes-specific complications at the time of diagnosis. Although FPG is the recommended screening test, OGTT may be necessary for the diagnosis of diabetes when FPG is normal. The ADA recommends screening all individuals >45 yr of age (American College of Endocrinology and American Association of Clinical Endocrinologists over 30 yr) every 3 yr and screening high-risk subjects at an earlier age. The major risk factors for type 2 diabetes are, according to the ADA *(69)*, having a family history of diabetes, being overweight as defined as a BMI ≥25 kg/m^2, being habitually physically inactive and belonging to a high-risk ethnic or racial group (e.g., Native Americans, African Americans, or Hispanics). Screening should also be considered in persons with previously identified IFG or IGT, hypertension, dyslipidemia, PCOS, history of GDM, or delivery of a baby weighing >4.1 kg (9 lb). A screening protocol is illustrated in Fig. 4.

SCREENING FOR TYPE 1 DIABETES

A series of autoantibodies have been identified that are predictive of development of type 1 diabetes. The most important ones are anti-islet cell autoantibodies, autoantibodies to GAD, anti-insulin autoantibodies, and autoantibodies to the amino acid residues of the intracellular domain on the protein IA-2 (ICA512/IA-2) *(70)*. Some studies proved that there is a significant increase in the risk of developing diabetes if an increased number of autoantibodies are present. The 5-yr risk of an individual with a first-degree relative with type 1 diabetes would be 68% if two antibodies are present and almost 100% if three are present *(71)*. However, because there is no potential treatment to slow or prevent the progression of the disease, using autoantibodies as a screening tool is not yet justified *(70)*.

Diagnostic Criteria and Screening for GDM

GDM is defined as any degree of glucose intolerance first recognized during pregnancy. The definition applies regardless of therapy or whether the condition persists after pregnancy. Gestational diabetes complicates about 4% of all pregnancies. Early diagnosis is very important in order to reduce perinatal morbidity and mortality *(35)*. In most women who develop GDM, onset of the disorder occurs in the third trimester of pregnancy *(31)*. At least 6 wk after pregnancy ends, women who have had GDM should receive an OGTT to be reclassified as having diabetes, normal glucose tolerance, IGT, or IFG *(72)*.

Risk assessment and testing for GDM should be undertaken at the first prenatal visit, but consideration of a woman's clinical characteristics allows more efficient and selective screening for gestational diabetes *(73)*. Women at high risk (*see* Table 6)

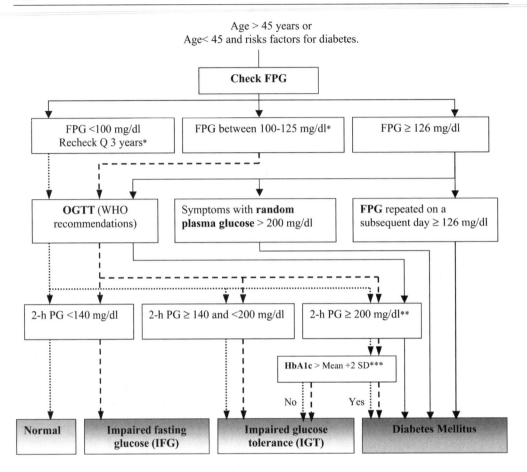

Fig. 4. Screening protocol for type 2 diabetes. *If the clinical suspicion is still very high, some investigators recommend performing an OGTT. In the Strong Heart Study in American Indians *(40)*, 4.7–6.9% of patients with normal FPG received a diagnosis of diabetes after OGTT. **Two values of 2-h plasma glucose (PG) need to be >200 mg/dL for diabetes to be diagnosed in healthy and IFG groups. ***In general, HbA1c is not recommended as a screening test (*see* text). Consider HbA1c in special populations (e.g., American Indians) and other situations in which FPG is <126 mg/dL but 2-h PG is ≥200 mg/dL. In these situations, HbA1c could be a potential tool, which could help diagnose diabetes. In The Strong Heart Study in American Indians *(40)*, 20% of those with IFG had diabetes after OGTT criteria.

should be screened as soon as feasible. If the initial screening is negative, they should undergo retesting at 24–28 wk. Women of average risk should have the initial screen performed at 24–28 wk. Women at low risk need not be screened for GDM in compliance with ADA *(31)* and American College of Obstetricians and Gynecologist guidelines (ACOG) *(74)*, although some clinicians still recommend universal screening *(75–77)*.

A FPG >126 mg/dL (7.0 mmol/L) or a casual glucose >200 mg/dL (11.1 mmol/L) establishes the diagnosis of diabetes if confirmed on a subsequent day and obviates the need for more glucose tolerance testing.

Women who require more formal testing should receive a 100-g oral glucose load with plasma glucose levels determined at baseline, 1 h, 2 h, and 3 h (Table 7), and the diagnosis of GDM is made if two or more of the plasma glucose values are equal to or higher than those listed in Table 5. This one-step approach may be cost-effective in high-risk patients *(31)*. A different approach recommended by ACOG is a two-step approach.

Table 6
Risk Assessment and Testing for GDM[a]

Group	Characteristics	Test
Low-risk group (all characteristics should be present)	• Age <25 yr • A normal body weight before pregnancy (BMI < 25 kg/m^2) • No family history • No history of abnormal glucose metabolism • No history of poor obstetric outcome • Not a member of an ethnic/racial group with a high prevalence of diabetes[b]	No screening test necessary
Average-risk group	• Age 25–45 yr • BMI 25–27 kg/m^2 before pregnancy • None of the conditions listed below	GCT (50 g glucose)[c]
High-risk group	• Age > 45 yr • A family history of diabetes, especially in first-degree relatives • A prepregnancy weight of ≥110% of ideal body weight or BMI > 27 kg/m^2 • A previously large baby, >4.1 kg (9 lb) • A history of abnormal glucose tolerance (IFG, IGT, or diabetes) • A member of an ethnic group with a higher than normal rate of type 2 diabetes • A previously unexplained perinatal loss or birth of a malformed child • A mother who was large at birth (>4.1 kg [9 lb]) • Maternal low birth weight (<2.7 kg [6 lb]) • Hypertension • Dyslipidemia • PCOS	Diagnostic OGTT (100 g glucose)[d]

[a]From refs. 31,35,73,74, and 76.
[b]Hispanic American, Native American, Asian, African American, Pacific Islander.
[c]Two-step approach: (1) perform an initial GCT (glucose challenge test) and (2) perform a diagnostic OGTT on that subset of women exceeding the glucose threshold value on the GCT.
[d]One-step approach may be cost-effective, by performing directly a diagnostic OGTT in high-risk patients or population (some Native American groups).

Table 7
Diagnosis of GDM With a 100-g Glucose Load[a]

Time	Plasma glucose	
	mg/dL	mmol/L
Fasting	≥95	≥5.3
1 h	≥180	≥10.0
2 h	≥155	≥8.6
3 h	≥140	≥7.8

[a]Two or more values must be met or exceeded for a diagnosis of diabetes to be made. The test should be done in the morning after an 8- to 14-h fast and after at least 3 d of unrestricted diet (≥150 g of carbohydrate/d). (Adapted from ref. 31, derived from the original work of O'Sullivan and Mahan, modified by Carpenter and Coustan.)

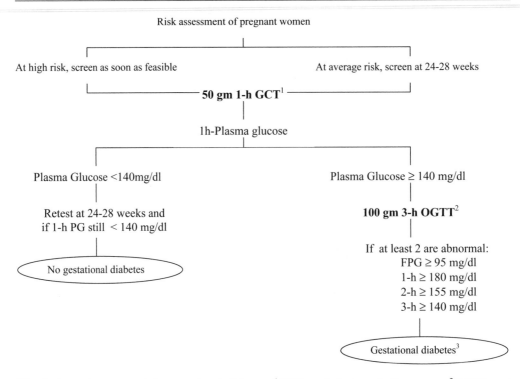

Fig. 5. Screening protocol for gestational diabetes. [1]GCT, oral glucose challenge test. [2]OGTT, oral glucose tolerance test. [3]At least 6 wk after the pregnancy ends, women who have had GDM should receive an OGTT and be reclassified as having diabetes, normal glucose tolerance, IGT, or IFG on the basis of the diagnostic criteria listed in Table 5. (Adapted from ref. *76*.)

After an initial 50-g oral glucose challenge test (GCT), the subset of women exceeding the glucose threshold of 140 mg/dL (7.8 mmol/L) will have a diagnostic 100-g OGTT *(74)*. Figure 5 illustrates screening protocol for gestational diabetes.

DIAGNOSING INSULIN RESISTANCE SYNDROME

This last part of the chapter focuses on IR, its clinical implications (metabolic syndrome), and the importance of recognizing IR as a risk factor of increasing importance for CVDs and type 2 diabetes. Clinical and biochemical definitions of IRS and IR are reviewed.

Introduction

The IRS (metabolic syndrome) has become a major health problem not only because of its high prevalence, but also because of the risks associated with this syndrome. Obesity, diabetes, hypertension, dyslipidemia, and accelerated atherosclerosis together contribute to increased morbidity and mortality. Obesity, and especially central obesity, is the main condition that predisposes to IR, while IR is the core metabolic abnormality underlying type 2 diabetes mellitus *(78)* (Fig. 1).

Definition

IR is a state of decreased sensitivity of tissues to insulin. To control circulating glucose level and maintain normal glucose metabolism, insulin secretion is increased (hyperinsulinemia). However, in the long term, in states of insulin resistance, circulating insulin concentrations cannot adequately promote peripheral glucose disposal, suppress hepatic glucose production, and inhibit very low-density lipoprotein output *(79)*.

The terms *insulin resistance syndrome, metabolic syndrome ("X"), Reaven's syndrome (80), and "dysmetabolic" syndrome* describe a cluster of related abnormalities associated with a state of IR and subsequent compensatory hyperinsulinemia. Considering the underlying pathophysiology, the most recent position statement of the American College of Endocrinology (ACE) suggests that *insulin resistance syndrome* is the term to be used *(81)*, and, thus, this is the term used herein.

The abnormalities included in the definition of IRS (*see* Table 8) are a group of disease states/risk factors that increase a subject's chance of developing CVD, type 2 diabetes, accelerated atherosclerosis, hypertension, stroke, or PCOS. Thus, CHAOS (Coronary artery disease, Hypertension, Atherosclerosis, Obesity, and Stroke) is an acronym coined for the IRS that describes the coexistence of these disorders in this syndrome.

Link Among Obesity, Type 2 Diabetes, and IRS

Not all obese individuals have IRS. So-called metabolically healthy, but obese individuals have normal insulin sensitivity, despite having a large amount of fat mass, possibly owing to low visceral fat *(82)*. Android/abdominal/visceral obesity has been clearly associated with insulin resistance and serves as a marker for developing the metabolic complications of obesity *(83)*.

IRS does not affect only those with frank obesity; it has also been reported in persons of normal weight *(84)*, but an increased amount of visceral fat or body-fat redistribution and lipodystrophic changes, such as those observed in the human immunodeficiency virus-associated metabolic syndrome or other types of genetic or acquired lipodystrophy.

IRS is usually considered an intermediate state between normality and diabetes, but although the majority of insulin-resistant subjects may not develop diabetes, they remain at increased risk of developing other clinical consequences of insulin resistance/compensatory hyperinsulinemia *(80,81)*.

Epidemiology

According to the third National Health and Nutrition Examination Survey (NHANES III) *(86,87)*, the overall prevalence of IRS increases with age (>40 yr), body weight (BMI > 25 kg/m^2), postmenopausal status, smoking, high-carbohydrate diet, no alcohol or excessive alcohol consumption, and physical inactivity. Non-Caucasian ethnicity; a family history of type 2 diabetes or IRS; high blood pressure (BP); CVD *(87)*; or a personal history of CVD, PCOS, GDM, and acanthosis nigricans increase the likelihood of developing IRS.

The prevalence of the disorder in the US population is very high (calculated up to 25% of the population). A recent epidemiological study showed that the age-adjusted prevalence in the United States is 23.9% (men: 24.2%; women: 23.5%) and likely increasing among US adults, using the National Cholesterol Education Program/the Adult Treatment Panel III (NCEP/ATP III) definition *(88)*. According to the ACE position statement on IRS, one in three or four US adults has IRS and 90% of patients with diabetes are insulin resistant and 10% of women have PCOS.

Diagnostic Criteria

CLINICAL CRITERIA

According to the NCEP/ATP III report *(89)* and the 2004 report from the National Heart, Lung, and Blood Institute and American Heart Association *(90)*, a diagnosis of metabolic syndrome can be made if a person has three or more of the following five features:

1. Android/abdominal obesity defined as increased WC ≥102 cm (40 in.) in men and ≥88 cm (35 in.) in women and a BMI ≥30 kg/m^2.
2. Elevated triglycerides (≥150 mg/dL or 1.7 mmol/L).
3. Decreased high-density lipprotein (HDL) cholesterol (<40 mg/dL for men, <50 mg/dL for women).
4. Blood pressure >130/85 mmHg or active treatment for hypertension.
5. Fasting glucose levels >100 mg/dL (5.6 mmol/L) and/or 2-h plasma glucose (PG) between 140 and 200 mg/dL (7.8–11.0 mmol/L) after a 75-g OGTT.

The following should also be noted when interpreting these criteria. Some genetically susceptible individuals may develop IRS only at slightly increased WC (between 94 and 102 cm [37–40 in.]) *(89)*. When the (W/H) ratio is used, android obesity is defined as a W/H ratio >0.95 in men, and >0.85 in women. The ACE has concluded, in a recent position statement, that BMI >30, rather than WC, is an appropriate index for obesity and an adequate estimate of IR. FPG levels are in compliance with the new 2003 ADA criteria for defining IFG *(32)*. In NCEP and ATP III criteria, FPG levels were >110 mg/dL, set as the former definition of IFG. However, although FPG is currently a good tool to diagnose diabetes, the 2-h PG after OGTT is a more sensitive measure/index of risk for IRS *(81,91)*.

The 1998 WHO criteria for diagnosis of IRS require hyperinsulinemia or FPG > 110 mg/dL or glucose intolerance (120-min postload glucose level between 140 and 200 mg/dL) plus the presence of at least two additional conditions (abdominal obesity, dyslipidemia, or high blood pressure) *(64)*.

Biochemical Definition and Methods for Assessing IR

Although the diagnosis of IRS should be based mainly on clinical grounds, as suggested by ACE and ATP III, it can be additionally confirmed or quantified by directly assessing insulin resistance. Insulin resistance can be estimated by several methods (Table 8), all based on the relationship between glucose and insulin measurements. However, use of these methods is not recommended as a routine clinical tool, because of lack of standardization and lack of clinical evidence that hyperinsulinemia *per se* can predict development of CVD.

The "gold standard" for assessing IR remains the euglycemic hyperinsulinemic clamp *(92)*. It involves raising the plasma insulin concentration and maintaining it at a fixed level, approx 100 μUI/mL, by a continuous iv insulin infusion. The plasma glucose concentration is held constant (clamped) at basal levels by a glucose infusion *(93)*. Because endogenous hepatic glucose production is inhibited by the high insulin concentration, the quantity of glucose infused per unit of time (milligrams/minute) to maintain euglycemia reflects the amount of glucose metabolized in the peripheral tissue (*M* value measured in milligrams/[kilogram/minute]) and is therefore an indirect index of sensitivity of target tissues to insulin. The higher the *M* value, the more sensitive the individual is to insulin. Conversely, the insulin-resistant patient requires less glucose to maintain basal plasma glucose level. Another index is insulin sensitivity (ISI), defined as the ratio of *M/I*, in which *M* is the rate of glucose infusion at steady state (i.e., when glucose infusion rate is stabilized) and *I* is the mean insulin level during the test (usually at time points between 15 and 120 min) *(78)*. However, because this technique is invasive, difficult to perform in a clinical setting, and time-consuming, its use is limited to research laboratories.

The second best technique for estimating insulin sensitivity is the frequently sampled iv glucose tolerance test (FSIVGTT). This technique requires determination of

Table 8
Methods for Measuring Insulin Resistance[a]

Index	Formula	Reported level
Insulin fasting level	N/A	<15 μUI/mL[b]
Insulin peak level during OGTT	N/A	<150 μUI/mL[b]
2-h Insulin level post-OGTT	N/A	<75 μUI/mL[b]
HOMA-IR	Fasting glucose (mmol/L) × Fasting insulin (μUI/mL)/22.5	2.1–2.7[b]
QUICKI	$1/[\log(\text{Ins } 0) + \log(\text{Glu } 0)]$	Mean value: 0.382 in lean subjects
Cederholm and Wibell (SI)	$[75{,}000 + (\text{Glu } 0 - \text{Glu } 2\text{ h}) \times 1.15 \times 180 \times 0.19 \times \text{BW}]/[120 \times \log(\text{mean Ins}) \times \text{mean Glu}]$	79 ± 14
Belfiore (ISI)	$2/[(\text{AUC insulin} \times \text{AUC glucose}) + 1]$	Over or about 1.0
Gutt ($\text{ISI}_{0,120}$)	$[75{,}000 + (\text{Glu } 0 - \text{Glu } 2\text{ h}) \times 0.19 \times \text{BW}]/[120 \times \log(\text{insulin } 0/2 + \text{insulin } 2\text{ h}/2) \times (\text{Glu } 0/2 + \text{Glu } 2\text{ h}/2]$	89 ± 39 lean controls 58 ± 23 obese controls
Matsuda (ISI composite)	$10{,}000/\sqrt{(\text{Ins } 0 \times \text{Glu } 0 \times \text{mean insulin} \times \text{mean glucose during OGTT})}$	—
Stumvoll (ISI)	$0.22 - 0.0032 \times \text{BMI} - 0.0000645 \times \text{Ins } 2\text{ h} - 0.0037 \times \text{Glu } 1.5\text{ h}$	—
Avignon (Si2h and SiM)	$\text{Si2h} = 10^{8}/(\text{Ins } 2\text{ h} \times \text{Glu } 2\text{ h} \times 150)$ $\text{SiM} = [0.137 \times 10^{8}/(\text{Ins } 0 \times \text{Glu } 0 \times 150) + \text{Si2h}]/2$	1.79 ± 0.33 1.71 ± 0.24
ITT	$K_{ITT} = 0.693/\text{plasma glucose}$ half time × 100	>2%/min
FSIVGTT insulin sensitivity (Si)	Si = glucose clearance rate per change in plasma insulin concentration	5–7 in nonobese; 2–3.5 min^{-1}/ (μU ·mL^{-1}) in obese subjects
Euglycemic hyperinsulinemic clamp	M value = glucose infused per unit of time	4.7–8.7 mg/kg/min)

[a]N/A, not applicable; BW, body weight; Ins 0 and 2 h, plasma insulin level at time 0 and 2 h after an OGTT, respectively; Glu 0 and 2 h, plasma glucose level at time 0 and 2 h after an OGTT, respectively; ISI/SiM, insulin sensitivity index; Si, insulin sensitivity; FSIVGTT, frequently sampled intravenous glucose tolerance test; AUC, area under the curve; ITT, insulin tolerance test; K_{ITT}, percentage of decline in plasma glucose concentration per minute. (From refs. 78,95–98,100–102, and 104.)

plasma glucose and insulin levels after administration of an iv glucose bolus of 0.3 g/kg of body weight, over a 3-h period (78). The glucose and insulin levels are then mathematically interpreted in order to calculate an index of insulin sensitivity, Si, which represents the glucose clearance rate per change in plasma insulin concentration (94). Results of this technique correlate well with clamp measurements but it is labor-intensive, invasive, and therefore not applicable to clinical practice (95).

Fasting levels of insulin >15 μUI/mL or >75 μUI/mL at 2 h post-OGTT and/or insulin peak level during OGTT >150 μUI/mL are considered hyperinsulinemic levels, which indicate insulin resistance (96). The cutoff value for fasting insulin, however,

Table 9
Components of IRS[a]

Insulin resistance
Decreased tissue insulin sensitivity
Compensatory hyperinsulinemia
Android obesity
BMI ≥ 30 kg/m²
WC of ≥102 cm (40 in.) in men and ≥88 cm (35 in.) in women
W/H ratio of >0.95 in men and >0.85 in women
Dyslipidemia
Triglycerides ≥ 150 mg/dL (1.7 mmol/L)
HDL cholesterol of <40 mg/dL for men <50 mg/dL for women
Smaller denser LDL cholesterol particles (type B pattern)
Postprandial accumulation of triglyceride-rich lipoproteins
Hemodynamic changes
BP > 130/85 mmHg or active treatment for hypertension
Hypersympathicotonia
Increased renal sodium retention
Glucose intolerance
FPG levels >100 mg/dL (5.6 mmol/L)
120-min postload glucose level between 140 and 200 mg/dL
Vascular abnormalities
Endothelial dysfunction
Increased urinary albumin excretion rate (>20 μg/min or albumin/creatinine ratio of >30 mg/g)
Abnormal uric acid metabolism
Hyperuricemia
Decreased renal clearance of uric acid
Prothrombotic factors/procoagulant state
Raised PAI-1
Increased plasma fibrinogen
Inflammatory markers/adipocytokines
TNF-α
Elevated level of CRP, IL-6
Increased Fibrinogen level
Decreased adiponectin level

[a]LDL, low-density lipoprotein. (Adapted from refs. *81* and *85*.)

differs from investigator to investigator because there is lack of standardization of the insulin assays used. Therefore, even if from a clinical perspective fasting insulin levels seem to be the most practical approach for assessing insulin sensitivity, the test is not recommended for routine screening *(92)*.

Mathematical models using the FPG-insulin ratio as screening tests are also available, and include the homeostasis assessment model (HOMA) *(97)* and the quantitative insulin sensitivity check index (QUICKI) *(98)*. HOMA is the most widely used test because it is relatively simple; it only requires measurements of FPG and insulin levels. Three samples for fasting plasma insulin should be drawn 5 min apart, and the mean concentration is to be used in order to avoid errors that may arise from pulsatile insulin secretion. IR is then quantified by calculating the index HOMA-IR: *HOMA-IR = Fasting insulin (μUI/mL) × Fasting glucose (mmol/L)/22.5.* The mean HOMA-IR for healthy subjects is approximately between 2.1 and 2.7; HOMA-IR increases with glycemia and insulinemia. In subject with IGT, it is approx 4.3–5.2 and in type 2 diabetes patients 8.3–9.5 *(85)*. In their original report, Matthews et al. *(97)* found HOMA-IR ranges lower than these, but further studies have reported higher HOMA-IR values *(99)*.

Insulin sensitivity can also be assessed by several other indexes based on OGTT (Table 9) *(100–103)*. These indexes correlate with the indexes of insulin sensitivity obtained from HOMA and from the euglycemic hyperinsulinemic clamp *(104)*, but because they do not offer additional advantages they are only rarely used.

OTHER PARAMETERS POTENTIALLY USEFUL IN DIAGNOSIS OF IRS

The metabolic syndrome has also been recognized as a proinflammatory, prothrombotic state associated with elevated levels of C-reactive protein (CRP), interleukin-6 (IL-6), plasminogen activator inhibitor-1(PAI-1), tumor necrosis factor-α (TNF-α), and other inflammatory markers *(105,106)*. Routine measurements of these parameters are not recommended for clinical purposes, although some investigators have suggested adding CRP as a clinical criterion for metabolic syndrome *(107)*. Although CRP has proved to be a predictor of coronary heart disease and adds clinically important prognostic information to metabolic syndrome *(108,109)*, whether CRP should be routinely measured remains a point of active research and discussion.

A urinary albumin excretion rate >20 µg/min or an albumin/creatinine ratio >30 mg/g, markers of endothelial dysfunction, and hyperuricemia are other features of IRS, but they are not necessary for diagnosis of the condition (Table 9). Adiponectin, an adipocytokine secreted mainly by the visceral adipose tissue, exerts insulin-sensitizing and antiatherogenic effects and is strongly and inversely correlated with IR *(110,111)*, but the clinical utility of measuring its level remains to be proven.

REFERENCES

1. Flier JS, Flier FE. Obesity. In: Kasper A, Longo DL, Braunwald E, Hauser SL, Jameson JL, eds. Harrison's Principle of Internal Medicine, 16th ed. McGraw-Hill, Medical Publisher Division, New York, 2005, pp. 422–430.
2. Obesity: Preventing and Managing the Global Epidemic. WHO Consultation on Obesity, Geneva, 1997.
3. Clinical guidelines on the identification, evaluation, and treatment of overweight and obesity in adults—the evidence report. National Institutes of Health. Obes Res 1998;6(Suppl 2)51S–209S.
4. Kuczmarski RJ, Ogden CL, Grummer-Strawn LM, et al. CDC growth charts: United States. Adv Data 2000;(314):1–27.
5. Committee on Nutrition Status During Pregnancy and Lactation, Institute of Medice. Nutrition During Pregnancy, Weight Gain and Nutrient Supplements; Part I: Weight Gain. National Academies Press, Washington, DC, 1990.
6. Abrams B, Altman SL, Pickett KE. Pregnancy weight gain: still controversial. Am J Clin Nutr 2000;71(Suppl 5):1233S–1241S.
7. Parker JD, Abrams B. Prenatal weight gain advice: an examination of the recent prenatal weight gain recommendations of the Institute of Medicine. Obstet Gynecol 1992;79(5)(Pt 1):664–669.
8. Linne Y, Dye L, Barkeling B, Rossner S. Weight development over time in parous women—the SPAWN study—15 years follow-up. Int J Obes Relat Metab Disord 2003;27(12):1516–1522.
9. Pai MP, Paloucek FP. The origin of the "ideal" body weight equations. Ann Pharmacother 2000;34(9):1066–1069.
10. Harrison GG. Height-weight tables. Ann Intern Med 1985;103(6)(Pt 2):989–994.
11. Pietrobelli A, Faith MS, Allison DB, Gallagher D, Chiumello G, Heymsfield SB. Body mass index as a measure of adiposity among children and adolescents: a validation study. J Pediatr 1998;132(2):204–210.
12. Maynard LM, Wisemandle W, Roche AF, Chumlea WC, Guo SS, Siervogel RM. Childhood body composition in relation to body mass index. Pediatrics 2001;107(2):344–350.
13. Hammer LD, Kraemer HC, Wilson DM, Ritter PL, Dornbusch SM. Standardized percentile curves of body-mass index for children and adolescents. Am J Dis Child 1991;145(3):259–263.

14. Must A, Dallal GE, Dietz WH. Reference data for obesity: 85th and 95th percentiles of body mass index (wt/ht2) and triceps skinfold thickness. Am J Clin Nutr 1991;53(4):839–846.

15. Rosner B, Prineas R, Loggie J, Daniels SR. Percentiles for body mass index in U.S. children 5 to 17 years of age. J Pediatr 1998;132(2):211–222.

16. Troiano RP, Frongillo EA Jr, Sobal J, Levitsky DA. The relationship between body weight and mortality: a quantitative analysis of combined information from existing studies. Int J Obes Relat Metab Disord 1996;20(1):63–75.

17. Calle EE, Thun MJ, Petrelli JM, Rodriguez C, Heath CW Jr. Body-mass index and mortality in a prospective cohort of U.S. adults. N Engl J Med 1999;341(15):1097–1105.

18. Lean ME, Han TS, Seidell JC. Impairment of health and quality of life using new US federal guidelines for the identification of obesity. Arch Intern Med 1999;159(8):837–843.

19. Janssen I, Katzmarzyk PT, Ross R. Body mass index, waist circumference, and health risk: evidence in support of current National Institutes of Health guidelines. Arch Intern Med 2002;162(18): 2074–2079.

20. Wong WW, Stuff JE, Butte NF, Smith EO, Ellis KJ. Estimating body fat in African American and white adolescent girls: a comparison of skinfold-thickness equations with a 4-compartment criterion model. Am J Clin Nutr 2000;72(2):348–354.

21. Van der Kooy K, Seidell JC. Techniques for the measurement of visceral fat: a practical guide. Int J Obes Relat Metab Disord 1993;17(4):187–196.

22. Bray GA. Clinical evaluation of the obese patient. Baillieres Best Pract Res Clin Endocrinol Metab 1999;13(1):71–92.

23. Bray GA, Ryan DH. Clinical evaluation of the overweight patient. Endocrine 2000;13(2):167–186.

24. McTigue KM, Harris R, Hemphill B, et al. Screening and interventions for obesity in adults: summary of the evidence for the U.S. Preventive Services Task Force. Ann Intern Med 2003;139(11): 933–949.

25. McTigue K, Harris R, Hemphill MB, et al. Screening and Interventions for Overweight and Obesity in Adults. File Inventory, Systematic Evidence Review Number 21. December 2003. Agency for Healthcare Research and Quality of Rockville, MD. www.ahrq.gov/clinic/prev/obesinv.htm.

26. Gray DS, Fujioka K. Use of relative weight and body mass index for the determination of adiposity. J Clin Epidemiol 1991;44(6):545–550.

27. Deurenberg P, Weststrate JA, Seidell JC. Body mass index as a measure of body fatness: age- and sex-specific prediction formulas. Br J Nutr 1991;65(2):105–114.

28. Knowler WC, Barrett-Connor E, Fowler SE, et al. Reduction in the incidence of type 2 diabetes with lifestyle intervention or metformin. N Engl J Med 2002;346(6):393–403.

29. Buchwald H, Avidor Y, Braunwald E, et al. Bariatric surgery: a systematic review and meta-analysis. JAMA 2004;292(14):1724–1737.

30. Report of the expert committee on the diagnosis and classification of diabetes mellitus. Diabetes Care 2003;26(Suppl 1):S5–S20.

31. American Diabetes Association. Diagnosis and classification of diabetes mellitus. Diabetes Care 2004;27(Suppl. 1):5–10.

32. Genuth S, Alberti KG, Bennett P, et al. Follow-up report on the diagnosis of diabetes mellitus. Diabetes Care 2003;26(11):3160–3167.

33. McCulloch DK. Definition and classification of diabetes mellitus. http://patients.uptodate.com/topic. asp?file=diabetes/9879.5-12-2004.

34. National Diabetes Data Group. Classification and diagnosis of diabetes mellitus and other categories of glucose intolerance. Diabetes 1979;28(12):1039–1057.

35. Myers J, Zonszein J. Diagnosis and epidemiology of diabetes. In: Poretsky L, ed. Principles of Diabetes Mellitus. Kluwer Academic, Norwell, MA, 2002, pp. 95–106.

36. Mooy JM, Grootenhuis PA, de Vries H, et al. Intra-individual variation of glucose, specific insulin and proinsulin concentrations measured by two oral glucose tolerance tests in a general Caucasian population: the Hoorn Study. Diabetologia 1996;39(3):298–305.

37. Feskens EJ, Bowles CH, Kromhout D. Intra- and interindividual variability of glucose tolerance in an elderly population. J Clin Epidemiol 1991;44(9):947–953.

38. McDonald GW, Fisher GF, Burnham C. Reproducibility of the oral glucose tolerance test. Diabetes 1965;14:473–480.

39. Ko GT, Chan JC, Woo J, et al. The reproducibility and usefulness of the oral glucose tolerance test in screening for diabetes and other cardiovascular risk factors. Ann Clin Biochem 1998;35(Pt 1): 62–67.

40. Wang W, Lee ET, Fabsitz R, Welty TK, Howard BV. Using HbA(1c) to improve efficacy of the American Diabetes Association fasting plasma glucose criterion in screening for new type 2 diabetes in American Indians: The Strong Heart Study. Diabetes Care 2002;25(8):1365–1370.

41. Masharani U, Karam JH. Pancreatic hormones & Diabetes mellitus. In: Greenspan FS, Gardner DG, eds. Basic & Clinical Endocrinology. McGraw-Hill, New York, 2001, 623–698.

42. Picardi A, Pozzilli P. Dynamic tests in the clinical management of diabetes. J Endocrinol Invest 2003;26(Suppl 7):99–106.

43. American Diabetes Association. Tests of glycemia in diabetes. Diabetes Care 2001;24(Suppl 1): S80–S82.

44. The Diabetes Control and Complications Trial Research Group. The effect of intensive treatment of diabetes on the development and progression of long-term complications in insulin-dependent diabetes mellitus. N Engl J Med 1993;329(14):977–986.

45. Kilpatrick ES, Maylor PW, Keevil BG. Biological variation of glycated hemoglobin: implications for diabetes screening and monitoring. Diabetes Care 1998;21(2):261–264.

46. Phillipou G, Phillips PJ. Intraindividual variation of glycohemoglobin: implications for interpretation and analytical goals. Clin Chem 1993;39(11)(Pt 1):2305–2308.

47. Klein R, Klein BE, Moss SE, Davis MD, DeMets DL. Glycosylated hemoglobin predicts the incidence and progression of diabetic retinopathy. JAMA 1988;260(19):2864–2871.

48. The relationship of glycemic exposure (HbA1c) to the risk of development and progression of retinopathy in the diabetes control and complications trial. Diabetes 1995;44(8):968–983.

49. American Diabetes Association. Standards of medical care for patients with diabetes mellitus. Diabetes Care 2001;24(Suppl 1):33–43.

50. Report of the Expert Committee on the Diagnosis and Classification of Diabetes Mellitus. Diabetes Care 1997;20(7):1183–1197.

51. American Diabetes Association. Postprandial blood glucose. Diabetes Care 2001;24(4):775–778.

52. Schnedl WJ, Krause R, Halwachs-Baumann G, Trinker M, Lipp RW, Krejs GJ. Evaluation of HbA1c determination methods in patients with hemoglobinopathies. Diabetes Care 2000;23(3):339–344.

53. Camargo JL, Gross JL. Conditions associated with very low values of glycohaemoglobin measured by an HPLC method. J Clin Pathol 2004;57(4):346–349.

54. Tran HA, Silva D, Petrovsky N. Case study: potential pitfalls of using hemoglobin A1c as the sole measure of glycemic control. Clin Diabetes 2004;22:141–143.

55. McCance DR, Hanson RL, Charles MA, et al. Comparison of tests for glycated haemoglobin and fasting and two hour plasma glucose concentrations as diagnostic methods for diabetes. BMJ 1994;308(6940):1323–1328.

56. Tsuji I, Nakamoto K, Hasegawa T, et al. Receiver operating characteristic analysis on fasting plasma glucose, HbA1c, and fructosamine on diabetes screening. Diabetes Care 1991;14(11):1075–1077.

57. Rohlfing CL, Little RR, Wiedmeyer HM, et al. Use of GHb (HbA1c) in screening for undiagnosed diabetes in the U.S. population. Diabetes Care 2000;23(2):187–191.

58. Little RR, England JD, Wiedmeyer HM, et al. Relationship of glycosylated hemoglobin to oral glucose tolerance. Implications for diabetes screening. Diabetes 1988;37(1):60–64.

59. Barr RG, Nathan DM, Meigs JB, Singer DE. Tests of glycemia for the diagnosis of type 2 diabetes mellitus. Ann Intern Med 2002;137(4):263–272.

60. Davidson MB, Schriger DL, Peters AL, Lorber B. Relationship between fasting plasma glucose and glycosylated hemoglobin: potential for false-positive diagnoses of type 2 diabetes using new diagnostic criteria. JAMA 1999;281(13):1203–1210.

61. Gerken KL, Van Lente F. Effectiveness of screening for diabetes. Arch Pathol Lab Med 1990; 114(2):201–203.

62. Guillausseau PJ, Charles MA, Paolaggi F, et al. Comparison of HbA1 and fructosamine in diagnosis of glucose-tolerance abnormalities. Diabetes Care 1990;13(8):898–900.

63. Intensive blood-glucose control with sulphonylureas or insulin compared with conventional treatment and risk of complications in patients with type 2 diabetes (UKPDS 33). UK Prospective Diabetes Study (UKPDS) Group. Lancet 1998;352(9131):837–853.

64. Alberti KG, Zimmet PZ. Definition, diagnosis and classification of diabetes mellitus and its complications. Part 1: diagnosis and classification of diabetes mellitus provisional report of a WHO consultation. Diabet Med 1998;15(7):539–553.

65. Glucose tolerance and mortality: comparison of WHO and American Diabetes Association diagnostic criteria. The DECODE study group. European Diabetes Epidemiology Group. Diabetes epidemiology: collaborative analysis of diagnostic criteria in Europe. Lancet 1999;354(9179):617–621.

66. Meigs JB, Nathan DM, D'Agostino RB Sr, Wilson PW. Fasting and postchallenge glycemia and car-diovascular disease risk: the Framingham Offspring Study. Diabetes Care 2002;25(10):1845–1850.

67. Harris MI, Hadden WC, Knowler WC, Bennett PH. Prevalence of diabetes and impaired glucose tol-erance and plasma glucose levels in U.S. population aged 20–74 yr. Diabetes 1987;36(4):523–534.

68. Harris MI, Klein R, Welborn TA, Knuiman MW. Onset of NIDDM occurs at least 4–7 yr before clinical diagnosis. Diabetes Care 1992;15(7):815–819.

69. American Diabetes Association. Screening for diabetes. Diabetes Care 2002;25:21–24.

71. Verge CF, Gianani R, Kawasaki E, Yu L, et al. Prediction of type I diabetes in first-degree relatives using a combination of insulin, GAD, and ICA512bdc/IA-2 autoantibodies. Diabetes 1996;45(7):926–933.

70. Goldfine AB. Diagnosis and management of diabetes. In: Hall J, Nieman L, eds. Handbook of Diagnostic Endocrinology. Humana, Totowa, NJ, 2003: pp. 157–177.

72. Reasner C, DeFronzo RA. Classification and Diagnosis of Diabetes Mellitus: Chapter 7. www.endo-text.com/diabetes/diabetes1/diabetesframe1.htm, 2003.

73. Naylor CD, Sermer M, Chen E, Farine D. Selective screening for gestational diabetes mellitus. Toronto Trihospital Gestational Diabetes Project Investigators. N Engl J Med 1997;337(22):1591–1596.

74. American College of Obstetrics and Gynecology (ACOG) Committee on Practice Bulletins–Obstetrics. Clinical management guidelines for obstetrician-gynecologists. Number 30, September 2001 (replaces Technical Bulletin Number 200, December 1994). Gestational diabetes. Obstet Gynecol 2001;98(3):525–538.

75. Jovanovic L, Pettitt DJ. Gestational diabetes mellitus. JAMA 2001;286(20):2516–2518.

76. Jovanovic L. Screening and Diagnosis of Gestational Diabetes Mellitus. http://patients. uptodate.com/topic.asp?file=diabetes/14302.2004. Last accessed April 26, 2005.

77. Jovanovic L. Achieving euglycaemia in women with gestational diabetes mellitus: current options for screening, diagnosis and treatment. Drugs 2004;64(13):1401–1417.

78. Monzillo LU, Hamdy O. Evaluation of insulin sensitivity in clinical practice and in research set-tings. Nutr Rev 2003;61(12):397–412.

79. Lebovitz HE. Insulin resistance: definition and consequences. Exp Clin Endocrinol Diabetes 2001; 109 (Suppl 2):S135–S148.

80. Reaven GM. Banting lecture 1988: role of insulin resistance in human disease. Diabetes 1988; 37(12):1595–1607.

81. Einhorn D, Reaven GM, Cobin RH, et al. American College of Endocrinology position statement on the insulin resistance syndrome. Endocr Pract 2003;9(3):237–252.

82. Karelis AD, St Pierre DH, Conus F, Rabasa-Lhoret R, Poehlman ET. Metabolic and body composition factors in subgroups of obesity: what do we know? J Clin Endocrinol Metab 2004;89(6): 2569–2575.

83. Frayn KN. Visceral fat and insulin resistance—causative or correlative? Br J Nutr 2000;83 (Suppl 1):71–77.

84. Ruderman N, Chisholm D, Pi-Sunyer X, Schneider S. The metabolically obese, normal-weight indi-vidual revisited. Diabetes 1998;47(5):699–713.

85. Lebovitz HE. Insulin resistance and the insulin resistance syndrome. In: Clinician's Manual on Insulin Resistance. Science Press, London, UK, 2002: pp. 1–15.

86. Ford ES, Giles WH, Dietz WH. Prevalence of the metabolic syndrome among US adults: findings from the third National Health and Nutrition Examination Survey. JAMA 2002;287(3):356–359.

87. Park YW, Zhu S, Palaniappan L, Heshka S, Carnethon MR, Heymsfield SB. The metabolic syn-drome: prevalence and associated risk factor findings in the US population from the Third National Health and Nutrition Examination Survey, 1988–1994. Arch Intern Med 2003;163(4):427–436.

88. Ford ES. Prevalence of the metabolic syndrome in US populations. Endocrinol Metab Clin North Am 2004;33(2):333–350.

89. Expert Panel on Detection, Evaluation, and Treatment of High Blood Cholesterol in Adults Executive Summary of the Third Report of the National Cholesterol Education Program (NCEP) (Adult Treatment Panel III). JAMA 2001;285(19):2486–2497.

90. Grundy SM, Brewer HB Jr, Cleeman JI, Smith SC Jr, Lenfant C. Definition of metabolic syndrome: report of the National Heart, Lung, and Blood Institute/American Heart Association conference on scientific issues related to definition. Circulation 2004;109(3):433–438.

91. Proceedings of the American College of Endocrinology Insulin Resistance Syndrome Conference. Washington, DC, USA. August 25-26, 2002. Endocr Pract 2003;9(Suppl 2):22–112.

92. Consensus Development Conference on Insulin Resistance. 5–6 November 1997. American Diabetes Association. Diabetes Care 1998;21(2):310–314.

93. DeFronzo RA, Tobin JD, Andres R. Glucose clamp technique: a method for quantifying insulin secretion and resistance. Am J Physiol 1979;237(3):214–223.

94. Pacini G, Bergman RN. MINMOD: a computer program to calculate insulin sensitivity and pancreatic responsivity from the frequently sampled intravenous glucose tolerance test. Comput Methods Programs Biomed 1986;23(2):113–122.

95. Ten S, Maclaren N. Insulin resistance syndrome in children. J Clin Endocrinol Metab 2004; 89(6):2526–2539.

96. Reaven GM, Chen YD, Hollenbeck CB, Sheu WH, Ostrega D, Polonsky KS. Plasma insulin, C-peptide, and proinsulin concentrations in obese and nonobese individuals with varying degrees of glucose tolerance. J Clin Endocrinol Metab 1993;76(1):44–48.

97. Matthews DR, Hosker JP, Rudenski AS, Naylor BA, Treacher DF, Turner RC. Homeostasis model assessment: insulin resistance and beta-cell function from fasting plasma glucose and insulin concentrations in man. Diabetologia 1985;28(7):412–419.

98. Katz A, Nambi SS, Mather K, et al. Quantitative insulin sensitivity check index: a simple, accurate method for assessing insulin sensitivity in humans. J Clin Endocrinol Metab 2000;85(7):2402–2410.

99. Yeni-Komshian H, Carantoni M, Abbasi F, Reaven GM. Relationship between several surrogate estimates of insulin resistance and quantification of insulin-mediated glucose disposal in 490 healthy nondiabetic volunteers. Diabetes Care 2000;23(2):171–175.

100. Belfiore F, Iannello S, Volpicelli G. Insulin sensitivity indices calculated from basal and OGTT-induced insulin, glucose, and FFA levels. Mol Genet Metab 1998;63(2):134–141.

101. Matsuda M, DeFronzo RA. Insulin sensitivity indices obtained from oral glucose tolerance testing: comparison with the euglycemic insulin clamp. Diabetes Care 1999;22(9):1462–1470.

102. Stumvoll M, Mitrakou A, Pimenta W, et al. Use of the oral glucose tolerance test to assess insulin release and insulin sensitivity. Diabetes Care 2000;23(3):295–301.

103. Mari A, Pacini G, Murphy E, Ludvik B, Nolan JJ. A model-based method for assessing insulin sensitivity from the oral glucose tolerance test. Diabetes Care 2001;24(3):539–548.

104. Gutt M, Davis CL, Spitzer SB, et al. Validation of the insulin sensitivity index (ISI(0,120)): comparison with other measures. Diabetes Res Clin Pract 2000;47(3):177–184.

105. Moon YS, Kim DH, Song DK. Serum tumor necrosis factor-alpha levels and components of the metabolic syndrome in obese adolescents. Metabolism 2004;53(7):863–867.

106. Festa A, D'Agostino R Jr, Howard G, Mykkanen L, Tracy RP, Haffner SM. Chronic subclinical inflammation as part of the insulin resistance syndrome: the Insulin Resistance Atherosclerosis Study (IRAS). Circulation 2000;102(1):42–47.

107. Ridker PM, Wilson PW, Grundy SM. Should C-reactive protein be added to metabolic syndrome and to assessment of global cardiovascular risk? Circulation 2004;109(23):2818–2825.

108. Ridker PM, Buring JE, Cook NR, Rifai N. C-reactive protein, the metabolic syndrome, and risk of incident cardiovascular events: an 8-year follow-up of 14 719 initially healthy American women. Circulation 2003;107(3):391–397.

109. Ridker PM, Koenig W, Fuster V. C-reactive protein and coronary heart disease. N Engl J Med 2004;351(3):295–298.

110. Chandran M, Phillips SA, Ciaraldi T, Henry RR. Adiponectin: more than just another fat cell hormone? Diabetes Care 2003;26(8):2442–2450.

111. Matsuda M, Shimomura I. Adipocytokines and metabolic syndrome—molecular mechanism and clinical implication. Nippon Rinsho 2004;62(6):1085–1090.

112. Center for Disease Control and Prevention (CDC). Prevalence of diabetes and impaired fasting glucose in adults—United States, 1999–2000. MMWR Morb Wkly Rep 2003;52:833–837.

113. Morton CJ, ed. Guidance for treatment of adult obesity, 2nd ed. Shape up America! and the American Obesity Association, Bethesda, MD, 1998.

9

Metabolic Syndrome

Rochelle L. Chaiken, MD
and Mary Ann Banerji, MD

CONTENTS

INTRODUCTION

In the last number of years, a great deal of attention has been given to a cluster of risk factors associated with the development of cardiovascular disease (CVD) identified as metabolic syndrome. Several organizations have issued definitions in an attempt to heighten awareness and identify patients who ultimately may be at increased risk for CVD *(1–4)*.

One of the key components of metabolic syndrome is insulin resistance, which historically was first identified by Himsworth and Kerr in the 1930s. They observed that obese subjects with diabetes had insulin insensitivity and did not respond normally to exogenous insulin *(5)*. However, it was not until the 1960s, with the development of the first insulin assay, that there could be a greater understanding of the relationship between circulating insulin levels and the stimulation of various metabolic processes, in particular glucose metabolism *(6,7)*. A logical observation that followed was that the maintenance of normal glucose tolerance in the context of insulin resistance resulted in the development of compensatory hyperinsulinemia *(7,8)*.

From: *Contemporary Diabetes: Obesity and Diabetes*
Edited by: C. S. Mantzoros © Humana Press Inc., Totowa, NJ

In the late 1980s, Modan and colleagues *(9,10)* described an association between hyperinsulinemia and atherogenic lipid profiles, impaired glucose tolerance (IGT), obesity, and hypertension. Reaven *(11)* put forth the concept that insulin resistance may play a central role in the pathogenesis of a variety of disease states such as type 2 diabetes, hypertension, and coronary artery disease, and described this constellation of clinical and laboratory findings as Syndrome X. Syndrome X was defined as (1) resistance to insulin-stimulated glucose uptake; (2) glucose intolerance; (3) hyperinsulinemia, (4) increased very-low-density lipoprotein (LDL) triglyceride; (5) decreased high-density lipoprotein (HDL) cholesterol; and (6) hypertension.

Since then, there have been many studies elucidating the association between insulin resistance and many risk factors for the development of cardiovascular disease. The clustering of these factors (with slight variation) has now been formally termed metabolic syndrome. This chapter will review the pathogenetic factors associated with metabolic syndrome and its association with disease.

DEFINITION OF METABOLIC SYNDROME

The definition of metabolic syndrome by several organizations has differed slightly, depending on their view of the major underlying pathophysiology. The National Heart, Lung, and Blood Institute and the American Heart Association issued the National Cholesterol Education Program's Adult Treatment Panel III (ATP III) report identifying abdominal obesity measured as increased waist circumference as the key driver of the syndrome. The presence of three of the five characteristics in Table 1 is required for the diagnosis of metabolic syndrome *(1)*. The World Health Organization (WHO) includes metabolic syndrome in its classification of diabetes and identifies insulin resistance as the major underlying pathophysiological abnormality. Insulin resistance is identified as type 2 diabetes, impaired fasting glucose or glucose intolerance, or a glucose uptake below the lowest quartile. This and the presence of two of five other characteristics in Table 1B render the metabolic syndrome diagnosis *(2)*. A combination of the WHO and ATP III criteria and clinical judgment are used in the American Association of Clinical Endocrinologists (AACE) definition *(3)*. In 2005, the International Diabetes Foundation (IDF) convened a consensus workshop to develop a new worldwide definition built on the ATP III and WHO definitions, Table 2 *(4)*. One of the key advances in these definitions is that they recognize different criteria for the definition of central obesity in different ethnic groups (*see* Table 3) *(4,12–13)*.

PATHOPHYSIOLOGY OF THE COMPONENTS ASSOCIATED WITH METABOLIC SYNDROME

Obesity, Regional Body Fat Distribution, and Insulin Resistance

Numerous studies have demonstrated a relationship between obesity and insulin resistance *(14–17)*. Many studies have also shown that weight reduction improves insulin sensitivity *(15–17,23)*. However, body mass index (BMI) and insulin sensitivity do not have a simple linear relationship. As early as in the 1950s, it was observed that body fat distribution, not just obesity, was important in understanding the diseases associated with obesity *(18)*. In recent years, several techniques to assess body composition and adipose tissue distribution have become available. Although waist circumference and waist-to-hip or waist-to-thigh ratios are used in large studies to assess visceral

Table 1
Clinical Identification of Metabolic Syndrome

A. ATP III

Risk factor	Defining level
Abdominal obesity, given as waist circumference	
Men	>102 cm (>40 in)
Women	>88 cm (>35 in)
Triglycerides	≥150 mg/dL
High-density lipoprotein cholesterol	
Men	<40 mg/dL
Women	<50 mg/dL
Blood pressure	≥130/≥85 mmHg
Fasting glucose	≥110 mg/dL[a]

B. WHO[b]

Glucose intolerance (IGT) or diabetes and/or insulin resistance and two or more of the following:
- Elevated arterial pressure ≥140/90 mmHg
- Elevated plasma triglycerides (≥1.7 mmol/L; 150 mg/dL) and/or low high-density lipoprotein cholesterol (<0.9 mmol/L, 35 mg/dL men; <1.0 mmol/L, 39 mg/dL women)
- Central obesity (males: waist-to-hip ratio >0.90; females: waist-to-hip ratio >0.85) and/or BMI >30 kg/m^2
- Microalbuminuria (urinary albumin excretion rate ≥20 µg/min or albumin:creatinine ratio ≥30 mg/g)
- Several other components of metabolic syndrome have been described (e.g., hyperuricaemia, coagulation disorders, raised PAI-1, and so on) but they are not necessary for the recognition of the condition.

[a]The American Diabetes Association has recently established a cutpoint of ≥100 mg/dL, above which persons have either prediabetes (impaired fasting glucose) or diabetes (12). This new cutpoint should be applicable for identifying the lower boundary to define an elevated glucose as one criterion for metabolic syndrome. Adapted from ref. 1.
[b]Adapted from ref. 2.

Table 2
International Diabetes Foundation (IDF) Definition of Metabolic Syndrome

According to the new IDF definition, for a person to be defined as having the metabolic syndrome they must have:

Central obesity (defined as waist circumference ≥94 cm for Europid men and ≥80 cm for Europid women, *with ethnicity-specific values for other groups*)

Plus any two of the following four factors:

- **Elevated triglyceride level:** ≥150 mg/dL (1.7 mmol/L*), or *specific treatment for this lipid abnormality*
- **Reduced high-density lipoprotein cholesterol**: <40 mg/dL (1.03 mmol/L*) in males and <50 mg/dL (1.29 mmol/L*) in females, *or specific treatment for this lipid abnormality*
- **Elevated blood pressure (BP):** systolic BP ≥130 or diastolic BP ≥85 mmHg, *or treatment of previously diagnosed hypertension*
- **Elevated fasting plasma glucose (FPG)**: ≥100 mg/dL (5.6 mmol/L), *or previously diagnosed type 2 diabetes*

*If above 5.6 mmol/L or 100 mg/dL, OGTT is strongly recommended but is not necessary to define presence of the syndrome.

Table 3
Criteria for the Definition of Central Obesity in Different Ethnic Groups

Country/ethnic group		Waist circumference*
Europids	Male	≥94 cm
In the USA, the ATP III values (102 cm male; 88 cm female) are likely to continue to be used for clinical purposes	Female	≥80 cm
South Asians	Male	≥90 cm
Based on a Chinese, Malay and Asian-Indian population	Female	≥80 cm
Chinese	Male	≥90 cm
	Female	≥80 cm
Japanese	Male	≥85 cm
	Female	≥90 cm
Ethnic South and Central Americans	Use South Asian recommendations until more specific data are available	
Sub-Saharan Africans	Use European data until more specific data are available	
Eastern Mediterranean and Middle East (Arab) populations	Use European data until more specific data are available	

adiposity, the most accurate measurements are made using computed tomography (CT) and magnetic resonance imaging, often together with dual-energy X-ray absorptiometry scanning *(19–22)*. These techniques have enabled an examination of the relationship between visceral adiposity and insulin resistance. This relationship may be present independently of the presence of obesity (BMI ≥30 kg/m^2) and may help explain why individuals who are seemingly of normal weight as assessed by BMI are insulin resistant, have a metabolic profile associated with insulin resistance, and may even have metabolic syndrome. In one study of a group of subjects who underwent significant weight loss, improvement in insulin sensitivity correlated with reduction in visceral fat *(23)*. In studies of African Americans with type 2 diabetes, insulin-sensitive and insulin-resistant variants have been characterized *(24)*. The insulin-resistant variant had more visceral adiposity and a lipid profile characteristic of metabolic syndrome as compared with the insulin-sensitive variant *(25–26)*. Moreover, in subjects with a BMI between 24.5 and 28.5 kg/m^2, the frequency of distribution of insulin action was bimodal with almost equal numbers having normal insulin action and insulin resistance (Fig. 1) *(27)*. In fact visceral fat correlated significantly with insulin-mediated glucose disposal, where as total or subcutaneous fat and gender did not (Fig. 2) *(26)*. Similar findings have been reported in nondiabetic populations as well *(28)*. In lean insulin-resistant, insulin-sensitive, and obese insulin-resistant subjects, visceral adipose tissue explained 54% of the variance in insulin sensitivity and leptin levels correlated strongly with subcutaneous fat *(29)*.

Longitudinal studies of Japanese American men have shown that accumulation of visceral adiposity predicts the development of insulin resistance and subsequent diabetes *(30,31)*. In a small study of 43 mildly obese postmenopausal women, those women who were metabolically normal (that is, with normal insulin sensitivity) had less visceral adiposity than the women who were metabolically abnormal (with insulin

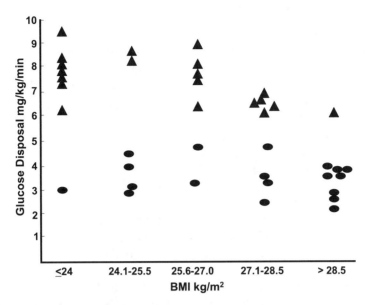

Fig. 1. The figure shows the relationship between the body mass index (BMI) and glucose disposal or insulin sensitivity. Among lean individuals (BMI <24 k/m^2), most subjects are normally insulin sensitive, and among obese individuals (BMI >28.5), most were insulin resistant. Note that between 24 and 28.5, there is no relationship between BMI and glucose disposal *(27)*.

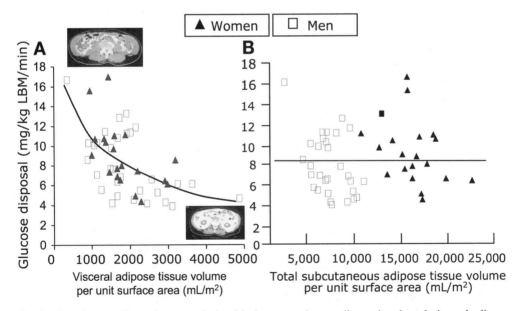

Fig. 2. There is a nonlinear inverse relationship between glucose disposal and total visceral adipose tissue volume ($p < 0.0001$) **(A),** whereas there is no relationship with glucose disposal and total sub-cutaneous adipose tissue volume **(B)**. **(A)** The inset shows high visceral adipose tissue area (bright white region) on a computed tomograph of an abdominal slice (lower right) and low visceral adipose tissue area (upper left) *(26)*.

resistance), despite the fact that the total adiposity was the same for both groups of women (32).

Furthermore, information highlighting the fact that adipose tissue is an active metabolic tissue capable of producing many proteins continues to emerge. Some of these proteins are preferentially secreted by adipose tissue in different compartments. Leptin, for example, a measure of sufficient energy stores, is secreted in larger amounts by subcutaneous than visceral adipose tissue (33). In contrast, adiponectin, another adipose tissue protein, is secreted in larger amounts by visceral as opposed to subcutaneous adipose tissue. Adiponectin has a strong inverse correlation with insulin resistance and emerges as a surrogate marker of insulin sensitivity (34).

Abnormal Glucose Metabolism

Studies in many populations have shown a relationship between the presence of obesity, and insulin resistance and the subsequent development of type 2 diabetes (35,36). Diabetes has long been associated with an increased risk of CVD. In a study of Finnish patients with type 2 diabetes, the 7-yr incidence rates for myocardial infarction with and without prior history of a myocardial infarction (MI) were 45% and 20.2%, respectively. In fact, the risk of death from coronary heart disease (CHD) in the patients with type 2 diabetes, but with no prior history of MI was no different from that in the patient without diabetes who had had a prior MI (37). Recent guidelines have recommended that diabetes is a risk equivalent for CVD and patients should be treated as though they have already had a cardiovascular event (38–40). In a 20-yr mortality study of nondiabetic, middle-aged men in three European cohorts, death from CVD was most common in those in the upper 2.5% of 2-h and fasting glucose distributions, the age-adjusted hazard ratios being 1.8 and 2.7, respectively (41). In the Norfolk cohort of the European Prospective Investigation into Cancer and Nutrition, an increase in hemoglobin A1c of 1%, in a nondiabetic male cohort was associated with a 28% ($p < 0.002$) increase in risk of death (42).

Atherogenic Dyslipidemia

A relationship between obesity and insulin resistance and an atherogenic lipid profile, usually identified as elevated serum triglycerides and low HDL cholesterol levels, has been previously demonstrated (43). More recent studies that have better characterized the lipid profile have shown that the relationship holds; is independent of ethnicity, gender, and glucose tolerance; and may correlate best with central adiposity, which, in turn, correlates well with insulin sensitivity. In one study of middle-aged men and women who were either lean and insulin sensitive or obese and insulin resistant, increasing visceral adiposity was associated with increased triglycerides, LDL cholesterol, and apolipoprotein B and decreased HDL cholesterol and LDL buoyancy (44). Other studies have shown normal LDL cholesterol studies, but the LDL particles are small and dense and can enter the arterial wall more easily, thus contributing to their being more atherogenic. Oxidized LDL has also been shown to be more atherogenic, and in a report in healthy older adults, those with metabolic syndrome had elevated oxidized LDL and showed a greater predisposition for MI (45).

Elevated Blood Pressure

Obesity has been associated with elevations in blood pressure (BP). In a recent analysis of the National Health and Nutrition Examination Survey (NHANES) data on trends in hypertension, about 2%, or more than half, of the increase in the prevalence of hypertension could be attributed to increases in BMI in the population *(46)*. Studies have also shown reduction of BP with modest weight loss. In fact, in some populations, insulin resistance and BP are linearly related. Furthermore, the relationship between elevated BP and risk of CVD is well known *(47)*.

Emerging Components

PROINFLAMMATORY AND PROTHROMBOTIC STATES

Inflammation is emerging as a key component in the development of atherosclerosis and cardiovascular disease. Almost all of the characteristics of metabolic syndrome have been associated with inflammation. The adipocyte produces a large number of proteins, including cytokines, cytokine-derived proteins, and proteins related to the fibrinolytic system, to name a few. Because obesity is a state of adipocyte excess, it would be expected that an elevation in inflammatory markers is present. An elevation of C-reactive protein, a marker of systemic inflammation, has been shown to be associated with hypertension, insulin resistance, and risk of CVD *(48,49)*. Prothrombotic factors such as plasminogen activator inhibitor-1 (PAI-1), are elevated in obesity and insulin resistance and have been shown to predict diabetes and CVD *(50)*.

MICROALBUMINURIA

Microalbuminuria is a marker of endothelial dysfunction and increasing mortality and is also associated with central obesity *(51)*. In one study of patients with type 2 diabetes, microalbuminuria was the criterion most predictive of metabolic syndrome based on the WHO criteria *(52)*.

PREVALENCE OF METABOLIC SYNDROME

Many studies have shown that metabolic syndrome occurs across a wide range of ethnic groups. With the recent data showing the increasing burden of obesity throughout the world, it can be expected that the rates of metabolic syndrome will be increasing. A number of factors increase the risk of developing metabolic syndrome, particularly weight gain and sedentary lifestyle. Middle-aged men participating in the Kuopio Ischemic Heart Disease Risk Factor Study from Eastern Finland who gained more than 10% of their youthful (age 20) weight by middle age were more likely to have metabolic abnormalities consistent with metabolic syndrome (such as hypertension, hyperinsulinemia, and dyslipidemia) as compared with those men whose weight remained stable over time *(53)*. In the Bruneck Study, a population-based survey on atherosclerosis and its risk factors in Bruneck (a small town in northeastern Italy), insulin resistance was present in 9.6% of the population as assessed by homeostasis assessment model. Interestingly, 5.1% of the population had normal weight and no metabolic abnormalities, but was insulin resistant. Hypertriglyceridemia and low HDL-cholesterol were as likely to accompany insulin resistance as was type 2 diabetes, whereas there was less of an association between hypertension, hypercholesterolemia, and hyperuricemia and insulin resistance *(54)*.

As reported recently from the third NHANES, the age-adjusted prevalence rate of metabolic syndrome, as defined by ATP III, was 23.7% in the United States. In general, age-adjusted rates for men and women were similar, but for both African-American and Hispanic groups, women had higher rates than men (Fig. 3) *(55)*. Moreover, the presence of metabolic syndrome has been shown to independently predict the risk for the development of diabetes *(56)*.

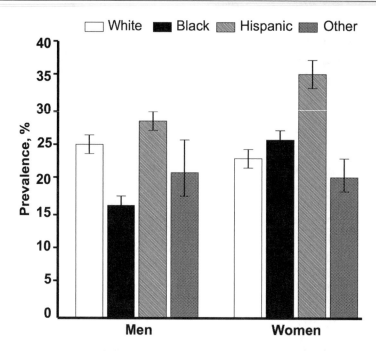

Fig. 3. The figure demonstrates the age-adjusted prevalence of metabolic syndrome among 8814 US adults aged at least 20 yr, by sex and race or ethnicity. (From the National Health and Nutrition Examination Survey III, 1988–1994 *[55]*).

METABOLIC SYNDROME IN CHILDREN AND EARLY LIFE DETERMINANTS

Recent reports show that the prevalence of overweight/obesity is increasing in children in the United States and so is the prevalence of type 2 diabetes in children *(57,58)*. Assessment of insulin resistance and clustering of metabolic abnormalities associated with metabolic syndrome in African-American children aged 5–10 yr without diabetes showed a positive correlation with insulin resistance, BP, triglycerides, and cholesterol. Girls were more insulin resistant than boys *(59)*. In an evaluation of almost 500 children and adolescents ranging from nonobese to severely obese, the prevalence of metabolic syndrome increased to 50% in the severely obese subjects *(60)*. Among both European and South Asian populations, an early determinant of adult metabolic syndrome and diabetes is maternal nutrient deprivation and intrauterine growth retardation followed by catch-up growth in childhood. Intrauterine growth retardation appears to alter nutrient partitioning, resulting in increased adult adiposity and glucose intolerance *(61–64)*. Nutrient deprivation during early gestation was associated with higher cardiovascular risk in adult life, and nutrient deprivation during late to mid-gestation was associated with reduced glucose tolerance.

THE METABOLIC SYNDROME AND CARDIOVASCULAR DISEASE

A large number of studies have evaluated the relationship between insulin resistance *(65–67)*; clustering of the other characteristics of metabolic syndrome, such as dyslipidemia and glucose intolerance *(54,68–71)*; and the development of CVD.

In the Botnia study, a large family study in Finland and Sweden, the presence of metabolic syndrome, as defined according the WHO definition, correlated with a three-fold increase in risk for CHD and stroke. Cardiovascular mortality was also markedly increased in those subjects with the syndrome (12.0 vs 2.2% [$p < 0.001$]) and microalbuminuria was the strongest predictor of cardiovascular death (68).

The prevalence of metabolic syndrome in the Kuopio Ischemic Heart Disease Risk Factor Study, a population-based prospective cohort study of 1209 Finnish men followed for approx 11.4 yr, was 8.8% to 14.3%, respectively, depending on whether it was defined according to ATP III or WHO. The presence of the syndrome, regardless of the definition used, resulted in an almost three- to fourfold increase in CVD and CHD and an almost twofold increase in allcause mortality (71).

In the Insulin Resistance Atherosclerosis Study (IRAS), a large epidemiological study evaluating a triethnic cohort (African American, Hispanics, and non-Hispanic whites) in four communities in the United States, insulin resistance measured by the frequently sampled intravenous glucose tolerance test (FSIVGTT) was associated with intimal medial thickness of the carotid arteries, a surrogate marker for cardiovascular risk, in Hispanic and non-Hispanics whites, but not in African Americans (69). When factors common to metabolic syndrome are included in the model, the association between insulin resistance and measures of atherosclerosis diminished, suggesting that the syndromes is components contribute to the development of atherosclerosis in the insulin-resistant state.

In a recent application of the ATP III metabolic syndrome criteria to the NHANES III subjects, the presence of the Syndrome was associated with a more than twofold increase in MI and stroke in both men and women. Moreover, insulin resistance, low HDL-cholesterol, hypertension, and hypertriglyceridemia all independently correlated with risk of MI and stroke (72). The absence of metabolic syndrome in the NHANES cohort correlated with a low age-adjusted prevalence of CHD (8.7%). It was similar to the prevalence in the subjects with diabetes who did not have the syndrome, although diabetes without metabolic syndrome was uncommon (13%). The prevalence of coronary heart disease in the presence of metabolic syndrome was 13.9% and 19.2% for those without and with diabetes, respectively (73).

POTENTIAL TREATMENTS

There is considerable uncertainty regarding the treatment of metabolic syndrome. The approach depends on whether the underlying cause should be treated or whether the individual components should be treated. There are considerable outcome data that address the treatment of the individual components. For example, drugs that raise HDL cholesterol levels (fibrates), lower BP, or are anti-inflammatory (aspirin) have been shown to improve mortality (74–76). There are no studies that target all of the components of metabolic syndrome in subjects with diabetes, and there is no consensus as to whether treatment of the components should be intensified in nondiabetic persons with metabolic syndrome (84). Finally there is a question as to whether the underlying abnormality of metabolic syndrome should be targeted. Assuming insulin resistance is the underlying cause, there is a rationale for its treatment in prediabetes and diabetes; diabetes can be prevented (with lifestyle modification, metformin, or thiazolidinediones) and hyperglycemia improved (77–79). However, there is no evidence for the pharmacological treatment of insulin resistance in individuals without glucose intolerance who have metabolic syndrome. Such individuals are clearly at risk of increased mortality and CVD, and treatment of this group is an area of active interest.

WEIGHT LOSS AND EXERCISE

The benefits of weight loss and increased physical activity have been demonstrated in several prospective studies showing a decrease in the development of type 2 diabetes and an improvement in other factors of the metabolic syndrome (77,78). Voluntary weight loss results in an improvement in insulin sensitivity (79). Increased physical activity has been shown to be beneficial in numerous clinical studies with end points being either mortality or metabolic syndrome (80,81). It is difficult to identify the precise mechanism(s) whereby lifestyle alterations improve outcomes, the effects may be multiple and but are likely to include decreases in adiposity, insulin resistance, and nutrient fluxes; altered intramyocelluar and intrahepatic metabolism; and increased adiponectin levels and skeletal muscle blood flow. The optimum dose of lifestyle change is not known.

Liposuction

Liposuction is a popular approach to decreasing adiposity in which large amounts of subcutaneous adipose tissue removed. A recent key study sheds some light on its metabolic effects (82). Despite a 44% decrease in abdominal subcutaneous adipose tissue, there was no effect on metabolic syndrome, including inflammatory markers, plasma adiponectin, lipid levels, and insulin sensitivity. This argues that the beneficial effects of usual weight loss are likely to be related to decreases in visceral adiposity and/or associated caloric restriction, but not to changes in subcutaneous adipose tissue.

Pharmacological Agents

Various pharmacological agents may also impact on one or more features of metabolic syndrome. Metformin improves metabolic syndrome either directly or indirectly (83). Metformin may decrease mortality in persons with diabetes, reduce the development of diabetes in prediabetes and in individuals with polycystic ovary syndrome, and reduce hyperandrogenism. The thiazolidinediones or peroxisome proliferator activator receptor agonists act at a nuclear level to improve glycemia, decrease insulin resistance and plasma triglyceride levels, and variably increase HDL cholesterol levels resultant modest increases in body weight represent increases of subcutaneous, not visceral, adipose tissue, and thus may not be deleterious. Ongoing studies will determine the potential for long-term benefit of the thiazolidinediones in metabolic syndrome. Decreasing the activity of the renin angiotensin system has been reported to decrease the development of diabetes and mortality. Other agents directly target weight change, including orlistat, which decreases GI fat absorption, and sibutramine, a combination of norepinephrine and dexfenfluramine which reduces appetite. To the extent that these agents sustain long-term weight loss, they are likely to decrease obesity related factors of metabolic syndrome. Numerous investigational approaches target relevant receptors and pathways including central appetite regulators (such as the cannabinoid-1 receptor antagonist, rimonabant), GI-neural pathways (ghrelin antagonists), and local increases in cortisol (antagonists of adipocyte 11β hydroxysteroid dehydrogenase type 1 activity).

SUMMARY

In summary, metabolic syndrome is defined by a cluster of risk factors associated with the development of cardiovascular disease. Obesity, in particular visceral adiposity, insulin resistance, and some degree of abnormal glucose metabolism coupled with dyslipidemia and abnormal BP are the hallmarks of the syndrome. A large body of epidemiological data correlates the presence of metabolic syndrome with an increased risk of CVD and overall mortality. Because obesity is an increasing global burden, it is expected that the number of individuals with metabolic syndrome will increase as will the rates of morbidity and mortality from CVD. Efforts are underway to better understand the pathophysiology of metabolic syndrome and explore opportunities for its prevention and treatment.

REFERENCES

1. Grundy SM, Brewer HB, Cleeman JI, Smith SC, Lenfant C, for the conference participants. Definition of metabolic syndrome, report of the National Heart, Lung, and Blood Institute/American Heart Association Conference on Scientific Issues Related to Definition. Circulation 2004;109: 433–438.
2. World Health Organization. Definition, Diagnosis, and Classification of Diabetes Mellitus and Its Complications: Report of a WHO Consultation. Part 1: Diagnosis and Classification of Diabetes Mellitus. WHO/NCD/NCS/99.2. World Health Organization, Department of Noncommunicable Disease Surveillance, Geneva, 1999.
3. Einhorn D, Reaven GM, Cobin RH, et al. American College of Endocrinology position statement on the insulin resistance syndrome. Endocr Pract 2003;9(3):237–252.
4. The International Diabetes Foundation. The IDF consensus worldwide definition of the metabolic syndrome. www.idf.org
5. Himsworth HP, Kerr RB. Insulin-sensitive and insulin-insensitive types of diabetes mellitus. Clin Sci 1939;4:119–152.
6. Cahill GF. Physiology of insulin in man. Diabetes 1971;20:785–799.
7. Bagdade JD, Bierman EL, Porte D Jr. The significance of basal insulin levels in the evaluation of the insulin response to glucose and non-diabetic subjects. J Clin Invest 1967;46:1549–1557.
8. Polonsky KS, Given BD, Hirsch L, et al. Quantitative study of insulin secretion and clearance in normal and obese subjects. J Clin Invest 1988;81:435–441.
9. Modan M, Halkin H, Fuchs Z, et al. Hyperinsulinemia—a link between glucose intolerance, obesity, hypertension, dyslipoproteinemia, elevated serum uric acid and internal cation imbalance. Diabetes Metab 1987;13:375–380.
10. Modan M, Halkin H, Lusky A, Segal P, Fuchs Z, Chetrit A. Hyperinsulinemia is characterized by jointly disturbed plasma VLDL, LDL, and HDL levels. A population-based study. Arteriosclerosis 1988;8:227–236.
11. Reaven GM. The role of insulin resistance in human disease. Diabetes 1988;37:1595–1607.
12. WHO Expert Consultation. Appropriate body mass index for Asian poipulations and its implications for policy and intervention strategies. Lancet 2004;363:157–163
13. Tan C-E, Na S, Wai D, Chew S-K, Tai E-S. Can we apply the National Cholesterol Education Program Adult Treatment Panel definition of the metabolic syndrome to Asians. Diabetes Care 2004;27:1182–1186.
14. Olefsky JM, Kolterman OG, Scarlett JA. Insulin action and resistance in obesity and non-insulin-dependent type 2 diabetes mellitus. Am J Physiol 1982;243:E15–E30.
15. Su HY, Sheu WH, Chin HM, Jeng CY, Reaven GM. Effect of weight loss on blood pressure and insulin resistance in normotensive and hypertensive obese individuals. Am J Hypertens 1995;8:1067–1071.
16. Niskanen L, Uusitupa M, Sarlund H, Siitonen O, Paljarvi L, Laasko M. The effects of weight loss on insulin sensitivity, skeletal muscle composition, and capillary density in obese non-diabetic subjects. Int J Obes 1996;20:154–160.
17. Muscelli E, Camastra S, Catalano C, et al. Metabolic and cardiovascular assessment in moderate obesity: effect of weight loss. J Clin Endocrinol Metab 1997;82:2937–2943.
18. Vague J. The degree of masculine differences of obesities: a factor determining predisposition to diabetes, atherosclerosis, gout, and uric calculous disease. Am J Clin Nutr 1956;4:20–34.
19. Kvist H, Sjostrom L, Tylen U. Adipose tissue volume determinations in women by computerized tomography: technical considerations. Int J Obesity 1986;10:53–67.

20. Kvist H, Chowdhury B, Grangard U, Tylen U, Sjostrom L. Total and visceral adipose tissue volume derived from measurements with computerized tomography in adult men and women: predictive equations. Am J Clin Nutr 1988;48:1351–1361.

21. Abate N, Burns D, Peshock RM, Garg, Grundy SM. Estimation of adipose tissue mass by magnetic resonance imaging: validation against dissection in human cadavers. J Lipid Res 1994;35:1490–1496.

22. Tataranni PA, Ravussin E. Use of dual X-ray absorptiometry in obese individuals. Am J Clin Nutr 1995;55:730–734.

23. Goodpaster BH, Kelley DE, Wing RR, Meier A, Thaete FL. Effects of weight loss on regional fat distribution and insulin sensitivity in obesity. Diabetes 1999;48:839–847.

24. Banerji MA, Lebovitz HE. Insulin-sensitive and insulin-resistant variants in NIDDM. Diabetes 1989;38:784–792.

25. Banerji MA, Chaiken RL, Gordon D, Kral JG, Lebovitz HE. Does intra-abdominal adipose tissue in black men determine whether NIDDM is insulin resistant or insulin-sensitive? Diabetes 1995;44:141–146.

26. Banerji MA, Lebowitz J, Chaiken RL, Gordon D, Kral J, Lebovitz HE. Relationships of visceral adipose tissue and glucose disposal is independent of sex in black NIDDM subjects. Am J Physiol 1997;273:E425–E432.

27. Banerji MA, Lebovitz HL. Insulin action in black Americans with NIDDM. Diabetes Care 1992;15:1295–1302.

28. Kahn SE, Prigeon RL, Schwartz RS, et al. Obesity, body fat distribution, insulin sensitivity and islet b-cell function as explanations for metabolic diversity. J Nutr 2001;131:354S–360S.

29. Cnop M, Landchild MJ, Vidal J, et al. The concurrent accumulation of intra-abdominal and subcutaneous fat explains the association between insulin resistance and plasma leptin concentrations: distinct metabolic effects of to fat compartments. Diabetes 2002;51:1005–1015.

30. Bergstrom RW, Newell-Morris LL, Leonetti DL. Association of elevated fasting C-peptide level and increased intra-abdominal fat distribution with development of NIDDM in Japanese-American men. Diabetes 1990;39:104–111.

31. Boyko EJ, Fujimoto WY, Leonetti DL, Newell-Morris L. Visceral adiposity and risk for type 2 diabetes: A prospective study among Japanese-Americans. Diabetes Care 2000;23:465–471.

32. Brochu M, Tchernof A, Dionne IJ, et al. What are the physical characteristics associated with a normal metabolic profile despite a high level of obesity in postmenopausal women? J Clin Endocrinol Metab 2001;86:1020–1025.

33. Kershaw EE, Flier JS. Adipose tissue as an endocrine organ. J Clin Endocrinol Metab 2004;89:2548–2556.

34. Chandran M, Phillips SA, Ciaraldi T, Henry RR. Adiponectin: more than just another fat cell hormone? Diabetes Care 2003;26:2442–2450.

35. Hanson RL, Narayan KMV, McCance DR, et al. Rate of weight gain, weight fluctuation, and incidence of NIDDM. Diabetes 1995;44:261–266.

36. Colditz GA, Willet WC, Stampfer MJ, et al. Weight as a risk factor for clinical diabetes in women. Am J Epidemiol 1990;132:501–513.

37. Haffner SM, Lehto S, Ronnemaa T, Pyorala K, Laasko M. Mortality from coronary heart disease in subjects with type 2 diabetes and in nondiabetic subjects with and without prior myocardial infarction. N Engl J Med 1998;339:229–234.

38. Grundy SM, Cleeman JI, Merz NB, et al., for the Coordinating Committee of the National Cholesterol Educational Program. Implications of the recent clinical trials for the National Cholesterol Educational Program Adult Treatment Panel III Guidelines Circulation 2004;110:227–239.

39. American Diabetes Association. Standards of medical care in diabetes. Diabetes Care 2004;27 (Suppl 1):S15–S35.

40. Snow V, Aronson MD, Hornbake ER, Mottur-Pilson C, Weiss KB for the Clinical Efficacy Assessment Subcommittee of the American College of Physicians. Lipid control in the management of type 2 diabetes mellitus: a clinical practice guideline from the American College of Physicians. Ann Intern Med 2004;140:644–649.

41. Balku B, Shipley M, Jarrett RJ, et al. High blood glucose concentration is a risk factor for mortality in middle-aged nondiabetic men. Diabetes Care 1998;21:360–367.

42. Khaw K, Wareham N, Luben R, et al. Glycated haemoglobin, diabetes, and mortality in men in Norfolk cohort of European Prospective Investigation of Cancer and Nutrition (EPIC-Norfolk). BMJ 2001;322:1–6.

43. Carr M, Brunzell J. Abdominal obesity and dyslipidemia in the Metabolic Syndrome: Importance of type 2 diabetes and familial combined hyperlipidemia in coronary artery disease risk. J Clin Endocrinol Metab 2004;89:2601–2607.

44. Nieves DJ, Cnop M, Retzlaff B, et al. The atherogenic lipoprotein profile associated with obesity and insulin resistance is largely attributable to intra-abdominal fat. Diabetes 2003;52:172–179.

45. Holvoet P, Kritchevsky SB, Tracy RP, et al. The metabolic syndrome, circulating oxidized LDL, and risk of myocardial infarction in well-functioning elderly people in the Health, Aging, and Body Composition Cohort. Diabetes 2004;53:1068–1073.

46. Hajjar I, Kotchen T. Trends in prevalence, awareness, treatment, and control of hypertension in the United States, 1988–2000. JAMA 2003;290:199–2051.

47. Reaven G. Insulin resistance/compensatory hyperinsulinemia, essential hypertension, and cardiovascular disease. J Clin Endocrinol Metab 2003;88:2399–2403.

48. Sesso H, Buring J, Rifai N, Blake G, Gaziano J, Ridker P. C-reactive protein and the risk of developing hypertension. JAMA 2003;290:2945–2951.

49. Visser M, Bouter L, McQuillan G, Wener M, Harris TB. Elevated C-reactive protein levels in overweight and obese adults. JAMA 1999;282:2131–2135.

50. Pradhan A, Manson J, Rifai N, Buring J, Ridker P. C-reactive protein, interleukin 6, and risk of developing type 2 diabetes mellitus. JAMA 2001;286:327–334.

51. Stehouwer CD, Gall MA, Twisk JW, Knudsen E, Emies JJ, Parving HH. Increased urinary albumin excretion, endothelial dysfunction and chronic low grade inflammation in type 2 diabetes: progressive, interrelated and independently associated with risk of death. Diabetes 2002;51:1157–1165.

52. Marchesini G, Forlani G, Cerrelli F, et al. WHO and ATP III proposals for the definition of the metabolic syndrome in patients with type 2 diabetes. Diab Med 2004;21:383–387.

53. Everson SA, Goldberg DE, Helmrich SP, et al. Weight gain and the risk of developing insulin resistance syndrome. Diabetes Care 1998;21:1637–1643.

54. Bonora E, Kiechl S, Willeit J, et al. Prevalence of insulin resistance in metabolic disorders. The Bruneck Study. Diabetes 1998;47:1643–1649.

55. Ford E, Giles W, Dietz W. Prevalence of the metabolic syndrome among US adults-Findings from the Third National Health and Nutrition Examination Survey. JAMA 2002;87:356–359.

56. Lorenzo C, Okoloise M, Williams K, Stern MP, Haffner SM. The metabolic syndrome as predictor of type 2 diabetes-The San Antonio Heart Study. Diabetes Care 2003;26:3153–3159.

57. Flegal KM. The obesity epidemic in children and adults: current evidence and research issues. Med Sci Sports Exer 1999;31(Suppl 11):S509–S514.

58. American Diabetes Association. Type 2 diabetes in children and adolescents (Consensus Statement) Diabetes Care 2000;23:381–389.

59. Young-Hyman D, Schlundt DG, Herman L, De Luca F, Counts D. Evaluation of the insulin resistance syndrome in 5- to 10-year-old overweight/obese African-American children. Diabetes Care 2001;24:1359–1364.

60. Weiss R, Dziura J, Burgert TS, et al. Obesity and the metabolic syndrome in children and adolescents. N Engl J Med 2004;350:2362–2374.

61. Yajnik CS, Fall CH, Coyaji KJ, et al. Neonatal anthropometry: the thin-fat Indian baby. The Pune Maternal Nutrition Study. Int J Obes Relat Metab Disord 2003;27:173–180.

62. Bhargava SK, Sachdev HS, Fall CH, et al. Relation of serial changes in childhood body-mass index to impaired glucose tolerance in young adulthood. N Engl J Med 2004;350(9):865–875.

63. Eriksson JG, Forsen T, Tuomilehto J, Osmond C, Barker DJ. Early adiposity rebound in childhood and risk of Type 2 diabetes in adult life. Diabetologia 2003;46:190–194.

64. Stern MP, Bartley M, Duggirala R, Bradshaw B. Birth weight and the metabolic syndrome: thrifty phenotype or thrifty genotype? Diabetes Metab Res Rev 2000;16:88–93.

65. Ducimetiere P, Eschwege E, Papoz L, Richard JL, Claude JR, Rosselin G. Relationship of plasma insulin levels to the incidence of myocardial infarction and coronary heart disease in middle aged men. Diabetologia 1980;19:205–210.

66. Fontbonne A, Charles MA, Thibult N, et al. Hyperinsulinemia as a predictor of coronary heart disease mortality in a healthy population: the Paris Prospective Study, 15-year follow-up. Diabetologia 1991;34:356–361.

67. Depres J-P, Lamarche B, Mauriege P, et al. Hyperinsulinemia as an independent risk factor for ischemic heart disease N Engl J Med 1996;334:952–957.

68. Isomaa B, Almgren P, Tuomi T, et al. Cardiovascular morbidity and mortality associated with the metabolic syndrome. Diabetes Care 2001;24:683–689.
69. Haffner SM, Mykkanen L, Festa A, Burke JP, Stern MP. Insulin-resistant prediabetic subjects have more atherogenic risk factors than insulin-sensitive prediabetic subjects. Circulation 2000;101:975–980.
70. Greenlund KJ, Valdez R, Casper ML, Rith-Najarian S, Croft JB. Prevalence and correlates of the insulin resistance syndrome among Native Americans. The Inter-Tribal Heart Project. Diabetes Care 1999;22:441–447.
71. Lakka HM, Laaksonen DE, Lakka TA, et al. The metabolic syndrome and total and cardiovascular disease mortality in middle-aged men. JAMA 2002;288:2709–2716.
72. Ninomiya JK, L' Italien G, Criqui MH, Whyte JL, Gamst A, Chen RS. Association of the metabolic syndrome with history of myocardial infarction and stroke in the Third National Health and Nutrition Examination Survey. Circulation 2004;109;42–46.
73. Alexander CM, Landsman PB, Teutsch SM, Haffner SM. NCEP-defined metabolic syndrome, diabetes, and prevalence of coronary heart disease among NHANES III participants age 50 years and older. Diabetes 2003;52:210–1214.
74. Robins SJ, Rubins HB, Faas FH, et al. Veterans Affairs HDL Intervention Trial (VA-HIT). Insulin resistance and cardiovascular events with low HDL cholesterol: the Veterans Affairs HDL Intervention Trial (VA-HIT). Diabetes Care 2003;26:1513–1517.
75. ALLHAT Officers and Coordinators for the ALLHAT Collaborative Research Group. The Antihypertensive and Lipid-Lowering Treatment to Prevent Heart Attack Trial. Major outcomes in moderately hypercholesterolemic, hypertensive patients randomized to pravastatin vs usual care: The Antihypertensive and Lipid-Lowering Treatment to Prevent Heart Attack Trial (ALLHAT-LLT). JAMA 2002;288:2998–3007.
76. Colwell JA and the American Diabetes Association Aspirin therapy in diabetes. Diabetes Care 2004;27(Suppl 1):S72–S73.
77. Tuomilehto J, Lindstrom J, Eriksson JG, et al., for the Finnish Diabetes Prevention Study Group. Prevention of type 2 diabetes mellitus by changes in lifestyle among subjects with impaired glucose tolerance. N Engl J Med 2001;344:1343–1350.
78. Diabetes Prevention Program Research Group. Reduction in the incidence of type 2 diabetes with lifestyle intervention or metformin. N Engl J Med 2002;346:393–403.
79. McAuley KA, Williams SM, Mann JI, et al. Intensive lifestyle changes are necessary to improve insulin sensitivity. Diabetes Care 2002;25:445–452.
80. Manson JE, Nathan DM, Krolewski AS, Stampfer MJ, Willett WC, Hennekens CH. A prospective study of exercise and the incidence of diabetes among US male physicians. JAMA 1992;268:63–67.
81. Laaksonen DE, Lakka HM, Salonen JT, Niskanen LK, Rauramaa R, Lakka TA. Low levels of leisure time physical activity and cardiorespiratory fitness predict the development of the Metabolic Syndrome. Diabetes Care 2002;25:1612–1618.
82. Klein S, Fontana L, Young VL, Coggan AR, Kilo C, Patterson BW, Mohammed BS. Absence of an effect of liposuction on insulin action and risk factors for coronary heart disease. N Engl J Med 2004;350:2549–2557.
83. Lebovitz HE, Banerji MA. Treatment of insulin resistance in diabetes mellitus. Eur J Pharmacol 2004;490:135–146.
84. Kahn R, Buse J, Ferrannini E, Stern M. The metabolic syndrome: time for a critical reappraisal. Diabetes Care 2005;28:2289–2304.

10 Obesity, Diabetes, and Hypertension

Anjanette S. Tan, MD,
Stephen A. Brietzke, MD, FACE,
David W. Gardner, MD, FACE,
and James R. Sowers, MD, FACE, FACP, FAHA

CONTENTS

INTRODUCTION

Obesity, the so-called killer of the 21st century, is a serious and pervading health problem in the industrialized world and developing countries. Its prevalence is on the rise, and its cost to health systems is astounding. The risk of death from all causes rises as body mass index (BMI) increases for both men and women in all age groups *(1)*. For example, a 20-yr-old Caucasian male with a BMI greater than 45 kg/m^2 is estimated to lose 13 yr of his life owing to obesity—a 17% reduction in life expectancy assuming a life expectancy of 78 yr *(2)*.

Concurrent with this increase in obesity, the prevalence of diabetes mellitus is also on the rise, with increasing trends being observed in all demographic groups: age, gender, and ethnicity *(3)*. The annual cost attributed to diabetes, directly or indirectly, amounts to $132 billion *(4)*.

Hypertension affects approx 50 million individuals in the United States and approx 1 billion individuals worldwide *(5)*. It is the most common primary diagnosis in the United States, leading to 35 million office visits annually.

In this chapter, we review the current knowledge, trends, and research in the field of hypertension in relation to type 2 diabetes and obesity. We explore the mechanisms, relationships, issues in management, and unique features of hypertension in persons with coexistent obesity and diabetes.

From: *Contemporary Diabetes: Obesity and Diabetes*
Edited by: C. S. Mantzoros © Humana Press Inc., Totowa, NJ

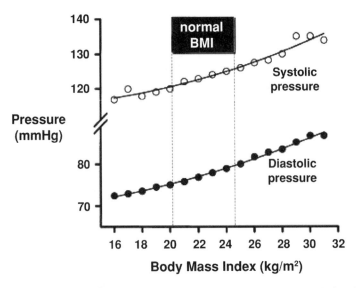

Fig. 1. Relationship of blood pressure to body mass index (BMI). The linear relationship exists even within the normal BMI range *(1)*.

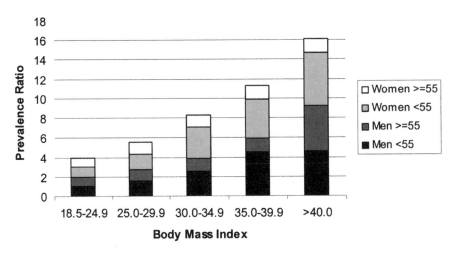

Fig. 2. Prevalence ratios of hypertension in relationship to body mass index (BMI). The prevalence of hypertension increases with increasing BMI *(7)*.

EPIDEMIOLOGY

Hypertension in Obesity

The association of obesity and hypertension is well recognized. Population studies demonstrate a good correlation between BMI and blood pressure (BP) in both normotensive and hypertensive individuals *(6)* (Fig. 1). Data from the National Health and Nutrition Examination Survey (NHANES) show a strong linear relationship between rise in BMI and systolic blood pressure (SBP), diastolic blood pressure (DBP), and pulse pressure *(7)* (Fig. 2). This relationship remains consistent even in obese children and adolescents *(8)*. The Framingham Heart Study showed that a weight gain of 5% increases the risk of hypertension by 30% in a 4-yr period *(9)*. In regression models corrected for age-related rise in BP, a gain of 1.7 kg/m^2 for men and 1.25 kg/m^2 for women in BMI or an increase of 4.5 cm for men and 2.5 cm for women in waist circumference is associated with an increase in BP of 1 mmHg *(10)*. It is important to note that there is considerable interindividual variability in the BP response to weight gain, and not all obese individuals become hypertensive *(11)*. The underlying reasons for this variability remain unclear, but genetic factors are thought to contribute *(11)*.

Body fat distribution in obesity has also been linked to hypertension. Visceral adiposity, measured using computed tomography, has been shown to increase the risk of hypertension *(12)*. Numerous studies have also used different measurements, such as subscapular skinfold thickness and waist circumference, to imply central obesity. These surrogate measurements have modestly correlated with increased BP *(13)*.

Diabetes in Obesity

It is estimated that 60–90% of individuals who have type 2 diabetes are obese. The reverse, however, is not true and the majority of patients who are obese do not become diabetic *(14)*. In the NHANES analysis of health burdens associated with overweight and obesity, the prevalence rate of type 2 diabetes was three- to fourfold greater in the overweight and the obese *(7)*. In this context, overweight is defined as a BMI of 25 kg/m^2 or more, and obesity as a BMI of 30 kg/m^2 or more *(2,7)*.

Hypertension in Diabetes

Hypertension is more common in patients with diabetes, and persons with hypertension are considerably more likely to develop diabetes than those without it *(15,16)*. Type 2 diabetes mellitus is 2.5 times as likely to develop in hypertensive individuals as in their normotensive counterparts *(16)*. Hypertensive individuals also generally have a greater BMI, waist-to-hip ratio, and higher fasting glucose and insulin levels, when compared with normotensive individuals *(16)*. This suggests a clustering of characteristics compatible with metabolic syndrome.

In type 1 diabetes, hypertension generally parallels the occurrence of renal disease *(15)*. In type 2 diabetes, hypertension often parallels the progression of metabolic abnormalities, with its onset being less dependent on the occurrence of renal disease *(15)*. A recent analysis of the database from the NHANES III population categorized adults over 50 yr of age by the presence of the National Cholesterol Education Program (NCEP)-defined metabolic syndrome, with or without diabetes. Risk factors for cardiovascular disease (CVD), specifically hypertension, were comparable in patients who had metabolic syndrome, whether or not they had diabetes *(17)*. These data strongly suggest the important role of the metabolic syndrome, much more than hyperglycemia, in mediating risk factors for CVD, including hypertension.

Cardiometabolic Syndrome, Obesity, and Risk of CVD

Cardiometabolic syndrome is a clustering of maladaptive characteristics that confers an increased risk of CVD events. Insulin resistance clusters with hypertension, diabetes, and dyslipidemia and occurs in isolation in less than 20% of the population. Approximately 44% of the US population over the age of 50 meets the NCEP Adult Treatment Panel criteria for metabolic syndrome *(18)*. It is likewise extremely common in type 2 diabetics; only about 13% of patients do not have metabolic syndrome *(17)*. These comorbidities are known to act synergistically to increase the risk of CVD. Even mild hyperglycemia (i.e., impaired fasting glucose), when associated with moderate hypertension (SBP of 140–149), significantly increases CVD mortality *(19)*.

MECHANISMS OF HYPERTENSION IN DIABETES AND OBESITY

Sympathetic Nervous System

Activation of the sympathetic nervous system (SNS) is well linked to the development of hypertension and age-associated obesity *(20)*. It is a major common pathway known to alter peripheral vasoreactivity and renal volume and pressure handling, which ultimately results in obesity-induced hypertension.

There is a tight association between norepinephrine (NE) levels and an elevation in BP during weight gain. Subjects with an elevation in BP accompanying weight gain have significantly higher plasma norepinephrine levels than those without an increase in BP, regardless of baseline BMI or BP *(20)*.

Sympathetic activity has also been directly assessed by regional NE spillover, microneurographic recording of muscle sympathetic nerve activity *(21)*, and immuno-histochemical labeling of central neuron proteins (*Fos* and *Fos*-like proteins) involved in the regulation of arterial pressure *(22)*. With these techniques, sympathetic hyperactivity has been demonstrated to occur when weight gain is accompanied by an elevation in BP. Moreover, it has been demonstrated that baroreflex-sympathetic modulation is impaired in obese subjects, such that when obesity and hypertension exist in the same patient, there is a particularly striking impairment of a major mechanism that restrains SNS activity *(23)*. Central regulation of SNS activity is complex and involves a number of pathways and interconnections among several neurotransmitters and neuromodulators. The role of leptin on the activation of the central SNS has been the best studied. Other mediators of central SNS activation, whether acting through leptin or alone, include the hypothalamic melanocortin system through melanocortin receptor 3 and 4 agonists and corticotropin-releasing factor *(24,25)*.

The increase in arterial pressure in response to a high-fat diet is also associated with increased tubular sodium reabsorption and subsequent positive sodium balance. This is completely attenuated by bilateral renal denervation, suggesting the significant role of the renal sympathetic nervous system (RSNA) in the development of hypertension *(26)*. A progressively defective baroreflex control, causing sustained increases in RSNA, has also been shown to contribute to the development of hypertension *(26)*.

Kidneys

The kidney is an organ rich in structures vulnerable to the metabolic insults brought about by diabetes and obesity. Both diabetes and obesity are well-recognized causes of renal structural and hemodynamic changes that independently predispose individuals to hypertension and nephropathy.

RENAL STRUCTURAL CHANGES IN DIABETES AND OBESITY

Hypertension often antedates and contributes to the development of nephropathy in many diabetic individuals. Diabetic nephropathy, which occurs after 15 yr of diabetes in 33% of people with type 1 diabetes and one-fifth of people with type 2 diabetes, is an important contributor to hypertension in persons with diabetes *(27)*.

The changes in kidney structure caused by diabetes are specific, creating a pattern not seen in other renal diseases. Type 1 and 2 diabetes differ in the degree of functional change relative to the severity of structural lesions *(28)*. Microalbuminuric type 2 diabetic patients generally have normal glomerular structure and less severe glomerular lesions than microalbuminuric type 1 diabetic patients *(28)*. The earliest pathological change seen in patients with diabetes is an increase in the thickness of the glomerular basement membrane, followed by an increase in the mesangial matrix. These changes result in a general increase in glomerular volume. Increases in volume in this low-compliance capsule raise interstitial pressure, which slows intrarenal and tubular flow rate, leading to increased sodium reabsorption *(29)*. Feedback mechanisms are then activated (i.e., increased glomerular filtration rate [GFR], stimulation of renin–angiotensin system [RAS]) to overcome this *(30)*. This hyperfiltration eventually increases glomerular wall stress and in the presence of other risk factors provokes glomerulosclerosis and loss of functional nephrons. These mechanisms involve a complex interplay of mechanical forces, vasoactive substances, cytokines, and growth factors *(29)* that ultimately contribute to hypertension.

RENAL HEMODYNAMIC CHANGES IN DIABETES AND OBESITY

Obese persons require an increased arterial pressure to maintain sodium balance. They often have an inappropriately small natriuretic response to a saline load and intraglomerular pressure. There is a shift in the pressure–natriuresis curve toward a higher pressure, leading to hyperfiltration. In fact, the early glomerular hyperfiltration in obesity is often as great as observed in uncontrolled type 1 diabetes *(30)*.

The hypertension accompanying obesity is often a salt-sensitive type. This abnormal renal sodium handling is due to the result of the RSNA promoting tubular reabsorption *(26)*, RAS activation *(29)*, decreased circulating atrial natriuretic peptide (ANP) *(31)*, and hyperinsulinemia through direct actions on the renal tubule *(30)*.

RENIN–ANGIOTENSIN–ALDOSTERONE SYSTEM

Plasma renin activity is increased in many obese subjects despite marked salt retention and increased extracellular fluid volume. Plasma renin activity is increased, in part, to SNS activation and as a response to reduced sodium delivery to the macula densa *(29)*. Angiotensin II (Ang II) exerts autocrine, paracrine, and endocrine effects to stimulate sodium reabsorption and to shift pressure natriuresis *(29)*. Increased levels of Ang II also upregulate the expression of transforming growth factor-β1 (TGF-β1), tumor necrosis factor-α (TNF-α), vascular cell adhesion molecule-1, and nuclear factor-κB (NF-κB) *(32)*. Ang II signals through the Ang I (AT1) receptor, which results in vasoconstriction, stimulation of growth, and activation of fibroblasts and myocytes *(33,34)*. Ang II also stimulates the generation of reactive oxygen species (ROS), which is reversed by AT1 receptor blockade *(33,34)*. Moreover, the angiotensinogen gene, which provides the precursor to Ang II production, is stimulated by NF-κB *(33)* and TNF-α *(35)*, thereby creating a self-perpetuating cycle of upregulation and damage.

Aldosterone also appears to have effects on the brain, heart, vasculature, and kidneys that lead to elevated BP via genomic and nongenomic effects. These changes include enhanced SNS activity, reduced vascular compliance and endothelial-derived vasorelaxation, increases in volume expansion and reduced serum potassium, and increases in left ventricular mass and cardiac output *(36)*. Aldosterone has been shown to contribute to the development of nephrosclerosis and renal fibrosis in models of diabetes and hypertension *(36)*. In the deoxycortisone acetate salt hypertensive rat model, exogenous administration of mineralocorticoids induced lesions of malignant hypertension and stroke *(37)*, while receptor blockade reduced proteinuria and nephrosclerotic lesions *(38)*.

ENDOTHELIAL DYSFUNCTION IN DIABETES: ITS EFFECT ON KIDNEYS

Albuminuria is associated with an increase in mortality, mostly attributable to CVD *(15)*. It is thought that microalbuminuria is a marker of generalized endothelial damage in patients with diabetes. This may help explain why diabetic glomerulosclerosis parallels diabetic atherosclerosis.

There are several major hypotheses as to how hyperglycemia and other metabolic abnormalities cause diabetic nephropathy and hypertension. Increased activity of growth factors such as TGF-β, connective-tissue growth factor, and platelet-derived growth factor (PDGF) causes mesangial hypertrophy *(39)*. Hyperglycemia causes *de novo* synthesis of diacylglycerol, leading to elevated protein kinase C activity *(40)*, and subsequent activation of phospholipase A2 and increased arachidonic acid metabolite production, which then enhances vascular tone and permeability. Hyperglycemia also accelerates the formation of nonenzymatic advanced glycation end products (AGEs), which accumulate irreversibly in vascular tissue. AGEs form crosslinks and generate oxygen-derived free radicals *(40)*. Glycosylation of collagen results in increased rigidity and decreased responsiveness to collagenase *(41)*. Diabetes has been associated with an increased generation of ROS, which may impair endothelium-dependent vasodilatation through inactivation of nitric oxide (NO) *(40)*. Activation of the polyol pathway results in the formation of sorbitol through aldose reductase, a reaction that utilizes nicotinamide adenine dinucleotide phosphate required for the production of NO synthase (NOS), cytochrome P450, and glutathione reductase, all of which have antioxidant activities *(40)*. These metabolic and structural abnormalities may lead to increased vascular rigidity and decreased compliance, characteristics of the hypertension accompanying obesity and diabetes.

Natriuretic Peptide System

The natriuretic peptide system is a major regulator of body fluid volumes and arterial pressure through several actions, including enhancement of natriuresis, inhibition of the RAAS, direct vasodilation, and possible inhibitory effects on arginine vasopressin and on the SNS *(42)*. It consists of ANP, brain natriuretic peptide (BNP), and C-type natriuretic peptide (CNP), each encoded by a separate gene (Fig. 3). These peptides, specifically ANP, act by binding to specific natriuretic peptide receptors (NPrs), either coupled (NPr-A and NPr-B) or uncoupled (NPr-C) with guanylyl cyclase activity *(42)*. NPr-A mediates most of the known activities of ANP, and the binding of ANP to this receptor is followed by an increase in plasma levels and urinary excretion of cyclic guanosine 5′-monophosphate. NPr-C, on the other hand, appears to mediate the clearance of circulating natriuretic peptides and is therefore known as the "clearance" receptor *(42)*.

Human and rat adipose tissue contain very high levels of NPr-C mRNA *(43,44)*, suggesting an increased clearance of natriuretic peptides in obese individuals. Data from the Framingham cohort demonstrate the inverse relationship between BMI and plasma natriuretic peptide levels *(45)*. Plasma levels of ANP in obese hypertensive individuals are also reported to be lower than in obese normotensive individuals, with concomitant increases in the expression of the clearance receptor in the former *(46)*.

The role of the natriuretic peptide system in diabetes remains unclear. ANP levels are found to be lower in patients with type 2 diabetes mellitus despite normal extracellular fluid volume *(47)*. These levels rise as renal function worsens, leading to increased glomerular filtration pressure, and are thus thought to contribute to the development of hyperfiltration and proteinuria in diabetic nephropathy *(48)*. Type 2 diabetes mellitus, along with hypertension, has also been associated with elevated ANP levels in the presence of normal renal function and normal or decreased plasma renin and aldosterone levels. In this setting, ANP levels are found to rise in parallel with mean arterial BP,

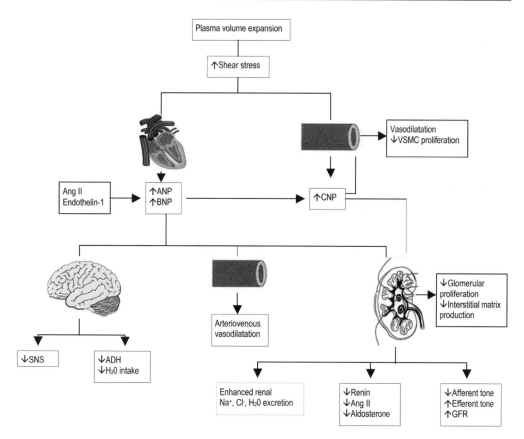

Fig. 3. Physiology of natriuretic peptides. ANP is synthesized in atrial myocytes and BNP in ventricular myocytes. CNP is synthesized in vascular endothelium. All are released in response to shear stress. ANP and BNP have endocrine effects via NPrs (NPr-A and NPr-B), while CNP largely acts via autocrine and paracrine effects. ADH, antidiuretic hormone. (Adapted from ref. *3*.)

suggesting a counterregulatory role *(42,48)*. Positive correlations between plasma levels of BNP and microalbuminuria, with significant correlations with albumin excretion rates, have also been found in patients with diabetes *(47)*. This infers that the elevated BNP levels are caused, in part, by the presence of nephropathy. In states of obesity, insulin resistance, and diabetes, there appears to be resistance to the action of natriuretic peptides *(42)*.

Endocrine System

ROLE OF INSULIN AND HYPERINSULINEMIA

Hyperinsulinemia accompanying insulin resistance has been debated as the link between obesity and hypertension. It is estimated that 40% of patients with essential hypertension have insulin resistance *(15)*. Several mechanisms may be responsible for the high prevalence of insulin resistance in patients with essential hypertension. Hyperinsulinemia/insulin resistance has been shown to increase renal tubular sodium reabsorption *(49)*, tissue renin–angiotensin–aldosterone system (RAAS) activation *(49)*, and SNS activation *(50)*. It also causes an elevation in intracellular calcium concentration in vascular smooth muscle cells (VSMCs), leading to vasoconstriction *(51)*, and causes proliferation of VSMCs and cardiac myocyte growth, leading to arteriolar narrowing and cardiac hypertrophy *(51)*. Associations between insulin concentration and hypertension have often been confounded by age and obesity *(52)*. The distinction between hyperinsulinemia and insulin resistance is also important to make. Administration of insulin in healthy nonobese, normotensive subjects induces vasodilatation and results in lowering of BP. These effects are blunted in obese, insulin-resistant hypertensive individuals *(53)*.

CORTISOL

Cushing's syndrome is associated with the development of metabolic syndrome, and even subtle degrees of cortisol excess demonstrated in patients with adrenal incidentalomas have been associated with increases in SBP and DBP and reduced insulin sensitivity when compared with control subjects *(54)*. Furthermore, patients with both overt and subclinical Cushing's syndrome have been demonstrated to have an increased risk of CVD *(55)*. Some variants of the glucocorticoid receptor gene *(GRL)* locus, *Bcl*I restriction fragment length polymorphism, have also been associated with an elevated BMI, abdominal obesity, increased leptin, and increased SBP *(56)*.

The hormone 11β-hydroxysteroid dehydrogenase (11β-HSD) may play an important role in linking obesity to hypertension. 11β-HSD1 regenerates active cortisol from inactive 11-keto forms. Transgenic mice, that have a relative amplification of 11β-HSD1 in white adipose tissue develop arterial hypertension, visceral obesity, diabetes, dyslipidemia, and insulin resistance *(57)*. These mice are salt sensitive and have elevated levels of angiotensinogen, Ang II, and aldosterone, causing hypertension that is attenuated by AT1 receptor antagonism. Thus, overexpression of 11β-HSD1 produces a salt-sensitive hypertension that is RAAS mediated. This hypertension is reflected by an appreciable hypertrophy and hyperplasia of the renal distal tubules, consistent with changes from chronic hypertension *(58)*. On the other hand, 11β-HSD1 deficiency, as demonstrated in 11β-HSD1 null mice, has been shown to alter beneficially adipose tissue distribution and function, improve insulin sensitivity, reduce lipolysis, and counteract the accumulation of visceral fat and its related metabolic abnormalities *(59)*. Furthermore, corticotropin-releasing hormone receptor (CRH-R) types 1 and 2 have been isolated in human adipose tissue *(60)*. These regulate adipocyte metabolism by downregulating 11β-HSD *(61)*.

THE ADIPOCYTE AND ITS ROLE IN DIABETES AND HYPERTENSION

The adipocyte has been increasingly recognized in recent years as an important organ that secretes a number of hormones and adipose-specific cytokines, termed *adipokines*, that mediate important homeostatic pathways involved in metabolism and are linked to hypertension (Fig. 4). Visceral fat accumulation is characterized by progressive infiltration of macrophages *(62)*, which then secrete several proinflammatory cytokines: TNF-α, interleukin-6 (IL-6), IL-1-β. Along with insulin resistance, obesity is increasingly being recognized as a chronic, low-level, inflammatory state that leads to hypertension; metabolic derangements; and, ultimately, coronary heart disease *(30,63)*. C-reactive protein (CRP), a predictor of CVD events in previous reports, is independently related to insulin sensitivity in nondiabetic insulin-resistant individuals *(64)*. A strong association likewise exists between CRP and BMI/waist circumference *(64)*. Abnormalities in humoral and cellular immunity and the complement system have also been implicated in the development of hypertension *(63)*. Whether these cytokines are produced as a result of ongoing atherosclerosis or insulin resistance or whether they

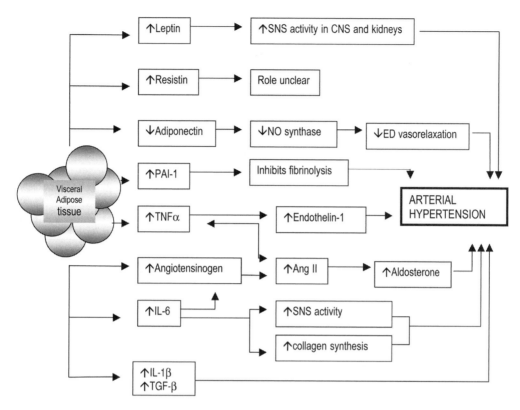

Fig. 4. Proposed role of adipose tissue in inflammatory mechanisms leading to hypertension. (Adapted from refs. *1*, *31*, and *42*.)

are primary occurrences in the cascade of events is still unclear and needs to be carefully studied.

Leptin. Leptin is a 167-amino acid protein that is expressed and secreted exclusively from adipocytes. It is mainly involved in the regulation of appetite, energy expenditure, and body weight *(65)*. Aside from the regulation of food intake, leptin has been shown to cause dose-dependent increases in SNS activity in brown adipose tissue, kidney, and adrenal gland in rats *(65)*. Leptin does not cause sympathoactivation in obese Zucker rats, which are known to possess a mutation in the gene for the leptin receptor. This suggests that the sympathetic action of leptin requires the presence of an intact leptin receptor. Central administration of leptin also increases catecholamine secretion, suggesting functions that are mediated by the central nervous system (CNS). Transgenic mice overexpressing leptin have elevated BP and urinary catecholamine levels that are abrogated by α1-adrenergic, sympathetic ganglionic, and nonselective β-adrenergic blockers *(66)*. Furthermore, peripheral leptin receptors are known to exist in vascular endothelial cells and the adrenal medulla, which may, in part, mediate leptin's hypertensive effects *(66)*.

Resistin. Resistin is a 17.5-kDa cysteine-rich protein molecule that is secreted during adipogenesis. It has been proposed to be the link between obesity and insulin resistance. Serum levels of resistin were found to be elevated in diet-induced and genetically obese mice, because they gain weight and develop insulin resistance *(67)*. However, human studies have provided conflicting results. Recent investigations on the role of resistin in the development of hypertension have been in the context of insulin resistance (68,69). A direct relationship between resistin and hypertension has not been elucidated and remains an area that requires further investigation.

Adiponectin. Adiponectin is a 244-amino acid protein that is the gene product of the adipose most abundant gene transcript-1 (apM1) and is secreted exclusively by adipocytes. Plasma adiponectin levels are negatively correlated with insulin sensitivity and fasting insulinemia, more closely than adiposity and glycemia (70). Adiponectin has also been found to be a modulator of vascular remodeling, attenuating the excessive inflammatory response in the vascular wall. Adiponectin-knockout (KO) mice have been found to have significantly reduced acetylcholine-induced vasorelaxation compared with controls (71). When fed a high-fat/high-sucrose/high-salt diet, body weight and SBP are significantly higher in adiponectin-KO mice compared with wild-type (WT) mice (71). In healthy nondiabetic individuals, adiponectin levels are independently associated with endothelium-dependent vasodilatation (72) and endothelium-independent vasodilatation (73). This association has been found to be weaker in patients with diabetes (72), suggesting a multifactorial etiology for endothelial dysfunction. It is also proposed that adiponectin may have direct vascular effects. Plasma adiponectin has been shown to accumulate rapidly in the subendothelial space of the injured human artery (74). Adiponectin also stimulates the phosphorylation and activation of endothelial NOS via phosphatidylinositol-3-kinase-dependent pathways in vascular endothelial cells (75).

Initial human studies on the direct relationship between adiponectin levels and essential hypertension were inconsistent, and oftentimes studied in the context of adiponectin's relationship to insulin sensitivity (76–78). Recent studies show that hypoadiponectinemia is an independent risk factor for hypertension (79). Plasma adiponectin levels are also significantly decreased with increases in BP, even in normotensive individuals without insulin resistance or diabetes (79).

Pasminogen Activator Inhibitor-1. Plasminogen activator inhibitor-1 (PAI-1) is a key regulator of fibrinolysis by inhibiting tissue plasminogen activator (80). PAI-1 is overexpressed in the adipose tissue of obese mice and humans (81). Along with CRP, elevated PAI-1 levels are independently associated with the development of type 2 diabetes in obese subjects (82).

PAI-1 is induced both in vitro and in vivo by Ang II via the AT1 receptor (83,84). Obesity results in increased activity and expression of the RAAS in adipocytes, which further upregulates PAI-1 expression (85). Compared with WT mice, high-fat diet-induced obesity, hyperglycemia, and hyperinsulinemia have been prevented in mice lacking PAI-1 (86). Obesity and insulin resistance are also attenuated by inhibition of angiotensin in WT controls, suggesting interactions of angiotensin and PAI-1 in both obesity and insulin resistance (86).

Tumor Necrosis Factor-α. TNF-α is another inflammatory adipocytokine that is implicated in the pathogenesis of insulin resistance. Genetically obese rodents are found to express a higher level of TNF-α in their adipose tissue (87). TNF-α levels are also positively correlated with BMI in humans up to a BMI of 45 kg/m^2, and levels are decreased with weight loss (88).

The independent role of TNF-α in hypertension has not been studied as extensively as in obesity and insulin resistance. TNF-α is known to increase endothelin-1 (ET-1) (89) and Ang II (90). Its production is, in turn, stimulated by Ang II (90). TNF-α production by the thick ascending tubule of the renal medulla has been found to be elevated in Ang II-dependent hypertensive rats.

Candidate gene investigations in hypertensive pedigrees of French-Canadian origin have also shown that the TNF-α gene locus contributes to the determination of obesity and obesity-associated hypertension *(91)*. A positive and independent correlation between TNF-α levels and SBP has been demonstrated in a Canadian cohort, paralleling the positive correlation of TNF-α and insulin resistance. Stable TNF receptor fractions (sTNFR1 and sTNFR2), which are proteolytically cleaved with TNF-α binding, have also been used as indicators of TNF-α activation. The ratio of these soluble receptors is positively correlated with SBP and DBP *(92)* and is significantly greater in patients with type 2 diabetes than in patients with type 1 diabetes and in control subjects *(63)*. Thus, enhanced TNF-α activation may contribute to the link among obesity, insulin resistance, and hypertension.

Interleukin-6. IL-6 is a multifunctional cytokine produced by immune cells, endothelial cells, fibroblasts, myocytes, and adipose tissue *(63)*. It is considered a major regulator in the production of acute-phase reactants, such as CRP, PAI-1, and fibrinogen, in the liver *(30)*.

Omental adipose tissue produces threefold more IL-6 than sc adipose tissue *(93)*. Mechanisms of action include SNS activation, increased collagen synthesis, and increased angiotensinogen expression, leading to hypertension. A positive association between different measures of obesity and plasma IL-6 levels has been described in men and postmenopausal women *(94,95)*. Studies relating hypertension and insulin resistance to IL-6 levels have yielded discordant results, with positive associations with hypertension observed in postmenopausal women *(95,96)* and with insulin resistance observed in men *(96)*. A polymorphism in the promoter region of the IL-6 gene has also been found to show divergent associations with BP *(97,98)*.

Cardiovascular System

Cardiac Muscle: Adaptations to Obesity and Hypertension

Obesity, and its resulting hypertension, have been shown to cause early intrinsic functional changes and long-term structural changes in the heart *(99)*. Diet-induced obese and hypertensive dogs have been found to express certain cardiac genes in both the atria and ventricles, which are known to be involved in multiple cell functions. These include extracellular matrix (ECM) remodeling, cytoskeletal, nuclear and sarcolemmal structural processes, energy metabolism, ionic flux, cell proliferation, stress response, and signal transduction, that eventually lead to left ventricular hypertrophy (LVH) *(99)*. Obese hypertensive rabbits have been found to have a reduced cardiac contractile response to β-stimulation using isoproterenol, and reduced diastolic compliance *(100)*. These findings link obesity and hypertension to both systolic and diastolic dysfunction.

Postmortem studies in healthy normotensive women demonstrate an increase in heart weight indexed to height (heart weight/height—g/m^2) over increasing tertiles of BMI and waist-to-hip ratio *(101)*. In the absence of hypertension, the obese heart is subject to chronic volume overload owing to an elevated cardiac output, resulting in left ventricular dilatation and an eccentric pattern of LVH *(102)*. Both concentric and eccentric LVH have been shown to increase the risk of systolic as well as diastolic dysfunction of the heart *(103)*. Obesity has been identified as an independent predictor of left ventricular diastolic dysfunction and symptomatic heart failure *(104)*. LVH in itself is a major CVD risk factor independent of both SBP and DBP *(105)*. Obesity is associated with an increased resting heart rate and with decreased heart rate variability *(106)*, a prognostic indicator of increased mortality *(107)*.

VASCULAR SYSTEM

Arterial stiffening occurs with aging and also results in higher SBP and widened pulse pressure. Accelerated arterial stiffness has been linked to diabetes, insulin resistance, and obesity *(15)*. Investigators have demonstrated consistent associations of arterial stiffness with visceral adiposity across all tertiles of body weight *(108)*.

Endothelial Dysfunction in Obesity and Diabetes. The hemodynamic changes that occur in hypertension, obesity, and diabetes are complicated further by the presence of endothelial dysfunction. The endothelium regulates vascular tone by releasing vasoactive substances such as ET-1 and NO. Both ET-1 and NO also have effects beyond their contributions to the regulation of vascular tone through the modulation of platelet activity, lipid oxidation, leukocyte chemotaxis, and local production of thrombotic factors as well as the growth and proliferation of VSMCs and mural fibroblasts. Imbalances in the actions of NO and ET-1 are therefore of potential importance beyond the acute regulation of vascular tone *(109)*.

Role of ET-1. The ETs are potent 21 amino acid vasoactive peptides that are produced by endothelial cells, smooth muscle cells of blood vessels, and adventitial fibroblasts and cardiomyocytes. ET-1 stimulates the production of growth factors such as vascular endothelial growth factor and basic fibroblast growth factor and potentiates the effects of TGF-β and PDGF *(110)*. Chronic ET-1 stimulation can result in myocardial fibrosis and hypertrophy and vascular fibrosis with ECM proliferation. ET-1 works through G protein-coupled ET receptors, ET_A and ET_B, on endothelial cells and smooth muscle cells (SMCs). ET_A receptors induce vasoconstriction, cellular proliferation, and cell hypertrophy by increasing intracellular calcium *(110)*. Endothelial ET_B receptors stimulate the production of NO and prostacyclin, eliciting vasorelaxation. The predominant physiological action varies in the different vascular beds. ET_A receptors are found in the medial smooth muscle layers of the blood vessels, and atrial and ventricular myocardium. ET_B receptors are localized on endothelial cells, SMCs, and macrophages. In normal states, the vasoconstrictive actions of the ET_A receptors are opposed by ET_B receptors. However, in pathological states, there could be upregulation of the ET_B receptors located on SMCs that function similarly to the ET_A receptors, which amplify the vasoconstrictive and mitogenic effects of ET-1 *(111)*. Wall stretch, ischemia, Ang II, low-density lipoprotein, thrombin, and glucose stimulate ET-1's production, whereas NO, prostacyclin, ANPs, and estrogens inhibit it *(110)*.

Plasma ET levels are usually normal in essential hypertension. Individuals who have hyperinsulinemic insulin resistance have relatively elevated circulating levels of ET-1 *(109)*. Both obese persons and those with type 2 diabetes have similar but greater effects of ET-1 blockade when compared with healthy control subjects, suggesting increased contributions of ET-1 to vasoconstrictor tone *(109)*. In subsequent studies, ET_A receptor blockade resulted in significant vasodilation in overweight and obese but not in lean hypertensive subjects or normotensive control subjects, suggesting a selective enhancement of ET_A-dependent vasoconstrictor tone in hypertensive patients with increased BMI *(112)*.

Role of NO. NO release from the endothelium plays an important role in the regulation of vascular tone, inhibition of both platelet and leukocyte aggregation and adhesion, and inhibition of cell proliferation. Obesity and diabetes have been independently found to affect several transcriptional and posttranscriptional regulatory pathways involved in the generation of NO. It is speculated that both calcium-dependent and -independent NO production is probably abnormal in the obese *(113)*. An increase in blood flow into the leg in response to methacholine, a muscarinic agent, is blunted in obese humans, with the degree of dilatation being inversely proportional to the degree of obesity *(114)*. There is reduced NO-dependent dilatation in patients with the metabolic syndrome, in those with impaired glucose tolerance, and in first-degree relatives of patients with diabetes *(115)*.

GENETICS

Hypertension is a complex multifactorial and polygenic disorder that results from an interaction between an individual's genetic background and various environmental factors *(116)*. An individual's capacity for a BP response to obesity might be modified by this complex interaction. The hypertensive effect of obesity is less in Pima Indians, Hispanic Americans, and African Americans than it is in Caucasians *(117)*. Even among Caucasians, not all obese individuals are hypertensive. Various gene candidate and genetic linkage studies have identified several polymorphisms in several substances that have been associated with the development of hypertension. These studies have been limited by size and ethnic variation. A large-scale association study in 1940 unrelated Japanese individuals found that two genetic polymorphisms (825CT in the G protein β3 subunit gene and 190GA in the CC chemokine receptor 2 gene) were significantly associated with hypertension in men, and one polymorphism (–238GA in the TNF gene) was significantly associated in women *(118)*. CC chemokine receptor 2 is a receptor for monocyte chemoattractant protein-1 (MCP-1) and closely related proteins (MCP-2, -3, -4, and -5), both implicated in the development of coronary artery disease (CAD) *(118)*.

TREATMENT OF HYPERTENSION IN OBESE PATIENTS WITH DIABETES

Initial evaluation of a hypertensive patient with diabetes should include a careful history and physical examination, focusing on his or her overall cardiovascular risk *(15)*. The degree of glucose control, presence of microvascular and macrovascular complications, and existence of end-organ damage from hypertension should be emphasized. A search for secondary causes of hypertension should also be part of a good history. Physical examination should focus on measuring BP in an appropriate manner, along with obtaining a BMI measurement, examining optic fundi, performing auscultation of the lungs and heart, palpating of the abdomen for bruits, and evaluating the extremities for edema and reductions in pedal pulse. Laboratory evaluation should include a complete blood count, as well as serum magnesium, potassium, calcium, blood urea nitrogen, creatinine, and uric acid levels. A fasting blood glucose, glycosylated hemoglobin (HbA1c), fasting lipid profile, as well as urinalysis should be obtained.

Several nonpharmacological and pharmacological modalities are available for the treatment and prevention of hypertension in the obese diabetic, which are discussed next.

Nonpharmacological Treatment

Nonpharmacological modalities should be emphasized to patients when they first present to the physician. Weight reduction, increased physical activity, and diet and lifestyle changes have been shown to provide benefit in ameliorating hypertension in the obese with diabetes.

EVIDENCE FOR BENEFIT OF WEIGHT LOSS ON HYPERTENSION

The Swedish Obese Subjects study is, to date, the largest prospective intervention study comparing the development of CVD risk factors in obese patients treated with gastric surgery vs matched severely obese control patients over a 10-yr period. A 23% maintained weight reduction for 2 yr resulted in a 2.5-fold reduction in the incidence of hypertension and a 32-fold reduction in the incidence of noninsulin-dependent diabetes mellitus *(119)*.

The effects of weight loss are also greatly limited by the fact that long-term nonsurgical results of weight loss are disappointing, with most people regaining most of the weight initially lost. Patients in weight-loss programs averaging 6 mo to 1 yr can achieve an average weight loss of 8% of baseline weight *(120)*. Several studies have therefore concentrated on the effects of modest weight loss on hypertension and risk of CVD.

The Trial of Antihypertensive Interventions and Management showed that a weight loss of 4.5 kg or more, equivalent to approx 5% of baseline weight, lowered DBP to the same extent as a single dose of antihypertensive medication *(121)*. Several studies have shown that a modest weight loss can lower or even discontinue the need for antihypertensive medication *(121)*. A weight loss ranging from 3.5 to 4.5 kg, or 4.1 to 5.8% of baseline body weight, achieved through diet and lifestyle change, significantly reduced the incidence and risk of hypertension *(122,123)*.

EVIDENCE FOR BENEFIT OF PHYSICAL ACTIVITY ON HYPERTENSION

Several clinical studies and cross-sectional studies have indicated that physical activity or aerobic exercise is inversely associated with BP *(124)*. Prospective studies have demonstrated that regular physical activity is associated with a significantly reduced risk of hypertension in men and women independent of age, education, smoking habits, alcohol intake, history of diabetes, BMI, and SBP at baseline *(125)*. The protective effect of physical activity is also consistent in both overweight and normal-weight subjects *(125)*. It has been hypothesized that increasing physical activity might reduce BP through decreased body weight or favorable changes in body fat distribution.

The Finnish Diabetes Prevention Study showed that overweight subjects with glucose intolerance who received intensified lifestyle intervention, which consisted of diet and moderate exercise for at least 30 min/d, resulted not only in a marked reduction in the risk of developing type 2 diabetes, but also in a significant drop in BP (4 mmHg for SBP and 2 mmHg for DBP compared with control subjects) *(126)*.

EVIDENCE FOR BENEFIT OF DIET ON HYPERTENSION

The Dietary Approaches to Stop Hypertension (DASH), a diet regimen rich in fruits and vegetables, and low-fat dairy products, has been proven to significantly reduce BP, and significantly more so in hypertensive individuals than in normotensive individuals *(127)*. Studies on the effects of the DASH diet on the pressure–natriuresis curve show that this diet lowers BP through a natriuretic/diuretic action *(128)*. These results emphasize the role of dietary interventions for the treatment of hypertension.

Because obesity hypertension is considered a salt-sensitive form of hypertension, sodium restriction has been a proposed treatment strategy. Some studies have shown a modest effect *(129)*, whereas others have observed dramatic reductions in BP *(130)*.

Pharmacological Treatment

To date, only a few randomized controlled trials have been conducted to address specifically pharmacological treatment in the obese population *(131,132)*. However, large randomized controlled trials have been conducted on hypertension in diabetic populations. The choice of pharmacological agents to treat obese patients with hypertension and diabetes has to take into account the effects on body weight, metabolic disturbances, and complications of diabetes and/or hypertension.

Major multicenter randomized controlled trials have proven the overwhelming benefits of good BP control in reducing CVD events *(133)*. The United Kingdom Prospective Diabetes Study (UKPDS) demonstrated a 24% reduction in diabetes-related end points, including micro- and macrovascular disease, in patients with tight BP control (<150/85 mmHg) vs less-tight control (<180/105 mmHg) *(134)*. The Hypertension Optimal Trial (HOT) found a 51% risk reduction in CVD events in individuals whose DBP was treated to <80 mmHg compared with those whose target was <90 mmHg *(135)*. The Seventh Report of the Joint National Committee on Prevention, Detection, Evaluation, and Treatment of High Blood Pressure (JNC VII) recommends a BP goal of <130/80 mmHg among individuals with diabetes *(5)*.

THIAZIDE DIURETICS

The Systolic Hypertension in the Elderly Program trial showed that chlorthalidone therapy (12.5–25 mg) was twice as effective in individuals with diabetes as in those without diabetes in reducing major CVD events *(136)*. The Antihypertensive and Lipid-Lowering Treatment to Prevent Heart Attack Trial (ALLHAT) of 33,357 hypertensive individuals, 36% of whom were diabetic, concluded that neither calcium channel blockers nor angiotensin-converting enzyme (ACE) inhibitors were superior to diuretics (chlorthalidone) in preventing major coronary events or in increasing survival *(133)*.

Early studies have shown that obese elderly patients with hypertension who required treatment with diuretics and β-blockers had a greater risk of developing type 2 diabetes than those who had normal BP *(137)*. ALLHAT also demonstrated a higher incidence of new diabetes in the chlorthalidone group compared with either the amlodipine or lisinopril groups *(133)*. The results on previous studies have not demonstrated any excess diabetogenic effects of thiazide diuretics *(138,140,141)*. A recent prospective study in a relatively large group of hypertensive patients (median follow-up period of 6 yr) demonstrated that baseline levels of plasma glucose and the use of diuretics (chlorthalidone or hydrochlorthiazide 12.5–25 mg daily) not only independently predicted the development of new-onset diabetes,but also carried a risk of subsequent CVD events similar to that for those who already had diabetes and hypertension at the onset of the study *(142)*. These data suggest that diuretics along with β-blockers need to be started cautiously in hypertensive patients who have impaired fasting glucose (≥100 mg/dL) *(143)*.

ACE INHIBITORS AND ANGIOTENSIN II RECEPTOR BLOCKERS

The JNC VII recommends that ACE inhibitor- or angiotensin receptor blocker (ARB)–based treatments have the added benefit of favorably affecting the progression of diabetic nephropathy and reducing albuminuria *(5)*. This recommendation is based on results of controlled clinical trials.

In the Heart Outcomes Prevention Evaluation (HOPE) trial, the use of ramipril in patients with diabetes lowered the risk of combined primary outcomes by 25%, myocardial infarction (MI) by 22%, stroke by 33%, CVD death by 37%, total mortality by 24%, and overt nephropathy by 24% *(144)*. All these were independent of the observed effects in BP *(144)*. Furthermore, there was a 30% decrease in the rate of development of diabetes *(144)*. The MICRO-HOPE study found that an ACE inhibitor provided protection against CVD events and attenuated the increase in proteinuria in patients with type 2 diabetes with microalbuminuria *(145)*.

ARBs have also been well documented to confer renoprotection in hypertensive patients with type 2 diabetes. The Reduction of Endpoints in NIDDM with the Angiotensin II Antagonist Losartan Study *(146)* and Irbesartan in Diabetic Nephropathy Trial *(147)* established reduction in proteinuria and renoprotection in patients with type 2 diabetes with microalbuminuria or nephropathy, independent of BP lowering. In multiple clinical trials, ARBs have also been shown to reduce the risk of new-onset diabetes. In the LIFE trial, a 25% reduction in the risk of new-onset diabetes was observed in the losartan group compared to β-blocker-based therapy *(148)*. The Study of Cognition and Prognosis in the Elderly trial with candesartan also showed a similar result *(149)*. The Candesartan in Heart Failure Assessment of Reduction in Mortality and Morbidity trial reported a 22% reduction in the risk of new-onset diabetes in patients with heart failure *(150)*. The recently concluded Valsartan Antihypertensive Long-Term Use Evaluation trial, although showing no significant difference in the primary end points in patients treated with valsartan vs those treated with amlodipine, also showed a significant (23%) risk reduction in new-onset diabetes *(151)*.

CALCIUM CHANNEL BLOCKERS

Calcium channel blockers are very efficacious in lowering BP and are metabolically neutral for glucose and lipid profiles *(152)*. Seventy-eight percent of patients in the HOT trial were taking felodipine, a long-acting dihydropyridine, along with an ACE inhibitor (41%) and β-blocker (28%) *(135)*.

The placebo-controlled Systolic Hypertension in Europe Trial analyzed the effect of nitrendipine in systolic hypertension in the elderly. Patients with diabetes comprised 10% of the total patients studied, and BP was lower in the nitrendipine group than in the placebo group. Nitrendipine reduced CVD events by 69%, CVD mortality by 76%, and overall mortality by 55%. These reductions were greater than those observed in the patients without diabetes *(153)*.

β-BLOCKERS

The use of β-blockers has generally been avoided as a first-line agent in patients with type 2 diabetes mellitus. In a large prospective cohort of 12,550 nondiabetic adults, it was found that hypertensive patients who were taking β-blockers had a 28% higher risk of diabetes than those taking no medication. Potential mechanisms by which β-blockers may contribute to the development of diabetes include weight gain, attenuation of the β-receptor-mediated release of insulin from pancreatic β-cells, and decreased blood flow through the microcirculation in skeletal muscle tissue, leading to decreased insulin sensitivity *(141)*. However, it is of note that in the UKPDS, despite being associated with greater weight gain, atenolol was as effective as captopril in protecting against vascular disease *(134)*. Carvedilol, a nonselective β-blocker, has been shown to reduce CVD mortality and microalbuminuria without adversely affecting glucose or lipid profiles *(154)*. β-Blockers have an important therapeutic role in patients with hypertension who have known CAD and in hypertensive patients who have diabetes, a population in which the prevalence of underlying coronary disease is very high.

ORAL DIABETIC AGENTS

Metformin, acarbose, and thiazolidinediones (TZDs) are diabetic oral agents that have been found to improve insulin sensitivity and lower BP *(155,156)*. Metformin has been found to produce a favorable CVD profile and to lower BP in a cohort of obese, hypertensive, nondiabetic women *(155)*. The mechanism that leads to BP lowering was initially attributed to the improvement in insulin sensitivity *(157)*. However, subsequent studies have proposed direct beneficial effects of metformin on decreasing intracellular calcium transients in the vascular smooth muscle *(158)* and inhibitory effects on the SNS *(159)*.

In the Study to Prevent Non-Insulin-Dependent Diabetes Mellitus (STOP-NIDOM) trial, acarbose was found to reduce significantly reduce the risk of new hypertension (>140/90 mmHg), MI and CVD events in patients with impaired glucose tolerance *(160)*. Acarbose was also associated with a small reduction in weight. However, this drug is poorly tolerated, mostly owing to gastrointestinal (GI) side effects, thereby limiting its use.

TZDs, high-affinity peroxisome proliferator-activated receptor γ (PPARγ) ligands, are known to improve insulin sensitivity and to lower BP in a variety of hypertensive animal models as well as in diabetic and nondiabetic hypertensive humans *(161)*. The mechanisms underlying their antihypertensive effects are not known. Recent studies have proposed that TZDs (pioglitazone) prevent hypertension by reducing free radical production and increasing NO production and availability *(161)*. Rosiglitazone has also been found to restore the function of dopamine D1A receptors in the proximal tubules of obese Zucker rats, increasing sodium excretion *(162)*. Unfortunately, TZDs also promote adipogenesis *(163)* and can cause increased adiposity both in animal models of insulin resistance and in humans with type 2 diabetes *(163)*. They are known to cause plasma volume expansion, leading to hemodilution and edema *(163)*. Caution is warranted against the use of these agents in patients who may have early underlying heart disease, as can exist in a large percentage of the diabetic population. In the studies by Dobrion et al. *(161)* and Trivedi et al. *(162)*, however, the antihypertensive effects of the occurred even with significant weight gain. Current work is focused on partial agonists to the PPARγ receptor that will differentially improve insulin resistance, yet curb weight gain and adiposity *(164)*.

WEIGHT LOSS AGENTS

Orlistat and sibutramine are two pharmacological agents that have been shown to result in a 5–10% sustained weight loss for up to a period of 2 yr *(165)*. Orlistat is a GI lipase inhibitor that reduces enteral fat absorption by about 30%. Reductions in BP and heart rate for a given weight achieved with orlistat treatment are similar to those expected with weight loss from lifestyle intervention *(165)*. Sibutramine, a serotonin- and norepinephrine-uptake inhibitor, leads to weight loss by reducing hunger and enhancing satiety. Increases in BP and heart rate judged to be clinically significant were reported in 1–3% of participants in clinical trials. However, weight loss is associated with a modest reduction in BP both in normotensive patients and in treated hypertensive patients. In general, the reduction in BP with sibutramine was about half of what might be expected for a given degree of weight loss *(165)*. Obese and hypertensive patients who were well controlled on an ACE inhibitor with or without a diuretic lost 5–10% of their body weight on sibutramine without significantly affecting their BP control *(166)*. This suggests that sibutramine is safe to use in obese patients with well-controlled hypertension. However, extreme caution should be exercised in those who have untreated or uncontrolled hypertension.

REFERENCES

1. Calle EE, Thun MJ, Petrelli JM, Rodriguez C, Heath CS. Body mass index and mortality in a prospective cohort of US adults. N Engl J Med 1999;341:1097–1105.
2. Fontaine KR, Redden DT, Wang C, Westfall AO, Allison DB. Years of life lost due to obesity. JAMA 2003;289(2):187–193.
3. National Center for Health Statistics. Healthy People 2010, Diabetes Progress Review. www.cdc.gov/nchs/hphome.htm. December 18, 2002.
4. Hogan P, Dall T, Nikolov P, American Diabetes Association. Economic costs of diabetes in the US in 2002. Diabetes Care 2003;26:917–932.
5. Chobanian AV, Bakris GL, Black HR, et al. The Seventh Report of the Joint National Committee on Prevention, Detection, Evaluation, and Treatment of High Blood Pressure: the JNC 7 Report. JAMA 2003;289(19):2560–2572.
6. Stamler R, Stamler J, Riedlinger WF, Algera G, Roberts RH. Weight and blood pressure: findings in hypertension screening of 1 million Americans. JAMA 1978;240:1607–1610.
7. Must A, Spadano J, Coakley EH, Field AE, Colditz G, Dietz WH. The disease burden associated with overweight and obesity. JAMA 1999;282(16):1523–1529.
8. Weiss R, Dziura J, Burgert TS, et al. Obesity and the metabolic syndrome in children and adolescents. N Engl J Med 2004;350:2362–2374.
9. Vasan RS, Larson MG, Leip EP, Kannel WB, Levy D. Assessment of frequency of progression to hypertension in non-hypertensive participants in the Framingham Heart Study: a cohort study. Lancet 2001;358:1682–1686.
10. Engeli S, Sharma AM. Emerging concepts in the pathophysiology and treatment of obesity-associated hypertension. Curr Opin Cardiol 2002;17:355–359.
11. Davy KP, Hall JE. Obesity and hypertension: two epidemics or one? Am J Physiol Regul Integr Comp Physiol 2004;286:R803–R813.
12. Hayashi T, Boyko EJ, Leonetti DL, et al. Visceral adiposity is an independent predictor of incident hypertension in Japanese Americans. Ann Intern Med 2004;140(12):992–1000.
13. Doll S, Paccaud F, Bovet P, et al. Body mass index, abdominal adiposity and blood pressure: consistency of their association across developing and developed countries. Int J Obes 2002;26:48–57.
14. Felber JP, Golay A. Pathways from obesity to diabetes. Int J Obes 2002;26(Suppl 2):S39–S45.
15. Sowers JR, Haffner S. Treatment of cardiovascular and renal risk factors in the diabetic hypertensive. Hypertension 2002;40:781–788.
16. Gress TW, Nieto FJ, Shahar E, Wofford MR, Brancati FL. Hypertension and antihypertensive therapy as risk factors for type 2 diabetes mellitus: Atherosclerosis Risk in Communities Study. N Engl J Med 2000;342:905–912.
17. Alexander CM, Landsman PB, Teutsch SM, Haffner SM. NCEP-defined metabolic syndrome, diabetes, and prevalence of coronary heart disease among NHANES III participants age 50 years and older. Diabetes 2003;52:1210–1214.
18. Expert Panel on Detection, Evaluation, and Treatment of High Blood Cholesterol in Adults. Executive summary of the third report of the National Cholesterol Education Program (NCEP) expert panel on detection, evaluation, and treatment of high blood cholesterol in adults (Adult Treatment Panel III). JAMA 2001;285:2486–2497.
19. Henry P, Thomas F, Benetos A, Guize L. Impaired fasting glucose, blood pressure and cardiovascular disease mortality. Hypertension 2002;40(4):458–463.
20. Seals DR, Bell C. Chronic sympathetic activation. Diabetes 2004;53(2):276–284.
21. Grassi G, Seravalle G, Cattaneo BM, et al. Sympathetic activation in obese normotensive subjects. Hypertension 1995;25:560–563.
22. Lohmeier TE, Warren S, Cunningham JT. Sustained activation of the central baroreceptor pathway in obesity hypertension. Hypertension 2003;42:96–102.
23. Grassi G, Seravalle G, Dell'Oro R, Turri C, Bolla GB, Mancia G. Adrenergic and reflex abnormalities in obesity-related hypertension. Hypertension 2000;36:538–542.
24. Kuo JJ, Da Silva AA, Tallam AS, Hall JE. Role of adrenergic activity in pressor responses to chronic melanocortin receptor activation. Hypertension 2004;43(Pt 2):370–375.
25. Correia MLG, Morgan DA, Mitchell JL, Sivitz WI, Mark AL, Haynes WG. Role of corticotrophin-releasing factor in effects of leptin on sympathetic nerve activity and arterial pressure. Hypertension 2001;38:384–388.
26. DiBona GF. The sympathetic nervous system and hypertension: recent developments. Hypertension 2004;43:147.

27. Sowers JR, Epstein M. Diabetes mellitus and associated hypertension, vascular disease and nephropathy. Hypertension 1995;26:869–879.
28. Caramori ML, Mauer M. Diabetes and nephropathy. Curr Opin Nephrol Hypertens 2003; 12:273–282.
29. Hall JE, Brands MW, Henegar Jr. Mechanisms of hypertension and kidney disease in obesity. Ann NY Acad Sci 1999;892:91–107.
30. El-Atat F, Aneja A, Mcfarlane S, Sowers J. Obesity and hypertension. Endocrinol Metab Clin North Am 2003;32:823–854.
31. Montani JP, Antic V, Yang Z, Abdul D. Pathways from obesity to hypertension: from the perspective of a vicious triangle. Int J Obes 2002;26(Suppl 2):S28–S38.
32. Klahr S, Morrissey JJ. Angiotensin II and gene expression in the kidney. Am J Kidney Dis 1998;31:171–176.
33. Klahr S, Morrissey JJ. The role of vasoactive compounds, growth factors and cytokines in the progression of renal disease. Kidney Int 2000;57(Suppl 75):S7–S14.
34. Sowers JR. Hypertension, angiotensin II, and oxidative stress. N Engl J Med 2002;346:1999–2001.
35. Brasier AR, Li J. Mechanisms for inducible control of angiotensinogen gene transcription. Hypertension 1996;27:465–475.
36. McFarlane SI, Sowers JR. Aldosterone function in diabetes mellitus: effects on cardiovascular and renal disease. J Clin Endocrinol Metab 2003;88:516–523.
37. Remuzzi G, Schieppati A, Ruggenenti P. Nephropathy in patients with type 2 diabetes. N Engl J Med 2002;346:1145–1151.
38. Rocha R, Chander PN, Zuckerman A, Stier CT Jr. Role of aldosterone in renal vascular injury in stroke-prone hypertensive rats. Hypertension 2002;33:232–237.
39. Abdel-Wahab N, Weston BS, Roberts T, Masson RM. Connective tissue growth factor and regulation of the mesangial cell cycle: role in cellular hypertrophy. J Am Soc Nephrol 2002; 13:2437–2445.
40. De Vriese AS, Verbeuren TJ, Van de Voorde J, Lameire NH, Vanhoutte PM. Endothelial dysfunction in diabetes. Br J Pharmacol 2000;130:963–974.
41. Vlassara H. Recent progress on the biologic and clinical significance of advanced glycosylation end products. J Lab Clin Med 1994;124:19–30.
42. McFarlane SI, Winer N, Sowers JR. Role of the natriuretic peptide system in cardiorenal protection. Arch Intern Med 2003;163(22):2696–2704.
43. Sarzani R, Dess-Fulgheri P, Paci MV, Espinosa E, Rappelli A. Expression of natriuretic peptide receptors in human adipose and other tissues. J Endocrinol Invest 1996;19:581–585.
44. Sarzani R, Paci MV, Dess-Fulgheri P, Espinosa E, Rappelli A. Comparative analysis of atrial natriuretic peptide receptor expression in rat tissues. J Hypertens 1993;11(Suppl 5):S214–S216.
45. Wang TJ, Larson MG, Levy D, et al. Impact of obesity on plasma natriuretic peptide levels. Circulation 2004;109:594–600.
46. Dessi-Fulgheri P, Sarzani R, Tamburrini P, et al. Plasma atrial natriuretic peptide and natriuretic peptide receptor gene expression in adipose tissue of normotensive and hypertensive obese patients. J Hypertens 1997;15:1695–1699.
47. Yano Y, Katsuki A, Gabazza AC, et al. Plasma brain natriuretic peptide levels in normotensive noninsulin-dependent diabetic patients with microalbuminuria. J Clin Endocrinol Metab 1999; 84:2353–2356.
48. Chattington PD, Anderson JV, Rees LH, Leese GP, Peters JR, Vora JP. Atrial natriuretic peptide in type 2 diabetes mellitus: response to a physiological mixed meal and relationship to renal function. Diabet Med 1998;15:375–379.
49. DeFronzo RA, Ferrannini E. Insulin resistance: a multifaceted syndrome responsible for NIDDM, obesity, hypertension, dyslipidemia and atherosclerotic cardiovascular disease. Diabetes Care 1991;14:173–194.
50. Anderson EA, Hoffman RP, Balon TW, Sinkey CA, Mark AL. Hyperinsulinemia produces both sympathetic neural activation and vasodilation in normal humans. J Clin Invest 1991; 87:2246–2252.
51. Sowers JR. Insulin resistance and hypertension. Mol Cell Endocrinol 1990;74:C87–C89.
52. Ferrannini E, Natali A, Capaldo B, Lehtovirta M, Jacob S, Yki-Järvinen H, for the European Group for the Study of Insulin Resistance (EGIR). Insulin resistance, hyperinsulinemia, and blood pressure: role of age and obesity. Hypertension 1997;30:1144–1149.
53. Heise T, Magnusson K, Heinemann L, Sawicki PT. Insulin resistance and the effect of insulin on blood pressure in essential hypertension. Hypertension 1998;32(2):243–248.

54. Terzolo M, Pia A, Al A, et al. Adrenal incidentaloma: a new cause of the metabolic syndrome? J Clin Endocrinol Metab 2002;87:998–1003.

55. Tauchmanovà L, Rossi R, Biondi B, et al. Patients with subclinical Cushing's syndrome due to adrenal adenoma have increased cardiovascular risk. J Clin Endocrinol Metab 2002;87:4872–4878.

56. Rosmond R, Chagnon YC, Holm G, et al. A glucocorticoid receptor gene marker is associated with abdominal obesity, leptin, and dysregulation of the hypothalamic-pituitary-adrenal axis. Obes Res 2000;8:211–218.

57. Masuzaki H, Paterson J, Shinyama H, et al. A transgenic model of visceral obesity and the metabolic syndrome. Science 2001;294:2166–2170.

58. Masuzaki H, Yamamoto H, Kenyon CJ, et al. Transgenic amplification of glucocorticoid action in adipose tissue causes high blood pressure in mice. J Clin Invest 2003;112(1):83–90.

59. Morton NM, Paterson JM, Masuzaki H, et al. Novel adipose tissue-mediated resistance to diet-induced visceral obesity in 11β-hydroxysteroid dehydrogenase type 1-deficient mice. Diabetes 2004; 53:931–938.

60. Seres J, Bornstein SR, Seres P, et al. Corticotropin-releasing hormone system in human adipose tissue. J Clin Endocrinol Metab 2004;89(2):965–970.

61. Friedberg M, Zoumakis E, Hiroi N, Bader T, Chrousos GP, Hochberg Z. Modulation of 11 β-hydroxysteroid dehydrogenase type 1 in mature human subcutaneous adipocytes by hypothalamic messengers. J Clin Endocrinol Metab 2003;88:385–393.

62. Weisberg SP, McCann D, Desnai M, et al. Obesity is associated with macrophage accumulation in adipose tissue. J Clin Invest 2003;112:1796–1808.

63. Fernandez-Real JM, Ricart W. Insulin resistance and chronic cardiovascular inflammatory syndrome. Endocr Rev 2003;24(3):278–301.

64. Festa A, D'Agostino R Jr, Howard G, Mykkänen L, Tracy RP, Haffner SM. Chronic subclinical inflammation as part of the insulin resistance syndrome: the Insulin Resistance Atherosclerosis Study (IRAS). Circulation 2000;102:42–47.

65. Haynes WG, Morgan DA, Walsh SA, Mark AL, Sivitz WI. Receptor-mediated regional sympathetic nerve activation by leptin. J Clin Invest 1997;100:270–278.

66. Aizawa-Abe M, Ogawa Y, Masuzaki H, et al. Pathophysiological role of leptin in obesity-related hypertension. J Clin Invest 2000;1059:1243–1252.

67. Steppan CM, Bailey ST, Bhat S, et al. The hormone resistin links obesity to diabetes. Nature 2001;409:307–312.

68. Zhang JL, Qin YW, Zheng X, Qiu JL, Zou DJ. Serum resistin level in essential hypertension patients with different glucose tolerance. Diabet Med 2003;20(10):828–831.

69. Furuhashi M, Ura N, Higashiura K, Murakami H, Shimamoto K. Circulating resistin levels in essential hypertension. Clin Endocrinol 2003;59(4):507–510.

70. Hotta K, Funahashi T, Arita Y, et al. Plasma concentrations of a novel, adipose-specific protein, adiponectin, in type 2 diabetic patients. Arterioscler Thromb Vasc Biol 2000;20:1595–1599.

71. Ouchi N, Ohishi M, Kihara S, et al. Association of hypoadiponectinemia with impaired vasoreactivity. Hypertension 2003;42:231–234.

72. Tan KCB, Xu A, Chow WS, et al. Hypoadiponectinemia is associated with impaired endothelium-dependent vasodilation. J Clin Endocrinol Metab 2004;89:765–769.

73. Fernandez-Real JM, Castro A, Vazquez G, et al. Adiponectin is associated with vascular function independent of insulin sensitivity. Diabetes Care 2004;27(3):739–745.

74. Okamoto Y, Arita Y, Nishida M, et al. An adipocyte-derived plasma protein, adiponectin, adheres to injured vascular walls. Horm Metab Res 2000;32:47–50.

75. Chen H, Montagnani M, Funahashi T, Shimomura I, Quon MJ. Adiponectin stimulates production of nitric oxide in vascular endothelial cells. J Biol Chem 2003;278:45,021–45,026.

76. Mallamaci F, Zoccali C, Cuzzola F, et al. Adiponectin in essential hypertension. J Nephrol 2002;15:507–511.

77. Adamczak M, Wiecedilcek A, Funahashi T, Chudek J, Kokot F, Matsuzawa Y. Decreased plasma adiponectin concentration in patients with essential hypertension. Am J Hypertens 2003;16:72–75.

78. Furuhashi M, Ura N, Hishiura K, et al. Blockade of renin-angiotensin system increases adiponectin concentration in patients with essential hypertension. Hypertension 2003;42:76–81.

79. Iwashima Y, Katsuya T, Ishikawa K, et al. Hypoadiponectinemia is an independent risk factor for hypertension. Hypertension 2004;43:1318–1323.

80. Devaraj S, Xu DY, Jialal I. C-reactive protein increases plasminogen activator inhibitor-1 expression and activity in human aortic endothelial cells: implications for the metabolic syndrome and atherothrombosis. Circulation 2003;107:398–404.

81. Alessi MC, Peiretti F, Morange P, Henry M, Nalbone G, Juhan-Vague I. Production of plasminogen activator inhibitor 1 by human adipose tissue: possible link between visceral fat accumulation and vascular disease. Diabetes 1997;46:860–867.

82. Festa A, D'Agostino R, Tracy RP, Haffner SM. Elevated levels of acute-phase proteins and plasminogen activator inhibitor-1 predict the development of type 2 diabetes: The Insulin Resistance Atherosclerosis Study. Diabetes 2002;51:1131–1137.

83. Kerins DM, Hao I, Vaughan DE: Angiotensin induction of PAI-1 expression in endothelial cells is mediated by hexapeptide angiotensin IV. J Clin Invest 1995;96:2515–2520.

84. Nakamura S, Nakamura I, Ma L-J, Vaughan DE, Fogo AB: Plasminogen activator inhibitor-1 expression is regulated by the angiotensin type 1 receptor in vivo. Kidney Int 2000;58:251–259.

85. Ailhaud G, Fukamizu A, Massiera F, Negrel R, Saint-Marc P, Teboul M. Angiotensinogen, angiotensin II and adipose tissue development. Int J Obes Relat Metab Disord 2000;24(Suppl 4): S33–S35.

86. MA LJ, Mao SL, Taylor KL, et al. Prevention of obesity and insulin resistance in mice lacking plasminogen activator inhibitor I. Diabetes 2004;53:336–346.

87. Hotamisligil GS, Shargill NS, Spiegelman BM. Adipose expression of tumor necrosis factor-alpha: direct role in obesity-linked insulin resistance. Science 1993;259(5091):87–91.

88. Kern PA, Saghizadeh M, Ong JM, Bosch RJ, Deem R, Simsolo RB. The expression of tumor necrosis factor in human adipose tissue: regulation by obesity, weight loss, and relationship to lipoprotein lipase. J Clin Invest 1995;95(5):2111–2119.

89. Winkler G, Lakatos P, Salamon F, Nagy Z, Speer G, Kovacs M. Elevated serum TNF-a level as a link between endothelial dysfunction and insulin resistance in normotensive obese patients. Diabet Med 1999;16:207–211.

90. Ferreri NR, Zhao Y, Takizawa H, McGiff JC. Tumor necrosis factor-α-angiotensin interactions and regulation of blood pressure. J Hypertens 1997;15:1481–1484.

91. Pausova Z, Deslauriers B, Gaudet D, et al. Role of tumor necrosis factor-α gene locus in obesity and obesity-associated hypertension in French Canadians. Hypertension 2000;36:14–19.

92. Fernandez-Real JM, Laínez B, Vendrell J, et al. Shedding of tumor necrosis factor-α receptors, blood pressure and insulin sensitivity in type 2 diabetes mellitus. Am J Physiol Endocrinol Metab 2002;282:E952–E959.

93. Fried SK, Bunkin DA, Greenberg AS. Omental and subcutaneous adipose tissues of obese subjects release interleukin-6: depot difference and regulation by glucocorticoid. J Clin Endocrinol Metab 1998;83:847–850.

94. Mohamed-Ali V, Goodrick S, Rawesh A, et al. Subcutaneous adipose tissue releases interleukin-6, but not tumor necrosis factor-α, in vivo. J Clin Endocrinol Metab 1997;82:4196–4200.

95. Straub RH, Hense HW, Andus J, Schölmerich J, Riegger AJ, Schunkert H. Hormone replacement therapy and interrelation between serum interleukin-6 and body mass index in postmenopausal women: a population-based study. J Clin Endocrinol Metab 2000;85:1340–1344.

96. Fernandez-Real JM, Vayreda M, Richart C, Gutierrez C, Broch M, Vendrell J, Ricart W. Circulating interleukin 6 levels, blood pressure, and insulin sensitivity in apparently healthy men and women. J Clin Endocrinol Metab 2001;86(3):1154–1159.

97. Humphries SE, Luong LA, Ogg MS, Hawe E, Miller GJ. The interleukin-6-174 G/C promoter polymorphism is associated with risk of coronary heart disease and systolic blood pressure in healthy men. Eur Heart J 2001;22:2243–2252.

98. Pola R, Flex A, Gaetani E, Pola P, Bernabei R. The –174 G/C polymorphism of the interleukin-6 gene promoter and essential hypertension in an elderly Italian population. J Hum Hypertens 2002;16:637–640.

99. Philip-Couderc P, Smih F, Pelat M, et al. Cardiac transcriptome analysis in obesity-related hypertension. Hypertension 2003;41:414–421.

100. Carroll JF, Summers RL, Dzielak DJ, Cockrell K, Montani JP, Mizelle HL. Diastolic compliance is reduced in obese rabbits. Hypertension 1999;33:811–815.

101. Kortelainen ML, Sarkioja T. Coronary atherosclerosis and myocardial hypertrophy in relation to body fat distribution in healthy women: an autopsy study on 33 violent deaths. Int J Obes 1997;21:43–49.

102. Hense HW, Gneiting B, Muscholl M, et al. The associations of body size and body composition with left ventricular mass: impacts for indexation in adults. J Am Coll Cardiol 1998;32:451–457.

103. Kuch B, Hense HW, Gneiting B, et al. Body composition and prevalence of left ventricular hypertrophy. Circulation 2000;102:405–410.

104. Alpert MA, Terry BE, Mulekar M, et al. Cardiac morphology and left ventricular function in normotensive morbidly obese patients with and without congestive heart failure, and effect of weight loss. Am J Cardiol 1997;80:736–740.

105. De Simone G, Verdecchia P, Pede S, Gorini M, Maggioni AP, on behalf of the MAVI Investigators. Prognosis of inappropriate left ventricular mass in hypertension: The MAVI Study. Hypertension 2002;40:470–476.

106. Verwaerde P, Senard JM, Galinier M, et al. Changes in short-term variability of blood pressure and heart rate during the development of obesity-associated hypertension in high-fat fed dogs. J Hypertens 1999;17:1135–1143.

107. Kikuya M, Hozawa A, Ohokubo T, et al. Prognostic significance of blood pressure and heart rate variabilities: the Ohasama study. Hypertension 2000;36:901–906.

108. Sutton-Tyrrell K, Newman A, Simonsick EM, et al, for the Health ABC Investigators. Aortic stiffness is associated with visceral adiposity in older adults enrolled in the study of health, aging, and body composition. Hypertension 2001;38:429–433.

109. Mather KJ, Mirzamohammadi B, Lteif A, Steinberg HO, Baron AD. Endothelin contributes to basal vascular tone and endothelial dysfunction in human obesity and type 2 diabetes. Diabetes 2002;51:3517–3523.

110. Rich S, McLaughlin VV. Endothelin receptor blockers in cardiovascular disease. Circulation 2003;108:2184–2190.

111. Haynes WG, Strachan FE, Webb DJ. Endothelin ETA and ETB receptors mediate vasoconstriction of human resistance and capacitance vessels in vivo. Circulation 1995;92:357–363.

112. Cardillo C, Campia U, Iantorno M, Panza JA. Enhanced vascular activity of endogenous endothelin-1 in obese hypertensive patients. Hypertension 2004;43:36–40.

113. Williams IL, Wheatcroft SB, Shah AM, Kearney MT. Obesity, atherosclerosis and the vascular endothelium: mechanisms of reduced nitric oxide bioavailability in obese humans. Int J Obes 2002;26:754–764.

114. Steinberg HO, Chaker H, Leaming R, Johnson A, Brechtel G, Baron AD. Obesity/insulin resistance is associated with endothelial dysfunction: implications for the syndrome of insulin resistance. J Clin Invest 1996;97:2601–2610.

115. Caballero AE, Arora S, Saouaf R, et al. Microvascular and macrovascular reactivity is reduced in subjects at risk for type 2 diabetes. Diabetes 1999;48(9):1856–1862.

116. Lifton RP, Gharavi AG, Geller DS. Molecular mechanisms of human hypertension. Cell 2001;104:545–556.

117. Mark AL, Correia M, Morgan DA, Shaffer RA, Haynes WG. Obesity-induced hypertension new concepts from the emerging biology of obesity. Hypertension 1999;33(Pt II):537–541.

118. Izawa H, Yamada Y, Okada T, Tanaka M, Hirayama H, Yokota M. Prediction of genetic risk for hypertension. Hypertension 2003;41:1035–1040.

119. Sjostrom CD, Lissner L, Wedel H, Sjostrom L. Reduction in incidence of diabetes, hypertension and lipid disturbances after intentional weight loss induced by bariatric surgery: the SOS Intervention Study. Obes Res 1999;7:477–484.

120. NHLBI Obesity Education Initiative Expert Panel on the Identification, Evaluation, and Treatment of Overweight and Obesity in adults. Clinical guidelines on the identification, evaluation, and treatment of overweight and obesity in adults: the evidence report. Obes Res 1998;6(Suppl 2):51S–210S.

121. Wassertheil-Smoller S, Blaufox D, Oberman AS, Langford HG, Davis BR, Wylie-Rosett J. The Trial of Antihypertensive Interventions and Management (TAIM) Study: adequate weight loss, alone and combined with drug therapy in the treatment of mild hypertension. Arch Intern Med 1992;152:131–136.

122. He J, Whelton PK, Appel LJ, Charleston J, Klag MJ. Long-term effects of weight loss and dietary sodium reduction on incidence of hypertension. Hypertension 2000;35:544–549.

123. The Trials of Hypertension Prevention Collaborative Research Group. Effects of weight loss and sodium reduction intervention on blood pressure and hypertension incidence in overweight people With high-normal blood pressure: the Trials of Hypertension Prevention, Phase II. Arch Intern Med 1997;157(6):657–667.

124. Whelton SP, Chin A, Xin X, He J. Effect of aerobic exercise on blood pressure: a meta-analysis of randomized, controlled trials. Ann Intern Med 2002;136:493–503.

125. Hu G, Barengo NC, Tuomilehto J, Lakka TA, Nissinen A, Jousilahti P. Relationship of physical activity and body mass index to the risk of hypertension: a prospective study in Finland. Hypertension 2004;43:25–30.

126. Tuomilehto J, Lindstrom J, Eriksson JG, et al. Prevention of type 2 diabetes mellitus by changes in lifestyle among subjects with impaired glucose tolerance. N Engl J Med 2001;344:1343–1350.

127. Sacks FM, Svetkey LP, Vollmer WM, et al. Effects on blood pressure of reduced dietary sodium and the dietary approaches to stop hypertension (DASH) diet. N Engl J Med 2001;344:3–10.

128. Akita S, Sacks FM, Svetkey LP, Conlin PR, Kimura G for the DASH-Sodium Trial Collaborative Research Group. Effects of the dietary approaches to stop hypertension (DASH) diet on the pressure-natriuresis relationship. Hypertension 2003;42:8–13.

129. Stevens VJ, Obarzanek E, Cook NR, et al. Long-term weight loss and changes in blood pressure: results of the the Trials of Hypertension Prevention, phase II. Ann Intern Med 2001;134:1–11.

130. Seals DR, Tanaka H, Clevenger CM, et al. Blood pressure reductions with exercise and sodium restriction in postmenopausal women with elevated systolic pressure: role of arterial stiffness. J Am Coll Cardiol 2002;38:506–513.

131. Reisin E, Weir MR, Falkner B, Hutchinson HG, Anzalone DA, Tuch ML. Lisinopril versus hydrochlorthiazide in obese hypertensive patients: a multicenter placebo-controlled trial. Treatment in Obese Patients with Hypertension (TROPHY) Study Group. Hypertension 1997;30:140–145.

132. Grassi G, Seravalle G, Dell'Oro R, et al. Comparative effects of candesartan and hydrochlorothiazide on blood pressure, insulin sensitivity, and sympathetic drive in obese hypertensive individuals; results of the CROSS study. J Hypertens 2003;21:1761–1769.

133. The ALLHAT Officers and Coordinators for the ALLHAT Collaborative Research Group. Major outcomes in high-risk hypertensive patients randomized to angiotensin-converting enzyme inhibitor or calcium channel blocker vs diuretic: The Antihypertensive and Lipid-Lowering Treatment to Prevent Heart Attack Trial (ALLHAT). JAMA 2002;288(23):2981–2997.

134. UKPDS 38 UK Prospective Diabetes Study Group. Tight blood pressure control and risk of macrovascular and microvascular complications in type 2 diabetes. BMJ 1998;317:703–713.

135. Hansson L, Zanchetti A, Carruthers SG, et al. Effects of intensive blood pressure lowering and low-dose aspirin in patients with hypertension: principal results of the Hypertension Optimal Treatment (HOT) randomized trial. Lancet 1998;351:1755–1762.

136. David CJ, Pressel SL, Cutler JA, et al. Effect of diuretic-based antihypertensive treatment on cardiovascular disease risk in older diabetic patients with isolated systolic hypertension. JAMA 1996;276(23):1886–1892.

137. Mykkanen L, Kuusisto J, Pyorala K, Laakso M, Haffner SM. Increased risk of non-insulin-dependent diabetes mellitus in elderly hypertensive subjects. J Hypertens 1994;12:1425–1432.

138. Fletcher AE. Adverse treatment effects in the trial of the European Working Party on High Blood Pressure in the Elderly. Am J Med 1991;90:42S–44S.

139. Neaton JD, Grimm RH Jr, Prineas RJ, Stamler J, Grandits GA, Elmer PJ. Treatment of mild hypertension study: final results. JAMA 1993;270:713–724.

140. Gress TW, Nieto FJ, Shahar E, Wofford MR, Brancati FL. Hypertension and antihypertensive therapy as risk factors for type 2 diabetes mellitus: Atherosclerosis Risk in Communities Study. N Engl J Med 2000;342(13):905–912.

141. Sowers JR, Bakris GL. Antihypertensive therapy and the risk of type 2 diabetes mellitus. N Engl J Med 2000;342(13):969, 970.

142. Verdecchia P, Borgioni C, Angeli F, et al. Adverse prognostic significance of new diabetes in treated hypertensive subjects. Hypertension 2004;43:963–969.

143. Bakris GL, Sowers JR. When does new onset diabetes resulting from antihypertensive therapy increase cardiovascular risk. Hypertension 2004;43:941, 942.

144. Yusuf S, Sleight P, Pogue J, Bosch J, Davies R, Dagenais G. Effects of an angiotensin-converting-enzyme inhibitor, ramipril, on cardiovascular events in high-risk patients: the Heart Outcomes Prevention Evaluation Study Investigators. N Engl J Med 2000;342:145–153.

145. Heart Outcomes Prevention Evaluation Study Investigators. Effects of ramipril on cardiovascular and microvascular outcomes in people with diabetes mellitus: results of the HOPE study and MICRO-HOPE substudy [published erratum appears in Lancet 2000;356:860]. Lancet 2000;355:253–259.

146. Brenner BM, Cooper ME, De Zeeuw D, et al., the RENAAL Study Investigators. Effects of losartan on renal and cardiovascular outcomes in patients with type 2 diabetes and nephropathy. N Engl J Med 2001;345:861–869.

147. Parving HH, Lehnert H, Brochner-Mortensen J, Gomis R, Andersen S, Arner P, the Irbesartan in Patients with Type 2 Diabetes and Microalbuminuria Study Group. The effect of irbesartan on the development of diabetic nephropathy in patients with type 2 diabetes. N Engl J Med 2001;345:870–878.

148. Lindholm LH, Ibsen H, Dahlof B, et al. for the LIFE Study Group. Cardiovascular morbidity and mortality in patients with diabetes in the Losartan Intervention for Endpoint reduction in hypertension study (LIFE): a randomised trial against atenolol. Lancet 2002; 359(9311): 1004–1010.

149. Lithell H, Hansson L, Skoog I, et al; SCOPE Study Group. The Study on Cognition and Prognosis in the Elderly (SCOPE): principal results of a randomized double-blind intervention trial. J Hypertens 2003;21(5):875–886.

150. Pfeffer MA, Swedberg K, Granger CB, et al. CHARM Investigators and Committees. Effects of candesartan on mortality and morbidity in patients with chronic heart failure: the CHARM-Overall programme. Lancet 2003;362(9386):759–766.

151. Julius S, Kjeldsen SE, Weber M, et al. for the VALUE trial group. Outcomes in hypertensive patients at high cardiovascular risk treated with regimens based on valsartan or amlodipine: the VALUE randomised trial. Lancet 2004;363:2022–2031.

152. Zanella MT, Kohlmann O Jr, Ribeiro AB. Treatment of obesity hypertension and diabetes syndrome. Hypertension 2001;38(Pt 2):705–708.

153. Tuomilehto J, Rastenyte R, Birkenhager WH, et al. Effects of calcium-channel blockade in older patients with diabetes and systolic hypertension. N Engl J Med 1999;340:677–684.

154. Jacob S, Balletshofer B, Henriksen EJ, et al. Beta-blocking agents in patients with insulin resistance: effects of vasodilating beta-blockers. Blood Press 1999;8:261–268.

155. Giugliano D, De Rosa N, Di Maro G, et al. Metformin improves glucose, lipid metabolism, and reduces blood pressure in hypertensive, obese women. Diabetes Care 1993;16:1387–1390.

156. Buchanan TA, Meehan WP Jeng YY, yang D, Chan TM, Nadler JL. Blood pressure lowering by pioglitazone: evidence for a direct vascular effect. J Clin Invest 1995;96:354–360.

157. Giugliano D, Quatraro A, Consoli G, et al. Metformin for obese, insulin-treated diabetic patients: improvement in glycaemic control and reduction of metabolic risk factors. Eur J Clin Pharmacol 1993;44:107–112.

158. Peuler JD, Miller JA, Bourghli M, Zammam HY, Soltis EE, Sowers JR. Disparate effects of antidiabetic drugs on arterial contraction. Metabolism 1997;46:1199–1205.

159. Muntzel MS, Hamidou I, Barrett S. Metformin attenuates salt-induced hypertension in spontaneously hypertensive rats. Hypertension 1999;33(5):1135–1140.

160. Chiasson J, Josse RG, Gomis R, Hanefeld M, Karasik A, Laakso M, for The STOP-NIDDM Trial Research Group. Acarbose for prevention of type 2 diabetes mellitus: the STOP-NIDDM randomised trial. Lancet 2002;359(9323):2072–2077.

161. Dobrian AD, Schriver SD, Khraibi AA, Prewitt RL. Pioglitazone prevents hypertension and reduces oxidative stress in diet-induced obesity. Hypertension 2004;43:48–56.

162. Trivedi M, Marwaha A, Lokhandwala M. Rosiglitazone restores G-protein coupling, recruitment, and function of renal dopamine D1A receptor in obese zucker rats. Hypertension 2004;43(Pt 2):376–382.

163. Reginato MJ, Lazar MA. Mechanisms by which thiazolidinediones enhance insulin action. Trends Endocrinol Metab 1999;10:9–13.

164. Berger JP, Petro AE, Macnaul KL, et al. Distinct properties and advantages of a novel peroxisome proliferator-activated proteinγ selective modulator. Mol Endocrinol 2003;17(4):662–676.

165. Pischon T, Sharma AM. Recent developments in the treatment of obesity-related hypertension. Curr Opin Nephrol Hypertens 2002;11(5):497–502.

166. McMahon FG, Weinstein SP, Rowe E, et al. Sibutramine is safe and effective for weight loss in obese patients whose hypertension is well controlled with angiotensin-converting enzyme inhibitors. J Hum Hypertens 2002;16:5–11.

11

Dyslipidemia Associated With Diabetes and Insulin Resistance Syndromes

Jody Dushay, MD and J. Peter Oettgen, MD

CONTENTS

INTRODUCTION

Type 2 diabetes is a coronary heart disease (CHD) risk equivalent, which means that the diagnosis of type 2 diabetes confers the same risk for CHD over a 10-yr period as a prior cardiovascular event. In addition to having markedly increased risk of CHD, patients with type 2 diabetes have much worse outcomes after a major cardiovascular event. Patients with diabetes who suffer a myocardial infarction (MI) have a 50% increased in-hospital mortality and a twofold increase in mortality 2 yr after the event *(1,2)*. Data from large epidemiological studies show that 70% of patients with type 2 diabetes will die of some form of cardiovascular disease (CVD). The accelerated atherosclerosis seen among patients with type 2 diabetes begins years to decades before the diagnosis of diabetes.

Whereas there is robust clinical evidence that tight glycemic control significantly reduces the incidence of microvascular disease in both type 1 and type 2 diabetes, there are no outcome studies showing that lowering hemoglobin A1C (HbA1C) reduces the incidence of macrovascular disease to the same degree *(3–5)*. The United Kingdom Prospective Diabetes Study, the largest prospective study examining the effects of tight glycemic control in patients with type 2 diabetes, showed that lowering HbA1C significantly reduced the frequency of microvascular disease, but the effect on macrovascular disease was not statistically significant *(6)*. In the absence of clinical trial data supporting a relationship between improved glycemic control and reduced risk of CHD, an understanding of the pathophysiology and treatment of other modifiable metabolic abnormalities that often cluster with type 2 diabetes and independently increase risk of CHD may help reduce the incidence of and mortality from CHD in this population. The

From: *Contemporary Diabetes: Obesity and Diabetes*
Edited by: C. S. Mantzoros © Humana Press Inc., Totowa, NJ

dyslipidemia associated with type 2 diabetes and insulin resistance is one such modifiable risk factor. Large interventional studies have shown that lowering low-density lipoprotein (LDL) cholesterol reduces cardiovascular risk by as much as 30% among patients with type 2 diabetes (7). Lowering triglyceride levels and raising high-density lipoprotein (HDL) levels are also associated with lower rates of CHD, although outcome studies of these lipid parameters are comparatively less robust than those for LDL cholesterol (8).

Obesity, in particular abdominal obesity, is commonly seen in patients with type 2 diabetes. Abdominal obesity poses an independent risk of CVD even in the absence of diabetes, however, because it causes insulin resistance and an overall proinflammatory state. The increased risk of CHD among patients with abdominal obesity has been demonstrated in studies focusing on individuals with metabolic syndrome.

Metabolic syndrome (also referred to as syndrome X or insulin resistance syndrome) is a cluster of metabolic abnormalities that together equal more than the sum of their parts in terms of cardiovascular risk and all-cause mortality (9). Several organizations have formulated criteria for diagnosing metabolic syndrome, including the World Health Organization, the European Group for the Study of Insulin Resistance, the American Association of Clinical Endocrinologists, and the National Cholesterol Education Program/Adult Treatment Panel III (NCEP/ATP III). The individual criteria for diagnosis are not uniform, but most include threshold values for lipids, blood pressure (BP), and glucose, as well as a measurement of insulin resistance, such as waist circumference.

Despite differences in individual diagnostic criteria, the common goal among these organizations is to identify individuals who will benefit from aggressive risk reduction and heightened surveillance for the development of diabetes or CVD, two common sequelae of metabolic syndrome. In large European cohorts, the diagnosis of metabolic syndrome increased risk of cardiovascular mortality by two- to threefold (10). A study examining carotid intima-media thickness, which is a proxy for overall atherogenesis, found that insulin resistance predicted the degree of atherogenesis as well as elevated LDL cholesterol in patients with metabolic syndrome and no history of diabetes (11). Similarly, the Women's Ischemia Syndrome Evaluation study found that the risk of an adverse outcome after a cardiac event was similar among women with metabolic syndrome and known coronary artery disease (CAD) and women with diabetes (12). The pathophysiological basis for increased atherogenicity in patients with type 2 diabetes and insulin resistance is an area of active investigation. Emerging data suggest that insulin resistance in muscle, fat cells, and liver causes many aspects of the dyslipidemia and increased risk of CHD in this population (13).

In the United States, the ATP III criteria are used most commonly for clinical diagnosis of metabolic syndrome (Table 1). According to these guidelines, individuals with three or more of the criteria carry the diagnosis of metabolic syndrome. Data from the Third National Health and Nutrition Examination Survey (NHANES III) show that 24% of the US population (47 million people) meets ATP III criteria for metabolic syndrome; the prevalence soars to 43% for adults age 60 and older (14). By comparison, 15% of nondiabetic adults in Europe have metabolic syndrome (10).

Although the ATP III criteria are helpful in identifying individuals at high risk of CVD and diabetes, there are several caveats. First, because a diagnosis of metabolic syndrome is made when an individual meets three or more of the criteria, the population of patients who carry this diagnosis is heterogeneous. Some patients have low HDL, high triglycerides, and an increased waist circumference, whereas others have

Table 1
NCEP/ATP III Diagnostic Criteria for Metabolic Syndrome[a]

Measurement	Value
Waist circumference	>88 cm for women, >102 cm for men
Fasting triglycerides	≥150 mg/dL
BP	≥130/85 mmHg
HDL cholesterol	≤50 for mg/dL for women, ≤40 mg/dL for men
Fasting glucose[b]	≥110 mg/dL

[a]Diagnosis is made when three or more of the criteria are present.
[b]This does not reflect the 2004 ADA criteria for impaired fasting glucose (100–125 mg/dL) and may change to ≥100 mg/dL.

hypertension, elevated fasting glucose, and dyslipidemia. Analysis of NHANES III data from 1988 to 1994 shows that 84% of those who met ATP III criteria for metabolic syndrome had obesity, 75% had hypertension, 75% had low HDL, 74% had elevated triglycerides, and 41% had elevated fasting glucose *(15)*. Emerging data suggest that the more criteria met, the greater the risk of CHD, but it remains to be determined which combinations of metabolic abnormalities confer greatest risk. Second, the quantitative thresholds for dyslipidemia do not take into account qualitative changes in lipoproteins that occur in the setting of type 2 diabetes and insulin resistance. As discussed later in this chapter, qualitative changes in lipoproteins may contribute significantly to increased cardiovascular risk. Third, the ATP III criteria may not apply uniformly across ethnic groups. There is some evidence that African Americans who are insulin resistant do not have hypertension or the same lipid abnormalities as Hispanics or non-Hispanic whites *(16)*. This population may therefore not meet the criteria commonly used for diagnosis of metabolic syndrome and, consequently, may not be screened as aggressively *(16)*.

This chapter focuses primarily on the dyslipidemia associated with type 2 diabetes and obesity as part of the insulin-resistant metabolic syndrome. We first provide an overview of the major lipoproteins and lipoprotein metabolism. We then present the characteristics and mechanisms of dyslipidemia associated with diabetes and obesity. Lipid goals according to the American Diabetes Association (ADA) and ATP III criteria are reviewed and lipid-lowering treatment options are discussed. We first discuss the benefits of lifestyle modification. Then we discuss the mechanisms of action of the lipid-lowering medications available in the United States and review clinical trial data relevant to the management of patients with diabetes and the metabolic syndrome. The lipid-lowering effects of oral hypoglycemics are addressed next, and we describe one agent under investigation that targets HDL cholesterol. At the end of the chapter, we briefly discuss dyslipidemia associated with type 1 diabetes (insulin deficiency) and with insulin-resistant states including human immunodeficiency virus (HIV) and polycystic ovary syndrome (PCOS).

OVERVIEW OF LIPOPROTEINS AND LIPOPROTEIN METABOLISM

The lipoproteins discussed in this chapter are chylomicrons, very low-density lipoproteins (VLDLs), intermediate-density lipoproteins (IDLs), LDLs, and HDLs (Fig. 1). The absolute and relative amounts of triglyceride and cholesterol in lipoprotein particles

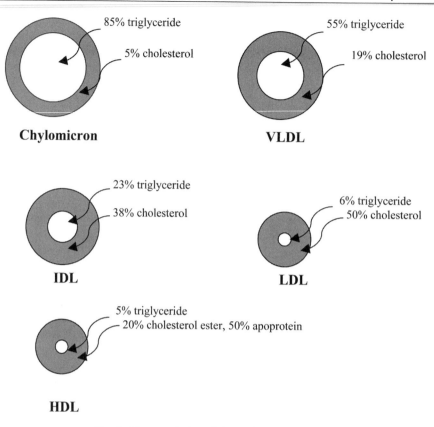

Fig. 1. Characteristics of the major lipoproteins.

assign them their individual characteristics and relative degrees of atherogenicity. Lipoprotein particle size also contributes to atherogenicity, because smaller, denser particles penetrate the blood vessel wall more easily. Once inside the blood vessel, lipid particles can be oxidized and integrated into the atheromatous plaque *(17)*.

The most triglyceride-rich lipoproteins are chylomicrons and VLDL particles. Chylomicrons (85% triglycerides, 5% cholesterol) are synthesized and secreted by the small intestine. Their role is to carry dietary triglycerides throughout the body and to deliver dietary cholesterol back to the liver. VLDL particles (55% triglycerides, 19% cholesterol) are synthesized and secreted by the liver. VLDL particles deliver triglycerides and cholesterol made in the liver to tissues throughout the body. IDL particles (23% triglycerides, 38% cholesterol) are produced when VLDL particles are partially hydrolyzed. LDL particles (6% triglycerides, 50% cholesterol) are commonly referred to as "bad cholesterol." They are the final product in the sequential breakdown of VLDL particles and are smaller and denser than VLDL and IDL particles. In the setting of elevated circulating triglycerides, LDL particles are hydrolyzed and become even smaller and denser. HDL particles (5% triglycerides, 20% cholesterol ester, 50% apoprotein) are made in both the liver and small intestine. HDL particles deliver cholesterol from peripheral tissues back to the liver for elimination via a process called reverse cholesterol transport. Reverse cholesterol transport is cardioprotective—peripheral tissues have no other way of removing excess cholesterol.

The major enzymes that regulate lipid metabolism are lipoprotein lipase (LPL), hepatic lipase (HL), hormone-sensitive lipase (HSL), and cholesterol ester transfer protein

Table 2
Actions of Major Enzymes Involved in Lipid Metabolism

Enzyme	Substrate	End product
LPL	Chylomicrons	FFAs, glycerol
	VLDL	IDL
	IDL	LDL
	Triglyceride-rich HDL	Buoyant HDL
HL	Buoyant LDL	Small, dense LDL
	Buoyant HDL	Small, dense HDL
	HDL	Cleared particles
HSL	Adipocytes	FFAs
CETP	VLDL	Triglyceride-rich LDL and HDL

(CETP). Table 2 summarizes the actions of these enzymes. LPL is a hydrolytic enzyme that is synthesized in adipocytes and myocytes. LPL resides on the luminal side of the capillary wall in most tissues and plays a key role in exogenous and endogenous lipid metabolism by converting chylomicrons into nonesterified fatty acids and glycerol and orchestrating the lipid depletion sequence that converts VLDL into IDL and then LDL *(18)*. An additional role for LPL is the conversion of dense, triglyceride-rich HDL particles into more buoyant, less atherogenic HDL particles *(18)*. HL, an enzyme synthesized by hepatocytes, adrenal cells, and gonadal cells, hydrolyzes triglycerides and phospholipids in LDL and HDL particles. Increased HL activity causes conversion of large, buoyant HDL and LDL particles into small, dense, and more atherogenic particles. HL may also play a role in the clearance of HDL particles and in the conversion of IDL into LDL *(19,20)*. HSL hydrolyzes adipocytes, causing the release of free fatty acids (FFAs). Increased HSL activity raises the amount of circulating FFA in the body. CETP exchanges antiatherogenic lipoprotein particles for proatherogenic particles in both HDL and LDL. The net effect of CETP activity is to reduce HDL levels and to decrease LDL particle size.

CHARACTERISTICS AND MECHANISMS OF DYSLIPIDEMIA IN DIABETES AND OBESITY

Patients with diabetes and obesity typically have an atherogenic dyslipidemia characterized by elevated triglycerides and low HDL levels as well as an increased proportion of small, dense LDL particles. Total LDL levels may be modestly increased but are comparable with those of the general population, although an individual with type 2 diabetes and a total LDL of 100 mg/dL may actually have many more circulating small, dense LDL particles than an individual with normal insulin sensitivity and the same LDL level. Individuals with diabetic dyslipidemia and significantly elevated LDL levels are considered to have a mixed dyslipidemia. As discussed later, mixed dyslipidemia poses particular challenges with respect to dietary counseling and may require pharmacological therapy with more than one medication.

Hypertriglyceridemia

Triglycerides come from the diet (exogenous) or are newly synthesized by the liver (endogenous) using dietary carbohydrate precursors and reesterified fatty acids

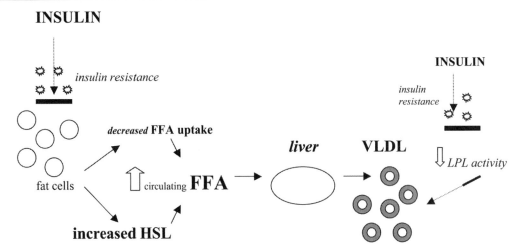

Fig. 2. Mechanism by which insulin resistance leads to hypertriglyceridemia. In the setting of insulin resistance, there is decreased FFA uptake by fat cells and increased HSL activity, both of which lead to increased FFA in the circulation. Increased FFA delivery to the liver causes increased secretion of triglyceride-rich VLDL particles. Impaired or reduced activity of LPL in the setting of insulin resistance leads to diminished lipolysis of VLDL particles, also contributing to hypertriglyceridemia.

absorbed from peripheral tissues. Exogenous triglycerides circulate as chylomicrons, while endogenous triglycerides combine with hepatic cholesterol to form VLDL particles, which are secreted into the circulation by hepatocytes.

Abnormalities of LPL activity, HSL activity, and fatty acid metabolism all contribute to baseline and often extreme postprandial hypertriglyceridemia associated with type 2 diabetes and insulin resistance (Fig. 2). Although fasting LPL levels are typically increased in the setting of obesity because of the large number of adipocytes, insulin resistance at the level of the fat cell causes decreased LPL activity and, therefore, an abnormal response of LPL to a glucose load *(21,22)*. Diminished LPL activity leads to an accumulation of atherogenic LDL precursors, such as VLDL, in the circulation *(18,22,23)*. HSL activity is increased in type 2 diabetes, which causes increased circulating FFA. In the setting of insulin resistance, adipocytes take up less circulating FFA. This situation, called reduced fatty acid trapping, allows excess FFA delivery to the liver, which, in turn, causes increased hepatic secretion of VLDL particles *(24)*. This is most pronounced and prolonged after a meal.

Decreased HDL

Reduced HDL leads to diminished clearance of cholesterol from peripheral tissues. The actions of CETP illustrate why hypertriglyceridemia and reduced HDL typically go hand in hand in patients with type 2 diabetes (Fig. 3). In the setting of elevated circulating triglycerides, CETP allows an increased influx of VLDL triglycerides into HDL particles. This occurs as an exchange reaction, with a simultaneous efflux of cholesteryl ester out of HDL particles. This process leads to reduced HDL levels owing to increased clearance of HDL particles. Triglyceride-rich HDL particles are preferentially broken down in the liver by HL and are stripped of an important structural protein called Apo A-1, which is cleared by the kidney. There is also reduced production of HDL particles in type 2 diabetes owing to abnormal LPL activity, causing decreased conversion of dense, triglyceride-rich HDL to more buoyant particles.

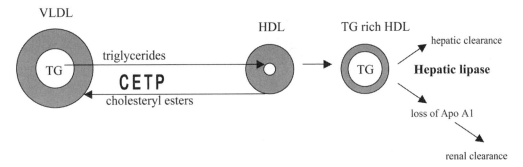

Fig. 3. Hypertriglyceridemia causes a reduction in HDL via actions of CETP. CETP exchanges triglycerides (TG) from VLDL particles with cholesteryl esters from HDL particles. The resulting triglyceride-rich HDL particles are small and dense and are substrates for HL.

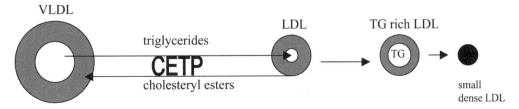

Fig. 4. Hypertriglyceridemia promotes a shift toward small, dense LDL via actions of CETP. CETP exchanges triglycerides from VLDL particles with cholesteryl esters from LDL particles. The triglyceride (TG)-rich LDL particles are then converted into small, dense LDL particles, which are more atherogenic.

Qualitative Changes in LDL: LDL Particle Size

As already mentioned, although the total LDL level may be normal or only modestly elevated in patients with type 2 diabetes and insulin resistance, there are frequently qualitative changes in LDL particles that confer increased risk of CHD. As individuals proceed from normal insulin sensitivity to insulin resistance, VLDL particles become larger and LDL particles become smaller. Individuals with type 2 diabetes have been shown to have smaller, denser LDL particles even after adjusting for elevated triglyceride levels and lower HDL levels *(25)*.

LDL particles are divided into two subclasses based on particle size and atherogenicity. Pattern A particles are buoyant and pattern B particles are small, dense, and more atherogenic. Pattern B molecules are formed by a lipid-exchange process similar to that that occurs in HDL particles in the setting of elevated triglycerides (Fig. 4). Through the actions of CETP, triglyceride from VLDL is exchanged with cholesteryl ester from LDL. Hydrolysis of the triglyceride-rich LDL particle produces smaller, denser LDL particles. Hypertriglyceridemia and increased circulating FFAs both provide a metabolic environment that favors LDL remodeling *(22)*.

Pattern B particles are considered more atherogenic than pattern A particles for several reasons: they adhere to and penetrate the arterial wall more easily, they are more toxic to endothelial cells, they exert a procoagulant effect by causing greater production of plasminogen activator inhibitor-1 by endothelial cells, and they are oxidized more easily *(22,26)*. Studies done in the general population and in diabetic populations have shown that individuals with elevated levels of pattern B particles are at higher risk of CHD *(26)*.

Table 3
Guidelines for Lipid Levels in Patients With Type 2 Diabetes

	ADA	ATP III
Total cholesterol	No specific goal	<200 mg/dL
LDL cholesterol	<100 mg/dL	<100 mg/dL
		<70 mg/dL if very high risk[a]
HDL cholesterol	>50 mg/dL in women	>45 mg/dL
	>40 mg/dL in men	
Triglycerides	<150 mg/dL	<150 mg/dL

[a]This is a therapeutic option published in the 2004 ATP III guidelines. Very high-risk individuals are those with known CHD, or a CHD risk equivalent plus one or more additional risk factors. Risk of CHD in this population is >20% over 10 yr.

Glycosylation of LDL

Epidemiological data have demonstrated that higher HbA1C levels are associated with higher rates of CHD (6). Severe hyperglycemia may worsen diabetic dyslipidemia via glycosylation of LDL particles. Glycosylated LDL particles are thought to have increased atherogenicity (27,28). Advanced glycation end products may modify LDL particles such that they have reduced affinity for hepatic LDL receptors and thereby a prolonged half-life (29,30). LDL particles that "live longer" may have a greater likelihood of becoming oxidized or taken up by macrophages, in turn leading to the formation of foam cells (29,30).

TREATMENT OF DYSLIPIDEMIA

Lipid Goals

The ATP III and the ADA have independently established lipid targets and treatment priorities for individuals with type 2 diabetes (Table 3). Both organizations endorse an LDL goal of <100 mg/dL for patients with type 2 diabetes, although the ATP III published guidelines in July 2004 that offered an optional LDL goal of <70 mg/dL for very high-risk individuals, which includes people with diabetes and known CHD (31). The ADA suggests initiating medical therapy if LDL is >100 mg/dL and there is known CHD or peripheral vascular disease, or if LDL is >130 mg/dL without known CHD (32). The ATP III guidelines similarly suggest starting pharmacotherapy if the LDL is >100 mg/dL and there is known CHD but also state that medical therapy is indicated if non-HDL cholesterol (total cholesterol minus HDL cholesterol) is >130 mg/dL and triglycerides are >200 mg/dL (31). Despite these evidence-based lipid goals, a worldwide survey of 2000 physicians found that although 91% of patients with type 2 diabetes are screened for lipid abnormalities, only about 50% achieve target lipid values (33). Patients with type 2 diabetes and known cardiovascular disease (CVD) tend to be treated more aggressively than those without known disease, but this large survey found that only 59% of physicians were aiming for LDL levels <100 mg/dL (33).

Therapeutic Strategies

The ATP III guidelines recommend therapeutic lifestyle changes, including weight loss, dietary modifications, and exercise, as the cornerstones of therapy for all components of metabolic syndrome. The ADA recommends similar lifestyle modifications (31,32).

WEIGHT LOSS

Studies examining lipid parameters after weight loss was achieved with or without prescription medication for weight reduction have yielded conflicting results. A small nonrandomized trial of sibutramine, one of the two available weight-lowering medications in the United States, showed that 12 mo of sibutramine treatment plus a low-calorie diet yielded significantly lower triglyceride levels and higher HDL levels, although LDL and total cholesterol levels did not change significantly *(34)*. Three months of treatment with orlistat plus a low-calorie diet resulted in significant reductions in total cholesterol, LDL cholesterol, LDL particle concentration, and insulin levels; this nonrandomized study did not show a significant increase in HDL levels *(35)*. A much larger, randomized, placebo-controlled study of orlistat treatment for 2 yr showed that BP and lipid parameters improved in both groups during the 4-wk placebo lead-in period and that the effect was sustained in the orlistat but not the placebo group *(36)*. LDL cholesterol was reduced 10 points in the orlistat group compared with 8 points in the placebo group, although there was no significant change in HDL or triglyceride levels *(36)*. Together these studies indicate that weight loss alone may not be sufficient for improving dyslipidemia in patients with morbid obesity.

DIETARY MODIFICATIONS

Both the ATP III and the American Heart Association (AHA) recommend a stepwise approach to lowering the relative amounts of dietary fat and cholesterol. The AHA Step 1 diet contains <30% total fat, <10% saturated fat, and <300 mg of total cholesterol. In general, the Step 1 diet can lower total cholesterol by 5–7%. The Step 2 diet, which is followed if Step 1 does not effectively modify the lipid profile, contains <30% total fat, <7% saturated fat, and <200 mg of total cholesterol. The Step 2 diet may lower cholesterol 3–7% beyond that achieved by the Step 1 diet.

It is important to recognize that dietary recommendations aimed primarily at lowering total cholesterol and LDL levels without attention to triglyceride or HDL levels may not be appropriate for patients with diabetic dyslipidemia. Neither epidemiological studies nor outcome studies have demonstrated a strong association between total fat intake and the risk of developing diabetes or CVD *(37)*. People typically reduce fat intake in an effort to lower cholesterol levels, but without appropriate nutritional counseling, individuals will often increase carbohydrate intake as they reduce dietary fat. Carbohydrates raise triglyceride levels and lower HDL levels, usually without an added effect on LDL.

Hu and Willett *(38)* have published a comprehensive review of epidemiological and clinical trial evidence regarding the optimal diet for CHD reduction. They summarized data from low-fat diets, diets high in polyunsaturated fat, diets with increased omega-3 fatty acids (discussed in greater detail later in this section), and what that they termed a *whole-diet* approach *(38)*. Low-fat diets (20–30% of calories from fat) had no significant effect on CHD event rates or total cholesterol. Diets high in polyunsaturated fat and low in saturated fat reduced CHD events by 25–44% in three large studies and total cholesterol by 13–15% in four large studies (both reductions were statistically significant). Diets high in omega-3 fatty acids reduced CHD events by 30% in two large studies. The whole-diet approach, which includes a high intake of fruits; vegetables; nuts; and olive, canola, or flaxseed oil, reduced CHD events by 40–70% in two large studies of male patients who have had an MI *(38)*.

By putting this clinical evidence into practice, it is found that a better strategy for individuals with elevated triglycerides and low HDL levels is to limit carbohydrate intake and replace saturated fat with mono- and polyunsaturated fat. The total fat content in this diet might be higher than that recommended in the AHA Step 1 or 2 diets, but the addition of "good" fats rather than excess carbohydrates more closely addresses the lipid abnormalities in diabetic dyslipidemia and the proven approaches to CHD reduction. Dietary counseling for patients with mixed dyslipidemia, including elevated triglycerides, low HDL levels, and frankly elevated LDL levels, is more challenging and should incorporate aspects of the Step 1 and 2 diets, increased intake of monounsaturated fats, and reduced amounts of carbohydrates. All nutrition counseling must also include attention to overall caloric reduction in order to achieve weight loss.

Modest alcohol intake has been shown to have cardioprotective effects *(39)*. This has been widely advertised and patients frequently ask about alcohol consumption. All types of alcohol appear to raise HDL levels by decreasing CETP activity. However, the recommendation of routine alcohol intake among individuals with type 2 diabetes should be offered very cautiously. Alcohol is preferentially oxidized in the liver, leaving circulating FFAs as available substrate for the synthesis of triglyceride. Even modest alcohol intake can dramatically raise serum triglycerides.

Another dietary intervention that has received popular attention is increased intake of omega-3 fatty acids, which include long-chain eicosapentaneoic acid (EPA) and docosahexanoic acid (DHA) and short-chain α-linolenic acid. Omega-3 fatty acids are found in soy, olive, flaxseed, and canola oils and in fatty fish. They may also be taken as a dietary supplement. Omega-3 fatty acids are thought to have several cardioprotective effects, including lowering of triglycerides, slowing of the growth of atherosclerotic plaque, reduction in thrombogenesis, and promotion of nitric oxide-induced endothelial relaxation *(40)*. Secondary prevention trials have shown that the addition of omega-3 fatty acid to the diet significantly reduced the incidence of fatal and nonfatal MI and stroke in patients with known CHD *(40–42)*. In 2002, the AHA published recommendations regarding fish, fish oil, and omega-3 fatty acid consumption. According to the AHA, people without CHD should eat fatty fish (salmon, mackerel, fresh tuna) at least twice weekly and to include oils and foods rich in α-linolenic acid in their diet. Those with known CHD should consume 1 g of long-chain omega-3 fatty acid daily (EPA + DHA), preferably from fish but alternatively from a dietary supplement. Individuals with hypertriglyceridemia should consume 2–4 g of EPA + DHA daily in capsule form under the supervision of a physician *(40)*.

EXERCISE

Daily aerobic exercise is an important lifestyle modification that can improve the lipid profile in patients with type 2 diabetes or insulin resistance, especially if exercise is combined with appropriate dietary recommendations to achieve weight loss. Independent of weight loss, however, exercise increases insulin sensitivity, raises HDL levels, and lowers triglycerides. The mechanisms through which these beneficial changes occur are essentially the opposite of those that go awry in diabetes and obesity. Exercise increases skeletal muscle LPL activity, which lowers triglyceride levels *(43)*. When circulating triglycerides are reduced, there is reduced CETP-mediated exchange of lipid from triglyceride-rich particles to HDL particles. HDL particles with lower triglyceride content are less vulnerable to clearance and, therefore, the HDL level increases. Exercise also causes increased formation of HDL cholesteryl esters and decreased hepatic lipase activity, both of which contribute to increased HDL levels *(43)*.

PHARMACOTHERAPY

Although attention to diet, weight loss, and exercise is essential for patients with diabetic dyslipidemia and insulin resistance, many are unable to attain desirable lipid profiles with lifestyle modification alone. ATP III guidelines recommend pharmacotherapy if the LDL goal is not met after a 3-mo trial of lifestyle modification alone (two follow-up visits scheduled 6 wk apart) *(44)*. In practice, treatment with lipid-lowering agents is common.

HMG-CoA Reductase Inhibitors. HMG-CoA reductase inhibitors, well known as "statins," competitively inhibit the rate-limiting step in cholesterol synthesis. LDL receptor activity is upregulated in the setting of reduced cholesterol synthesis, leading to a reduction in LDL cholesterol level. Statins also reduce the formation and entry of LDL and IDL into the circulation *(45)*. The effect of statins on triglycerides and HDL levels is less robust than their LDL-lowering effect. The ADA and ATP III endorse statins as first-line lipid-lowering therapy for patients with type 2 diabetes. The American College of Physicians published recommendations in April 2004 stating that statins should be used at moderate doses for primary prevention in all patients with type 2 diabetes who have one or more additional cardiac risk factors and for secondary prevention in all patients with type 2 diabetes and known CAD, regardless of baseline LDL levels *(46)*.

The statins available in the United States include lovastatin, pravastatin, fluvastatin, atorvastatin, and simvastatin. The most potent for LDL reduction are simvastatin and atorvastatin. At maximal dosing, these medications can lower LDL cholesterol 45–55% and decrease triglycerides 20–45% *(45,47)*. Greater triglyceride reduction is seen when initial triglyceride levels are markedly elevated. Statins can raise HDL levels by 5–10% but are not first-line therapy for raising HDL, particularly if initial HDL levels are <40 mg/dL. In terms of dose titration, doubling the dose of a statin above the minimal effective dose generally decreases LDL concentration by an additional 6% *(45)*.

One potential side effect of statins is myositis, which occurs in roughly 0.1% of patients. Creatine kinase (CK) levels may increase to more than 10 times the normal value and patients may experience muscle soreness, weakness, and fatigue *(45)*. On occasion, patients may have symptoms of myositis with only mild elevations in CK. Rarely, rhabdomyolysis can occur, and myoglobinuria associated with rhabdomyolysis can put patients at risk of renal failure. Statins should be prescribed with caution for patients with diabetic nephropathy and for elderly patients, who may have significantly diminished glomerular filtration rates (GFRs) even with creatinine levels in the normal range. Statins cause elevations in transaminases in 1 to 2% of patients, but this is generally not clinically significant and typically does not require discontinuation of the medication. Significant hepatotoxicity from statins is extremely rare *(45)*. Statins do not adversely affect glycemic control.

In 2002, the American College of Cardiology (ACC), AHA, and National Heart, Lung, and Blood Institute (NHLBI) established guidelines for statin use, which include checking baseline transaminases and CK levels prior to starting the medication *(48)*. If transaminases are less than three times the upper limit of normal, statins are not contraindicated. If symptoms of myositis develop, CK level should be checked. If it is less than three times the upper limit of normal, the statin may be continued, but a lower dose should be considered and CK levels should be monitored. If the CK level is greater than 10 times normal, the statin should be discontinued. Asymptomatic patients with elevated CK levels may continue to take statins but should have CK levels checked periodically *(48)*.

Several large, randomized clinical trials have shown convincingly that statins reduce risk of CHD and improve outcomes when used for primary or secondary prevention of CHD in patients with type 2 diabetes. The 2004 ATP III guidelines show a log-linear relationship between LDL levels and relative risk (RR) of CHD, such that for every 1%

reduction in LDL levels, RR for major CHD events is reduced by 1%. This relationship appears to hold for LDL levels well below 100 mg/dL, suggesting that there is no lower threshold for LDL reduction *(31)*. Subgroup analyses of patients enrolled in the Scandanavian Simvastatin Survival Study (4S), the Heart Protection Study (HPS), and the Cholesterol and Recurrent Events (CARE) trial show that statins reduce the incidence of CHD events by 25–50% in patients with type 2 diabetes *(7,49–51)*.

The first large, randomized, placebo-controlled trial focusing on primary prevention of CHD exclusively in patients with type 2 diabetes is the Collaborative Atorvastatin Diabetes Study study. This trial examined the effects of 10 mg of atorvastatin vs placebo on risk of CHD. The study was stopped nearly 2 yr early because of the significant difference in CHD events in the treatment group. Patients who received 10 mg of atorvastatin daily had a 37% reduction in all major cardiovascular events, including acute MI, stroke, angina, or revascularization. The reduction in stroke risk was even greater, with 48% fewer patients in the atorvastatin group experiencing a stroke *(52)*. At study entry, 25% of patients had LDL cholesterol levels <100 mg/dL, suggesting that even when LDL levels are at goal, there may be significant benefit to statin therapy among patients with type 2 diabetes.

Bile Acid-Binding Resins. Resins bind bile acids in the small intestine and interrupt their enterohepatic circulation. When fewer bile acids are returned to the liver, there is increased conversion of hepatic cholesterol into bile acids. This, in turn, leads to a relative depletion of hepatic cholesterol pools, an upregulation of hepatic LDL receptors, and an overall reduction in LDL levels *(45)*. However, when hepatic cholesterol stores are decreased, hepatic synthesis of cholesterol increases, which results in increased secretion of VLDL particles into the circulation. The elevation in circulating triglycerides that occurs with resins mitigates their LDL-lowering effect *(45)*. Additional adverse effects of these medications include bloating and constipation.

Bile acid-binding resins include cholestyramine, colestipol, and colesevelam. Cholestyramine is available only as a powder, limiting palatability and compliance. Colestipol and colesevelam are available as tablets, but the number of pills necessary to achieve maximal dosing ranges from 6 to 30. At maximal doses of cholestyramine (24 g/d) or colestipol (30 g/d), LDL levels may be reduced by approx 25% *(45)*. Reduction in LDL is slightly less for colesevelam. Given the tendency for patients to comply poorly with dosing levels and/or regimens, these agents achieve the greatest LDL-lowering effect when used in combination with a statin.

Fibrates. Fibrates, such as gemfibrozil and fenofibrate, are fibric acid derivatives that work through activation of peroxisome proliferator-activated receptor α (PPARα), a nuclear transcription factor. Activation of PPARα has pleiotropic effects, including upregulation of LDL cholesterol and apolipoprotein AI genes and increased LPL expression. Activation of PPAR leads to increased oxidation of fatty acids in both liver and muscle. In liver, this causes increased formation of ketones and decreased secretion of triglyceride-rich lipoproteins. In muscle, increased oxidation of fatty acids is associated with an increase in LPL activity and fatty acid uptake. Fibrates also cause increased buoyancy of LDL particles and are thought to have an anti-inflammatory effect at the level of endothelial cells *(45)*.

Fibrates are generally well tolerated. When used alone or in combination with other lipid-lowering medications, fibrates reduce triglyceride levels and increase HDL. The combination of a fibrate, particularly gemfibrozil, and a statin increases the risk of myopathy to approx 1% *(53)*. Gemfibrozil, but not fenofibrate, interferes with glucuronidation and, therefore, clearance of most statins, but both gemfibrozil and fenofibrate may reduce clearance of statins by adversely affecting liver function *(53)*. Fibrates and statins are cleared renally and should be used very cautiously in combination if there is renal impairment. Renal function, best measured by estimated GFRs, should determine initial dosing and dose titration. Baseline liver function tests and CK levels are recommended prior to initiating a fibrate, and the previously mentioned 2002 ACC/AHA/NHLBI guidelines for statin use also apply to fibrate/statin combination therapy *(48)*. Fibrates do not adversely affect glycemic control.

Two large randomized, placebo-controlled studies have examined the effects of fibrates on risk of CHD in patients with type 2 diabetes and insulin resistance. The Helsinki Heart Study showed a 68% reduction in CHD events among patients with diabetes treated with gemfibrozil; however, this result was not statistically significant owing to the small number of diabetic patients enrolled *(54,55)*. The Veterans Affairs-High-Density Lipoprotein Cholesterol Intervention Trial, a large secondary prevention study, showed a significant 24% reduction in CHD events over 5 yr among patients with diabetes treated with gemfibrozil *(56)*. The Diabetes Atherosclerosis Intervention Study, which used angiography to assess the rate of progression of CAD in patients treated with a fibrate vs placebo, found a 40% reduction in the progression of local atherosclerosis among patients treated with fenofibrate *(57)*. There is a large ongoing primary prevention trial examining the effects of fenofibrate on cardiovascular mortality among 9000 patients with diabetes and average cholesterol levels, the results of which will contribute significantly to outcome data on the use of fibrates in this population.

Niacin. Niacin, a form of nicotinic acid, inhibits mobilization of FFA from peripheral tissues (primarily fat), in turn reducing hepatic production and secretion of triglycerides *(45)*. Niacin also causes a shift from small, dense to large, buoyant LDL particles and increases HDL levels through either increased HDL synthesis or reduced hepatic clearance of apolipoprotein A-1, a major structural protein on HDL particles *(45,58)*. In patients with significantly elevated triglycerides and modestly elevated LDL, 2 g of niacin daily can lower triglycerides by 20–50% and LDL by 20% *(58)*.

The most common adverse effect of niacin is flushing, which usually occurs 30 min after taking the medication and can last for up to 60 min. This may be ameliorated by taking an aspirin 30 min prior to taking niacin. Additional adverse effects include gastric irritation; elevation of transaminases; and hyperuricemia, which can precipitate a gouty flare. Case reports and relatively small studies have demonstrated worsening glycemia in patients with and without type 2 diabetes treated with niacin *(58)*. This has led clinicians to be particularly cautious about using niacin in patients with impaired fasting glucose or impaired glucose tolerance (IGT), out of concern that the medication may lead to frank diabetes in this population. However, recent studies have shown that elevations of blood glucose in patients treated with extended-release niacin decrease over time and that the effect on HbA1C is minimal in patients with type 2 diabetes *(59,60)*.

Sterol Inhibitors. Ezetimibe, a relatively new cholesterol-lowering agent, acts on the intestinal wall to inhibit absorption of cholesterol and the glucuronide metabolite *(61)*. The medication undergoes enterohepatic circulation and is repeatedly delivered back to the gut. Ezetimibe can lower LDL cholesterol by approx 17%, making it comparable to resins as adjuvant LDL-lowering therapy *(61)*. This medication could be used as first-line therapy in patients who have only mildly elevated LDL levels and cannot tolerate statins. The effect of ezetimibe on HDL cholesterol and triglycerides is less than that of fibrates or niacin; it is generally not used as first-line therapy for raising HDL or lowering triglyceride levels *(61)*.

Combination Therapies. Combination therapy may be necessary if LDL reduction is not achieved with a statin alone, if triglycerides are markedly elevated, or if HDL is significantly reduced. Titrating the dose of a statin from 40 to 80 mg daily is associated with a threefold increase in liver toxicity and myopathy (with the exception of extended-release fluvastatin), whereas the addition of a fibrate, a resin, or the sterol inhibitor ezetimibe to a statin can lower LDL an additional 18% *(62)*. This reduction in LDL is comparable with that achieved by tripling the dose of a statin.

One comparison of the lipid-lowering effects of atorvastatin, fenofibrate, or both in patients with type 2 diabetes showed that the atorvastatin-fibrate combination led to a 46% reduction in LDL cholesterol, 50% reduction in triglycerides, and 22% increase in HDL *(63)*. These changes were significantly better than those achieved with either drug used as monotherapy *(63)*. Similarly, a larger multicenter study showed that a simvastatin-fibrate combination reduced total cholesterol, non-HDL, VLDL, and triglyceride levels significantly more than simvastatin or fenofibrate alone *(64)*. Finally, subgroup analysis of patients with metabolic syndrome enrolled in the HDL-Atherosclerosis Treatment Study, a 3-yr, double-blind trial examining the effect of niacin, simvastatin, and antioxidants on lipid profiles and progression of stenosis, found that simvastatin plus niacin had the greatest effect on raising HDL and increasing the percentage of less atherogenic LDL particles *(65)*. Progression of stenosis decreased by 90%, and rates of coronary death, nonfatal MI, stroke, and revascularization were reduced by 40% in patients receiving simvastatin plus niacin *(65)*.

Oral Hypoglycemics. Because the vast majority of patients with type 2 diabetes are treated for years with oral hypoglycemics, the effect of these medications on diabetic dyslipidemia is of interest. The most commonly prescribed oral hypoglycemics in the United States include second-generation sulfonylureas (glyburide, glipizide, and glimepiride), glinides (repaglinide and nateglinide), α-glucosidase inhibitors (acarbose and miglitol), biguanides (glucophage) and thiazolidenediones (TZDs) (rosiglitazone and pioglitazone). On the whole, studies examining the effects of individual oral hypoglycemics on lipid parameters have been relatively small, although some have shown statistically significant improvements in lipid parameters.

Buse et al. *(66)* published a comprehensive review of the effects of oral hypoglycemics on lipid parameters. They conclude that studies examining the effects of sulfonylureas and glinides have not consistently demonstrated statistically significant effects on lipid profiles *(66)*. The effects of α-glucosidase inhibitors on lipid profiles have been studied only in small numbers of patients. Statistically significant but clinically modest reductions in LDL levels have been shown with this class of medication *(66)*. Glucophage, the most commonly prescribed biguanide in the United States, has been shown in some, but not all, studies to reduce total cholesterol levels significantly when dosed maximally. Its effect on LDL, HDL, and triglyceride is inconsistent across studies, but the trend is toward modest improvement in each of the lipid parameters *(66)*.

The most clinical trial data are emerging for TZDs. There appear to be small differences between the two available agents in this class, pioglitazone and rosiglitazone, with pioglitazone showing a slightly more favorable effect on the lipid profile overall. Pioglitazone has been shown to increase both LDL and HDL levels, with an inconsistent effect on total cholesterol levels *(66)*. The qualitative increase in LDL seen with both pioglitazone and rosiglitazone treatment is thought to be owing to increased LDL particle size and buoyancy and may therefore exert a positive effect on lipid profile. In a large observational trial, pioglitazone reduced triglycerides and increased HDL levels to the same degree as either statins or fibrates *(67)*.

Two large, multicenter, randomized clinical trials have examined lipid profiles after adding pioglitazone to metformin or sulfonylureas. Pioglitazone added to either medication decreased triglyceride levels by 20% and increased HDL levels by 22% *(68)*. LDL levels decreased slightly when pioglitazone was added to a sulfonylurea and increased slightly when pioglitazone was added to metformin *(68)*. The add-on effects of pioglitazone occurred independent of glycemic control. The results of three large ongoing studies examining the effects of pioglitazone vs sulfonylureas on cardiovascular events and mortality as well as one study comparing ramipril, rosiglitazone, both, or neither on carotid intima thickness should add to the understanding of the nonhypoglycemic effects of TZDs. Combination therapies of TZDs plus statins or fibrates (PPARα/γ therapy) are currently being investigated for potentially additive effects on lipid parameters.

Future Therapies: CETP Antagonists. If a very low HDL level is the primary, or even only, lipid abnormality in a patient with diabetes and obesity, highly effective therapeutic options are limited. A potentially promising therapeutic target for primarily raising HDL levels is CETP. As shown in Fig. 3, when HDL and VLDL particles collide in the circulation, CETP exchanges VLDL with cholesteryl ester. The triglyceride-rich HDL particles are more vulnerable to clearance and the net effect is lower HDL levels. Torcetrapib is a recently developed inhibitor of CETP. Early studies have examined the effects of torcetrapib used alone or in combination with atorvastatin on HDL levels *(69)*. At a low dose, torcetrapib alone increased HDL levels by 46%, and at a higher dose HDL levels increased by 106% *(69)*. The higher dose of torcetrapib also resulted in a 26% reduction in triglycerides *(69)*. The quantitative effect on LDL cholesterol was modest, but there were significant qualitative changes in LDL particles. Torcetrapib alone at low and high doses increased levels of pattern A LDL particles by 257 and 294%, respectively *(69)*. Additional studies of this CETP inhibitor, including outcome studies examining effects of the medication on CHD events, are under way.

OTHER INSULIN-DEFICIENT AND -RESISTANT STATES

Type 1 Diabetes Mellitus

Type 1 diabetes is an insulin-deficient state, but some patients have significant insulin resistance in addition to insulin deficiency. The prevalence of dyslipidemia in type 1 diabetes is less than that in type 2 diabetes. The Wisconsin Epidemiological Study of Diabetic Retinopathy found that among 801 subjects with type 1 diabetes, 17% had hypercholesterolemia (defined as total cholesterol >240 mg/dL) and 29% had border-line high cholesterol (200–239 mg/dL) *(5)*. The Diabetes Control and Complications Trial included a larger population of patients with type 1 diabetes and found that lipids and lipoprotein profiles were similar to those found in nondiabetic subjects *(3)*. However, when type 1 diabetes is poorly controlled or untreated, patients may have markedly elevated triglycerides, especially postprandially.

Hypertriglyceridemia is primarily owing to insulin resistance and increased dietary triglycerides in type 2 diabetes, but hyperglycemia is thought be the underlying cause of hypertriglyceridemia in type 1 diabetes. Hyperglycemia causes hepatic overproduction of VLDL and reduced LPL activity, leading to decreased VLDL clearance *(47)*. Insulin therapy improves glycemia and normalizes LPL activity *(47)*. In fact, intensive insulin therapy can actually *overcorrect* dyslipidemia and produce low triglyceride levels;

the clinical significance of hypotriglyceridemia is not known. HDL levels may be normal or even elevated in type 1 diabetes, but as with type 2 diabetes, normal lipoprotein levels may be misleading. Patients with type 1 diabetes may have qualitative lipoprotein abnormalities, including cholesterol enrichment of VLDL and chylomicron remnants and glycosylation of LDL particles if there have been periods of severe hyperglycemia (47). The clinical significance of qualitative lipid abnormalities in type 1 diabetes is less well understood than in type 2 diabetes.

HIV Lipodystrophy and Dyslipidemia

Patients with HIV who are treated with antiretroviral medications, in particular protease inhibitors but also several other antiretroviral medications, often have a metabolic profile characterized by severe hypertriglyceridemia, modest hypercholesterolemia, decreased HDL, hyperinsulinemia and insulin resistance, and lipodystrophy (sc lipoatrophy of the face, extremities, and gluteal region and lipohypertrophy of the abdomen, dorsocervical area, and breasts) (70). Some patients also have IGT. Early HIV literature describes elevated triglycerides and VLDL levels in HIV patients not treated with highly active antiretroviral therapy (HAART), suggesting that the disease itself may also contribute to dyslipidemia. Subsequent observational studies have found multiple risk factors for HIV lipodystrophy, including interactions between the HIV itself and HAART (70,71).

Recognition and treatment of HIV-associated dyslipidemia is increasingly important in an era when patients are achieving sustained virological suppression and living longer. Studies are beginning to show that dyslipidemia as a risk factor for CHD applies to the HIV population, just as it does to the general population. A cross-sectional Norwegian study of 700 HIV-positive patients treated with HAART found that 12% of patients receiving HAART but only 5% of control subjects had a 10-yr CHD risk of >20% (which is the same 10-yr risk as for someone with diabetes or known CHD) (72). Smoking, increased total cholesterol, and decreased HDL all contributed to the significantly increased risk of CHD among this group of HIV patients (72).

Hypertriglyceridemia is the most common lipid abnormality associated with the use of protease inhibitors. Triglyceride levels are typically elevated by 200–300%, but there have been reports of even greater increases, putting patients at risk of pancreatitis (70,71). By comparison, total cholesterol levels tend to be increased by 30–40% (70,71). There are several proposed mechanisms by which protease inhibitors cause hyperlipidemia, including alteration of gene regulation within the adipocyte (reduced adipogenesis and increased lipolysis), competitive binding to LDL receptor-related protein, downregulation of the LDL receptor, and stimulation of hepatic triglyceride synthesis (70,71). In addition, elevated cytokine levels in HIV patients may lead to downregulation of LPL, HL, and CETP, leading to elevated triglyceride and decreased HDL levels (70,71). Recommendations for screening and treatment of patients with HIV dyslipidemia include routine monitoring of lipid profiles in all patients receiving antiretroviral therapy as well as ensuring a proper diet, getting regular exercise, stopping smoking, restricting alcohol intake, and monitoring for hypertension.

Pharmacotherapy should be initiated if lifestyle modifications are not effective, but choosing a lipid-lowering agent is complicated by the interaction between protease inhibitors and several of the statins. Simvastatin and lovastatin are both cleared hepatically via cytochrome P450 mechanisms, as are protease inhibitors. Simultaneous use of these medications may lead to increased toxicity through decreased clearance of the statin. Pravastatin is cleared via non-P450 mechanisms and is preferred, but atorvastatin, which has reduced interaction with protease inhibitors, may also be used with careful monitoring. In a small placebo-controlled randomized study of HIV patients taking protease inhibitors, pravastatin led to reductions in total LDL levels, small LDL particles, and small VLDL particles and also improved endothelial function, as measured by flow-mediated vasodilation *(73)*.

If the most significant metabolic abnormality is hypertriglyceridemia, first-line therapy may be a fibrate, which can lower triglycerides by 40%. A small randomized trial showed that fenofibrate led to significant reductions in triglycerides, total cholesterol, and non-HDL cholesterol and a significant increase in HDL cholesterol *(74)*. In this study, fenofibrate also increased LDL particle size and enhanced LDL resistance to oxidation *(74)*. Fibrate metabolism is not affected to the same degree as statins by protease inhibitors. Resins would not be a good choice for patients with HIV/HAART-associated dyslipidemia owing to their triglyceride-raising effects, and niacin may similarly not be a good choice in HIV patients with IGT *(71)*.

TZDs are being investigated for their effect on insulin resistance in HIV lipodystrophy. Initial results are conflicting. Small studies have shown that rosiglitazone increased peripheral sc fat in patients with HIV lipodystrophy, but a fairly large randomized study showed that 48 wk of rosiglitazone therapy did not improve any HIV lipodystrophy end point and caused asymptomatic hypertriglyceridemia and hypercholesterolemia *(75,76)*. Novel therapies, including recombinant human growth hormone, leptin, and protease inhibitors that do not cause dyslipidemia, are currently in the clinical trial stage.

Polycystic Ovary Syndrome

Women with PCOS typically have insulin resistance and hyperinsulinemia, both of which lead to reproductive and metabolic abnormalities. Obese women with PCOS often meet the criteria for metabolic syndrome, because they frequently also have hypertension and glucose intolerance. Not all studies have found that women with PCOS have significant lipid abnormalities, however, and those that have suggest that the dyslipidemia associated with PCOS is much more heterogeneous than that associated with type 2 diabetes. The lack of a characteristic lipid profile among women with PCOS is probably owing to the fact that a heterogeneous group of women carries this diagnosis. Troglitazone, a TZD no longer available in the United States, can improve insulin sensitivity, ovulatory function, and hirsutism among women with PCOS, but it has not been shown to affect lipid profiles in this population *(77)*. Moreover, retrospective studies have not shown that women with PCOS have increased risk of CHD above that of the general population.

REFERENCES

1. Miettinen H, Lehto S, Salomaa V, et al. Impact of diabetes on mortality after the first myocardial infarction: the FINMONICA myocardial infarction register study group. Diabetes Care 1998;21:69–75.
2. Haffner SM, Lehto S, Ronnemaa T, et al. Mortality for coronary heart disease in subjects with Type 2 diabetes and in nondiabetic subjects with and without prior myocardial infarction. N Engl J Med 1998;339:229–234.
3. DCCT Research Group. The effect of intensive treatment of diabetes on the development and progression of long-term complications in IDDM. N Engl J Med 1993;329:977–986.
4. Ohkubo Y, Kishikawa H, Araki E, et al. Intensive insulin therapy prevents the progression of diabetic microvascular complications in Japanese patients with noninsulin dependent diabetes mellitus: a randomized prospective 6 year study. Diabetes Res Clin Pract 1995;28:103–117.
5. Klein R, Klein BE, Moss SE. Relation of glycemic control to diabetic microvascular complications in diabetes mellitus. Ann Intern Med 1996;124:90–96.

6. UK Prospective Diabetes Study (UKPDS) Group. Intensive blood-glucose control with sulphony-lureas or insulin compared with conventional treatment and risk of complications in patients with type 2 diabetes (UKPDS 33). Lancet 1998;352:837–853.

7. Collins R, Armitage J, Parish S, et al. Heart Protection Study Collaborative Group. MRC/BHF Heart Protection Study of cholesterol-lowering with simvastatin in 5963 people with diabetes: a randomized placebo-controlled trial. Lancet 2003;361:2005–2016.

8. Dean BB, Borenstein JE, Henning JM, et al. Can change in high-density lipoprotein cholesterol levels reduce cardiovascular risk? Am Heart J 2004;147:966–976.

9. Lakka HM, Laaksonen DE, Lakka TA, et al. The metabolic syndrome and total and cardiovascular disease mortality in middle-aged men. JAMA 2002;288:2709–2716.

10. Hu G, Qiao Q, Tuomilehto J, et al. Prevalence of the metabolic syndrome and its relation to all-cause and cardiovascular mortality in nondiabetic European men and women. Arch Intern Med 2004; 164:1066–1076.

11. Wang PW, Liou CW, Wang ST, et al. Relative impact of low-density lipoprotein-cholesterol concentration and insulin resistance on carotid wall thickening in nondiabetic, normotensive volunteers. Metabolism 2002;51:255–259.

12. Marroquin OC, Kip KE, Kelly DE, et al. Metabolic syndrome modifies the cardiovascular risk associated with angiographic coronary artery disease in women: a report from the Women's Ischemia Syndrome Evaluation. Circulation. 2004;109:714–21.

13. Nieves DJ, Cnop M, Retzlaff B, et al. The atherogenic lipid profile associated with obesity and insulin resistance is largely attributable to intra-abdominal fat. Diabetes 2003;52:172–179.

14. Ford ES, Giles WH, Dietz WH. Prevalence of the metabolic syndrome among US adults. JAMA 2002;287:356–359.

15. Jacobson TA, Case CC, Roberts S, et al. Characteristics of US adults with the metabolic syndrome and therapeutic implications. Diabetes Obes Metab 2004;27:788–793.

16. Palaniappan L, Carnethon MR, Wang Y, et al. Predictors of the incident metabolic syndrome in adults: the Insulin Resistance Atherosclerosis Study. Diabetes Care 2004;27:788–793.

17. Libby P. Current concepts of the pathogenesis of the acute coronary syndromes. Circulation 2001; 104:365–372.

18. Eckel RH. Lipoprotein lipase. N Engl J Med 1989;320:1060–1068.

19. Ginsberg HN. Lipoprotein physiology in nondiabetic and diabetic states: relationship to atherogenesis. Diabetes Care 1991;12:839–855.

20. Zambon A, Hokanson JE, Brown BG, Brunzell JD. Evidence for a new pathophysiological mechanism for coronary artery disease regression: hepatic lipase mediated changes in LDL density. Circulation 1999;99:1959–1964.

21. Panarotto D, Remillard P, Bouffard L, Maheux P. Insulin resistance affects the regulation of lipoprotein lipase in the postprandial period and in an adipose-tissue specific manner. Eur Clin Invest 2002;32:84–92.

22. Krentz AJ. Lipoprotein abnormalities and their consequences for patients with type 2 diabetes. Diabetes Obes Metab 2003;5:S19–S27.

23. Garber AJ, Vinik AI, Crespin SR. Detection and management of lipid disorders in diabetic patients: a commentary for clinicians. Diabetes Care 1992;15:1068–1074.

24. Sniderman AD, Scantlebury T, Cianflone K. Hypertriglycedemic hyperapoB: the unappreciated atherogenic dyslipoproteinemia in type 2 diabetes mellitus. Ann Intern Med 2001;135:447–459.

25. Haffner SM. Management of dyslipidemia in adults with diabetes: position statement. Diabetes Care 1998;21:179–182.

26. St Pierre AC, Ruel IL, Cantin B, et al. Comparison of various electrophoretic characteristics of LDL particles and their relationship to the risk of ischemic heart disase. Circulation 2001;104:2295–2299.

27. Bowie A, Owens D, Collins P, et al. Glycosylated low density lipoprotein is more sensitive to oxidation: implications for the diabetic patient? Atherosclerosis 1993;102:63–67.

28. Matsui J, Onuma T, Tamasawa N, Suda T. Effects of advanced glycation endproducts on the generation of macrophage-mediated oxidized low-density lipoprotein. J Diabetes Complications 1997; 11:338–342.

29. Knott HM, Brown BE, Davies MJ, Dean RT. Glycation and glycoxidation of low-density lipoproteins by glucose and low-molecular mass aldehydes: formation of modified and oxidized particles. Eur J Biochem 2003;270:3572–3582.

30. Jinnouchi Y, Sano H, Nagai R, Hakamata H, et al. Glycoaldehyde-modified low density lipoprotein leads macrophages to foam cells via the macrophage scavenger receptor. J Biochem 1998;123:1208–1217.

31. Grundy SM, Cleeman JI, Bairey Merz CN, et al. Implications of recent clinical trials for the National Cholesterol Education Program Adult Treatment Panel III guidelines. Circulation 2004;110:227–239.
32. Haffner SM. Management of dyslipidemia in adults with diabetes: position statement. Diabetes Care 2003;26:S83–S86.
33. Leiter LA, Betteridge DJ, the AUDIT investigators. The AUDIT study: a worldwide survey of physician attitudes about diabetic dyslipidemia. Abstract 1170-P, American Diabetes Association Scientific Sessions, June 2004.
34. Sabuncu T, Ucar E, Birden F, Yasar O. The effect of 1 year sibutramine treatment on glucose tolerance, insulin sensitivity and serum lipid profiles in obese subjects. Diabetes Nutr Metab 2004;17:103–107.
35. Brook RD, Bard RL, Glazewski L, et al. Effect of short-term weight loss on the metabolic syndrome and conduit vascular endothelial function in overweight adults. Am J Cardiol 2004;93:1012–1016.
36. Davidson MH, Hauptman J, DiGiorlamo M, et al. Weight control and risk factor reduction in obese subjects treated for 2 years with orlistat: a randomized controlled trial. JAMA 1999;281:235–242.
37. Maki KC. Dietary factors in the prevention of diabetes mellitus and coronary artery disease associated with the metabolic syndrome. Am J Cardiol 2004;93S:12C–17C.
38. Hu FB, Willett WC. Optimal diets for prevention of coronary heart disease. JAMA 2002;288:2569–2578.
39. Mukamal KJ, Kronmal RA, Mittleman MA, et al. Alcohol consumption and carotid atherosclerosis in older adults: the Cardiovascular Health Study. Arterioscl Thromb Vasc Biol 2003;23:2252–2259.
40. Kris-Etherton PM, Harris WS, Appel LJ. American Heart Association Nutrition Committee. Fish consumption, fish oil, omega-3 fatty acids and cardiovascular disease. Circulation 2003;106:2747–2757.
41. GISSI-Prevenzione Investigators. Dietary supplementation with n-3 polyunsaturated fatty acids and vitamin E after myocardial infarction: results of the GISSI-Prevenzione trial. Lancet 1999; 354:447–455.
42. Lee KW, Lip GY. The role of omega-3 fatty acids in the secondary prevention of cardiovascular disease. QJM 2003;96:465–480.
43. Gill HM, Hardman AE. Exercise and postprandial lipid metabolism: an update on potential mechanisms and interactions with high-carbohydrate diets. J Nutr Biochem 2003;14:122–132.
44. Expert Panel on Detection, Evaluation and Treatment of High Blood Cholesterol in Adults. Executive summary of the third report of the National Cholesterol Education Program (NCEP) expert panel on detection, evaluation and treatment of high blood cholesterol in adults (adult treatment panel III). JAMA 2001;285:2486–2497.
45. Knopp RH. Drug treatment of lipid disorders. N Engl J Med 1999;341:498–511.
46. Snow V, Aronson MD, Hornbake ER, et al. Lipid control in the management of Type 2 diabetes mellitus: a clinical practice guideline from the American College of Physicians. Ann Intern Med 2004;140:644–649.
47. Ginsberg HN. Diabetic Dyslipidemia in Therapy for Diabetes Mellitus and Related Disorders, 4th ed. American Diabetes Association, 2004, pp. 293–309.
48. Jones PH. Statins as the cornerstone of drug therapy for dyslipidemia: monotherapy and combination therapy options. Am Heart J 2004;148:S9–S13.
49. Haffner SM, Alexander CM, Cook TJ, et al. Reduced coronary events in simvastatin-treated patients with coronary heart disease and diabetes or impaired fasting glucose levels: subgroup analyses in the Scandinavian Simvastatin Survival Study. Arch Intern Med 1999;159:2661–2667.
50. Goldberg RB, Mellies MJ, Sacks FM, et al. Cardiovascular events and their reduction with pravastatin in diabetic and glucose-intolerant myocardial infarction survivors with average cholesterol levels: subgroup analyses in the Cholesterol and Recurrent Events (CARE) trial. The CARE investigators. Circulation 1998;98:2513–2519.
51. Heart Protection Study Collaborative Group. MRC/BHF Heart protection study of cholesterol lowering with simvastatin in 20,536 high-risk individuals: a randomized, placebo-controlled trial. Lancet 2002;360:7–22.
52. Colhoun HM, Betteridge J, Durrington PN, et al. Primary prevention of cardiovascular disease with atorvastatin in type 2 diabetes in the Collaborative Atorvastatin Diabetes Study: multicentre randomized placebo-controlled clinical trial. Lancet 2004;364:685–696.
53. Jamal SM, Eisenberg MJ, Christopoulos S. Rhabdomyolysis associated with hydroxymethylglutaryl-coenzyme A reductase inhibitors. Am Heart J 2004;147:956–965.
54. Manninen V, Elo O, Frick MH, et al. Lipid alerations and decline in the incidence of coronary heart disease in the Helsinki Heart Study. JAMA 1988;260:641–651.
55. Koskinen P, Manttari M, Manninen V, et al. Coronary heart disease incidence in NIDDM patients in the Helsinki Heart Study. Diabetes Care 1992;15:820–825.

56. Rubins HB, Robins SJ, Collins D, et al. Gemfibrozil for the secondary prevention of coronary heart disease in men with low levels of high-density lipoprotein cholesterol: Veterans Affairs High-Density Lipoprotein Cholesterol Intervention Trial (VA-HIT) Study Group. N Engl J Med 1999;341:410–418.

57. Diabetes Atherosclerosis Intervention Study Investigators: Effect of fenofibrate on progression of coronary-artery disease in type 2 diabetes: the Diabetes Atherosclerosis Intervention Study, a randomized study. Lancet 2001;357:905–910.

58. Garg A, Grundy SM. Nicotinic acid as therapy for dyslipidemia in non-insulin dependent diabetes mellitus. JAMA 1990;264:723.

59. Grundy SM, Vega GL, McGovern ME, et al. Efficacy, safety and tolerability of once-daily niacin for the treatment of dyslipidemia associated with Type 2 diabetes. Arch Intern Med 2002;162:1568–1576.

60. Grundy SM, Vega GL, McGovern CF, et al. Comparative effects on lipids and glycemic control of niacin extended-release/lovastatin or fenofibrate in patients with diabetic dyslipidemia. Abstract 29-LB, American Diabetes Association Scientific Sessions, June 2004.

61. Davidson MH. Ezetimibe: a novel option for lowering cholesterol. Expert Rev Cardiovasc Ther 2003;1:11–21.

62. Davidson MH. Emerging therapeutic strategies for the management of dyslipidemia in patients with the metabolic syndrome. Am J Cardiol 2004;93S:3C–11C.

63. Athyros V, Papageorgiou A, Athyrou V, et al. Atorvastatin and micronized fenofibrate alone and in combination in Type 2 diabetes with combined hyperlipidemia. Diabetes Care 2002;25:1198–1202.

64. Grundy SM, Vega GL, Yuan Z, et al, for the SAFARI study group. Treatment of combined hyperlipidemia with simvastatin plus fenofibrate. Abstract 534-P, Am Diabetes Association Scientific Sessions, June 2004.

65. Brown BG, Zhao XQ, Chait A, et al. Simvastatin and niacin, antioxidant vitamins or the combination for the prevention of coronary disease. N Engl J Med 2001;354:1583–1592.

66. Buse JB, Tan MH, Prince MJ, Erickson PP. The effects of oral anti-hyperglycemic medications on serum lipid profiles in patients with type 2 diabetes. Diabetes Obes Metab 2004;6:133–156.

67. Schofl C, Luebben G. Pioglitazone improves diabetic dyslipidaemia in patients with type 2 diabetes mellitus with and without lipid-lowering therapy. Abstract 675-P, American Diabetes Association Scientific Sessions, June 2004.

68. Mariz S, Urquhart R, Moules I, et al. Effects of pioglitazone addition to metformin or sulfonylurea therapy on serum lipids in patients with type 2 diabetes mellitus: 2-year data. Abstract 578-P, American Diabetes Association Scientific Sessions, June 2004.

69. Brousseau ME, Schaefer EJ, Wolfe ML, et al. Effects of an inhibitor of cholesterol ester transfer protein on HDL cholesterol. N Engl J Med 2004;350:1505–1515.

70. Leow MKS, Addy CL, Mantzoros CS. Human immunodeficiency virus/highly active antiretroviral therapy-associated metabolic syndrome: clinical presentation, pathophysiology and therapeutic strategies. J Clin Endocrinol Metab 2003;88:1961–1976.

71. Koutkia P, Grinspoon S. HIV-Associated lipodystrophy: pathogenesis, prognosis, treatment and controversies. Ann Rev Med 2004;55:303–317.

72. Bergersen BM, Sandvik L, Bruun JN, Tonstad S. Elevated Framingham risk score in HIV-positive patients on highly active antiretroviral therapy: results from a Norwegian study of 721 subjects. Eur J Clin Microbiol Infect Dis. [abstract] July 2004 (Epublication).

73. Stein JH, Merwood MA, Bellehumeur JL, et al. Effects of pravastatin on lipoproteins and endothelial function in patients receiving human immunodefiency virus protease inhibitors. Am Heart J 2004;147:713.

74. Badiou S, De Boever CM, Dupuy AM, et al. Fenofibrate improves the atherogenic lipid profile and enhances LDL resistance to oxidation in HIV positive adults. Atherosclerosis 2004;172:273–279.

75. Carr A, Workman C, Carey D, et al. No effect of rosiglitazone for treatment of HIV-1 lipoatrophy: a randomized, double-blind, placebo-controlled trial. Lancet 2004;363:429–438.

76. Hadigan C, Yawetz S, Thomas A, et al. Metabolic effects of rosiglitazone in HIV lipodystrophy. Ann Intern Med 2004;140:786–794.

77. Azziz R, Ehrmann D, Legro RS, et al. Troglitazone improves ovulation and hirsutism in the polycystic ovary syndrome: a multicenter, double blind, placebo-controlled trial. J Clin Endocrinol Metab 2001;86:1626–1632.

12 Obesity, Diabetes, and Endothelial Dysfunction

Geetha R. Soodini, MD, Edward S. Horton, MD, and Osama Hamdy, MD, PhD

CONTENTS

INTRODUCTION

The prevalence of obesity is increasing globally and is associated with an increased risk of coronary artery disease (CAD), hypertension, dyslipidemia, and type 2 diabetes. The coexistence of obesity, hypertension, dyslipidemia, and insulin resistance or impaired glucose metabolism has been termed the *metabolic syndrome*. Many studies have shown that people with metabolic syndrome or type 2 diabetes are more likely to experience cardiovascular events even in the absence of baseline evidence of cardiovascular disease (CVD). This increased risk of CVD is owing to a complex interplay of many risk factors, one of which is endothelial dysfunction. Endothelial dysfunction is an early event in atherogenesis and has been shown to precede by several years the development of clinically detectable atherosclerotic plaques in the coronary arteries. Recent evidence points to adipose tissue as a complex and active endocrine tissue whose secretory products, including free fatty acids (FFAs), leptin, adiponectin, tumor necrosis factor-α (TNF-α), interleukin-6 (IL-6), resistin, and other cytokines, play a major role in the regulation of human metabolic and vascular biology. As a result, adipocytes are now claimed to be the missing link between insulin resistance and CVD. Lifestyle modification in the form of caloric restriction and increased physical activity is the most common approach used for improving endothelial and/or adipose-tissue functions with the expectation that this may reduce cardiovascular events in obese individuals with either the metabolic syndrome or type 2 diabetes.

OBESITY

Obesity is defined as having an excess amount of fat in relation to lean body mass as indicated by a body mass index (BMI) of 30 kg/m^2 or higher, and a BMI between

From: *Contemporary Diabetes: Obesity and Diabetes*
Edited by: C. S. Mantzoros © Humana Press Inc., Totowa, NJ

25 and 30 kg/m^2 indicates being overweight. The prevalence of obesity is increasing globally *(1–5)* and there is a parallel increase in type 2 diabetes *(6)*. A number of studies have shown that cardiovascular complications account for most of the morbidity and mortality associated with diabetes and the metabolic syndrome. It has also been shown that the risk of developing a myocardial infarction (MI) in diabetic patients with no prior history of coronary heart disease is equivalent to the risk observed in nondiabetic survivors with a prior MI *(7)*.

ENDOTHELIAL DYSFUNCTION

The vascular endothelium is no longer viewed as an inert lining of blood vessels. It plays a vital role in vascular homeostasis, vascular tone regulation, vascular smooth muscle cell proliferation, leukocyte migration, thrombosis, and thrombolysis *(8,9)*. In response to various mechanical, autonomic, and chemical stimuli, endothelial cells synthesize and release a large number of vasoactive substances, growth modulators, and other factors that mediate these functions. Endothelial dysfunction is described as a state in which factors that favor a vasoconstrictive, growth-promoting, procoagulant, and proinflammatory state become predominant over mediators that facilitate a vasodilator, growth-inhibiting, anticoagulant, and anti-inflammatory state *(10)*. It has been established that endothelial dysfunction is one of the earliest steps in the process of atherosclerosis. A number of studies have demonstrated endothelial dysfunction in patients with diabetes and obesity *(11–13)*. Caballero et al. *(14)* found that endothelial dysfunction is not only abnormal in the diabetic population but also in subjects with impaired glucose tolerance (IGT) and in healthy glucose-tolerant first-degree relatives of type 2 patients with diabetes.

Endothelial function can be evaluated by various methods, one of which is assessment of its ability to produce nitric oxide (NO). The release of NO occurs continuously under basal conditions and can be increased through activation of muscarinic receptors, as well as by changes in vascular shear forces associated with increased flow in the blood vessels. This vasodilatory effect in response to stimuli that are known to increase NO production is termed *endothelium-dependent vascular reactivity*. Invasive and noninvasive techniques, such as catheterization, ultrasound, positron emission tomography, laser Doppler flowmetry, and plethysmography, are the various methods used to evaluate vascular reactivity. The use of high-resolution ultrasound to assess brachial artery vasodilatory response is widely used owing to its noninvasive nature. This method can evaluate the flow-mediated dilation in the brachial artery, which represents the endothelium-dependent function, and also the vasodilatory response to sublingual nitroglycerine, which represents the endothelium-independent vasodilation related to vascular smooth muscle function. It has been found that endothelial dysfunction in the brachial artery correlates with endothelial dysfunction in the coronary circulation *(15)*.

Currently, atherosclerosis is viewed as an inflammatory process *(16)*. Metabolic disturbances such as obesity, hyperglycemia, dyslipidemia, and smoking are considered proinflammatory triggers, which cause chronic subclinical inflammation. This inflammatory process is started by adhesion of circulating monocytes to the endothelial surface via the adhesion molecules expressed on the endothelial surface. The normal endothelium expresses these molecules in limited amounts while dysfunctional endothelium, as seen in obesity and diabetes *(8)*, expresses these molecules in excess. The major increased adhesion molecules in these patients include selectins, intercellular adhesion molecule-1 (ICAM-1) and vascular cell adhesion molecule-1 (VCAM-1) *(8)*, which can be used as an indicator of endothelial function. Monocytes penetrate through the dysfunctional endothelium and transform to macrophages that have capabilities to engulf oxidized low-density lipoprotein (LDL) particles and transform to foam cells that form the atheromatous plaque.

Although the exact pathogenesis of endothelial dysfunction in these populations is not yet fully understood, multiple mechanisms are likely to be involved. Several components of the metabolic syndrome such as dyslipidemia, insulin resistance, hyperinsulinemia, hyperglycemia, and hypertension may be central to the development of endothelial dysfunction *(17)*. It has been hypothesized that endothelial dysfunction could be a consequence of either decreased synthesis of NO, increased inactivation of NO, or decreased responsiveness to NO. There is some evidence that decreased NO production results from diabetes-related endothelial cell injury *(18,19)*. Similarly, there is evidence that degradation of NO by oxygen-derived free radicals and advanced glycation end products may be augmented in the hyperglycemic state *(20,21)*.

The mechanisms linking obesity, insulin resistance, and endothelial function are increased FFAs, various cytokines, and altered body fat distribution or a combination of these. Increased FFAs acids from the insulin-resistant adipose tissue, particularly the visceral fat, lead to decreased insulin action in liver and skeletal muscle, through mechanisms that may affect the intracellular insulin-signaling cascade and are also associated with impaired vascular reactivity *(22,23)*. The adipocytokines have been closely linked to endothelial dysfunction and subclinical inflammation in obesity. Local infusion of TNF-α impairs endothelium-dependent vasodilation *(24)*. At a molecular level, TNF-α has been shown to increase monocyte adhesion to the vascular endothelium *(25)*, activate κB-dependent proinflammatory pathways *(26)*, induce endothelial expression of the adhesion molecule VCAM-1 *(27)*, and induce smooth muscle expression of matrix metalloproteinases, thus contributing to endothelial dysfunction and plaque destabilization *(28)*.

IL-6 has also been linked to endothelial dysfunction and subclinical inflammation. It is the major cytokine regulator of hepatic production of C-reactive protein (CRP), which, in turn, may have deleterious effects on the vascular wall *(29)*. The interlink between these two proinflammatory cytokines is complex: whereas TNF-α stimulates IL-6 production and, consequently, CRP production, IL-6 exerts a feedback inhibitory effect on TNF-α *(30)*. Interventions that mainly increase IL-6, such as exercise, paradoxically may have an anti-inflammatory effect through suppression of TNF-α, which is a major inducer of inflammation *(31)*.

Leptin has effects on energy expenditure, satiety, and neuroendocrine function. Leptin improves insulin sensitivity indirectly through satiety and body weight regulation, and in a more direct way by affecting insulin signaling in muscle *(32)*. Leptin also has some direct vasodilatory effects *(33)*. Conversely, adiponectin improves insulin sensitivity by enhancing intracellular insulin signaling and also has some direct vasodilatory and anti-inflammatory effects *(34,35)*.

Effect of Lifestyle Modification on Endothelial Function

Many studies have shown that exercise improves endothelial function *(36–39)*. The endothelial response to exercise training in humans appears to depend on the pretraining level of endothelial function. Individuals with initially impaired endothelial function at baseline, such as the elderly, patients with CAD, and those with risk factors for CVD, appear to be more responsive to exercise training than healthy individuals. Our group has recently demonstrated that a 6-mo program of lifestyle modification in the form of calorie restriction and moderate-intensity physical exercise in obese subjects with insulin resistance significantly improved endothelium-dependent vasodilation of the brachial artery *(40)*. This improvement was observed across the entire spectrum of glucose tolerance and was strongly associated with the percentage of weight reduction. This effect was also associated with a significant reduction in the plasma levels of sICAM. The latter change is consistent with a similar recent observation by Ziccardi et al. *(41)* in obese premenopausal women after 1 yr of weight reduction. A similar effect of combined energy-restricted diet and physical activity on endothelial function was also observed in obese healthy women using acetylcholine-stimulated vasodilation *(42)* and by measuring the response of blood pressure (BP) and platelet aggregation to an iv bolus of L-arginine, the natural precursor of NO *(43)*.

It is not yet clear whether the effect of lifestyle modification on endothelial function is predominantly related to the increased physical activity or is just an outcome of the metabolic changes associated with weight loss through diet restriction. In an effort to determine the origin of this effect, Sakamoto et al. *(44)* investigated the effect of exercise training and food restriction in two groups of Otsuka Long-Evans Tokushima Fatty rats, a genetic model of obesity and diabetes, in comparison to a matched group of sedentary rats. Interestingly, they found that exercise training, but not food restriction, prevents endothelial dysfunction in type 2 diabetic rats, although both interventions significantly suppressed plasma levels of glucose, insulin, and cholesterol; reduced the accumulation of abdominal fat; and improved insulin sensitivity to a comparable extent. This study also found that urinary excretion of nitrite was significantly decreased in sedentary and food-restricted rats compared with nondiabetic rats and was significantly increased in exercise-trained rats. Based on these findings, the investigators concluded that the improvement in endothelial function in exercised rats is the result of an exercise-induced increase in the production of NO *(44)*. Similar studies in humans are still lacking, and the currently available data are inconclusive.

Balkestein et al. *(45)* evaluated the effect of 3 mo of weight reduction with and without exercise on vessel-wall properties of the brachial and common carotid arteries in obese healthy men. Using a vessel-wall movement detector, they showed that weight loss increased carotid artery distensibility but found no additional benefit from adding an exercise component to the weight loss program. In contrast to this study, improvement in macrovascular endothelium-dependent vasodilation was reported after acute *(46)* and chronic exercise programs in two studies *(47,48)* that did not include a weight reduction component. The first *(47)* found that 3 mo of physical training enhanced brachial artery flow-mediated dilation in patients with the metabolic syndrome, and the second *(48)* observed that 12 wk of aerobic and resistance training improved brachial artery flow-mediated dilation in subjects with type 2 diabetes. A similar favorable effect of exercise training on flow-mediated dilation was recently seen in a group of patients with long-standing type 1 diabetes *(49)*.

In a recent study, Raitakari et al. *(50)* found that a very low-calorie diet for 6 wk improved endothelial function and reduced plasma glucose concentration independent of changes in weight, serum lipids, oxidized LDL, CRP, adiponectin, BP, and insulin. They thought that this improvement was related to the reduction in plasma glucose concentration and that changes in glucose metabolism may determine endothelial vasodilatory function in obesity. In another study *(51)* the effects of weight loss and glycemic control on endothelial dysfunction were compared using ICAM, endothelin-1 (ET-1) and E-selectin as outcome markers. Obese subjects had significant weight loss induced by bariatric surgery, and they showed a significant decrease in blood glucose, HbA1c, and all the aforementioned chemokines, whereas a small cohort who had weight loss induced by diet did not show any significant changes in the chemokines despite a significant reduction in blood glucose and HbA1c. These data indicate that weight loss is more important than glycemic control in regulating circulating levels of ICAM, ET-1, and E-selectin, which are expressed by the endothelium.

It is of particular interest that macronutrient modifications may also have an impact on endothelial function. Carluccio et al. *(52)* found that olive oil at nutritionally relevant concentrations transcriptionally inhibits endothelial adhesion molecule expression, thus partially explaining atheroprotection from Mediterranean diets. In addition, Yildirir et al. *(53)* found that a soy protein diet significantly improves endothelial function, as judged by flow-mediated endothelium-dependent dilatation and plasma thrombomodulin levels.

Several studies *(54–56)* have now shown that lifestlye modification programs focusing on weight reduction and increased physical activity significantly decrease the development of type 2 diabetes in high-risk individuals with IGT. However the effects of these programs on improving endothelial function in the short term or reducing CVD events in the long term have not been determined. It is also not known how long the beneficial effects of these lifestyle modification programs will last after these interventions have been discontinued.

REFERENCES

1. Flegal KM, Carroll MD, Ogden CL, Johnson CL. Prevalence and trends in obesity among US adults, 1999–2000. JAMA 2002;288:1723–1727.
2. Mokdad AH, Serdula MK, Dietz WH, et al. The spread of the obesity epidemic in the United States, 1991–1998. JAMA 1999;282:1519–1522.
3. Mokdad AH, Bowman BA, Ford ES, et al. The continuing epidemics of obesity and diabetes in the United Sates. JAMA 2001;286:1195–1200.
4. Mokdad AH, Ford ES, Bowman BA, et al. Prevalence of obesity, diabetes and obesity-related health risk factors, 2001. JAMA 2003;289:76–79.
5. Caballero B. Obesity in developing countries: biological and ecological factors. J Nutr 2001; 131:866S–870S.
6. Must A, Spadano J, Coakley EH, et al. The disease burden associated with overweight and obesity. JAMA 1999;282:1523–1529.
7. Haffner SM, Lehto S, Ronnemaa T, et al. Mortality from coronary heart disease in subjects with type 2 diabetes and in nondiabetic subjects with and without prior myocardial infarction. N Engl J Med 1998,339:229–234.
8. Dandona P. Endothelium, inflammation, and diabetes. Curr Diabetes Rep 2002;2:311–315.
9. Caballero AE. Endothelial dysfunction in obesity and insulin resistance: a road to diabetes and heart disease. Obes Res 2003;11:1278–1289.
10. McVeigh G, Cohn J. Endothelial dysfunction and the metabolic syndrome. Curr Diabetes Rep 2003;3:87–92.
11. Hogikyan RV, Galecki AT, Pitt B, et al. Specific impairment of endothelium-dependent vasodilation in subjects with type 2 diabetes. J Clin Endocrinol Metab 1998;83:1946–1952.
12. Williams SB, Cusco JA, Roddy MA, et al. Impaired nitric oxide-mediated vasodilation in patients with non-insulin-dependent diabetes mellitus. J Am Coll Cardiol 1996;27:567–574.
13. Tomiyama H, Kimura Y, Okazaki R, et al. Close relationship of abnormal glucose tolerance with endothelial dysfunction in hypertension. Hypertension 2000;36:245–249.
14. Caballero AE, Arora S, Saouaf R, et al. Micro vascular and macro vascular reactivity is reduced in subjects at risk for type 2 diabetes. Diabetes 1999;48:1856–1862.
15. Anderson TJ, Uehata A, Gerhard MD, et al. Close relation of endothelial function in the human coronary and peripheral circulations. J Am Coll Cardiol 1995;26:1235–1241.
16. Libby P, Ridker PM, Maseri A. Inflammation and atherosclerosis. Circulation 2002;105:1135–1143.

17. Tooke JE, Hannemann MM. Adverse endothelial function and the insulin resistance syndrome. J Intern Med 2000;247(4):425–431.

18. Chowienczyk PJ, Barnes DJ, Brett SE, Cockcroft JR, Viberti GC, Ritter JM. Correction of impaired NO-mediated vasodilation by L-arginine in non-insulin dependent diabetes. Endothelium 1995;3:955 (abstract).

19. Wascher TC, Graier WF, Dittrich P, et al. Effects of low-dose L-arginine on insulin-mediated vasodilation and insulin sensitivity. Eur J Clin Invest 1997; 27:690–695.

20. Ting HH, Timimi FK, Boles KS, Creager SJ, Ganz P, Creager MA. Vitamin C improves endothelium dependent vasodilation in patients with non-insulin-dependent diabetes mellitus. J Clin Invest 1996;97:22–28.

21. Bucala R, Tracey KJ, Cerami A. Advanced glycosylation products quench nitric oxide and mediate defective endothelium-dependent vasodilatation in experimental diabetes. J Clin Invest 1991;87:432–438.

22. Griffin ME, Marcucci MJ, Cline GW, et al. Free fatty acid induced insulin resistance is associated with activation of protein kinase C theta and alterations in the insulin signaling cascade. Diabetes 1999;48:1270–1274.

23. Steinberg HO, Baron AD. Vascular function, insulin resistance and fatty acids. Diabetologia 2002;45:623–634.

24. Patel JN, Jager A, Schalkwijk C, et al. Effects of tumor necrosis factor-alpha in the human forearm: blood flow and endothelin-1 release. Clin Sci (Lond) 2002;103(4):409–415.

25. Zeng M, Zhang H, Lowell C, He P. Tumor necrosis factor-alpha-induced leukocyte adhesion and microvessel permeability. Am J Physiol Heart Circ Physiol 2002;283(6):H2420–H2430.

26. Ashton AW, Ware GM, Kaul DK, Ware JA. Inhibition of tumor necrosis factor alpha-mediated NFkappaB activation and leukocyte adhesion, with enhanced endothelial apoptosis, by G protein-linked receptor (TP) ligands. J Biol Chem 2003;278(14):11,858–11,866.

27. Park SH, Park JH, Kang JS, Kang YH. Involvement of transcription factors in plasma HDL protection against TNF-alpha-induced vascular cell adhesion molecule-1 expression. Int J Biochem Cell Biol 2003;35(2):168–182.

28. Uzui H, Harpf A, Liu M, et al. Increased expression of membrane type 3-matrix metalloproteinase in human atherosclerotic plaque: role of activated macrophages and inflammatory cytokines. Circulation 2002;106(24):3024–3030.

29. Yudkin JS, Kumari M, Humphries M, Mohamed-Ali V, on behalf of the University College London Interleukin-6 group. Interleukin-6: a pro-inflammatory cytokine linking inflammation, obesity, stress, ethnicity, and coronary heart disease? Atherosclerosis 2000;148:209–214.

30. Suzuki K, Nakaji S, Yamada M, et al. Systemic inflammatory response to exhaustive exercise. Cytokine Kinet. Exerc Immunol Rev 2002;8:6–48.

31. Starkie R, Ostrowski SR, Jauffred S, et al. Exercise and IL-6 infusion inhibit endotoxin-induced TNF-alpha production in humans. FASEB J 2003;17:884–886.

32. Kim YB, Uotani S, Perozz DD, et al. In vivo administration of leptin activates signal transduction directly in insulin sensitive tissues: overlapping but distinct pathways from insulin. Endocrinology 2000;141:2328–2339.

33. Lembo G, Vecchione C, Fratta L, et al. Leptin induces direct vasodilation through distinct endothelial mechanisms. Diabetes 2000;49:293–297.

34. Chen H, Montagnani M, Funahashi T, et al. Adiponectin stimulates production of nitric oxide in vascular endothelial cells. J Biol Chem 2003;278:45,021–45,026

35. Matsuda M, Shimomura I, Sata M, et al. Role of adiponectin in preventing vascular stenosis: the missing link of adipo-vascular axis. J Biol Chem 2002;277(40):37,487–37,491.

36. Moyna NM, Thompson PD. The effect of physical activity on endothelial function in man. Acta Physiol Scan 2004;180:113–123.

37. Maiorana A, O'Driscoll G, Taylor R, Green D. Exercise and the nitric oxide vasodilator system. Sports Med 2003;33:1013–1035.

38. Higashi Y, Yoshizumi M. Exercsie and endothelial function: role of endothelium-derived nitric oxide and oxidative stress in healthy subjects and hypertensive patients. Pharmacol Ther 2004;102:87–96.

39. Woo KS, Chook P, Yu CW, et al. Effects of diet and exercise on obesity related vascular dysfunction in children. Circulation 2004,109:1981–1986.

40. Hamdy O, Ledbury S, Mullooly C, et al. Lifestyle modification improves endothelial function in obese subjects with the insulin resistance syndrome. Diabetes Care 2003;26(7):2119–2125.

41. Ziccardi P, Nappo F, Giugliano G, et al. Reduction of inflammatory cytokine concentrations and improvement of endothelial functions in obese women after weight loss over one year. Circulation 2002;105(7):804–809.

42. Ridker PM, Hennekens CH, Roitman-Johnson B, Stampfer MJ, Allen J. Plasma concentration of soluble intercellular adhesion molecule 1 and risks of future myocardial infarction in apparently healthy men. Lancet 1998;10:351(9096):88–92.

43. Sciacqua A, Candigliota M, Ceravolo R, et al. Weight loss in combination with physical activity improves endothelial dysfunction in human obesity. Diabetes Care 2003;26(6):1673–1678.

44. Sakamoto S, Minami K, Niwa Y, et al. Effect of exercise training and food restriction on endothelium-dependent relaxation in the Otsuka Long-Evans Tokushima Fatty rat, a model of spontaneous NIDDM. Diabetes 1998;47(1):82–86.

45. Balkestein EJ, van Aggel-Leijssen DP, van Baak MA, Struijker-Boudier HA, Van Bortel LM. The effect of weight loss with or without exercise training on large artery compliance in healthy obese men. J Hypertens 1999;17(12 Pt 2):1831–1835.

46. Gaenzer H, Neumayr G, Marschang P, Sturm W, Kirchmair R, Patsch JR. Flow-mediated vasodilation of the femoral and brachial artery induced by exercise in healthy nonsmoking and smoking men. J Am Coll Cardiol 2001;38(5):1313–1319.

47. Lavrencic A, Salobir BG, Keber I. Physical training improves flow-mediated dilation in patients with the polymetabolic syndrome. Arterioscler Thromb Vasc Biol 2000;20(2):551–555.

48. Maiorana A, O'Driscoll G, Cheetham C, et al. The effect of combined aerobic and resistance exercise training on vascular function in type 2 diabetes. J Am Coll Cardiol 2001;38(3):860–866.

49. Fuchsjager-Mayrl G, Pleiner J, Wiesinger GF, et al. Exercise training improves vascular endothelial function in patients with type 1 diabetes. Diabetes Care 2002;25(10):1795–1801.

50. Raitakari M, Ilvonen T, Ahotupa M, et al. Weight reduction with very low calorie diet and endothelial function in overweight adults: role of plasma glucose. Arterioscl Thromb Vasc Biol 2004;24:124–128.

51. Pontiroli AE, Pizzocri P, Koprivec D, et al. Body weight and glucose metabolism have a different effect on circulating levels of ICAM-1, E-selectin, and endothelin-1 in humans. Eur J Endocrinol 2004;150:195–200.

52. Carluccio MA, Siculella L, Ancora MA, et al. Olive oil and red wine antioxidant polyphenols inhibit endothelial activation: antiatherogenic properties of Mediterranean diet phytochemicals. Arterioscl Thromb Vasc Biol 2003;23(4):622–629.

53. Yildirir A, Tokgozoglu SL, Oduncu T, et al. Soy protein diet significantly improves endothelial function and lipid parameters. Clin Cardiol 2001;24(11):711–716.

54. Diabetes Prevention Program Research Group. Reduction in the incidence of type 2 diabetes with lifestyle intervention or metformin. N Engl J Med 2002;346(6):393–403.

55. Pan XR, Li GW, Hu YH, et al. Effects of diet and exercise in preventing NIDDM in people with impaired glucose tolerance: the Da Quing IGT and Diabetes Study. Diabetes Care 1997;20:537–544.

56. Tuomilehto J, Lindstrom J, Eriksson JG, et al., Finnish Diabetes Prevention Study Group. Prevention of type 2 diabetes mellitus by changes in lifestyle among subjects with impaired glucose tolerance. N Engl J Med 2001;344(18):1343–1350.

13

Atherosclerosis and Peripheral Vascular Disease

Sequelae of Obesity and Diabetes

Satish N. Nadig, MD *and Allen Hamdan,* MD

CONTENTS

INTRODUCTION
ATHEROSCLEROSIS IN THE OBESE PATIENT WITH DIABETES
METABOLIC SYNDROME AND PVD
PVD IN THE PATIENT WITH DIABETES
PERIPHERAL VASCULAR DISEASE
CONCLUSIONS
REFERENCES

INTRODUCTION

Over the past 10 yr, the disease of obesity has been described as an "epidemic" and a "pathogen." The increase in populations of the developed world exceeding a body mass index (BMI) of 25, rendering them overweight, is alarming. In 1999, in the United States 61% of adults fell into the first category and 27% were considered obese *(1)*. The medical ramifications of obesity include, but are certainly not limited to, conditions such as type 2 diabetes mellitus, hypertension, osteoarthritis, ischemic heart disease, cardiomyopathy, and dyslipidemia, as well as peripheral vascular disease (PVD). There are approx 14 million individuals with type 2 diabetes in the United States, and the risk of developing type 2 diabetes is directly proportional to an increasing BMI *(1–3)*. PVD in the diabetic population can be more advanced at the time of presentation than in the nondiabetic patient. The effects of sensory and motor neuropathy may mask subtle changes in perfusion and underlying infections secondary to advanced atherosclerosis. In fact, the diabetic patient population has a rate of lower-extremity amputation that is 15 times higher than that of the nondiabetic population *(4)*. Currently, no data exist regarding the rates of PVD for patients harboring both comorbidities of obesity and diabetes concomitantly. Using the obese and diabetic patient as a paradigm, this chapter discusses the pathophysiology of atherosclerosis and the clinical presentation, diagnosis, and treatment of PVD.

From: *Contemporary Diabetes: Obesity and Diabetes*
Edited by: C. S. Mantzoros © Humana Press Inc., Totowa, NJ

ATHEROSCLEROSIS IN THE OBESE PATIENT WITH DIABETES

Atherosclerosis is the degenerative and regenerative disease of the vasculature that primarily affects the intima (innermost layer) of vessels and eventually the media (intermediate layer) at the bifurcations of predominantly major arteries. *Athero* and *sclerosis*, from the Greek roots *gruel* and *induration*, respectively, consist of plaques made up of a necrotic base with a hardened fibrotic cap. These lesions comprise three fundamental components: (1) cholesterol esters; (2) smooth muscle cells (SMCs); and (3) connective tissue made up of collagen, elastin, and glycosaminoglycans *(5)*.

Many theories of atherogenesis have been postulated. Five such theories as enumerated by Tegos et al. *(5)* are presented in the following sections.

The Lipid Theory

The lipid theory is based on the well-documented observation of increased cholesterol esters of the low-density lipoprotein (LDL) subtype in the arterial intima. Increases in plasma LDL concentrations are thought to alter the permeability of cholesterol esters in the intima of arteries, mediated by vesicular transport. This event causes the intima to retain the LDL molecules and stymies the transport of LDL from intima to media.

The Hemodynamic Theory

The hemodynamic theory is based on the hypothesis that low and oscillating hemodynamic shear forces delay the clearance of potentially toxic substances and allow for prolonged contact with the arterial intima, which leads to endothelial injury. The altered hemodynamics may also affect endothelial permeability to LDL, allowing transport to the intima. This theory is evidenced by the affinity of atheromatous lesions to occur at arterial branching sites where there is relative turbulent and stagnant flow.

The Fibrin Incrustation Theory

The Fibrin incrustation theory was first proposed in the 19th century and postulates that as fibrinogen is converted into fibrin on the arterial luminal surface the thrombus is actively incorporated into the atheroma. The assimilation of the thrombus converts the appearance of the plaque to fibrous tissue. The pertinence of this older theory is that the formation of thrombi in atheromatous plaques leads to their instability.

The Nonspecific Mesenchymal Hypothesis

A stimulus to the arterial wall (i.e., shear stress or vasoactive agents) induces smooth muscle or mesenchymal cells to migrate from the media to the intima, where they proliferate and produce connective tissue, leading to the formation of atheroma.

The Response to Injury Hypothesis

As the endothelium of arteries is denuded by injurious stimuli (i.e., hemodynamic, chemical, physical, viral, or external factors, to name a few), platelets begin to adhere to the injured area, consistent with Virchow's triad, and release platelet-derived growth factor (PDGF). PDGF, also released by arterial endothelium, stimulates mesenchymal movement from media to intima, where the SMCs proliferate and form connective tissue or atheromas.

The response to injury hypothesis has been further studied to show that as the vascular endothelium is injured, expression of substances such as vascular cell adhesion molecule-1 and monocyte chemoattractant protein-1 is altered, aiding in the recruitment of monocytes to the injured site. Monocytes attach themselves to the endothelium and migrate to the arterial intima, where they constitute activated macrophages. Simultaneously, as LDL molecules traverse the endothelium they are oxidized by oxygen free radicals produced by the endothelium. These LDLs form complexes with the extracellular matrix proteins (collagen, elastin, and proteoglycans) and after they are oxidized and move to the intima of the artery interact as a ligand to specialized receptors on the aforementioned macrophages, which subsequently phagocytize the oxidized LDL. These lipid-laden macrophages, or foam cells, are the pathological hallmark of atheromatous lesions. Once atheromatous lesions are formed, these plaques may grow to cause luminal stenosis or may incorporate calcium as hydroxyapetite crystals. Further, the adventitia (externalmost layer) of arteries may induce neovascularization into the thrombus itself, leading to eventual hemorrhage (5). It is likely that a combination of these theories that best explains the complex process of atherogenesis. In addition, there is currently no evidence to suggest that the macrovascular disease seen in diabetes or obesity is any different from that of other conditions such as smoking.

METABOLIC SYNDROME AND PVD

The dyslipidemia of obesity includes an increase in LDL molecules, and this coupled with the hyperlipidemia associated with diabetes places patients who harbor both of these characteristics in a high-risk category for the formation of atheroma. The constellation of these features has been termed *metabolic syndrome*.

Central obesity is the cornerstone of metabolic syndrome, characterized by insulin resistance leading to hyperinsulinemia, dyslipidemia, hypertension, type 2 diabetes, and an increased risk of cardiovascular events (6). As part of metabolic syndrome, patients who are obese (BMI > 30) have high triglyceride and LDL levels. The small LDL molecules are rich with atherogenic apolipoprotein B particles, leading to the formation of plaque and diffuse atherosclerosis (7). It has been shown that patients with the constellation of metabolic syndrome have an 85% higher prevalence of PVD (8).

PVD IN THE PATIENT WITH DIABETES

Over the past 20 yr, there has been an evolution of thought regarding the distribution of atheromatous disease in the diabetic patient population. Forty-five to fifty years ago it was a popular belief that the patient with diabetes was the model for "microvascular disease." That is, the small distal arteries of the foot and ankle were the most affected by atherosclerotic occlusive disease (9). The predominance of this theory obviated the utility of distal arterial reconstruction in an attempt to save the diabetic foot. Distal revascularization procedures were not done on diabetics secondary to lack of target quality.

Since then, however, many studies have shown that although there are differences in the distribution and severity of diabetic atherosclerotic disease, the concept of "small vessel occlusive disease" is false—especially in the arteries of the foot. Although there is no specific microvascular occlusion, there is a significant difference in the pathobiology of the diabetic patient, particularly seen in the foot.

Atherosclerotic disease in the patient with diabetes may present at a younger age and evolve into occlusive disease at a more rapid pace than that of the patient without diabetes. The acceleration of disease may be accounted for by underlying endothelial dysfunction in the walls of the diabetic vessel. Vasodilatory reactivity is impaired in the diabetic patient and has been shown to normalize with oral hypoglycemic treatment in the patient with occult diabetes *(10)*. The impairment of endothelial-dependent vasodilatation at the level of the diabetic foot causes a reduced expression of endothelial nitric oxide synthase (NOS). Decreased levels of NOS result in reduced endoneurial blood flow and increased vascular resistance, ultimately leading to symptoms of neuropathy *(11)*.

Previously, the treatment protocol for diabetic patients with PVD did not include arterial reconstruction. This often resulted in a situation in which gangrene in a diabetic patient led to major amputation without any attempt at limb salvage. The distribution of arterial occlusion is unique in the diabetic patient in that it generally affects the infrageniculate arteries of the calf, namely, the anterior tibial, posterior tibial, and peroneal arteries, but spares the proximal superficial femoral, popliteal, and more important, distal dorsalis pedis—allowing for a potential target on the foot itself *(12)*.

The theory of microcirculatory occlusion impeded distal revascularization techniques early on; however, by using the spared superficial femoral artery (SFA) or popliteal as inflow, the dorsalis pedis artery has become a preferred target for distal reperfusion. Protocols now include more aggressive control of blood sugar, infection, and identification of pedal arteries suitable for distal bypass.

PERIPHERAL VASCULAR DISEASE

Clinical Presentation

The spectrum of atherosclerotic PVD spans three general categories: claudication, rest pain, and tissue loss. In the diabetic patient population, however, this "normal" continuum is altered by the effects of diabetes itself, namely, motor and sensory neuropathy (polyneuropathy), intrinsic muscle atrophy, and accelerated rate of infection. This altered pathobiology makes the clinical presentation of the diabetic patient much less uniform. To clarify the complicated presentation of the obese and diabetic patient, a thorough history and physical examination is still the "gold standard."

Claudication, or leg pain secondary to functional ischemia, commonly presents as intermittent and cramping calf pain precipitated by exercise and alleviated by rest. Claudication may be quantified and tracked by the *initial claudication distance*, or the distance one can walk prior to the onset of symptoms. In the nondiabetic patient, the symptoms of ischemic lower-extremity pain usually occur as a consequence of multivessel (more than two vessels affected) occlusion secondary to the rich vascularity of the leg. However, the diabetic patient population is much more susceptible to experience symptoms secondary to single-vessel occlusive disease because of these patients' sensitivity to even small changes in tissue perfusion. The relative risk of claudication in patients with diabetes has been shown to be 3.5 in men and 8.6 in women *(13)*. With the use of a detailed history, the extent and progression of claudication may be evaluated and followed with time.

Although intermittent claudication can be stable over a number of years, approx 25% of patients with symptoms of ischemic leg pain progress to rest pain or tissue loss. When PVD becomes more severe, patients develop symptoms of rest pain, characterized by a constant burning or painful sensation of the forefoot or metatarsal head. Again, a careful history aids in the diagnosis of rest pain. Most commonly, rest pain occurs at night and is alleviated by dependent positioning of the affected extremity. In the diabetic patient, rest pain can be easily confused with the pain of peripheral neuropathy, leading to a delay in diagnosis.

Tissue loss, characterized by ulceration or gangrene, is the most severe presentation of PVD. In almost all situations, ulceration in the diabetic patient involves some component of vascular compromise. In addition, because the structure of the foot is changed by atrophy of the intrinsic musculature related to motor neuropathy, a characteristic "claw" formation with pressure points now located beneath the metatarsal heads is formed (malperferous ulcers.) Furthermore, sensory neuropathy can render the diabetic foot insensate, accounting for chronic ulceration and penetration of foreign bodies leading to infection, the so-called silent-needle neuropathy (14). The cause of ulceration in the diabetic patient population is multifactorial; thus, all diabetic patients presenting with tissue loss warrant a thorough assessment for PVD.

When the symptoms of PVD progress even further, the picture of gangrene develops. The hallmark signs of gangrene are typically extremities that appear black and are insensate and lack motor function. Gangrene usually appears the same in both the individual with diabetes and the individual without diabetes alike; however, when an infection is superimposed (wet gangrene) the usual systemic response of fever and leukocytosis is sometimes blunted in the immunocompromised diabetic patient. Systemic infection in the setting of wet gangrene constitutes a surgical emergency and may only manifest as an increased insulin requirement or hyperglycemia. In fact, systemic infection may also occur in the setting of foot ulceration in the diabetic patient. These infections are aggressive, are most often polymicrobial, and are the leading cause of amputation in the diabetic population.

Diagnosis

As mentioned before, the physician's history and physical examination are still the foundation of a complete assessment for PVD. The evaluation of pedal pulses is the primary step in diagnosing the extent of occlusive disease. The absence of either palpable or Dopplerable pedal pulses points toward advanced disease and must be worked up further. The second step in the diabetic foot examination is evaluation of the presence and extent of tissue loss or gangrene. This includes assessment of the toes and web spaces along with evaluation of shoes for pressure points. When an ulcer is found and can be probed to bone, the diagnosis of osteomyelitis is made and no further imaging is necessary. Once the patient is evaluated at the bedside, many diagnostic techniques can be used to quantify the extent and location of occlusive disease. Noninvasive modalities include ankle-brachial indices (ABIs), pulse-volume recordings (PVR), and transcutaneous O_2 measurements. Finally, the invasive technique of digital subtraction angiography (DSA) is a modification of conventional angiography and is considered to be the "gold standard" in the diagnosis of PVD, allowing anatomic evaluation of occlusive disease. Computed tomographic angiography (CTA) and magnetic resonance angiography (MRA) are two limited noninvasive techniques that may be used when patients have contrast allergies or advanced renal impairment, two contraindications to the heavy dye load associated with DSA.

Noninvasive modalities are extremely useful in discerning the extent and location of occlusive disease in the nondiabetic patient; however, these studies can be limited in the diabetic and obese patient.

ABIs, which are part of the office exam, are measured by comparing the systolic pressures of the upper extremities with those of the lower extremities using a Doppler probe and a sphygmomenometer cuff. The higher of the dorsalis pedis and anterior tibial artery measurements is used as the numerator and divided by the higher of the brachial artery measurements (right vs left) in the ABI ratio. An index of <0.9 translates to impaired perfusion to the lower extremities and is the criterion most studies use in the initial diagnosis of PVD. In the diabetic population, however, diffuse calcification of the arterial wall causes decreased compressibility and falsely elevated, unreliable measurements. In the obese patient, blood pressure cuffs of the appropriate size are crucial but are rarely used, also causing a false reading. Thus, although generally a useful test, the ABI in the diabetic and obese patient can be misleading.

PVRs use a series of plethysmography cuffs placed along the leg in order to measure changes in diameter during systole and diastole. These measurements relate to the dilatation of the lower-extremity vasculature and are recorded as a waveform. In the normal leg, a triphasic waveform is recorded from the thigh down; however, in the extremity afflicted with occlusive disease, the triphasic wave is dampened to a monophasic or flat waveform, a qualitative rather than quantitative measurement of disease. Although the PVR is not the lone determinant of disease severity, the PVR in the diabetic population can be illustrative because it is not affected by calcifications within the arterial wall.

Tissue perfusion using transcutaneous O_2 measurements is a controversial method of evaluating the extent of occlusive disease. Using an O_2 measurement probe over an existing ulcer, surgical wound, or potential wound, the healing potential of the affected tissue may be assessed by attempting to quantify the amount of perfusion after equilibrating to environmental temperature. Although there are some reports that show transcutaneous O_2 measurements to be lower in the diabetic population than in the nondiabetic population with the same disease severity *(15)*, the results are largely variable and often difficult to interpret.

With the advent of conventional angiography, and later DSA, occlusive disease in the diabetic, obese, and nondiabetic patient may be more accurately quantified as to extent and level. By subtracting out the bone and soft-tissue background, an interpreter may clearly follow the contrast load coursing through the vasculature of the lower extremity over time. In addition, specific images may be selected for bypass target evaluation and/or percutaneous treatment, and levels of occlusion may be more accurately identified. A common mistake made by inexperienced radiographers is the incomplete angiogram, wherein the exam is terminated prematurely and the pedal vessels are not visualized. In the diabetic patient, occlusion of the tibial and peroneal vessels is commonly misconceived as unreconstructable disease. Therefore, even if tibial and peroneal vessels are found to be occluded, care must be taken to continue the exam distally to the foot and ankle for preferred target visualization. To prevent contrast-induced renal compromise, adequate iv hydration combined with pre- and postangiography treatment with oral *N*-acetylcysteine is recommended *(16)*. Both MRA and CTA have been studied as alternatives to DSA; however, the inability to visualize the patency of pedal vessels, often owing to institutional variability, using both modalities hampers the utility of CTA/MRA in the diabetic patient.

The complexity of the obese/diabetic patient calls for treatment protocols that require hypervigilence on the part of the physician with aggressive diagnostic and therapeutic schemes.

Treatment (Medical/Surgical)

Management of PVD in the diabetic patient requires a careful balance between early diagnosis and prevention of disease progression with medical therapies. When the extent of occlusive disease has become more severe than manageable with conservative therapies, the aggressive use of surgical debridement, bypass, and/or amputation is warranted.

When patients present early with the symptoms of intermittent claudication as described earlier, the management is twofold, involving risk factor modification and medical treatment. Murabito et al. *(17)* showed that more than 90% of patients who are referred to vascular clinics for evaluation of PVD in the United States have a history of smoking. Furthermore, patients with vascular disease who continue to smoke cigarettes have a 40–50% 5-yr mortality and an increased risk of amputation *(17,18)*. Therefore, it is obvious that the physician's first line of defense in the prevention of progressing disease is to encourage smoking cessation, clearly an important risk factor in the development of PVD. Obesity as part of metabolic syndrome leading to hypertension, diabetes, and dyslipidemia must be addressed in the initial work-up of a patient with intermittent claudication. The use of angiotensin-converting enzyme inhibitors as antihypertensive treatment may be particularly beneficial in patients with PVD owing to the vasoprotective effects of this class of drug *(19)*. The utility of HMG-CoA reductase inhibitors, particularly in the setting of cardiac prevention, has also been shown through various clinical trials to improve mildly the symptoms of claudication *(20–22)*. Finally, weight loss through exercise is unmatched in reducing cardiovascular risk as well as decreasing the symptoms of claudication. Walking 35–50 min approx three to five times per week at a pace that reproduces claudication has been shown to improve markedly a patient's initial claudication distance *(23,24)*. However, best results are seen with structured exercise programs, but these often are not covered by insurance.

Along with risk factor modification, the use of certain medical therapies, namely antiplatelet and phosphodiesterase type III (PDE III) inhibitors, may stymie the evolution of occlusive disease. Although there is an increased risk of bleeding, the use of aspirin and an adenosine diphosphate receptor antagonist such as clopidogrel together has been shown to be efficacious in lowering the risk of cardiovascular disease in patients with occlusive vessel disease *(25)*. In addition, cilostazol, a PDE III inhibitor, is an effective treatment for reducing symptoms of claudication. Cilostazol alleviates the pain of claudication by increasing vasodilatation through upregulation of cyclic adenosine monophosphate. The vascular benefits of cilostazol are also related to the drug's inhibition of the formation of thrombi, platelet aggregation, and vascular smooth muscle proliferation *(26)*. In a meta-analysis of eight randomized, placebo-controlled trials of 2702 patients with varying degrees of claudication, Thompson et al. *(27)* showed an increase of up to 67% in the initial claudication distance in patients with symptoms of 24 wk of duration with the use of cilostazol.

Patients with diabetes and obesity are in a high-risk category for progression of disease. Thus, treatment protocols for this patient population differ from those of the nondiabetic patient.

The management of diabetic patients with PVD must be deliberate and algorithmic. In the first step, any area of infection or necrotic tissue must be thoroughly drained and/or debrided, even if the infected area is ischemic. The common signs of infection might not exist in the diabetic patient. Therefore, one must aggressively evaluate and remove infected areas with a goal of complete eradication of septic foci. This may require multiple debridements over several days and possibly open-foot or -toe amputation. Local anesthetic is often not necessary in severe cases secondary to advanced neuropathy. After all areas of infection are eliminated, the affected extremity must be assessed for ischemia even in the face of infection. As stated previously, the pulse exam is crucial in deciphering the extent of ischemia. If a dorsalis pedis or posterior tibial pulse is not palpable, arteriography is essential.

After a patient is adequately hydrated and medicated with *N*-acetylcysteine, angiography will aid in the search for a "target" vessel to restore perfusion in the affected extremity. Even if peroneal and tibial arteries are occluded, pedal vessels must be visualized. The ultimate goal of any revascularization procedure is to restore pulsatile blood flow to the foot. Angiography allows the assessment of a suitable distal vessel. After a patient has undergone angiography and a patent distal vessel is identified, a bypass or percutaneous procedure is the next step, assuming the site of anastomosis is free of infection or necrosis. In addition, if calcifications in the dorsalis pedis artery are seen on plain films of the foot, this should not be considered a contraindication to reconstruction. The presence of calcifications does not equate to vascular occlusion.

To perform the bypass procedure itself, autogenous vein graft is the only appropriate conduit for bypass to the dorsalis pedis artery. Our experience, however, has indicated that the outcome of bypass is not influenced by the use of *in situ (28)*, reversed, translocated *(29)*, or nonreversed vein grafts. As previously mentioned, the spared superficial femoral or popliteal arteries may be used as a source for inflow, an uncommon route for nondiabetic patients. The use of these vessels for inflow results in a shorter vein graft and avoids the need for groin incisions, which are a major source of morbidity in the obese patient. The fundamental goal of the distal anastomosis is to restore perfusion to the foot. This may be achieved with a bypass to the anterior or posterior tibial artery, with runoff to the foot, or directly to a vessel on the foot itself, most often the dorsalis pedis. If a bypass is done to an isolated popliteal segment or to the peroneal artery, maximal perfusion to the foot will not be achieved, even though the circulation to the foot will improve. The preference at our institution is to bypass to the dorsalis pedis because it is easily accessible, provides maximum perfusion to the foot, and has equivalent or better patency than a tibial bypass *(30)*.

SURGICAL TECHNIQUE

Pedal bypass in the diabetic and obese patient can be a lengthy, tedious, and technically demanding procedure. All procedures are performed under magnification with ×2.5 or ×3.5 power binocular loupes with finely tooled instruments to improve proficiency.

Vein preparation has been improved by use of angioscope, particularly for *in situ* grafts. Autogenous vein is the only appropriate conduit for bypass to the dorsalis pedis artery. Beyond this, however, there is room for a great deal of flexibility on the part of the surgeon. Using an *in situ* graft minimizes size mismatch, eliminates the need to mobilize and harvest the vein completely, and avoids concerns about tunneling and twisting. The drawback of the *in situ* technique is that it requires two parallel incisions on the foot, one to harvest the distal vein and one to expose the dorsalis pedis artery, which creates a bridge of skin and SC tissue at the ankle between the incisions. To minimize problems with skin necrosis, common in the obese and diabetic patient population, the distal portion of the saphenous vein is mobilized and brought subcutaneously, anterior to the tibia, and proximal to the skin bridge, so that the conduit does not actually pass under the bridge. In addition, fine sutures are used instead of staples for skin closure of the incisions at the ankle and foot. Staples tend to gather excess skin and create unnecessary tension, which may lead to necrosis and dehiscence—two complications that are exacerbated by obesity and diabetes.

Distal anastomosis is initiated by exposing the dorsalis pedis artery through a longitudinal incision on the foot. The artery lies beneath the dense fascial layer and is usually found immediately lateral to the extensor hallucis longus tendon. The most suitable area for bypass is in the portion of the vessel located between the lateral tarsal artery and bifurcation of the dorsalis pedis artery into its metatarsal branches. Arteries with internal diameters of as little as 0.8 mm are acceptable for bypass.

Our Experience

At the Beth Israel Deaconess Medical Center, 90% of patients are diabetic, and the majority of revascularization procedures (30%) performed on this population are to the dorsalis pedis artery. Recently, we reviewed our experience of more than 1000 distal bypasses to the dorsalis pedis performed for failing previous bypass grafts or limb-threatening ischemia over the past 10 yr. In these patients 80% were affected with non-healing foot ulcers, 30% of which were infected. The use of the preferred ipsilateral saphenous vein graft or, alternatively, the contralateral leg vein, arm vein, or composite resulted in 5-yr secondary patency rates that were actually better in patients with diabetes than in those without diabetes (65.9 vs 56.3%) *(31)*. Prosthetic graft was avoided whenever possible. Furthermore, the use of saphenous vein was clearly more beneficial for 5-yr patency when compared to all other conduit options, at a rate of 67.6 vs 46.3%.

As discussed previously, the superficial location of the graft itself aids in the postoperative management of the patient. The extent of revascularization of the graft is monitored closely by direct palpation and duplex ultrasound. Patients are also instructed on monitoring the graft pulse by direct palpation over the dorsum of the foot. Routine surveillance is carried out via graft palpation and ultrasound every 3 mo for the first year, every 6 mo for the second year, and annually thereafter. Lesions of the affected foot and/or secondary revisions may be addressed after successful revascularization has been achieved.

Obesity/Diabetes

The physiological goal of energy expenditure is to maintain a homeostasis in the face of an environment with variablities in nutrition and energy demands *(32)*.

With increasing girth, in an abdominal fat distribution *(33)*, the prevalence of clinical manifestations of metabolic syndrome increases and there is a larger free fatty acid load on the hepatic uptake of insulin, leading to hyperinsulinemia and hyperlipidemia and peripheral insulin resistance, causing pancreatic β-cells to fail. As the body begins to retain more triglycerides, there is an increase in the population of LDLs that contain a higher concentration of the highly atherogenic apolipoprotein B subtype *(1)*. Increased atherogenesis then goes on to cause complications of peripheral vasculature, leading to the previously discussed sequelae.

Along with the management techniques that we have discussed, preoperatively all diabetic patients must have their insulin regimen adjusted for NPO status, and blood glucose must be tightly controlled pre- and postoperatively to reduce the rate of post-operative complications including wound infections. All obese patients should be offered larger beds for convenience, and postoperative ambulation is a must in order to reduce the risk of deep venous thrombosis (DVT). In addition, all patients in this population should receive 5000 U of sc heparin three times daily for effective DVT prophylaxis.

CONCLUSIONS

Obesity is quickly becoming the largest threat to the health of the developed world. Obesity brings with it the perils of many other disorders affecting almost all organ systems, from skin to vascular. The association with diabetes in the obese population creates a patient group that is very complex and requires close monitoring in the perioperative setting. Overall, in 2000, the prevalence of obesity in the United States was 19.8% and that of diabetes was 7.3%. The prevalence of patients with both diabetes and morbid obesity was 2.9% *(34)*.

The pathophysiology of diabetes in the obese patient must be kept in mind during initial evaluation, diagnosis, and treatment regimens. The most important measure taken by patients and primary care physicians to prevent PVD is the aggressive control of risk factors (i.e., smoking, weight gain, and hypertension). Early control of these predisposing factors stymies the development of long-term complications such as insulin resistance, dyslipidemia, essential hypertension, stroke/myocardial infarcts, and central obesity—components of metabolic syndrome. Furthermore, direct communication between the primary care physician and surgeon is essential when treating patients with PVD in order to direct specific diagnostic and therapeutic options.

With the advancement in knowledge and improvements in angiography, aggressive distal reconstruction has become effective therapy for limbsalvage in the diabetic patient. In our practice, 25% of all bypass grafts in patients with diabetes are to the dorsalis pedis artery. Using this procedure, there has been a true decline in our incidence of major amputation. With careful control of blood sugar and infection, distal grafts, particularly to the dorsalis pedis artery, have proven to be a safe and effective approach to distal arterial reconstruction. With a meticulous and methodical approach to infection control, complete angiography, and arterial revascularization, the likelihood of limbsalvage in the obese and diabetic patient should rival or exceed that of the weight-controlled nondiabetic patient.

REFERENCES

1. O'Brien PE, Dixon JB. The extent of the problem of obesity. Am J Surg 2002;184:4S–8S.
2. Colditz GA, Willett WC, Rotnitzky A, Manson JE. Weight gain as a risk factor for clinical diabetes mellitus in women. Ann Intern Med 1995;122:481–486.
3. Colditz GA, Willett W, Stampfer MJ, et al. Weight as a risk factor for clinical diabetes in women. Am J Epidemiol 1990;132:501–513.
4. Armstrong DG, Lavery LA. Diabetic foot ulcers: prevention, diagnosis and classification. Am Fam Physician 1998;57:1325–1332.
5. Tegos TJ, Kalodiki E, Sabetai MM. The genesis of atherosclerosis and risk factors: a review. Angiology 2001;52:89–98.
6. Reaven GM. Role of insulin resistance in human disease (syndrome X): an expanded definition. Annu Rev Med 1993;44:121–131.
7. Lamarche B, Tchernof A, Moorjani S, et al. Small, dense low-density lipoprotein particles as a predictor of the risk of ischemic heart disease in men: prospective results from the Quebec Cardiovascular Study. Circulation 1997;95:69–75.
8. Costa LA, Canani LH, Lisboa HR, Tres GS, Gross JL. Aggregation of features of the metabolic syndrome is associated with increased prevalence of chronic complications in Type 2 diabetes. Diabet Med 2004;21(3):252–255.
9. Goldenberg SG, Alex M, Joshi RA, et al. Nonatheromatous peripheral vascular disease of the lower extremity in diabetes mellitus. Diabetes 1959;8:261–273.
10. Akbari CM, Saouaf R, Barnhill DF, et al. Endothelium-dependent vasodilatation is impaired in both microcirculation and macrocirculation during acute hyperglycemia. J Vasc Surg 1998;28:687–694.
11. Veves A, Akbari CM, Primavera J, et al. Endothelial dysfunction and the expression of endothelial nitric oxide synthetase in diabetic neuropathy, vascular disease and foot ulceration. Diabetes 1998;47:457–463.
12. Conrad MC. Large and small artery occlusion in diabetics and nondiabetics with severe vascular disease. Circulation 1967;36:83–91.
13. Beckman JA, Creager MA, Libby P. Diabetes and atherosclerosis: epidemiology, pathophysiology, and management. JAMA 2002;287(19):2570–2581.

14. Nadig SN, Deibler AR, Marlow TJ, Wiley KM, Schabel SI. Retained needle fragments in patients with diabetic neuropathy. JAMA 2000;283(23):3072.

15. Rooke TW, Osmundson PJ. The influence of age, sex, smoking, and diabetes on lower limb transcutaneous oxygen tension in patients with arterial occlusive disease. Arch Intern Med 1990;150: 129–132.

16. Tepel M, Van der Giel M, Schwarzfeld C, et al. Prevention of radiographic-contrast-agent-induced reductions in renal function by acetylcysteine. N Engl J Med 2000;343:210–212.

17. Murabito JM, D'Agostino RB, Silbershatz H, Wilson WF. Intermittent claudication: a risk profile from the Framingham Heart Study. Circulation 1997;96(1):44–49.

18. Powell JT, Edwards RJ, Worrell PC, Franks PJ, Greenhalgh RM, Poulter NR. Risk factors associated with the development of peripheral arterial disease in smokers: a case-control study. Atherosclerosis 1997;129(1):41–48.

19. Yusuf S, Sleight P, Pogue J, Bosch J, Davies R, Dagenais G. Effects of an angiotensin-converting-enzyme-inhibitor, ramipril, on cardiovascular events in high-risk patients. The Heart Outcomes Prevention Evaluation Study Investigators. N Engl J Med 2000;342(3):145–153.

20. Mohler III ER, Hiatt WR, Creager MA. Cholesterol reduction with atorvastatin improves walking distance in patients with peripheral arterial disease. Circulation 2003;108(12):1481–1486.

21. Mondillo S, Ballo P, Barbati R, et al. Effects of Simvastatin on walking performance and symptoms of intermittent claudication in hypercholesterolemic patients with peripheral vascular disease. Am J Med 2003;114(5):359–364.

22. Aronow WS, Nayak D, Woodworth S, Ahn C. Effect of simvastatin versus placebo on treadmill exercise time until the onset of intermittent claudication in older patients with peripheral arterial disease at six months and at one year after treatment. Am J Cardiol 2003;92(6):711, 712.

23. Gardner AW, Poehlman ET. Exercise rehabilitation programs for the treatment of claudication pain: A meta-analysis. JAMA 1995;274(12):975–980.

24. Stewart KJ, Hiatt WR, Regensteiner JG, Hirsch AT. Exercise training for claudication. N Engl J Med 2002;347(24):1941–1951.

25. Yusuf S, Zhao F, Mehta SR, et al. The CURE Trial Investigators. Effects of Clopidogrel in addition to aspirin in patients with acute coronary syndromes without ST-segment elevation. N Engl J Med 2001;345(7):494–502.

26. Crouse JR III, Allan MC, Elam MB. Clinical manifestation of atherosclerotic peripheral arterial disease and the role of Cilostazol in treatment of intermittent claudication. J Clin Pharmacol 2002;42(12):1291–1298.

27. Thompson PD, Zimet R, Forbes WP, Zhang P. Meta-analysis of results from eight randomized, placebo-controlled trials on the effect of cilostazol on patients with intermittent claudication. Am J Cardiol 2002;90(12):1314–1319.

28. Leather RP, Powers SR, Karmody AM. A reappraisal of the in situ saphenous vein arterial bypass: its use in limb salvage. Surgery 1979;86:453–461.

29. Thompson RW, Mannick JA, Whittemore AD. Arterial reconstruction at divers sites using nonreversed autogenous vein. Ann Surg 1987;205:747–751.

30. Schneider JR, Walsh DB, McDaniel MD, Zwolek RM, Besso SR, Cronenwett JL. Pedal bypass versus tibial bypass with autogenous vein: a comparison of outcome and hemodynamic results. J Vasc Surg 1993;17:1029–1040.

31. Pomoposelli FB Jr, Kansal N, Hamdan AD, et al. A decade of experience with dorsalis pedis artery bypass: analysis of outcome in more than 1000 cases. J Vasc Surg 2003;37(2):307–315.

32. Flier JS. Obesity wars: molecular progress confronts an expanding epidemic. Cell 2004;116:337–350.

33. Planas A, Clara A, Pou JM, et al. Relationship of obesity distribution and peripheral arterial occlusive disease in elderly men. Int J Obesity Relat Metab Disord: J Int Assoc Study Obesity 2001;25(7): 1068–1070.

34. Mokdad AH, Bowman BA, Ford ES, Vinicor F, Marks J, Koplan JP. The continuing epidemics of obesity and diabetes in the United States. JAMA 2001;286(10):1195–1200.

14 Obesity, Diabetes, and Risk of Cancer

A Review of Epidemiological Studies

Susanna C. Larsson, LicMedSci,
Hans-Olov Adami, MD, PhD,
and Alicja Wolk, DrMedSci

CONTENTS

INTRODUCTION
REVIEW OF EPIDEMIOLOGICAL STUDIES
BIOLOGICAL MECHANISMS OF ALTERED CANCER RISK ASSOCIATED
    WITH OBESITY AND TYPE 2 DIABETES
CONCLUSIONS
REFERENCES

INTRODUCTION

Risk of cancer is affected by a number of environmental and lifestyle factors and by an interplay between these factors and genetic susceptibility. Over the past three decades, the prevalence of obesity and type 2 diabetes has been increasing in both developed countries and less developed areas along with an adoption of a Westernized lifestyle (*see* Chapter 2). It is well recognized that obesity dramatically increases the risk of type 2 diabetes. Moreover, there is an extensive body of epidemiological evidence that excess body weight considerably increases the risk of cancers at multiple sites *(1)*. Herein we summarize the mounting epidemiological studies linking overweight, obesity, and diabetes with cancer incidence and mortality.

In view of the large number of epidemiological studies relating overweight and obesity to the risk of cancer, this chapter is based primarily on data from previous comprehensive reviews and meta-analyses, including (1) a quantitative review and meta-analysis by Bergström et al. *(2)*, who summarized the epidemiological literature published between 1966 and 1997 investigating body mass index (BMI) (the weight in kilograms divided by the square of height in meters) in relation to the risk of developing cancer; (2) a comprehensive report by the International Agency for Research on Cancer (IARC) in 2002 *(1)*; and (3) the Cancer Prevention Study II *(3)*, a large prospective cohort study investigating the association of BMI with cancer mortality during 16 yr of follow-up of more than 900,000 adults in the United States.

From: *Contemporary Diabetes: Obesity and Diabetes*
Edited by: C. S. Mantzoros © Humana Press Inc., Totowa, NJ

In the review and meta-analysis by Bergström et al. *(2)*, "normal weight" was defined as a BMI of 20–24.9 kg/m^2, "overweight" as a BMI of 25–29.9 kg/m^2, and "obesity" as a BMI of 30.0 kg/m^2 or more. In the Cancer Prevention Study II *(3)*, BMI was categorized as follows: "normal weight" as 18.5–24.9 kg/m^2, "overweight" as 25.0–29.9 kg/m^2, "grade 1 overweight" as 30.0–34.9 kg/m^2, "grade 2 overweight" as 35.0–39.9 kg/m^2, and "grade 3 overweight" as 40.0 kg/m^2 or more, according to the recommendation by the World Health Organization *(4)*.

REVIEW OF EPIDEMIOLOGICAL STUDIES
Overall Cancer
OVERWEIGHT AND OBESITY

Overweight and obesity have been associated with overall cancer incidence and mortality. In a Swedish population-based cohort of 28,129 hospitalized patients with any discharge diagnosis of obesity, there was an overall 33% excess incidence of cancer in obese individuals (25% in men and 37% in women) in comparison with the general population *(5)*. In addition, the National Enhanced Cancer Surveillance System, a large Canadian population-based case–control study, showed that compared with normal-weight individuals (BMI < 25 kg/m^2), those who were overweight (BMI between 25 and 30 kg/m^2) had a 9% increased risk of cancer overall; obese individuals (BMI ≥30 kg/m^2) had a 34% increased risk *(6)*. The association of overweight and obesity with overall cancer mortality as well as mortality from specific cancers was examined in the American Cancer Prevention Study II *(3)* (see Tables 1 and 2). During 16 yr of follow-up of 900,000 participants, there were a total of 57,145 deaths from cancer. Compared with men with normal weight, the death rates from all cancers combined were 9% higher in men with a BMI between 30.0 and 34.9 kg/m^2 (grade 1 overweight), 20% higher for men with a BMI between 35.0 and 39.9 kg/m^2 (grade 2 overweight), and 52% higher for men with a BMI of 40.0 kg/m^2 or more (grade 3 overweight). The corresponding figures for women were 23, 32, and 62%.

DIABETES

In a Swedish cohort of 144,427 hospitalized diabetic patients, a total of 4919 men and 4742 women died from cancer during an average follow-up of 6.7 yr *(7)*. This study showed that overall cancer mortality was approx 50% higher among the diabetic patients compared with the general population. However, because the analysis was not adjusted for obesity, the association between diabetes and overall cancer risk independent of the effect of obesity on cancer risk could not be distinguished.

Breast Cancer
OVERWEIGHT AND OBESITY

Breast cancer is the leading type of cancer in women both worldwide (21% of all cancers) *(8)* and in the United States (32% of all cancers) *(9)*. The first epidemiological evidence of an association between excess body weight and increased breast cancer risk was obtained from a Dutch cohort study in 1974 *(10)*. Findings from many subsequent epidemiological studies indicate that the relationship between excess body weight and risk of breast cancer varies by menopausal status *(1)*. Whereas a positive association between body weight and risk of breast cancer has been observed in most studies of postmenopausal women, an inverse association has been noted in studies of premenopausal women *(1)*.

Table 1

Relative Risk and 95% Confidence Interval of Mortality From Selected Cancers
According to BMI in Men in the American Cancer Prevention Study II[a]

Type of cancer[b]	18.4–24.9[d]	25.0–29.9	BMI (kg/m²)[c] 30.0–34.9	35.0–39.9	≥40.0
All cancers					
No. of deaths	13,855	15,372	2683	350	43
RR (95% CI)	1.0	0.97 (0.94–0.99)	1.09 (1.05–1.14)	1.20 (1.08–1.34)	1.52 (1.13–2.05)
Colorectal cancer					
RR (95% CI)	1.0	1.20 (1.12–1.30)	1.47 (1.30–1.66)	1.84 (1.39–2.41)	
Esophageal cancer					
RR (95% CI)	1.0	1.15 (0.99–1.32)	1.28 (1.00–1.63)	1.63 (0.95–2.80)	
Gallbladder cancer					
RR (95% CI)	1.0	1.34 (0.97–1.84)	1.76 (1.06–2.94)		
Kidney cancer					
RR (95% CI)	1.0	1.18 (1.02–1.37)	1.36 (1.06–1.74)	1.70 (0.99–2.92)	
Leukemia					
RR (95% CI)	1.0	1.14 (1.02–1.28)	1.37 (1.13–1.67)	1.70 (1.08–2.66)	
Liver cancer					
RR (95% CI)	1.0	1.13 (0.94–1.34)	1.90 (1.46–2.47)	4.52 (2.94–6.94)	
Multiple myeloma					
RR (95% CI)	1.0	1.18 (1.01–1.39)	1.44 (1.10–1.89)	1.71 (0.93–3.14)	
Non-Hodgkin's lymphoma					
RR (95% CI)	1.0	1.08 (0.96–1.21)	1.56 (1.29–1.87)	1.49 (0.93–2.39)	

(Continued)

235

Table 1 (Continued)

Type of cancer[b]	BMI (kg/m²)[c]				
	18.4–24.9[d]	25.0–29.9	30.0–34.9	35.0–39.9	≥40.0
Pancreatic cancer					
RR (95% CI)	1.0	1.13 (1.03–1.25)	1.41 (1.19–1.66)	1.49 (0.99–2.22)	
Prostate cancer					
RR (95% CI)	1.0	1.08 (1.01–1.15)	1.20 (1.06–1.36)	1.34 (0.87–1.83)	

[a]Adapted from ref. 3.
[b]RR, relative risk; CI, confidence interval.
[c]The highest BMI category examined varies for different types of cancers; the highest categories have been combined when necessary because of small number of deaths.
[d]Reference group for all comparisons.

Table 2
Relative Risk and 95% Confidence Interval of Mortality From Selected Cancers According to BMI in Women in the American Cancer Prevention Study[a]

Type of cancer[b]	BMI (kg/m²)[c]				
	18.4–24.9[d]	25.0–29.9	30.0–34.9	35.0–39.9	≥40.0
All cancers					
No. of deaths	14,779	7107	2254	517	185
RR (95% CI)	1.0	1.08 (1.05–1.11)	1.23 (1.18–1.29)	1.32 (1.20–1.44)	1.62 (1.40–1.87)
Breast cancer					
RR (95% CI)	1.0	1.34 (1.23–1.46)	1.63 (1.44–1.85)	1.70 (1.33–2.17)	2.12 (1.41–3.19)
Cervical cancer					
RR (95% CI)	1.0	1.38 (0.97–1.96)	1.23 (0.71–2.13)	3.20 (1.77–5.78)	
Colorectal cancer					
RR (95% CI)	1.0	1.10 (1.01–1.19)	1.33 (1.17–1.51)	1.36 (1.06–1.74)	1.46 (0.94–2.24)

Cancer					
Endometrial cancer RR (95% CI)	1.0	1.50 (1.26–1.78)	2.53 (2.02–3.18)	2.77 (1.83–4.18)	6.25 (3.75–10.42)
Esophageal cancer RR (95% CI)	1.0	1.20 (0.86–1.66)	1.39 (0.86–2.25)		
Gallbladder cancer RR (95% CI)	1.0	1.12 (0.86–1.47)	2.13 (1.56–2.90)		
Kidney cancer RR (95% CI)	1.0	1.33 (1.08–1.63)	1.66 (1.23–2.24)	1.70 (0.94–3.05)	4.75 (2.50–9.04)
Leukemia RR (95% CI)	1.0	1.05 (0.91–1.21)	1.12 (0.89–1.42)	0.93 (0.58–1.49)	
Liver cancer RR (95% CI)	1.0	1.02 (0.80–1.31)	1.40 (0.97–2.00)	1.68 (0.93–3.05)	
Multiple myeloma RR (95% CI)	1.0	1.12 (0.93–1.34)	1.47 (1.13–1.91)	1.44 (0.91–2.28)	
Non-Hodgkin's lymphoma RR (95% CI)	1.0	1.22 (1.06–1.40)	1.20 (0.95–1.51)	1.95 (1.39–2.72)	
Ovarian cancer RR (95% CI)	1.0	1.15 (1.02–1.29)	1.16 (0.96–1.40)	1.51 (1.12–2.02)	
Pancreatic cancer RR (95% CI)	1.0	1.11 (1.00–1.24)	1.28 (1.07–1.52)	1.41 (1.01–1.99)	2.76 (1.74–4.36)

[a] Adapted from ref. 3.

[b] RR, relative risk; CI, confidence interval.

[c] The highest BMI category examined varies for different types of cancers; the highest categories have been combined when necessary because of small number of deaths.

[d] Reference group for all comparisons.

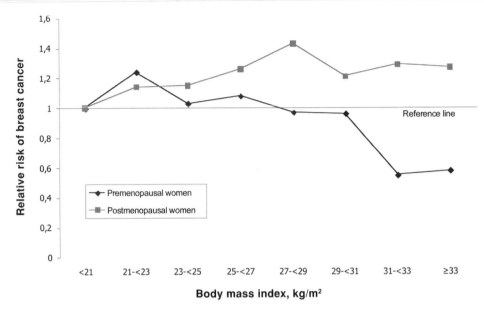

Fig. 1. Relative risk of breast cancer according to body mass index (BMI) of Pooling Project of Prospective Studies of Diet and Cancer. The reference group for all comparisons is women with a BMI <21 kg/m². (From ref. *11*.)

In a meta-analysis, Bergström et al. *(2)* estimated that there is a 2% reduction in premenopausal risk of breast cancer and a 2% increase in postmenopausal risk of breast cancer per unit increment in BMI (corresponding to an increase of 3 kg of body wt for women with a height of 1.64 m). Overweight women were estimated to have a 12% and obese women a 25% greater risk of breast cancer compared with women of normal weight *(2)*.

The Pooling Project of Prospective Studies of Diet and Cancer *(11)* also examined the association between BMI and risk of breast cancer. Using data from seven prospective cohort studies—comprising 337,819 women, including 4385 incident invasive breast cancer cases—the Pooling Project *(11)* confirmed a dual effect of obesity (Fig. 1). In premenopausal women, those with a BMI >31 kg/m² had a 46% reduced risk of breast cancer compared with women with a BMI <21 kg/m². In postmenopausal women, the risk of breast cancer did not continue to increase when BMI exceeded 28 kg/m², at which level the risk was 26% higher compared with women with a BMI of <21 kg/m². The positive association between BMI and risk of breast cancer was stronger and significant only among women who never used hormone replacement therapy (HRT), suggesting that the increased risk of breast cancer associated with excess body weight may be mediated through an elevation in endogenous estrogen production in heavier women (*see* Biological Mechanisms of Altered Cancer Risk Associated with Obesity and Type 2 Diabetes). The European Prospective Investigation into Cancer and Nutrition *(12)*, a follow-up study of 176,886 women among whom 1879 developed invasive breast cancer, confirmed that the relationship between BMI and postmenopausal risk of breast cancer is modified by the use of HRT. Among nonusers of HRT, obese women (BMI >30 kg/m²) had a 31% excess risk of breast cancer compared with women with a BMI <25 kg/m². Among HRT users, who already were at an increased risk of breast cancer owing to HRT, high BMI did not further increase risk of breast cancer.

In the Cancer Prevention Study II of 495,477 women including 2755 breast cancer deaths *(3)*, BMI showed a linear positive association with mortality from postmenopausal breast cancer (Table 2). Compared with women having normal weight, the risk of death from breast cancer was 63% higher for women with a BMI between 30.0 and 34.9 kg/m^2 and 70% higher for women with a BMI between 35.0 and 39.9 kg/m^2; women with a BMI of 40.0 kg/m^2 or higher (grade 3 overweight) had more than twofold increased risk.

In summary, there is an extensive body of epidemiological data showing that obesity has a dual effect on risk of breast cancer. Whereas obesity modestly reduces the risk of breast cancer in premenopausal women, obesity in postmenopausal women significantly increases the risk, in particular among nonusers of HRT.

DIABETES

Epidemiological studies concerning the relationship between diabetes and risk of breast cancer are not as consistent. A large prospective cohort study of US nurses *(13)* found that women with diabetes had an approx 20% elevated risk of breast cancer compared with women without diabetes independent of obesity and other risk factors for breast cancer. The increased risk associated with diabetes was only observed among postmenopausal women. Similar findings were obtained from a Swedish cohort study *(14)* and a large multicenter case–control study in Italy *(15)* showing a 30–50% increased risk of breast cancer associated with diabetes only in older or postmenopausal women. In the large American Cancer Prevention Study II *(16)*, diabetic women had a significantly elevated risk of fatal breast cancer (27%) compared with nondiabetic women; this association was not explained by high BMI and other known and possible risk factors for breast cancer. Other studies indicated no significant association between diabetes and risk of breast cancer *(17–22)*. However, several of these studies were limited in size and, therefore, did not have enough statistical power to observe associations.

In summary, although four large studies have shown an association between diabetes and increased risk of breast cancer independent of obesity other studies are nonsupportive. More large studies are needed before any conclusion can be drawn on this relationship.

Endometrial Cancer

OVERWEIGHT AND OBESITY

Endometrial cancer is the seventh most common malignancy in women worldwide *(8)* and the fourth most common in women in the United States *(9)*. Excess body weight appears to be a strong and consistent predictor of risk of endometrial cancer in both pre- and postmenopausal women, with overweight women having an approximate two- to threefold increased risk of endometrial cancer *(1)*. In most studies, risk of endometrial cancer increased approximately linearly in women with a BMI >25 kg/m^2, whereas a few studies suggested a threshold effect, with an increased risk observed only among women with a BMI of about 30 kg/m^2 or higher *(1)*.

In a review by Bergström et al. *(2)*, all but 1 of 14 studies showed a positive association between BMI and risk of endometrial cancer. Four of those 14 studies provided enough information to be included in a meta-analysis, which predicted a 10% increase in the risk of endometrial cancer per unit increment in BMI; the estimates implied an increase in risk by 59% for overweight and 152% for obese women compared with women of normal weight.

In the Cancer Prevention Study II *(3)*, risk of death from endometrial cancer increased in a stepwise manner with increasing BMI (Table 2). Women with a BMI of ≥40 kg/m^2 (grade 3 overweight) experienced greater than sixfold increased risk of endometrial cancer compared with women of normal weight.

DIABETES

A history of diabetes has frequently emerged across studies as a risk factor for endometrial cancer *(23)*, even after controlling for BMI and other established risk factors *(16,24–26)*. Most studies have observed a 30–400% excess risk of endometrial cancer for diabetic women compared with nondiabetic women *(14,16,24–28)*. In some studies *(26–28)*, but not all *(24,25,29)*, the positive association was more pronounced among obese women than among nonobese.

Ovarian Cancer

OVERWEIGHT AND OBESITY

Cancer of the ovary is the sixth most common malignancy in women worldwide *(8)* and the fifth most common in women in the United States (comprises 4% of all cancers) *(9)*. In contrast to epidemiological data on endometrial and postmenopausal breast cancer, studies linking excess body weight to ovarian cancer risk are inconclusive. Although a number of studies reported a positive association between overweight or obesity and ovarian cancer incidence or mortality *(3,5,6,30–35)*, other studies were nonsupportive *(36–43)*. The inconsistent results may be owing to the complex relationship between obesity and steroid hormones, depending on age and menopausal status. Studies that addressed the association between excess body weight and risk of ovarian cancer separately for pre- and postmenopausal women observed a positive association only in premenopausal women *(30,44)*.

In a Norwegian cohort study of approx 1.1 million women followed for an average of 25 yr, women who were overweight and obese in adolescence or in young adulthood had a significantly increased risk of ovarian cancer *(45)*. Likewise, several other studies *(31,36–38,45)* but not all *(32)*, have found a positive association between BMI in adolescence or early adulthood and risk of ovarian cancer.

In the Cancer Prevention Study II *(3)*, risk of death from ovarian cancer was increased for overweight women (Table 2). Compared with normal-weight women, those with a BMI of ≥35.0 kg/m^2 had a 51% increased risk of death from ovarian cancer.

In summary, a relatively large number of epidemiological studies have examined the relation between obesity and risk of ovarian cancer. Although the findings are not consistent, the most informative studies suggest that obesity in adolescence/young adulthood and in premenopausal women may increase the subsequent risk of ovarian cancer.

DIABETES

Diabetes was not observed to be associated with an increased risk of ovarian cancer in case-control *(19,29,46–48)* or cohort studies *(16,17,49–51)*.

Prostate Cancer

OVERWEIGHT AND OBESITY

Prostate cancer is the leading cancer in men in the United States (33% of all cancers) *(9)* and the fourth most common malignancy in men worldwide *(8)*. Although some studies have suggested an association between excess body weight and increased or decreased risk of prostate cancer, most studies have found no association *(1)*. A meta-analysis by Bergström et al. *(2)* estimated that compared with a man of normal weight, an overweight man had a 6% and an obese man a 12% increase in the risk of prostate cancer. In addition, the Cancer Prevention Study II of 404,576 men including

4004 prostate cancer deaths *(3)* found that obesity was associated with a 20–34% higher risk of fatal prostate cancer (Table 1). Overall, however, epidemiological data suggest the absence of a strong association between excess body weight and incidence of prostate cancer.

DIABETES

Epidemiological studies relating diabetes to risk of prostate cancer have yielded equivocal results. Small studies have generally not observed an association between diabetes and prostate cancer *(29,50–52)*. Larger studies have been either null *(16,53,54)* or showed an inverse association *(17,55–58)*. The American Cancer Prevention Study II found no association between diabetes at baseline and incidence of prostate cancer *(53)*. However, men who had diabetes for 5 yr or more had a significantly higher incidence of prostate cancer (56%) compared with men who did not have diabetes. These findings are in contrast to those from the Health Professionals Follow-Up Study, which showed an overall 25% reduction in risk of prostate cancer among diabetic patients, after controlling for high BMI and other potential confounders *(56)*. When time since diagnosis was taken into account, risk of prostate cancer was not reduced in the first 5 yr after diagnosis but was lower in the next 5 yr (33% lower risk) and lowest after 10 yr (46% lower risk). Likewise, in the Physicians' Health Study *(58)*, men who had been diagnosed with diabetes more than 10 yr prior to their diagnosis of prostate cancer had a 41% reduced risk of prostate cancer, relative to men without diabetes.

In a large population-based cohort study in Sweden *(55)*, patients hospitalized with diabetes had a significantly lower risk of prostate cancer (9%) in comparison with the general population. There was no consistent trend in risk related to age at first hospitalization or to duration of follow-up, but the risk reduction was more pronounced among patients who had been hospitalized for diabetes complications *(55)*. Similarly, in a population-based case–control study in the United States *(57)*, a history of diabetes was associated with a significantly decreased risk of prostate cancer (36%). As in the Swedish cohort, the inverse association of diabetes with risk of prostate cancer was somewhat stronger for those men experiencing complications *(57)*.

In summary, there is no evidence that diabetes increases the risk of prostate cancer. By contrast, some studies suggest that diabetic men may be less likely to develop prostate cancer.

Colorectal Cancer

OVERWEIGHT AND OBESITY

Colorectal cancer comprises 10% of all cancers worldwide and 22% of all cancers in the United States *(9)*. Many studies have shown that a high BMI is related to an increased risk of colorectal cancer in men, whereas this relationship has not been as consistent in studies of women *(1)*. Studies have suggested that the association between BMI and risk of colorectal cancer may vary by menopausal status and that the association is stronger for, or perhaps limited to, premenopausal women. In addition, several studies have reported a stronger association for cancer of the colon than of the rectum, and the distal colon appears more affected than the proximal colon *(1)*. A meta-analysis by Bergström et al. *(2)* predicted that each unit increment in BMI corresponds to a 3% increase in the risk of colon cancer. Overweight subjects were estimated to have a 15% and obese subjects a 33% increased risk of colon cancer compared with subjects having a normal weight.

In the Cancer Prevention Study II *(3)*, the risk of mortality from colorectal cancer increased approximately linearly with increasing BMI in both men and women, although the association was somewhat stronger in men (Table 1). In men, those with a BMI of ≥35.0 kg/m^2 had an 84% increased risk of mortality from colorectal cancer compared with normal-weight men. In women, compared with those of normal weight, the risk of mortality from colorectal cancer was increased by 36% for those having a BMI of 35.0–39.9 kg/m^2 and by 46% for those having a BMI of ≥40 kg/m^2. This lower risk in women may be owing to increased endogenous estrogen concentrations in obese postmenopausal women. The Women's Health Initiative (59), a randomized controlled trial in postmenopausal women, found that women who received estrogen (plus progestin) had a significantly decreased risk of colorectal cancer compared with women not receiving estrogen. Thus, estrogen may partly offset the deleterious effect of obesity on risk of colorectal cancer in postmenopausal women.

Overall, an increased risk of colorectal cancer with increasing BMI has been observed in most studies. The findings have been more consistent for colon than for rectal cancer. In addition, the association with BMI appears to be stronger for men than for women.

DIABETES

Most studies (16,29,60–64), but not all (65), have found a history of diabetes to be related to an increased risk of colon or colorectal cancer. In the Nurses' Health Study, Hu et al. (63) reported that diabetic women independent of obesity had a 43% increased risk of colorectal cancer compared with nondiabetic women. The association was most apparent for advanced colorectal cancer, with a risk being 240% higher for diabetic women (63). In addition, women whose diabetes had been diagnosed 11–15 yr earlier had a 230% greater risk of colorectal cancer compared with nondiabetic women (63). The positive association was stronger for colon cancer than for rectal cancer (63). The American Cancer Prevention Study II (16) reported that men and women with a history of diabetes had a significantly higher risk of fatal colon cancer (about 20%) compared with those without diabetes; this association was not explained by high BMI and other risk factors for colon cancer. Diabetes was not associated with mortality from cancer of the rectum (16).

In summary, available data indicate that diabetes independently from the effect of high BMI is a risk factor for colorectal cancer. The evidence is too limited to allow any conclusion on whether the relation between diabetes and risk of colorectal cancer is restricted to a specific subsite in the large bowel.

Kidney Cancer

OVERWEIGHT AND OBESITY

Kidney cancers account for about 2% of cancers both worldwide (8) and in the United States (9). Epidemiological studies have consistently identified a positive association of BMI with risk of kidney (mainly renal cell) cancer (1). Bergström et al. (66) summarized the epidemiological literature published between 1966 and 1998. Of the 14 studies included in a meta-analysis, all but one showed a positive association with obesity, and the association was significant in all but four studies (66). The meta-analysis showed a 7% increase in risk of kidney cancer per unit of increment in BMI. Compared with individuals of normal weight (BMI of 20–24.9 kg/m^2), those with a BMI of ≥40 kg/m^2 had a 240% increased risk of kidney cancer (Fig. 2). Besides a positive association between BMI and kidney cancer, repeated weight changes (weight cycling) has been associated with an almost fourfold increase in the risk of renal cell cancer in women (67).

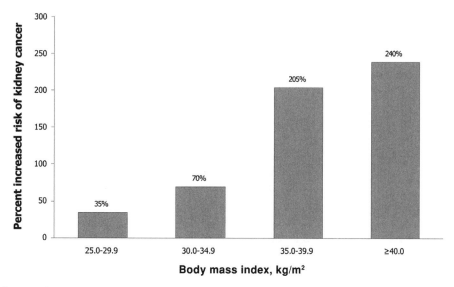

Fig. 2. Association between body mass index (BMI) and risk of kidney cancer. The reference group for all comparisons is individuals of normal weight (BMI between 20 and 25 kg/m²). (From ref. *66*.)

In the Cancer Prevention Study II *(3)*, the risk of death from kidney cancer was increased by 70% for men with a BMI of ≥35.0 kg/m² compared with men of normal weight (Table 1). In women, those with a BMI of ≥40 kg/m² had a nearly fivefold higher risk of death from kidney cancer compared with normal-weight women.

DIABETES

The evidence regarding the relationship between diabetes and risk of kidney cancer is conflicting. Whereas some case-control studies found no relation between a history of diabetes and risk of kidney cancer *(19,68,69)*, others showed a nonsignificant positive association *(70,71)* or a significant positive association *(72)*, or observed an increased risk restricted to women *(29,73–75)*. Three cohort studies found an increased risk of kidney cancer among patients with diabetes *(17,49,76)*. None of those three studies controlled for high BMI, and, thus, the effect of diabetes independent of that of obesity could not be addressed. In the large American Cancer Prevention Study II *(16)*, in which high BMI and other potential confounders were adjusted for, there was no evidence of an association between a history of diabetes and risk of kidney cancer in men or women. Furthermore, other cohort studies observed no relationship between diabetes and risk of kidney cancer *(50,77)*.

Pancreatic Cancer

OVERWEIGHT AND OBESITY

Cancer of the pancreas accounts for only about 2% of new cases of cancer worldwide *(8)* and in the United States *(9)*. Owing to its high fatality, pancreatic cancer is one of the leading causes of cancer-related death. In the United States, pancreatic cancer accounts for about 5% of cancer deaths in men and 6% in women *(9)*. Epidemiological studies pertaining to the association between excess body weight and risk of pancreatic cancer have not been consistent. Case–control studies published in the 1990s suggested little or no association of overweight or obesity with risk of pancreatic cancer *(78)*. Subsequently, a fairly consistent positive association has emerged from several prospective cohort studies in which weight was assessed before the diagnosis of pancreatic cancer *(3,6,79–81)*.

Berrington de Gonzalez et al. *(78)* conducted a meta-analysis of six case–control and eight cohort studies published from 1966 to 2003. The summary analysis predicted a 2% increase in risk of pancreatic cancer per-unit increment in BMI. This per unit increase translates into a 19% higher risk for obese individuals (BMI > 30 kg/m^2) compared with that for normal weight (BMI < 25 kg/m^2). In the Cancer Prevention Study II *(3)*, risk of death from pancreatic cancer was increased by 49% in men with a BMI of ≥35.0 kg/m^2 compared with men having a normal weight (Table 1). Women with a BMI of 35.0–39.9 kg/m^2 had a 41% and women with a BMI of ≥40 kg/m^2 had a 276% elevated risk of mortality from pancreatic cancer in comparison with normal-weight women.

In summary, data on obesity and risk of pancreatic cancer are not entirely consistent. The most informative studies, however, have indicated an association between obesity and increased risk of pancreatic cancer.

DIABETES

The weight of the evidence indicates an increased risk of pancreatic cancer associated with a history of diabetes. In a meta-analysis of 11 case–control and 9 cohort studies published between 1975 and 1994 *(82)*, an overall doubling of the risk of developing pancreatic cancer was noted for diabetic patients compared with nondiabetic individuals; this association remained when the data were restricted to subjects who had developed diabetes at least 5 yr before the diagnosis of pancreatic cancer.

In the Cancer Prevention Study II *(83)*, a history of diabetes was related to about a 50% elevated risk of fatal pancreatic cancer in both men and women. The death rate from pancreatic cancer was twice as high in individuals with diabetes as in those without during the second and third year of follow-up but only about 40% higher in yr 9–12.

Esophageal and Gastric Cardia Cancer

OVERWEIGHT AND OBESITY

Cancer of the esophagus, although relatively uncommon (4% of all cancers), is an important cause of cancer-related mortality *(8,84)*. The incidence rates of esophageal adenocarcinoma have been rapidly rising over the last three decades in the United States and western Europe *(85–87)*. Devesa et al. *(85)* noted a 350% increase in the incidence of adenocarcinoma of the esophagus in the United States between 1976 and 1994. Similar but less striking trends have been observed for adenocarcinomas of the gastric cardia *(85)*. By contrast, the incidence rates for squamous cell carcinoma of the esophagus and noncardia gastric adenocarcinoma have remained stable or declined slightly during the same period *(85)*.

Excess body weight has emerged as a strong and independent risk factor for esophageal adenocarcinoma and, albeit to a lesser extent, for gastric cardia, with risk rising steadily with increasing BMI *(88–94)*. In a large US multicenter population-based case–control study, Chow et al. *(90)* showed that compared with individuals in the lowest BMI quartile, those in the highest had a fourfold increased risk of adenocarcinoma of the esophagus and an approximate doubling of risk of gastric cardia adenocarcinoma. Similar findings emerged from a large population-based case–control study in Sweden, wherein Lagergren et al. *(91)* observed that subjects in the highest quartile of BMI had nearly an eightfold excess risk of esophageal adenocarcinoma in comparison with those in the lowest BMI quartile. This risk increased to 16-fold when obese subjects (BMI > 30 kg/m^2) were compared with subjects having a BMI <22 kg/m^2. Like the US study, the results for gastric cardia adenocarcinoma were weaker than those for esophageal adenocarcinoma, with a risk 2.3-fold higher for the top compared with the bottom quartile and 4.3-fold higher for a BMI >30 kg/m^2 vs a BMI <22 kg/m^2. Other case–control studies have also reported a positive association of BMI with risk of esophageal adenocarcinoma and gastric cardia adenocarcinoma, with a two- to sixfold increased risk for those in the highest vs lowest BMI categories *(88,89,92–94)*. Excess body weight has not been related to risk of esophageal squamous cell carcinoma *(90,91)*.

DIABETES

In the American Cancer Prevention Study II *(16)*, a history of diabetes was not significantly associated with risk of esophageal or stomach cancer, but additional studies are needed to assess this association accurately.

Other Cancer Sites

Regarding organ sites other than those discussed, the epidemiological literature is sparse and inconclusive. In the American Cancer Prevention Study II *(3)*, significant positive linear trends between BMI and death rates were observed for cancers of the gallbladder, liver, cervix, non-Hodgkin's lymphoma, leukemia (only in men), and multiple myeloma (Tables 1 and 2). Similarly, overweight and obesity were related to significant increased risk of non-Hodgkin's lymphoma, leukemia, and multiple myeloma in the Canadian National Enhanced Cancer Surveillance System *(6)*.

Population-Attributable Risk Percent for Cancer

The proportion of any disease owing to a risk factor in a population is determined by both the magnitude of the increased risk and the prevalence of the risk factor in the population. That proportion is often expressed as the population-attributable risk percent, meaning the percentage of disease incidence or mortality that would be eliminated if the risk factor were removed. The population-attributable risk percent for excess body weight in relation to certain cancers has been estimated for Europe *(2)*, Canada *(6)*, and the United States *(3,95)* (Fig. 3).

Bergström et al. *(2)* estimated the proportion of all cases of cancer at six sites (endometrium, breast in postmenopausal women, colon, kidney, gallbladder, and prostate) that might be avoided in the European Union (15 countries) if the population maintained a BMI in the normal range (i.e., between 20.0 and 24.9 kg/m^2). The estimates were based on the prevalence of overweight and obesity in European populations. Overall, excess body weight was estimated to account for 5% of all cancers, 6% in women and 3% in men, corresponding to 45,000 female and 27,000 male cancer cases occurring each year. Regarding specific cancer sites, the analysis showed that about 40% of endometrial cancers, almost 25% of kidney cancers, approx 25% of gallbladder cancers, about 10% of postmenopausal breast cancers, and >10% of colon cancers could be prevented by maintaining a healthy body weight with a BMI <25 kg/m^2.

Pan et al. *(6)* estimated the proportion of overall cancer and some specific cancers attributable to excess body weight in Canada by using data from the National Enhanced Cancer Surveillance System. Overweight and obesity together accounted for about 8% of all cancers (10% in men and 6% in women). Regarding specific cancer sites, the

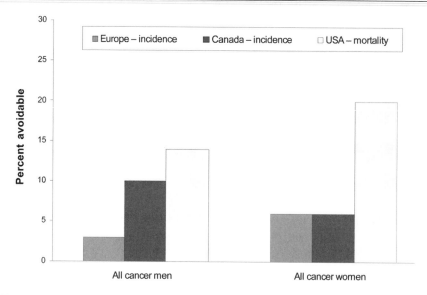

Fig. 3. Percentage of Cancer in Europe, Canada, and United States that is potentially preventable if population maintains body mass index in normal range. (From refs. *2*, *3*, and *6* for Europe, United States, and Canada, respectively.)

analysis showed that overweight and obesity were responsible for approx 41% of kidney cancers, 24% of colon cancers, 20% of rectal cancers, 20% of leukemia, 16% of ovarian cancers, 13% of postmenopausal breast cancers, and 11% of non-Hodgkin's lymphoma *(6)*. (Data for endometrial cancer were not available.)

Based on data from a large US multicenter population-based case–control study of cancers of the esophagus and stomach, Engel et al. *(95)* estimated that BMI above the lowest quartile (i.e., >23.1 kg/m^2) is responsible for about 40% of esophageal adenocarcinomas and about 20% of gastric cardia adenocarcinomas.

Using data from the Cancer Prevention Study II, Calle et al. *(3)* estimated the proportion of all cancer deaths in the United States that might be avoided if the adult population (age 50 yr and older) maintained a BMI in the normal range (i.e., between 18.5 and 24.9 kg/m^2). Current patterns of overweight and obesity were estimated to account for 20% of all deaths from cancer in women and 14% of all deaths from cancer in men *(3)*. In absolute numbers, more than 90,000 deaths from cancer could be prevented yearly in the United States if everyone in the adult population could maintain normal weight throughout life.

BIOLOGICAL MECHANISMS OF ALTERED CANCER RISK ASSOCIATED WITH OBESITY AND TYPE 2 DIABETES

The positive relationship between overweight and obesity and cancer risk suggests that an excess energy intake relative to energy expenditure or its consequences is implicated in carcinogenesis. For decades, laboratory researchers have known that restricting energy intake of experimental animals not only increases life span but also reduces spontaneous tumor occurrence *(96)*. There is also evidence that physical activity may reduce the risk of some cancers, including colon, breast, and perhaps endometrial *(1)*. Positive energy balance and obesity are associated with multiple metabolic changes that may subsequently affect cancer development. Several biological mechanisms have been put forth to explain the relationship between excess body weight and risk of cancer. Certainly the best studied factors to date involve endogenous hormones (steroid hormones and insulin) and the insulin-like growth factor (IGF) system.

Steroid Hormones and Sex Hormone-Binding Globulin

Steroid hormones, including androgens, estrogens, and progesterone, are involved in regulation of the balance among cellular differentiation, proliferation, and apoptosis (programmed cell death) and may favor the selective growth of preneoplastic and neo-plastic cells (97,98). Both overall and central adiposity have been associated with dif-ferences in total and bioavailable steroid hormones. A metabolic consequence of obesity, especially central adiposity, is the development of insulin resistance. Insulin resistance leads to a compensatory increase in insulin secretion from the pancreas, with consequent hyperinsulinemia. Chronic hyperinsulinemia results in an increase in IGF-1 bioavailability through a decrease in some of its binding proteins (IGF-binding protein-1 [IGFBP-1] and IGFBP-2) (99,100). Insulin and increased bioavailable IGF-1, in turn, suppress the hepatic synthesis of sex hormone-binding globulin (SHBG) (101–103). Lower SHBG concentrations consequently lead to an increase in the amount of unbound bioactive steroid hormones. Insulin and IGF-1 also stimulate the synthesis of steroid hormones, particularly androgens (100). Finally, in men and postmenopausal women, adipose tissue is a major site for the synthesis of estrogens through aromatization of androgenic precursors (104).

The risks of cancers of the breast, endometrium, and ovary are associated with factors such as early menarche, late menopause, age at first pregnancy, parity, and use of post-menopausal HRT and oral contraceptives, suggesting an important role of hormones in the etiology of these cancers.

For breast cancer, there is strong evidence that risk is increased in postmenopausal women who have high circulating estrogen concentrations (105), particularly in combi-nation with high progesterone concentrations (106,107). Risk is further increased in postmenopausal women who have low concentrations of SHBG and in those with ele-vated concentrations of total and bioavailable estrogens and androgens (108,109). In premenopausal women, obesity may lead to anovulation and decreased progesterone levels (110) and, thus, may explain, at least in part, why obesity appears to be inversely related to risk of breast cancer in premenopausal women.

With respect to endometrial cancer, the predominant hypothesis is that risk is increased in women who have normal to high concentrations of bioavailable estrogens but low concentrations of progesterone (111). This theory is supported by observations that risk of endometrial cancer is increased in women who use postmenopausal hor-mone replacements containing only estrogens, or those who take oral contraceptives with about 16 d of estrogen use followed by <10 d of progestin use (112–114). Studies in vitro have demonstrated that estrogens stimulate the proliferation of normal endome-trial tissue and endometrial tumor cells, and that this effect may, at least partly, be mediated through an increase in local IGF-1 concentrations (115). Progesterone, on the other hand, can increase the concentrations of IGFBP-1 in endometrium and thus reduce bioactive IGF-1 concentrations (115). Low circulating concentrations of SHBG and elevated concentrations of androgens have been related to increased risk of endometrial cancer in both pre- and postmenopausal women (116–118).

The etiology of ovarian cancer remains poorly understood. It has been hypothesized that risk of ovarian cancer may be increased by factors associated with excess androgenic stimulation of ovarian epithelial cells and may be decreased by factors related to greater progesterone stimulation *(119)*. As noted earlier, obesity may lead to anovulation and decreased progesterone concentrations *(110)*. Hence, if progesterone is protective *(119)*, then obesity might increase the risk of ovarian cancer in premenopausal women by reducing the concentrations of progesterone. Indeed, epidemiological studies have generally reported a positive association between obesity and risk of ovarian cancer only in premenopausal women and in women who were overweight or obese in adolescence or early adulthood.

Insulin and the IGF System

As noted earlier, a major metabolic consequence of obesity is related to hyperinsulinemia and an increase in bioactive IGF-1. Besides the effects on circulating total and bioavailable steroid hormones, insulin and IGF-1 may be directly involved in carcinogenesis. Insulin and IGF-1 play a crucial role in the regulation of cellular proliferation and apoptosis of normal and neoplastic cells of many types *(99,120–122)*. In addition, both hormones have effects on cellular differentiation *(120,123)* and angiogenesis *(124)*. Several studies have supported an association of elevated insulin production and insulin concentrations with an increased risk of developing colorectal cancer *(125–128)*. Furthermore, high circulating concentrations of IGF-1 have been associated with an increased risk of several cancers, including cancers of the breast, prostate, and colon *(99,129)*. The association between type 2 diabetes and risk of cancer may be explained, biologically, by hyperinsulinemia and its consequences.

Other Mechanisms

In addition to the effects on steroid hormones and on insulin and the IGF system, there are several other potential mechanisms by which excess body weight may confer an increased risk of cancer. For example, obesity may increase the risk of cancer by increasing the circulating concentration of several adipose tissue-secreted proteins, the best studied of which is leptin, a hormone closely related to the percentage and amount of adipose tissue *(130,131)*. Leptin in mice is involved in the regulation of blood pressure, angiogenesis, and wound healing *(132,133)*, and experimental studies have shown that leptin may stimulate growth of colonic epithelial cells *(134,135)*. Two case–control studies reported an increased risk of colon cancer associated with high circulating leptin concentrations *(136,137)*, but other studies did not observe any significant association between circulating leptin concentrations and risk of leukemia or cancers of the breast *(138)*, endometrium *(139)*, and prostate *(140,141)*.

Adiponectin is another adipocyte-secreted hormone that holds promise as a link between obesity and diabetes, and cancer. A strong and consistent inverse association between adiponectin and both insulin and inflammatory states has been established *(142)*. Circulating concentrations of adiponectin are reduced in conditions associated with insulin resistance such as obesity and type 2 diabetes *(143)*. Low concentrations of adiponectin have emerged as being implicated in cancers of the breast *(138,144)* and endometrium *(145,146)* independent of the possible effect of obesity and other known and potential risk factors for these cancers. A recent case–control study *(145)* reported that women with a high BMI and low plasma adiponectin had a 6.5-fold increased risk of endometrial cancer compared with women with the opposite characteristics. Noteworthy, some studies *(26–28)* have found that the association between diabetes and risk of endometrial cancer is stronger among women with a high BMI. This might suggest that diabetes and obesity may have multiplicative effects in endometrial carcinogenesis.

CONCLUSIONS

Ample evidence indicates that overweight and obesity are associated with increased incidence of and mortality from most cancers. A review in 2002 by IARC concluded that there is sufficient evidence of a cancer-preventive effect of avoidance of weight gain for cancers of the endometrium, breast (in postmenopausal women), and colon (especially in men); renal cell carcinoma; and esophageal adenocarcinoma (1). Since that review, a large cohort study (the Cancer Prevention Study II) along with other cohort and case–control studies, has provided evidence that obesity possibly may be a risk factor for other cancers as well, including those of the prostate, ovary, pancreas, and gallbladder; multiple myeloma; leukemia; and non-Hodgkin lymphoma. Overall, the current patterns of overweight and obesity in the United States have been estimated to account for 20% of all deaths from cancer in women and 14% in men.

An accumulating body of evidence further shows an association between diabetes and increased risk of certain forms of cancers such as endometrial and colon independent of obesity. The dramatically increasing prevalence of overweight and obesity and type 2 diabetes in most parts of the world underscores the importance of learning more about the relationship among excess body weight, diabetes, and risk of cancer and of clarifying the underlying mechanisms involved. In view of the high proportion of cancer cases that could be prevented if the population maintained a healthy body weight, efforts to promote physical activity and healthful dietary practices are of substantial relevance for maintaining public health.

REFERENCES

1. International Agency for Research on Cancer. IARC Handbooks of Cancer Prevention: Weight Control and Physical Activity. (Vaino, H and Bianchini, F, eds). IARC Press, Lyon, France, 2002.
2. Bergström A, Pisani P, Tenet V, Wolk A, Adami HO. Overweight as an avoidable cause of cancer in Europe. Int J Cancer 2001;91:421–430.
3. Calle EE, Rodriguez C, Walker-Thurmond K, Thun MJ. Overweight, obesity, and mortality from cancer in a prospectively studied cohort of U.S. adults. N Engl J Med 2003;348:1625–1638.
4. Physical status: the use and interpretation of anthropometry: report of a WHO Expert Committee. World Health Organ 1995;854:1–452.
5. Wolk A, Gridley G, Svensson M, et al. A prospective study of obesity and cancer risk (Sweden). Cancer Causes Control 2001;12:13–21.
6. Pan SY, Johnson KC, Ugnat AM, Wen SW, Mao Y. Association of obesity and cancer risk in Canada. Am J Epidemiol 2004;159:259–268.
7. Weiderpass E, Gridley G, Nyren O, Pennello G, Landstrom AS, Ekbom A. Cause-specific mortality in a cohort of patients with diabetes mellitus: a population-based study in Sweden. J Clin Epidemiol 2001;54:802–809.
8. Parkin DM, Pisani P, Ferlay J. Estimates of the worldwide incidence of 25 major cancers in 1990. Int J Cancer 1999;80:827–841.
9. Jemal A, Tiwari RC, Murray T, et al. Cancer statistics, 2004. CA Cancer J Clin 2004;54:8–29.
10. de Waard F, Baanders-van Halewijn EA. A prospective study in general practice on breast-cancer risk in postmenopausal women. Int J Cancer 1974;14:153–160.
11. van den Brandt PA, Spiegelman D, Yaun SS, et al. Pooled analysis of prospective cohort studies on height, weight, and breast cancer risk. Am J Epidemiol 2000;152:514–527.
12. Lahmann PH, Hoffmann K, Allen N, et al. Body size and breast cancer risk: findings from the European prospective investigation into cancer and nutrition (EPIC). Int J Cancer 2004;111: 762–771.

13. Michels KB, Solomon CG, Hu FB, et al. Type 2 diabetes and subsequent incidence of breast cancer in the Nurses' Health Study. Diabetes Care 2003;26:1752–1758.

14. Weiderpass E, Gridley G, Persson I, Nyren O, Ekbom A, Adami HO. Risk of endometrial and breast cancer in patients with diabetes mellitus. Int J Cancer 1997;71:360–363.

15. Talamini R, Franceschi S, Favero A, Negri E, Parazzini F, La Vecchia C. Selected medical conditions and risk of breast cancer. Br J Cancer 1997;75:1699–1703.

16. Coughlin SS, Calle EE, Teras LR, Petrelli J, Thun MJ. Diabetes mellitus as a predictor of cancer mortality in a large cohort of US adults. Am J Epidemiol 2004;159:1160–1167.

17. Wideroff L, Gridley G, Mellemkjaer L, et al. Cancer incidence in a population-based cohort of patients hospitalized with diabetes mellitus in Denmark. J Natl Cancer Inst 1997;89:1360–1365.

18. Weiss HA, Brinton LA, Potischman NA, et al. Breast cancer risk in young women and history of selected medical conditions. Int J Epidemiol 1999;28:816–823.

19. La Vecchia C, Negri E, Franceschi S, D'Avanzo B, Boyle P. A case-control study of diabetes mellitus and cancer risk. Br J Cancer 1994;70:950–953.

20. Kopp S, Tanneberger S, Mohner M, Kieser R. Diabetes and breast cancer risk. Int J Cancer 1990;46: 751, 752.

21. Moseson M, Koenig KL, Shore RE, Pasternack BS. The influence of medical conditions associated with hormones on the risk of breast cancer. Int J Epidemiol 1993;22:1000–1009.

22. Sellers TA, Sprafka JM, Gapstur SM, et al. Does body fat distribution promote familial aggregation of adult onset diabetes mellitus and postmenopausal breast cancer? Epidemiology 1994;5:102–108.

23. Grady D, Ernster V. Endometrial cancer. In: Schottenfeld D, Fraumeni J, eds. Cancer Epidemiology and Prevention, 2nd ed. Oxford University Press, New York, 1996, pp. 1058–1108.

24. Weiderpass E, Persson I, Adami HO, Magnusson C, Lindgren A, Baron JA. Body size in different periods of life, diabetes mellitus, hypertension, and risk of postmenopausal endometrial cancer (Sweden). Cancer Causes Control 2000;11:185–192.

25. Parazzini F, La Vecchia C, Negri E, et al. Diabetes and endometrial cancer: an Italian case-control study. Int J Cancer 1999;81:539–542.

26. Anderson KE, Anderson E, Mink PJ, et al. Diabetes and endometrial cancer in the Iowa women's health study. Cancer Epidemiol Biomarkers Prev 2001;10:611–616.

27. Salazar-Martinez E, Lazcano-Ponce EC, Lira-Lira GG, et al. Case-control study of diabetes, obesity, physical activity and risk of endometrial cancer among Mexican women. Cancer Causes Control 2000;11:707–711.

28. Shoff SM, Newcomb PA. Diabetes, body size, and risk of endometrial cancer. Am J Epidemiol 1998;148:234–240.

29. O'Mara BA, Byers T, Schoenfeld E. Diabetes mellitus and cancer risk: a multisite case-control study. J Chronic Dis 1985;38:435–441.

30. Purdie DM, Bain CJ, Webb PM, Whiteman DC, Pirozzo S, Green AC. Body size and ovarian cancer: case-control study and systematic review (Australia). Cancer Causes Control 2001;12:855–863.

31. Lubin F, Chetrit A, Freedman LS, et al. Body mass index at age 18 years and during adult life and ovarian cancer risk. Am J Epidemiol 2003;157:113–120.

32. Schouten LJ, Goldbohm RA, van den Brandt PA. Height, weight, weight change, and ovarian cancer risk in the Netherlands cohort study on diet and cancer. Am J Epidemiol 2003;157:424–433.

33. Farrow DC, Weiss NS, Lyon JL, Daling JR. Association of obesity and ovarian cancer in a case-control study. Am J Epidemiol 1989;129:1300–1304.

34. Lew EA, Garfinkel L. Variations in mortality by weight among 750,000 men and women. J Chronic Dis 1979;32:563–576.

35. Garfinkel L. Overweight and cancer. Ann Intern Med 1985;103:1034–1036.

36. Dal Maso L, Franceschi S, Negri E, et al. Body size indices at different ages and epithelial ovarian cancer risk. Eur J Cancer 2002;38:1769–1774.

37. Fairfield KM, Willett WC, Rosner BA, Manson JE, Speizer FE, Hankinson SE. Obesity, weight gain, and ovarian cancer. Obstet Gynecol 2002;100:288–296.

38. Anderson JP, Ross JA, Folsom AR. Anthropometric variables, physical activity, and incidence of ovarian cancer: the Iowa Women's Health Study. Cancer 2004;100:1515–1521.

39. Tornberg SA, Carstensen JM. Relationship between Quetelet's index and cancer of breast and female genital tract in 47,000 women followed for 25 years. Br J Cancer 1994;69:358–361.

40. Byers T, Marshall J, Graham S, Mettlin C, Swanson M. A case-control study of dietary and nondietary factors in ovarian cancer. J Natl Cancer Inst 1983;71:681–686.

41. Moller H, Mellemgaard A, Lindvig K, Olsen JH. Obesity and cancer risk: a Danish record-linkage study. Eur J Cancer 1994;30A:344–350.

42. Jonsson F, Wolk A, Pedersen NL, et al. Obesity and hormone-dependent tumors: cohort and co-twin control studies based on the Swedish Twin Registry. Int J Cancer 2003;106:594–599.

43. Lukanova A, Toniolo P, Lundin E, et al. Body mass index in relation to ovarian cancer: a multi-centre nested case-control study. Int J Cancer 2002;99:603–608.

44. Kuper H, Cramer DW, Titus-Ernstoff L. Risk of ovarian cancer in the United States in relation to anthropometric measures: does the association depend on menopausal status? Cancer Causes Control 2002;13:455–463.

45. Engeland A, Tretli S, Bjorge T. Height, body mass index, and ovarian cancer: a follow-up of 1.1 million Norwegian women. J Natl Cancer Inst 2003;95:1244–1248.

46. Parazzini F, Moroni S, La Vecchia C, Negri E, dal Pino D, Bolis G. Ovarian cancer risk and history of selected medical conditions linked with female hormones. Eur J Cancer 1997;33:1634–1637.

47. Weiderpass E, Ye W, Vainio H, Kaaks R, Adami HO. Diabetes mellitus and ovarian cancer (Sweden). Cancer Causes Control 2002;13:759–764.

48. Adler AI, Weiss NS, Kamb ML, Lyon JL. Is diabetes mellitus a risk factor for ovarian cancer? A case-control study in Utah and Washington (United States). Cancer Causes Control 1996;7:475–478.

49. Adami HO, McLaughlin J, Ekbom A, et al. Cancer risk in patients with diabetes mellitus. Cancer Causes Control 1991;2:307–314.

50. Kessler II. Cancer mortality among diabetics. J Natl Cancer Inst 1970;44:673–686.

51. Ragozzino M, Melton LJ 3rd, Chu CP, Palumbo PJ. Subsequent cancer risk in the incidence cohort of Rochester, Minnesota, residents with diabetes mellitus. J Chronic Dis 1982;35:13–19.

52. Smith GD, Egger M, Shipley MJ, Marmot MG. Post-challenge glucose concentration, impaired glucose tolerance, diabetes, and cancer mortality in men. Am J Epidemiol 1992;136:1110–1114.

53. Will JC, Vinicor F, Calle EE. Is diabetes mellitus associated with prostate cancer incidence and survival? Epidemiology 1999;10:313–318.

54. Tavani A, Gallus S, Bosetti C, et al. Diabetes and the risk of prostate cancer. Eur J Cancer Prev 2002;11:125–128.

55. Weiderpass E, Ye W, Vainio H, Kaaks R, Adami HO. Reduced risk of prostate cancer among patients with diabetes mellitus. Int J Cancer 2002;102:258–261.

56. Giovannucci E, Rimm EB, Stampfer MJ, Colditz GA, Willett WC. Diabetes mellitus and risk of prostate cancer (United States). Cancer Causes Control 1998;9:3–9.

57. Coker AL, Sanderson M, Zheng W, Fadden MK. Diabetes mellitus and prostate cancer risk among older men: population-based case-control study. Br J Cancer 2004;90:2171–2175.

58. Zhu K, Lee IM, Sesso HD, Buring JE, Levine RS, Gaziano JM. History of diabetes mellitus and risk of prostate cancer in physicians. Am J Epidemiol 2004;159:978–982.

59. Rossouw JE, Anderson GL, Prentice RL, et al. Risks and benefits of estrogen plus progestin in healthy postmenopausal women: principal results from the Women's Health Initiative randomized controlled trial. JAMA 2002;288:321–333.

60. La Vecchia C, D'Avanzo B, Negri E, Franceschi S. History of selected diseases and the risk of colorectal cancer. Eur J Cancer 1991;27:582–586.

61. Nilsen TI, Vatten LJ. Prospective study of colorectal cancer risk and physical activity, diabetes, blood glucose and BMI: exploring the hyperinsulinaemia hypothesis. Br J Cancer 2001;84:417–422.

62. Will JC, Galuska DA, Vinicor F, Calle EE. Colorectal cancer: another complication of diabetes mellitus? Am J Epidemiol 1998;147:816–825.

63. Hu FB, Manson JE, Liu S, et al. Prospective study of adult onset diabetes mellitus (type 2) and risk of colorectal cancer in women. J Natl Cancer Inst 1999;91:542–547.

64. Le Marchand L, Wilkens LR, Kolonel LN, Hankin JH, Lyu LC. Associations of sedentary lifestyle, obesity, smoking, alcohol use, and diabetes with the risk of colorectal cancer. Cancer Res 1997;57:4787–4794.

65. Kune GA, Kune S, Watson LF. Colorectal cancer risk, chronic illnesses, operations, and medications: case control results from the Melbourne Colorectal Cancer Study. Cancer Res 1988;48:4399–4404.

66. Bergström A, Hsieh CC, Lindblad P, Lu CM, Cook NR, Wolk A. Obesity and renal cell cancer—a quantitative review. Br J Cancer 2001;85:984–990.

67. Lindblad P, Wolk A, Bergstrom R, Persson I, Adami HO. The role of obesity and weight fluctuations in the etiology of renal cell cancer: a population-based case-control study. Cancer Epidemiol Biomarkers Prev 1994;3:631–639.

68. Wynder EL, Mabuchi K, Whitmore WF Jr. Epidemiology of adenocarcinoma of the kidney. J Natl Cancer Inst 1974;53:1619–1634.

69. McLaughlin JK, Gao YT, Gao RN, et al. Risk factors for renal-cell cancer in Shanghai, China. Int J Cancer 1992;52:562–565.

70. Asal NR, Geyer JR, Risser DR, Lee ET, Kadamani S, Cherng N. Risk factors in renal cell carcinoma. II. Medical history, occupation, multivariate analysis, and conclusions. Cancer Detect Prev 1988;13:263–279.

71. McCredie M, Stewart JH. Risk factors for kidney cancer in New South Wales, Australia. II. Urologic disease, hypertension, obesity, and hormonal factors. Cancer Causes Control 1992;3:323–331.

72. Schlehofer B, Pommer W, Mellemgaard A, et al. International renal-cell-cancer study. VI. The role of medical and family history. Int J Cancer 1996;66:723–726.

73. Mellemgaard A, Niwa S, Mehl ES, Engholm G, McLaughlin JK, Olsen JH. Risk factors for renal cell carcinoma in Denmark: role of medication and medical history. Int J Epidemiol 1994;23: 923–930.

74. Kreiger N, Marrett LD, Dodds L, Hilditch S, Darlington GA. Risk factors for renal cell carcinoma: results of a population-based case-control study. Cancer Causes Control 1993;4:101–110.

75. Goodman MT, Morgenstern H, Wynder EL. A case-control study of factors affecting the development of renal cell cancer. Am J Epidemiol 1986;124:926–941.

76. Lindblad P, Chow WH, Chan J, et al. The role of diabetes mellitus in the aetiology of renal cell cancer. Diabetologia 1999;42:107–112.

77. Coughlin SS, Neaton JD, Randall B, Sengupta A. Predictors of mortality from kidney cancer in 332,547 men screened for the Multiple Risk Factor Intervention Trial. Cancer 1997;79:2171–2177.

78. Berrington de Gonzalez A, Sweetland S, Spencer E. A meta-analysis of obesity and the risk of pancreatic cancer. Br J Cancer 2003;89:519–523.

79. Coughlin SS, Calle EE, Patel AV, Thun MJ. Predictors of pancreatic cancer mortality among a large cohort of United States adults. Cancer Causes Control 2000;11:915–923.

80. Gapstur SM, Gann PH, Lowe W, Liu K, Colangelo L, Dyer A. Abnormal glucose metabolism and pancreatic cancer mortality. JAMA 2000;283:2552–2558.

81. Michaud DS, Giovannucci E, Willett WC, Colditz GA, Stampfer MJ, Fuchs CS. Physical activity, obesity, height, and the risk of pancreatic cancer. JAMA 2001;286:921–929.

82. Everhart J, Wright D. Diabetes mellitus as a risk factor for pancreatic cancer: a meta-analysis. JAMA 1995;273:1605–1609.

83. Calle EE, Murphy TK, Rodriguez C, Thun MJ, Heath CW Jr. Diabetes mellitus and pancreatic cancer mortality in a prospective cohort of United States adults. Cancer Causes Control 1998;9:403–410.

84. Pisani P, Parkin DM, Bray F, Ferlay J. Estimates of the worldwide mortality from 25 cancers in 1990. Int J Cancer 1999;83:18–29.

85. Devesa SS, Blot WJ, Fraumeni JF Jr. Changing patterns in the incidence of esophageal and gastric carcinoma in the United States. Cancer 1998;83:2049–53.

86. Blot WJ, Devesa SS, Fraumeni JF Jr. Continuing climb in rates of esophageal adenocarcinoma: an update. JAMA 1993;270:1320.

87. Hansson LE, Sparen P, Nyren O. Increasing incidence of both major histological types of esophageal carcinomas among men in Sweden. Int J Cancer 1993;54:402–407.

88. Vaughan TL, Davis S, Kristal A, Thomas DB. Obesity, alcohol, and tobacco as risk factors for cancers of the esophagus and gastric cardia: adenocarcinoma versus squamous cell carcinoma. Cancer Epidemiol Biomarkers Prev 1995;4:85–92.

89. Brown LM, Swanson CA, Gridley G, et al. Adenocarcinoma of the esophagus: role of obesity and diet. J Natl Cancer Inst 1995;87:104–109.

90. Chow WH, Blot WJ, Vaughan TL, et al. Body mass index and risk of adenocarcinomas of the esophagus and gastric cardia. J Natl Cancer Inst 1998;90:150–155.

91. Lagergren J, Bergstrom R, Nyren O. Association between body mass and adenocarcinoma of the esophagus and gastric cardia. Ann Intern Med 1999;130:883–890.

92. Cheng KK, Sharp L, McKinney PA, et al. A case-control study of oesophageal adenocarcinoma in women: a preventable disease. Br J Cancer 2000;83:127–132.

93. Wu AH, Wan P, Bernstein L. A multiethnic population-based study of smoking, alcohol and body size and risk of adenocarcinomas of the stomach and esophagus (United States). Cancer Causes Control 2001;12:721–732.

94. Ji BT, Chow WH, Yang G, et al. Body mass index and the risk of cancers of the gastric cardia and distal stomach in Shanghai, China. Cancer Epidemiol Biomarkers Prev 1997;6:481–485.

95. Engel LS, Chow WH, Vaughan TL, et al. Population attributable risks of esophageal and gastric cancers. J Natl Cancer Inst 2003;95:1404–1413.

96. Kritchevsky D. Caloric restriction and experimental carcinogenesis. Toxicol Sci 1999;52:13–16.

97. Liao DJ, Dickson RB. Roles of androgens in the development, growth, and carcinogenesis of the mammary gland. J Steroid Biochem Mol Biol 2002;80:175–189.

98. Dickson RB, Thompson EW, Lippman ME. Regulation of proliferation, invasion and growth factor synthesis in breast cancer by steroids. J Steroid Biochem Mol Biol 1990;37:305–316.

99. Yu H, Rohan T. Role of the insulin-like growth factor family in cancer development and progression. J Natl Cancer Inst 2000;92:1472–1489.

100. Kaaks R, Lukanova A. Energy balance and cancer: the role of insulin and insulin-like growth factor-I. Proc Nutr Soc 2001;60:91–106.

101. Nestler JE. Obesity, insulin, sex steroids and ovulation. Int J Obes Relat Metab Disord 2000;24 (Suppl 2):S71–S73.

102. Crave JC, Lejeune H, Brebant C, Baret C, Pugeat M. Differential effects of insulin and insulin-like growth factor I on the production of plasma steroid-binding globulins by human hepatoblastoma-derived (Hep G2) cells. J Clin Endocrinol Metab 1995;80:1283–1289.

103. Pugeat M, Crave JC, Elmidani M, et al. Pathophysiology of sex hormone binding globulin (SHBG): relation to insulin. J Steroid Biochem Mol Biol 1991;40:841–849.

104. Siiteri PK. Adipose tissue as a source of hormones. Am J Clin Nutr 1987;45:277–282.

105. Bernstein L, Ross RK. Endogenous hormones and breast cancer risk. Epidemiol Rev 1993;15:48–65.

106. Magnusson C, Baron JA, Correia N, Bergstrom R, Adami HO, Persson I. Breast-cancer risk following long-term oestrogen- and oestrogen-progestin-replacement therapy. Int J Cancer 1999;81:339–344.

107. Ross RK, Paganini-Hill A, Wan PC, Pike MC. Effect of hormone replacement therapy on breast cancer risk: estrogen versus estrogen plus progestin. J Natl Cancer Inst 2000;92:328–332.

108. Key TJ. Serum oestradiol and breast cancer risk. Endocr Relat Cancer 1999;6:175–180.

109. Hankinson SE, Willett WC, Manson JE, et al. Plasma sex steroid hormone levels and risk of breast cancer in postmenopausal women. J Natl Cancer Inst 1998;90:1292–1299.

110. Pike MC, Krailo MD, Henderson BE, Casagrande JT, Hoel DG. 'Hormonal' risk factors, 'breast tissue age' and the age-incidence of breast cancer. Nature 1983;303:767–770.

111. Key TJ, Pike MC. The dose-effect relationship between 'unopposed' oestrogens and endometrial mitotic rate: its central role in explaining and predicting endometrial cancer risk. Br J Cancer 1988;57:205–212.

112. Persson I, Weiderpass E, Bergkvist L, Bergstrom R, Schairer C. Risks of breast and endometrial cancer after estrogen and estrogen-progestin replacement. Cancer Causes Control 1999;10:253–260.

113. Weiderpass E, Adami HO, Baron JA, Magnusson C, Lindgren A, Persson I. Use of oral contraceptives and endometrial cancer risk (Sweden). Cancer Causes Control 1999;10:277–284.

114. International Agency for Research and Cancer, Hormonal Contraception and Post-Menopausal Hormonal Therapy. IARC Monographs on the Evaluation of the Carcinogenic Risks to Humans. Lyon, France, 1999.

115. Rutanen EM. Insulin-like growth factors in endometrial function. Gynecol Endocrinol 1998;12:399–406.

116. Potischman N, Hoover RN, Brinton LA, et al. Case-control study of endogenous steroid hormones and endometrial cancer. J Natl Cancer Inst 1996;88:1127–1135.

117. Grady D, Ernster V. Endometrial cancer. In: Schottenfeld D, Fraumeni J, eds. Cancer Epidemiology and Prevention, 2nd ed. Oxford University Press, New York, 1996, pp. 1058–1089.

118. Lukanova A, Lundin E, Micheli A, et al. Circulating levels of sex steroid hormones and risk of endometrial cancer in postmenopausal women. Int J Cancer 2004;108:425–432.

119. Risch HA. Hormonal etiology of epithelial ovarian cancer, with a hypothesis concerning the role of androgens and progesterone. J Natl Cancer Inst 1998;90:1774–1786.

120. Werner H, LeRoith D. The role of the insulin-like growth factor system in human cancer. Adv Cancer Res 1996;68:183–223.

121. Wang HS, Chard T. IGFs and IGF-binding proteins in the regulation of human ovarian and endometrial function. J Endocrinol 1999;161:1–13.

122. Rosen CJ. Serum insulin-like growth factors and insulin-like growth factor-binding proteins: clinical implications. Clin Chem 1999;45:1384–1390.

123. Khandwala HM, McCutcheon IE, Flyvbjerg A, Friend KE. The effects of insulin-like growth factors on tumorigenesis and neoplastic growth. Endocr Rev 2000;21:215–244.

124. Kluge A, Zimmermann R, Munkel B, et al. Insulin-like growth factor I is involved in inflammation linked angiogenic processes after microembolisation in porcine heart. Cardiovasc Res 1995;29:407–415.

125. Ma J, Giovannucci E, Pollak M, et al. A prospective study of plasma C-peptide and colorectal cancer risk in men. J Natl Cancer Inst 2004;96:546–553.

126. Kaaks R, Toniolo P, Akhmedkhanov A, et al. Serum C-peptide, insulin-like growth factor (IGF)-I, IGF-binding proteins, and colorectal cancer risk in women. J Natl Cancer Inst 2000;92:1592–1600.

127. Palmqvist R, Stattin P, Rinaldi S, et al. Plasma insulin, IGF-binding proteins-1 and -2 and risk of colorectal cancer: a prospective study in northern Sweden. Int J Cancer 2003;107:89–93.

128. Schoen RE, Tangen CM, Kuller LH, et al. Increased blood glucose and insulin, body size, and incident colorectal cancer. J Natl Cancer Inst 1999;91:1147–1154.

129. Renehan AG, Zwahlen M, Minder C, O'Dwyer ST, Shalet SM, Egger M. Insulin-like growth factor (IGF)-I, IGF binding protein-3, and cancer risk: systematic review and meta-regression analysis. Lancet 2004;363:1346–1353.

130. Hassink SG, Sheslow DV, de Lancey E, Opentanova I, Considine RV, Caro JF. Serum leptin in children with obesity: relationship to gender and development. Pediatrics 1996;98:201–203.

131. Considine RV, Sinha MK, Heiman ML, et al. Serum immunoreactive-leptin concentrations in normal-weight and obese humans. N Engl J Med 1996;334:292–295.

132. Sierra-Honigmann MR, Nath AK, Murakami C, et al. Biological action of leptin as an angiogenic factor. Science 1998;281:1683–1686.

133. Ahima RS, Flier JS. Adipose tissue as an endocrine organ. Trends Endocrinol Metab 2000; 11:327–332.

134. Hardwick JC, Van Den Brink GR, Offerhaus GJ, Van Deventer SJ, Peppelenbosch MP. Leptin is a growth factor for colonic epithelial cells. Gastroenterology 2001;121:79–90.

135. Attoub S, Noe V, Pirola L, et al. Leptin promotes invasiveness of kidney and colonic epithelial cells via phosphoinositide 3-kinase-, rho-, and rac-dependent signaling pathways. FASEB J 2000; 14:2329–2338.

136. Stattin P, Palmqvist R, Soderberg S, et al. Plasma leptin and colorectal cancer risk: a prospective study in Northern Sweden. Oncol Rep 2003;10:2015–2021.

137. Stattin P, Lukanova A, Biessy C, et al. Obesity and colon cancer: does leptin provide a link? Int J Cancer 2004;109:149–152.

138. Mantzoros C, Petridou E, Dessypris N, et al. Adiponectin and breast cancer risk. J Clin Endocrinol Metab 2004;89:1102–1107.

139. Petridou E, Belechri M, Dessypris N, et al. Leptin and body mass index in relation to endometrial cancer risk. Ann Nutr Metab 2002;46:147–151.

140. Lagiou P, Signorello LB, Trichopoulos D, Tzonou A, Trichopoulou A, Mantzoros CS. Leptin in relation to prostate cancer and benign prostatic hyperplasia. Int J Cancer 1998;76:25–28.

141. Hsing AW, Chua S Jr, Gao YT, et al. Prostate cancer risk and serum levels of insulin and leptin: a population-based study. J Natl Cancer Inst 2001;93:783–789.

142. Kershaw EE, Flier JS. Adipose tissue as an endocrine organ. J Clin Endocrinol Metab 2004; 89:2548–2556.

143. Gale SM, Castracane VD, Mantzoros CS. Energy homeostasis, obesity and eating disorders: recent advances in endocrinology. J Nutr 2004;134:295–298.

144. Miyoshi Y, Funahashi T, Kihara S, et al. Association of serum adiponectin levels with breast cancer risk. Clin Cancer Res 2003;9:5699–5704.

145. Dal Maso L, Augustin LS, Karalis A, et al. Circulating adiponectin and endometrial cancer risk. J Clin Endocrinol Metab 2004;89:1160–1163.

146. Petridou E, Mantzoros C, Dessypris N, et al. Plasma adiponectin concentrations in relation to endometrial cancer: a case-control study in Greece. J Clin Endocrinol Metab 2003;88:993–997.

15 Polycystic Ovary Syndrome and Its Metabolic Complications

Emilia P. Liao, MD and Leonid Poretsky, MD

CONTENTS

INTRODUCTION
PATHOPHYSIOLOGY
METABOLIC COMPLICATIONS
TREATMENT
CONCLUSIONS
REFERENCES

INTRODUCTION

Polycystic ovary syndrome (PCOS) is a complex disorder with multiple potential etiologies and variable clinical presentations whose pathogenesis remains poorly understood. PCOS is characterized by clinical and/or biochemical hyperandrogenism and chronic anovulation. This syndrome is also associated with insulin resistance, obesity, increased risk of diabetes mellitus and, possibly, cardiovascular disease (CVD).

Background

In 1935, Stein and Leventhal *(1)* described a syndrome of amenorrhea and polycystic ovaries that was commonly associated with obesity, hyperandrogenism, and infertility. Laparotomy revealed enlarged ovaries with thickened tunica and multiple (20–100/ ovary) cysts. Resection of one-half to three-fourths of ovarian tissue resulted in normal menstrual function *(1)*.

In 1976, Kahn et al. *(2)* solidified the association of hyperandrogenism, polycystic ovaries, or ovarian hyperthecosis with insulin resistance and acanthosis nigricans in their description of adolescent girls with mutations of the insulin receptor gene. In 1980, hyperinsulinemia in "garden-variety" PCOS was confirmed by Burghen and Kitabchi *(3)*, who reported a linear correlation between circulating insulin levels and androgen levels in women with PCOS, suggesting etiological significance of hyperinsulinemia in the development of the disorder. Demonstration of insulin receptors in the human ovary in 1984 clearly established the ovary as a target for insulin action *(4,5)*.

During the past two decades, it became evident that PCOS held metabolic, in addition to reproductive, importance for the affected women.

From: *Contemporary Diabetes: Obesity and Diabetes*
Edited by: C. S. Mantzoros © Humana Press Inc., Totowa, NJ

Table 1
Prevalence of Clinical Features in PCOS

Feature	Prevalence in PCOS (%)
Hirsutism *(11,22)*	66–72
Acne *(11,22)*	15–35
Obesity (BMI $\geq$ 30 kg/m^2) *(22)*	60
Infertility *(11,22)*	33–40
Impaired glucose tolerance *(112)*	35
Type 2 diabetes *(112)*	10

Epidemiology

PCOS is the most common endocrinopathy affecting women of reproductive age, with a prevalence ranging from 5 to 10%. In prospective studies, the prevalence of PCOS was found to be 4.7% among Caucasian women in the southeastern United States *(6)*; 6.8% in Greeks in the island of Lesbos *(7)*; and 6.5% in Caucasians in Madrid, Spain *(8)*. In one study, the prevalence of PCOS among premenopausal women with type 2 diabetes mellitus was found to be 26.7% *(9)*.

Clinical Manifestations

The presentation of PCOS is variable. The classic symptoms of menstrual irregularity, polycystic ovaries, obesity, and hirsutism usually develop during adolescence but do not all need to be present for diagnosis (Table 1).

MENSTRUAL IRREGULARITY

Menstrual irregularity owing to oligo- or anovulation is the hallmark of PCOS. Normal or delayed menarche may be followed by regular cycles, which become irregular with the development of weight gain and hyperandrogenism. Women with PCOS usually have sufficient estrogen owing to peripheral conversion from androgens but are deficient in progesterone, leading to chronic stimulation of the endometrium, leading, in turn, to increased risk of endometrial hyperplasia and endometrial cancer, as well as dysfunctional uterine bleeding.

HYPERANDROGENISM

Hyperandrogenism is most commonly manifested as hirsutism, followed by acne *(10)*. Other manifestations include male-pattern balding, deepening of the voice, and increased muscle mass. Hirsutism is defined as excess terminal body hair in a male distribution and can be measured using the Ferrimen-Gallwey score *(11)*. Many women with PCOS, especially women of East Asian origin, do not exhibit hirsutism *(12)*.

Venous catheterization studies and dexamethasone suppression tests have proved the ovaries to be the primary source of androgens in women with PCOS *(13)*. Serum free testosterone concentration is usually increased, whereas serum sex hormone-binding globulin (SHBG) concentration is often low, owing to hyperinsulinemia. Total serum testosterone concentration varies depending on the level of SHBG. Although the ovary is the main source of excess androgen, circulating adrenal androgen levels can also be elevated, usually to a mild degree, with 40–60% of women with PCOS exhibiting elevations of serum concentrations of dehydroepiandrosterone sulfate (DHEA-S) *(13)*.

Table 2
Clinical and Biochemical Features of Obese vs Nonobese
Patients With PCOS

Feature	Obese	Nonobese
Hirsutism (11)	++	+
SHBG (17)	↓	Normal
Free testosterone (17)	↑↑	↑
Oligomenorrhea/anovulation (11,17)	++	+
Infertility (11)	++	+
Acanthosis nigricans (17)	++	+
Insulin resistance (17)	++	+
Increased GH/IGF system activity (109)	+	++
Dyslipidemia (124)	++	+
Impaired glucose homeostasis (112)	++	+
Risk of endometrial carcinoma (152)	++	+

HYPOTHALAMIC–PITUITARY ABNORMALITIES

Many women with PCOS exhibit elevated mean serum leutinizing hormone (LH) concentrations, owing to increased LH pulse frequency and amplitude. Follicle-stimulating hormone (FSH) concentration in the serum is usually normal or low, resulting in an elevated LH/FSH ratio. Because LH secretion is pulsatile, a single measurement may not be reliable. Furthermore, because FSH may be elevated owing to sporadic ovulation, LH/FSH ratio may be normal. Finally, overweight women with PCOS tend to have lower basal LH and LH pulse amplitude than lean women with PCOS (13). This variability makes LH/FSH ratio a relatively insensitive indicator of PCOS.

POLYCYSTIC OVARIES

Classically, PCOS ovaries contain 8–10 small (2- to 8-mm) follicles arranged peripherally, in a single-plane view, around an increased amount of stroma (13). This finding, however, is not unique to PCOS and has been observed in different settings and with varying prevalence, depending on the population studied: 92% of women with idiopathic hirsutism, 87% with oligomenorrhea, 82% of premenopausal women with type 2 diabetes mellitus, 82% of women with congenital adrenal hyperplasia (CAH), 40% of women with a history of gestational diabetes, and 22% of healthy volunteers (13–15).

OBESITY

Body mass index (BMI) > 25 kg/m^2 is present in at least 35–50% of women with PCOS (13,16). The type of obesity seen in PCOS is central, or android, with increased waist-to-hip ratio (>0.85). Obese women with PCOS are more likely to be hirsute and have menstrual disorders than nonobese women with PCOS. Infertility rates can be up to 40% higher in women with PCOS whose BMI is >30 kg/m^2 than in those whose BMI is <30 kg/m^2 (10). Serum SHBG concentrations are also lower in obese women with PCOS, and circulating SHBG is inversely related to insulin concentration (16) (Table 2).

INSULIN RESISTANCE

Both lean and obese women with PCOS demonstrate insulin resistance and hyperinsulinemia, although obese women with PCOS have a higher degree of insulin resistance than lean women with PCOS (16).

DIAGNOSIS

A 1990 National Institutes of Health (NIH) conference on PCOS developed the following diagnostic criteria for disease: (1) menstrual irregularity owing to oligo- or anovulation; and (2) evidence of hyperandrogenism, clinical or biochemical, with the exclusion of other causes of hyperandrogenism and ovulatory dysfunction *(17)*. More recently, in 2003, a consensus group agreed in Rotterdam to broaden the diagnostic criteria to include presence of polycystic ovary morphology as a third component *(18)*. Any two of the three components are sufficient to diagnose PCOS.

The most serious conditions to rule out in the differential diagnosis are virilizing tumors of the ovary or adrenal glands. Patients with tumors usually have rapid progression of masculinizing symptoms with very high circulating testosterone levels (>250 ng/mL), but occasionally testosterone values can be normal *(19)*. Although women with PCOS often have modest elevations of serum DHEA concentrations, markedly elevated DHEA levels point to an adrenal source. Another rare condition to rule out is Cushing's syndrome, which can present with hirsutism, weight gain, and oligomenorrhea.

Adrenal hyperandrogenism owing to CAH can result in hirsutism and menstrual irregularities. Classic forms of CAH are usually diagnosed at birth or in childhood and can present with varying degrees of hyperandrogenism with or without salt wasting. Nonclassic, or late onset, CAH is usually caused by 21-hydroxylase deficiency. Women with nonclassic CAH can present with mild hyperandrogenism during adolescence, similar to PCOS. Morning serum concentrations of 17-hydroxyprogesterone <2 ng/mL effectively rule out CAH, whereas higher values require further investigation with an adrenocorticotropic hormone (ACTH) stimulation test. ACTH-stimulated values of 17-hydroxyprogesterone >10 ng/mL are consistent with, although not necessarily diagnostic of, CAH *(20)*.

In a large study including 873 women with hyperandrogenism, the prevalence of androgen-secreting tumors was 0.2%, CAH was 0.6%, nonclassic CAH was 1.6%, idiopathic hirsutism was 4.7%, hyperandrogenic insulin-resistant acanthosis nigricans syndrome was 3.1%, and PCOS was 82% *(21)*.

PATHOPHYSIOLOGY

The etiology of PCOS is unknown, but there is a strong genetic component. Although familial clustering of hyperandrogenism with a high prevalence (46–55%) of PCOS among siblings is consistent with autosomal pattern of inheritance *(22–24)*, given the heterogeneity of the disease, etiology is likely to be multigenic, affecting a host of genes and their cellular responses.

Prevailing Hypotheses

Three main hypotheses for the pathogenesis of PCOS have been proposed, each based on the stated primary biochemical abnormality: (1) central hypothesis, (2) ovarian hypothesis, and (3) insulin hypothesis.

CENTRAL HYPOTHESIS

Excessive LH secretion leading to theca cell hyperplasia and androgen secretion by the ovaries is the basis of the central hypothesis. In women with PCOS, pituitary gonadotropes exhibit increased sensitivity to exogenous gonadotropin-releasing hormone (GnRH) *(25)*. Administration of GnRH agonists and/or pulsatile GnRH improves symptoms of hyperandrogenism and can induce ovulation in 40–72% of women with PCOS *(26,27)*. However, abnormalities in gonadal function often persist, and circulating testosterone levels may remain elevated despite LH suppression *(28)*. Thus, it is not clear whether excess LH is owing to increased GnRH secretion or to abnormal sex steroid feedback. Furthermore, the central hypothesis does not account for PCOS in those women who do not demonstrate excess LH.

OVARIAN HYPOTHESIS

The ovarian hypothesis postulates a primary intrinsic defect in the ovary leading to abnormal secretion of both androgens and estrogens. Ovarian resection, the initial intervention proposed by Stein and Leventhal *(1)*, results in reduction of androgen levels and resumption of menses, presumably by removing the androgen-producing tissue. Theca cell (where ovarian androgen production primarily occurs) hypertrophy and widespread overexpression of steroidogenic enzymes are characteristic of the polycystic ovary *(29)*. Furthermore, theca cells from PCOS ovaries produce increased amounts of progesterone and 17-hydroxyprogesterone compared with theca cells from normal ovaries *(30)*. Exaggerated responses of 17-hydroxyprogesterone and androstenedione to GnRH agonist and LH *(31)* suggest increased 17α-hydroxlyase activity, involving 17,20 lyase. These findings have led to a proposal that dysregulation of cytochrome P450c17α (which comprises both 17α-hydroxylase and 17,20 lyase activities) is the primary disorder in ovarian steroidogenesis in PCOS. Subsequently, the gene encoding P450c17α, *CYP17*, was investigated as the prime candidate gene for disease-carrying mutations or polymorphisms; however, results are conflicting *(32)*. An alternative view is that increased steroidogenesis in the ovary is simply the result of increased theca cell mass *(33)*.

Excessive serine phosphorylation of P450c17α has been shown to stimulate selectively 17,20 lyase activity, offering yet another mechanism of abnormal steroidogenesis in PCOS *(34)*. Interestingly, excessive serine phosphorylation of the insulin receptor has been reported in approx 50% of women with PCOS and proposed as a mechanism for insulin resistance *(35)*.

INSULIN HYPOTHESIS

Although not included among the 1990 NIH-sponsored consensus of diagnostic criteria for the disease, insulin resistance and compensatory hyperinsulinemia are prominent features of PCOS. The theory that hyperinsulinemia causes hyperandrogenism is supported by, among other findings, the fact that insulin sensitizers improve hyperandrogenism, while antiandrogens do not significantly improve insulin resistance. Hyperinsulinemia contributes to the pathogenesis of PCOS not only by directly increasing theca cell androgenesis, but also by increasing the bioavailability of androgens, and by contributing to the development of morphological changes in the ovary.

In vitro studies show that insulin stimulates 17α-hydroxylase activity in ovarian theca cells *(36)*, a finding not clearly confirmed by in vivo studies *(37,38)*. Insulin also acts synergistically with LH, augmenting theca cell response of androgenesis to LH *(39,40)*. Administration of human chorionic gonadotropin (hCG) causes the formation of ovarian follicular cysts in rats, which is augmented with the additional administration of insulin (Fig. 1) *(41)*. The mechanism of this synergism is unclear but may involve increasing LH receptor number *(42)*. Insulin suppresses circulating SHBG by inhibiting its production in the liver, resulting in increased free or bioavailable androgens *(43,44)*.

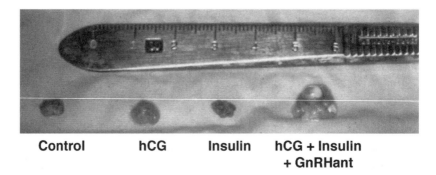

**Control   hCG   Insulin   hCG + Insulin
+ GnRHant**

Fig. 1. Effects of 23 d of daily injections of saline (control), hCG, insulin, and GnRH antagonist (GnRHant) on formation of ovarian cysts in rats. Female Sprague-Dawley rats were randomized to the following treatment groups: control, hCG, insulin, GnRHant, hCG + GnRHant, insulin + GnRHant, insulin + hCG, or hCG + insulin + GnRHant. Ovarian morphology in the group treated with insulin + hCG (not shown) did not differ from that seen in the group treated with hCG + insulin + GnRHant. (Reprinted from ref. *41* with permission from Elsevier.)

Circulating levels of SHBG correlate negatively with insulin levels *(45)*, and low serum SHBG concentration may be a marker for insulin resistance *(46)*.

Role of Obesity

The mechanisms by which obesity may contribute to the pathogenesis of PCOS are complex.

AROMATASE

Estrogen production by the ovaries and adipose tissue is increased in obesity, probably owing to increased aromatase activity, which correlates positively with adiposity *(47)*. Treatment with aromatase inhibitors can be used to induce ovulation *(48)*, and metformin and troglitazone, both of which inhibit aromatase, reduce hyperandrogenism *(49,50)*.

An alternate view is that ovarian aromatase activity in PCOS is decreased, disrupting the androgen–estrogen balance, favoring increased androgens *(51)*. The small follicles typical of PCOS ovaries have lower aromatase activity (which is a function of follicular size *[52]*) and, thus, lower concentrations of estradiol in the follicular fluid *(53)*. Aromatase knockout mice develop intra-abdominal obesity, decreased lean body mass, and hyperinsulinemia *(54)*, and women with aromatase gene mutations also exhibit polycystic ovaries and hirsutism *(55)*.

Thus, the role of aromatase in the pathogenesis of PCOS remains controversial. The issue is complicated by the possibility that aromatase activity may be increased peripherally (in the adipose tissue) while decreased in ovarian tissue.

LEPTIN

Leptin is a hormone synthesized in adipocytes, whose synthesis is regulated by many factors, including nutritional status, as well as multiple hormonal influences *(56)*.

Studies investigating circulating leptin concentrations in women with PCOS show no difference compared to levels in healthy women of similar adiposity *(57–60)*. Serum leptin levels also do not appear to correlate with androgen levels *(57,58)*. Studies comparing leptin and insulin levels, as well as leptin and LH levels, in women with PCOS produced conflicting results *(58–61)*.

CORTISOL

Plasma cortisol concentrations in obese subjects are often lower than in lean individuals *(62,63)*. However, there are no consistent differences between obese and nonobese subjects in cortisol response either to ACTH stimulation *(64)* or to hypoglycemia *(65)*. The number and affinity of glucocorticoid receptors on mononuclear leukocytes in women with PCOS, obese or nonobese, do not differ from those in control women *(66)*.

Some investigators have proposed that cortisol metabolism may be affected in patients with PCOS because of abnormal activity of 11β-hydroxysteroid dehydrogenase (11β-HSD). 11β-HSD exists in two isoforms: Type 1 is expressed in liver, gonads, and adipose tissue and in vivo acts as a reductase, generating active cortisol from inactive cortisone. Type 2 is responsible for the reverse reaction (cortisol to cortisone) and is predominantly present in mineralocorticoid target tissues, such as the placenta and kidney.

In an intriguing study by Masuzaki et al. *(67)*, transgenic mice overexpressing type 1 11β-HSD in adipocytes developed visceral obesity, insulin-resistant diabetes, and hyperlipidemia. The transgenic mice also had increased concentrations of corticosterone in adipose tissue, but not in serum, suggesting increased local conversion of cortisol into corticosterone *(67)*. Type 1 11β-HSD activity has also been found to be elevated in adipose tissue of obese humans *(68)* and may be the link explaining the phenotypic similarities between Cushing's syndrome and central obesity, in spite of normal circulating cortisol concentrations in obesity *(69)*.

OBESITY AND INSULIN RESISTANCE

Women with PCOS exhibit central obesity, which is associated with a higher risk of diabetes, hypertension, hyperlipidemia, atherosclerosis, and insulin resistance *(70)* than peripheral obesity *(71)*. In addition, increased upper-body fat correlates with significantly reduced clearance of insulin, which further contributes to hyperinsulinemia *(72)*. Euglycemic clamp studies also indicate that basal hepatic glucose production and the ED_{50} value of insulin needed to suppress hepatic glucose production are significantly increased only in obese women with PCOS *(73)*.

Free fatty acids (FFAs) and tumor necrosis factor-α (TNF-α) may play causative roles in the relationship between obesity and insulin resistance. FFAs are released from triglycerides in adipose tissue via lipolysis and are the key mediators of impaired insulin sensitivity. Increased FFA flux into the liver decreases hepatic insulin extraction and increases gluconeogenesis, resulting in hyperinsulinemia *(74)*. High circulating FFA concentrations also lead to peripheral insulin resistance by reducing glucose uptake by skeletal muscle *(75)*. Elevated circulating levels of FFA have been reported in women with PCOS *(76)*, and increased catecholamine-induced lipolysis has been demonstrated in vitro in visceral adipocytes from women with PCOS *(77)*.

TNF-α is produced by adipose tissue and leads to insulin resistance by stimulating phosphorylation of serine residues of insulin receptor substrate-1 (IRS-1), thereby inhibiting tyrosine kinase activity of the insulin receptor *(78)*. Serum TNF-α concentrations have been shown to be high in hyperandrogenic women, including women with PCOS *(79)*.

Role of Insulin Resistance and Hyperinsulinemia in Pathogenesis of PCOS

Endogenous insulin has a half-life of 3–5 min, with a circulating concentration of approx 10 μU/mL in the fasting state and 50 μU/mL postprandially. In insulin-resistant

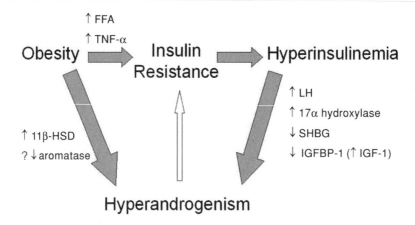

Fig. 2. Relationship among obesity, insulin, and androgens. Obesity, especially central obesity, is associated with insulin resistance and leads to compensatory hyperinsulinemia. High serum concentrations of insulin, in turn, lead to hyperandrogenism. Hyperandrogenism can cause mild insulin resistance, but not of the same magnitude as seen in PCOS (open arrow). The contributions of obesity to hyperandrogenism, in addition to insulin resistance/hyperinsulinemia, may involve alterations in the activities of 11β-HSD and aromatase. (*See* text for details.)

conditions, such as PCOS or type 2 diabetes, circulating insulin concentrations can be as high as 35 μU/mL fasting and 180 μU/mL after a glucose load *(80)*. In syndromes of extreme insulin resistance, circulating insulin levels can be increased more than 100-fold *(81)*.

Although androgens can induce mild insulin resistance, administration of androgen does not produce insulin resistance of the same magnitude as that seen in PCOS *(82,83)*. Oophorectomy *(84)*, GnRH agonists *(85)*, or antiandrogens *(86)*, which all eliminate hyperandrogenism in patients with PCOS, do not produce a significant change in insulin sensitivity.

The cause of insulin resistance in PCOS is not known, but the defects appear to involve abnormal postreceptor insulin signaling and glucose transport and are distinct from defects seen in type 2 diabetes *(87)*. Proposed mechanisms include (1) a reduced number of glucose transporter 4 *(88)*; (2) excessive serine phosphorylation of the insulin receptor, or decreased tyrosine phosphorylation of unknown cause *(35)*; and (3) excessive serine phosphorylation of IRS-1 that results in an inhibition of phosphatidylinositol-3 kinase *(89)*, a key enzyme in glucose transport. Increased basal insulin secretion *(90)* and decreased hepatic insulin clearance *(91)* in PCOS also contribute to hyperinsulinemia.

There is significant evidence to support the hypothesis that hyperinsulinemia leads to hyperandrogenism (Fig. 2). Hyperandrogenism commonly develops in women with syndromes of extreme insulin resistance, in which severe insulin resistance is clearly the primary event, caused by insulin receptor mutations or insulin receptor antibodies *(2,92)*. In addition, insulin can stimulate ovarian estrogen, androgen, and progesterone secretion in vitro *(93)*.

Insulin in high concentrations can mimic insulin-like growth factor-1 (IGF-1) actions by crossreacting with the type 1 IGF receptor and stimulating ovarian steroidogenesis via this pathway. Type 1 IGF receptors are present in the ovary *(94)*, and IGF-1 is produced by human ovarian tissue. In addition, ovarian IGF-1-binding sites may be upregulated by hyperinsulinemia *(95)*. However, studies have shown that ovarian sensitivity to insulin may be preserved in insulin-resistant states *(96,97)* because of activation of nonclassic insulin receptor signaling pathways *(98,99)*. Involvement of alternate pathways of insulin action and the upregulation of type 1 IGF receptors by hyperinsulinemia may explain why the ovary remains sensitive to insulin even when classic target organs of insulin action (liver, fat, muscle) are insulin resistant *(100,101)*.

The activity of IGFs is modulated by low molecular weight binding proteins, called IGF-binding proteins (IGFBPs), which bind IGFs with high affinity. Synthesis of IGFBP-1 is inhibited by insulin *(102)*, and its circulating levels correlate negatively with insulin levels in women with PCOS *(103)*. Low intrafollicular levels of IGFBP-1 owing to hyperinsulinemia may lead to increased intraovarian concentration of unbound IGFs and therefore contribute to stimulation of steroidogenesis. Increased ovarian androgen production may cause follicular atresia, resulting in the presence of multiple, small follicles, with no follicle reaching preovulatory dominance *(104)*.

In addition, production of IGF-1 by the liver is increased in PCOS owing to excessive growth hormone (GH) stimulation *(81,105)*. This mechanism is particularly important in nonobese patients with PCOS, in whom increased GH amplitude has been reported *(106)*. On the contrary, obese patients show reduced GH pulse amplitude and 24-h mean circulating GH levels *(107)*, and increased GH clearance, which further contributes to decreased GH/IGF system activity *(108)*. Therefore, although both hyperinsulinemia and an excessively activated IGF system contribute to the development of PCOS, the IGF system may play a larger role in the pathogenesis of PCOS in lean women, whereas hyperinsulinemia may be more important in the development of PCOS in obese patients *(107)*.

METABOLIC COMPLICATIONS

Women with PCOS are at increased risk of developing type 2 diabetes, CVD, hypertension, and obstructive sleep apnea. Much of the increased risk of these conditions is probably owing to long-standing insulin resistance and obesity, although the sex steroid hormones may also play a role.

Type 2 Diabetes Mellitus

Women with PCOS have a seven-fold increased risk of developing type 2 diabetes *(109)*, with age of onset 30 yr younger than the general population *(89)*. Large case-control series have reported a prevalence of diabetes approx 10% in women with PCOS of reproductive age, with another 30–35% exhibiting impaired glucose tolerance (IGT) *(110)*. In women with PCOS, type 2 diabetes initially manifests itself with postprandial hyperglycemia, while fasting glucose and hemoglobin A1c may be normal *(111)*. In a study by Ehrmann et al. *(110)*, only 9% of patients with PCOS had impaired fasting glucose (IFG), whereas 35% had IGT. The investigators also demonstrated that women with PCOS who have IGT convert to type 2 diabetes at an accelerated rate. Family history and obesity were also contributing factors.

Studies regarding pregnancy outcome in women with PCOS are small, with conflicting results. Haakova et al. *(112)* and Vollenhoven et al. *(113)* did not find significant differences in pregnancy complications, including gestational diabetes mellitus (GDM) and pregnancy-induced hypertension. However, Mikola et al. *(114)* found a 20% prevalence of GDM in their PCOS study group vs 8.9% in unselected control women. Women

Table 3
Components of Metabolic Syndrome

Central obesity
    Increased waist circumference (>100 cm in men, >88 cm in women)[a]
    Increased waist to hip ratio (>0.90 in men, >0.85 in women)[b]
Hypertension
    BP ≥ 130/85 mmHg[a,b]
    BP ≥ 140/90 mmHg[b]
Elevated triglycerides ≥ 150 mg/dL[a–c]
Low HDL
    <40 mg/dL in men, < 50 mg/dL in women[a,b]
    <35 mg/dL in men, < 39 mg/dL in women[b]
Impaired glucose homeostasis
    Fasting glucose ≥ 110 mg/dL[a]
    IFG (110–125 mg/dL)[b] or IGT (140–200 mg/dL)[b]
    Frank diabetes, IFG, or IGT[b]

[a]Adult Treatment Panel III definition: metabolic syndrome requires the presence of three criteria (117).

[b]American Association of Clinical Endocrinologists definition: insulin resistance syndrome requires the presence of risk factor for CVD and two additional components (119).

[c]World Health Organization definition: metabolic syndrome requires the presence of IFG, IGT, or type 2 diabetes mellitus, plus two additional components (118).

with PCOS had a higher BMI, which was found to be the strongest predictor for GDM (adjusted odds ratio [OR] = 5.1), and the presence of PCOS was a smaller predictor (OR = 1.9) (114). Finally, Radon et al. (115) and Bjercke et al. (116) found increased risks of GDM and preeclampsia in women with PCOS.

Cardiovascular Disease

Insulin resistance and obesity are associated with several risk factors for CVD. Insulin resistance syndrome, also known as metabolic syndrome, is a constellation of characteristics that are associated with insulin resistance and may predict CVD (Table 3). Patients with PCOS often have one or more of the components of metabolic syndrome and, therefore, are at risk of developing metabolic syndrome and its purported consequences. A recent study demonstrated that young women (<35 yr) with PCOS had increased left ventricular mass compared with weight-matched control women. This finding was also present in lean women with PCOS who had lipid profiles similar to those of weight-matched control subjects (120).

Although PCOS may confer increased risk factors for CVD, at this time there is insufficient evidence to indicate that women with PCOS have an earlier onset of atherosclerosis, an increased mortality owing to CVD, or an increased number of cardiovascular events.

Hypertension

Several studies concluded that blood pressure (BP) is generally in the normal range in young women with PCOS (121,122). Many studies showing an increase in systolic blood pressure (SBP) in patients with PCOS were not adjusted for BMI (122). However, only one study showed an increase in 24-h mean SBP in women with PCOS that persisted after adjustment for BMI, insulin sensitivity, and body fat distribution (122).

Dyslipidemia

Dyslipidemia may be the most common metabolic abnormality in PCOS. Elevated circulating levels of triglycerides, very low-density lipoprotein, and total cholesterol, accompanied by low levels of high-density lipoprotein (HDL), have been reported in PCOS *(122)*. Studies comparing obese and nonobese patients with PCOS usually find more pronounced lipid abnormalities in the obese groups *(122)*. Low HDL and high triglyceride levels are the most common findings *(123)*. In one study, the prevalence of HDL <35 mg/dL was 78% in obese women with PCOS *(124)*. Elevated apolipoprotein B and decreased apolipoprotein A1 concentrations are also commonly present. In nonobese women with PCOS, HDL and triglyceride levels may be normal *(125)*; however, markedly lower circulating HDL concentrations, especially the HDL2 subfraction, have been observed in lean women with PCOS, when compared with weight-matched control women *(122,123)*.

Hyperlipidemia is thought to be owing to altered activity of lipoprotein lipase and hepatic lipase, combined with decreased cholesterol ester transfer protein activity. Elevated circulating levels of androgens, particularly testosterone, may contribute to dyslipidemia, by inhibiting lipoprotein lipase activity in abdominal fat cells *(123)*. Indeed, elevated triglyceride and decreased HDL levels correlate with elevated testosterone levels *(125)*. However, suppression of testosterone using a GnRH agonist in 31 hyperandrogenic women did not normalize their lipid profiles *(123)*, suggesting that lipoprotein abnormalities are more closely related to insulin resistance than to hyperandrogenism.

Coagulation and Fibrinolytic Factors

Higher plasma fibrinogen and plasminogen activator inhibitor-1 (PAI-1) concentrations have been associated with a higher risk of CVD *(122)*. Atheromas from patients with type 2 diabetes contain markedly increased concentrations of PAI-1 compared with atheromas from nondiabetic, otherwise comparable individuals *(123)*. In one study, patients with PCOS were found to have PAI-1 concentrations that were even higher than those typically seen in type 2 diabetes *(123)*. However, not all studies confirm this finding *(122)*.

Elevated homocysteine levels have also been implicated as a significant risk factor for CVD, and increased levels of homocysteine have been positively associated with circulating insulin levels *(126)*. Schachter et al. *(127)* found that insulin-resistant women with PCOS had significantly higher plasma homocysteine levels than non-insulin-resistant patients with PCOS, regardless of BMI. The effects of elevated PAI-1 concentrations may be enhanced by elevated homocysteine levels and contribute to endothelial dysfunction and CVD.

Sleep Apnea

Recently, an association of PCOS with obstructive sleep apnea has been reported *(128)*. Women with PCOS were 30 times more likely to suffer from sleep-disordered breathing than control women. Women with PCOS who required treatment for their sleep disorder had significantly higher fasting insulin levels than those with PCOS who did not require treatment. Even lean subjects with PCOS had a higher prevalence of sleep apnea than the weight-matched control subjects, and obese patients with PCOS did have a higher prevalence of sleep apnea than their nonobese counterparts. The

Table 4
Effects of Various Treatment Modalities for PCOS

Treatment	Free testosterone	SHBG	Insulin sensitivity	Menses
Weight loss	↓(16)	↑(16)	↑(16)	Restoration (16)
Oral contraceptive agents	↓(135,136,139)	↑(135,136,139)	No effect (139)/↓ (138)	Restoration
Antiandrogens	↓(132)	↑(132)	No effect (133)/↑(134)	Restoration (132)
Insulin sensitizers	↓(140)	↑(140)	↑(8 studies)/ no effect (4 studies) (140)	Restoration (140)

investigators concluded that insulin resistance is a stronger risk factor than BMI or testosterone concentration for sleep-disordered breathing in women with PCOS.

TREATMENT

There are several treatment options for each of the manifestations of PCOS. The choice of treatment depends on the woman's goals, especially if pregnancy is desired. Many of the symptoms of PCOS can be reversed by losing weight and by reducing insulin resistance (Table 4).

Weight Loss

There is consistent evidence that weight loss improves clinical, hormonal, and menstrual parameters in obese patients with PCOS. These benefits appear to be related to the improvement in insulin sensitivity that occurs with weight loss.

Several studies have demonstrated a beneficial impact of weight loss on hyperinsulinemia in women with PCOS. Hypocaloric diets (<1500 kcal/d) resulted in rapid weight loss and significant reductions in insulin levels as measured by fasting insulin, fasting and glucose-challenged insulin, and euglycemic clamp (129,130). Huber-Buchholz et al. (131) showed that even a modest weight loss of 2–5% from lifestyle modification improves insulin sensitivity. Maintenance of weight loss, which remains a challenge, is an issue that was not addressed by these studies.

The available evidence suggests that weight loss has a beneficial effect on sex steroid levels, with a reduction in testosterone (21–36%) and an increase in SHBG (18–26%) seen in most studies. Restoration of normal LH pulsatility has not been demonstrated, although some studies show a reduction in baseline LH levels. Restoration of menses and ovulation may also occur, with rates approaching 50% (129).

Antiandrogens

Antiandrogens, such as spironolactone and flutamide, compete with testosterone and dihydrotestosterone in binding to the androgen receptor. Antiandrogens improve symptoms of hyperandrogenism and may also ameliorate insulin resistance and dyslipidemia that are associated with PCOS. De Leo et al. (132) reported significant reductions in circulating levels of LH, androstenedione, and free and total testosterone; an increase in serum SHBG; and resumption of regular menses after 6 mo of flutamide treatment. Diamanti-Kandarakis et al. *(133)* reported that treatment with flutamide (500 mg/d) for 12 wk resulted in a significant reduction (23%) in low-density lipoprotein (LDL)/HDL ratio, as well as significant reductions in total cholesterol, LDL, and triglycerides. These effects on lipid profile were not associated with changes in weight, glucose tolerance, or insulin sensitivity *(133)*. In a study of hyperandrogenic patients treated with any one of three agents (spironolactone, flutamide, or buserelin), Moghetti et al. *(134)* found an improvement in insulin sensitivity, with lean patients responding better than obese patients.

Oral Contraceptive Agents

Oral contraceptive agents have been used extensively in the treatment of PCOS. They are effective in improving the androgen profile of patients with PCOS and also prevent endometrial hyperplasia by inducing regular menses. Studies investigating treatment with ethinyl estradiol plus cyproterone acetate or desogestrel consistently show an improvement in hirsutism, a reduction in free testosterone levels, and an increase in SHBG as well as HDL and triglycerides *(135,136)*. A regimen of ethinyl estradiol plus drospirenone, which is structurally similar to spironolactone, also has been shown to be effective in improving clinical and hormonal features of PCOS *(137)*. The changes in lipoprotein associated with oral contraceptive use are attributed to the estrogen component of treatment, and changes in LDL have not been consistent.

Although oral contraceptives are believed to reduce insulin sensitivity slightly *(138)*, studies examining the effect of oral contraceptives on insulin sensitivity report conflicting results, from no effect *(137,139)* to unfavorable effects *(138)*.

Insulin Sensitizers

METFORMIN

Metformin, which belongs to the biguanide class of oral antihyperglycemic agents, has been shown to improve the metabolic, hormonal, and menstrual parameters in obese women with PCOS.

Multiple studies confirm metformin's effect on improving insulin sensitivity: reductions in area under the insulin curve during oral glucose tolerance test (OGTT) have been reported after metformin treatment (1500–1700 mg/d). However, not all studies show consistent improvement in insulin sensitivity with metformin therapy *(140)*. This discrepancy may be owing to variability in the doses of metformin used, as well as the variable effect of metformin on BMI.

Metformin has been shown to improve menstrual parameters in PCOS. Treatment with metformin for 3–6 mo in women with PCOS and irregular menses resulted in normalization of menses in 25–50% *(140)*. Based on a study in adolescents with PCOS, Ibanez et al. *(141)* reported that 4–6 mo of treatment with metformin is required before ovulatory menses occur.

Adrenal steroidogenesis can also be affected by metformin, suggesting that hyperinsulinemia may contribute to the increased adrenal androgen production in PCOS. Mean basal and peak (after ACTH or leuprolide stimulation) serum concentrations of 17-hydroxyprogesterone decreased by 38–51% after treatment with metformin. Velazquez et al. reported metformin-induced reductions of free testosterone by 52%, total testosterone by 44%, DHEA-S by 21%, and LH by 35%. Concurrently, circulating SHBG concentration increased by 33% and FSH by 95% *(140)*.

The use of metformin in combination with one or more of the treatments discussed in the previous sections is becoming increasingly common in the treatment of PCOS.

Although oral contraceptives and antiandrogens are effective in improving hirsutism, their metabolic effects are less established. Studies with metformin in combination with oral contraceptive agents and flutamide show synergistic effects on the reduction of serum testosterone and an increase in SHBG, along with a sustained beneficial effect on insulin sensitivity *(143,144)*. Metformin in combination with a hypocaloric diet resulted in more pronounced reductions in weight and BMI, as well as reductions in the concentrations of total testosterone, and fasting and glucose-stimulated insulin *(145)*. Gambineri et al. *(143)* also showed a synergistic effect of hypocaloric diet with combined metformin and flutamide therapy on reducing serum testosterone and increasing serum HDL.

In summary, treatment with metformin in most studies was associated with an improvement in insulin sensitivity. Improved insulin sensitivity, in turn, was associated with a reduction in circulating androgen levels and improvement in menstrual symptoms and ovulatory function. Metformin used in conjunction with weight loss appears to produce a more consistent effect on insulin sensitivity and androgen profile than metformin without weight loss.

THIAZOLIDINEDIONES

The thiazolidinediones (TZDs) are a group of insulin-sensitizing medications commonly used in the treatment of type 2 diabetes mellitus. Initial studies of the effects of TZDs in PCOS showed that troglitazone improved insulin sensitivity, reduced free testosterone and LH concentrations, and increased circulating SHBG levels *(140)*.

Preliminary findings of a randomized, double-blind, controlled study using rosiglitazone and metformin in lean patients with PCOS showed a greater increase in ovulation with metformin alone vs rosiglitazone alone, with no greater benefit with combination therapy. Serum free testosterone decreased in both groups *(146)*. Rosiglitazone (4 mg/d) for 3 mo was shown to improve insulin resistance parameters, reduce IGF-1 and LH concentrations, and normalize menses, although serum SHBG, androgens, and BMI remained unchanged *(147)*. Rosiglitazone (2 mg/d and 4 mg/d) for 8 mo in nonobese, insulin-resistant women with PCOS resulted in improved insulin sensitivity, decreased LH and free testosterone concentrations, and increased estradiol concentration. Response appeared to be dose-dependent, as the 4 mg group achieved greater improvements than the 2 mg group and a higher rate of ovulation (85 vs 70%) by 8 mo *(148)*.

Pioglitazone added to metformin in obese women with PCOS who were not optimally responsive to metformin resulted in a further decline in circulating concentrations of insulin and DHEA-S, improved menses, and a rise in circulating HDL *(149)*. Pioglitazone (30 mg/d) for 3 mo resulted in an improvement in insulin sensitivity, a rise in serum SHBG, and a decline in LH *(150)*. Pioglitazone (45 mg/d) appeared to be more effective in hyperinsulinemic women than normoinsulinemic women with PCOS (defined by OGTT), resulting in higher rates of menses restoration; reduction in LH; and significant improvements in insulin secretion, sensitivity, and clearance after 6 mo of treatment *(151)*. Although it is thought that the improvement in ovarian androgen secretion is owing to a reduction of circulating insulin concentrations by TZDs, direct effect of TZD on the ovarian steroidogenesis may also contribute. Human ovarian cells cultured in pioglitazone or rosiglitazone showed enhanced progesterone production and less testosterone and estradiol production. Both TZDs also abolished insulin-induced stimulation of testosterone and estradiol, and stimulated insulin-independent IGFBP-1 production *(152)*.

In summary, it appears that TZDs have beneficial effects in obese women with PCOS. Because troglitazone has been removed from the market because of liver toxicity, definitive studies with other TZDs need to be completed. Differences in results among studies are probably owing to variation in treatment dose and duration.

D-CHIRO-INOSITOL

Inositolphosphoglycans are involved in mediating insulin action *(144)*. It has been proposed that a deficiency in D-chiro-inositolphosphoglycan mediators may contribute to insulin resistance in PCOS and that repletion of D-chiro-inositol stores would lead to improved insulin sensitivity. Obese women with PCOS who were given 1200 mg of D-chiro-inositol daily for 6–8 wk demonstrated a significant reduction in the mean area under the insulin curve after oral glucose load, a decline in free testosterone and DHEA-S, a reduction in circulating triglyceride levels, and an increase in circulating SHBG concentrations. The placebo group demonstrated none of these changes. In addition, 86% of the women treated with D-chiro-inositol ovulated vs only 27% in the placebo group *(145)*. Recently, women with PCOS who were treated with metformin for 8 wk were shown to have increased insulin-mediated secretion of D-chiro-inositol-containing inositolphosphoglycans *(153)*. These observations offer one potential mechanism of metfomin-induced increase in insulin sensitivity and support the hypothesis that some individuals with insulin resistance may be deficient in D-chiro-inositolphosphoglycan mediators.

CONCLUSIONS

PCOS is a common disorder that in all likelihood, is etiologically diverse. Obesity is present in approx 50% of patients with PCOS. The differences in clinical manifestations between obese and nonobese patients with PCOS are mostly quantitative in nature (Table 2). Obesity contributes to the manifestations of PCOS by increasing the magnitude of hyperandrogenism and the rates of anovulatory cycles and infertility.

The pathophysiological mechanisms by which obesity makes these contributions to the clinical picture of PCOS appear to be related to hyperinsulinemia, which is caused by insulin resistance. Although insulin resistance is present in both obese and nonobese patients with PCOS, the magnitude of both insulin resistance and hyperinsulinemia is greater in obese women with PCOS. Hyperinsulinemia impacts ovarian function and morphology not only by stimulating ovarian androgen production directly and in synergism with gonadotropins, but also by activating the ovarian IGF system (specifically, by inducing expression of ovarian type 1 IGF receptors and by inhibiting IGFBP-1 production in both liver and ovary), by inhibiting SHBG production in the liver, and by contributing to ovarian growth and the formation of cysts. Therapeutic modalities directed at the reduction of hyperinsulinemia ameliorate symptoms of PCOS and restore normal ovarian function in obese women with PCOS.

ACKNOWLEDGMENTS

This work was supported, in part, by Gerald J. Friedman Foundation, Empire Clinical Research Investigator Program Grant from New York State Department of Health, and NIH grant no. R01-MH60563.

REFERENCES

1. Stein IF, Leventhal ML. Amenorrhea associated with bilateral polycystic ovaries. Am J Obstet Gynecol 1935;29:181–191.
2. Kahn CR, Flier JS, Bar RS, et al. The syndromes of insulin resistance and acanthosis nigricans: insulin-receptor disorders in man. N Engl J Med 1976;294:739–745.

3. Burghen GA, Given JR, Kitabchi AE. Correlation of hyperandrogenism with hyperinsulinism in polycysitc ovarian disease. J Clin Endocrinol Metab 1980;50:113–116.

4. Poretsky L, Smith D, Seibel M, Pazianos A, Moses AC, Flier JS. Specific insulin binding sites in human ovary. J Clin Endocrinol Metab 1984;59:809–811.

5. Poretsky L, Grigorescu F, Moses AC, Flier JS. Distribution and characterization of the insulin and IGF-I receptors in the human ovary. J Clin Endocrinol Metab 1985;61:728–734.

6. Azziz R, Woods KS, Reyna R, Key TJ, Knochenhauer ES, Yildiz BO. The prevalence and features of the polycystic ovary syndrome in an unselected population. J Clin Endocrinol Metab 2004;89:2745–2749.

7. Diamanti-Kandarakis E, Kouli CR, Bergiele AT. A survey of the polycystic ovary syndrome in the Greek island of Lesbos: hormonal and metabolic profile. J Clin Endocrinol Metab 1999;84: 4006–4011.

8. Asuncion M, Calvo RM, San Millan JL. A prospective study of the prevalence of the polycystic ovary syndrome in unselected Caucasian women from Spain. J Clin Endocrinol Metab 2000;85:2434–2438.

9. Peppard HR, Marfori, J, Iuorno MJ, Nestler JE. Prevalence of polycystic ovary syndrome among premenopausal women with type 2 diabetes. Diabetes Care 2001;24:1050–1052.

10. Balen AH, Conway GS, Kaltsas G, et al. Polycystic ovary syndrome: the spectrum of the disorder in 1741 patients. Hum Reprod 1995;10:2107–2111.

11. Ferrimen D, Gallwey JD. Clinical assessment of body hair growth in women. J Clin Endocr 1961;21:1440–1447.

12. Carmina E, Koyama T, Chang L, Stanczyk FZ, Lobo RA. Does ethnicity influence the prevalence of adrenal hyperandrogenism and insulin resistance in polycystic ovary syndrome? Am J Obstet Gynecol 1992;167:1807–1812.

13. Lewis V. Polycystic ovary syndrome: a diagnostic challenge. Obstet Gynecol Clin North Am 2001;28:1–20.

14. Conn JJ, Jacobs HS, Conway GS. The prevalence of polycystic ovaries in women with type 2 diabetes mellitus. Clin Endocrinol 2000;52:81–86.

15. Koivunen RM, Juutinen J, Vauhkonen I. Metabolic and steroidogenic alterations related to increased frequency of polycystic ovaries in women with a history of gestational diabetes. J Clin Endocrinol Metab 2001;86:25,912–25,919.

16. Hoeger K. Obesity and weight loss in polycystic ovary syndrome. Obstet Gynecol Clin North Am 2001;28:85–97.

17. Zawadzki JK, Dunaif A. Diagnostic criteria for polycystic ovary syndrome: towards a rational approach. In: Dunaif A, Givens JR, Haseltine FP, Meriiam GR, eds. (Series ed.: Hershman SM). Polycystic Ovary Syndrome. Current Issues in Endocrinology and Metabolism, vol. 4, Blackwell Scientific, Boston, 1992, pp. 377–384.

18. The Rotterdam ESHRE/ASRM-Sponsored PCOS Consensus Workshop Group. Revised 2003 consensus on diagnostic criteria and long-term health risks related to polycystic ovary syndrome. Fertil Steril 2004;81:19–25.

19. Meldrum DR, ABraham GE. Peripheral and ovarian venous concentrations of various steroid hormones in virilizing ovarian tymors. Obstet Gynecol 1979;53:36–43.

20. Azziz R, Dewailly D, Owerbach D. Nonclassic adrenal hyperplasia: current concepts. J Clin Endocrinol Metab 1994;78: 810–815.

21. Azziz R, Sanchez LA, Knochenhauer ES, et al. Androgen excess in women: experience with over 1000 consecutive patients. J Clin Endocrinol Metab 2004;89:453–462.

22. Simpson JL. Elucidating the genetics of polycystic ovary syndrome. In: Dunaif, Givens JR, Hasetline FP, Merriam GR, eds. Polycystic Ovary Syndrome: Current issues in Endocrinology and Metabolism. Blackwell Scientific, Boston, 1992, pp. 59–69.

23. Govind A, Obhrai MS, Clayton RN: Polycystic ovaries are inherited as an autosomal dominant trait: analysis of 29 polycystic ovary syndrome and 10 control families. J Clin Endocrinol Metab 1999;84(1):38–43.

24. Legro RS, Dirscoll D, Strauss JF, et al. Evidence for a genetic basis for hyperandrogenemia in polycystic ovary syndrome. Proc Natl Acad Sci USA 1998;95:14,956–14,960.

25. Rebar R, Judd HL, Yen SSC, Rakoff J, Vandenberg G, Naftolin F. Characterization of the inappropriate gonadotropin secretion in polycystic ovary syndrome. J Clin Invest 1976;57:1320–1329.

26. Gill S, Taylor AE, Martin KA, et al. Specific factors predict the response to pulsatile gonadotropin-releasing hormone therapy in polycystic ovary syndrome. J Clin Endocrinol Metabl 2001;86: 2428–2436.

27. Filicori M, Campaniello E, Michelacci L, et al. Gonadotropin-releasing hormone (GnRH) analog suppression renders polycystic ovarian disease patients more susceptible to ovulation induction with pulsatile GnRH. J Clin Endocrinol Metab 1988;66:327–333.

28. Filicori M, Flamigni C , Campaniello E, et al. The abnormal response of polycystic ovarian disease patients to exogenous pulsatile gonadotropin-releasing hormone: characterization and management. J Clin Endocrinol Metab 1989;69:825–831.

29. Rosenfield RL. Ovarian and adrenal function in polycystic ovary syndrome. Endocrinol Metab Clin North Am 1999;28:265–293.

30. Gilling-Smith C, Willis DS, Beard RW, et al. Hypersecretion of androstenedione by isolated thecal cells from polycystic ovaries. J Clin Endocrinol Metab 1994;79:1158–1165.

31. Rosenfield RL. Studies of the nature of 17-hydroxyprogesterone hyperresponsiveness to gonadotropin-releasing hormone agonist challenge in functional ovarian hyperandrogenism. J Clin Endocrinol Metab 1994;79:1686–1692.

32. Carey AH, Waterworth D, Patel K, et al. Polycystic ovaries and premature male pattern baldness are associated with one allel of the steroid metabolism gene CYP 17. Hum Mol Genet 1994;3:1873–1876.

33. Franks S. The 17a-hydroxylase, 17,20 lyase gene (CYP 17) and polycystic ovary syndrome. Clin Endocrinol 1997;46:135,136.

34. Zhang LH, Rodriguez H, Ohno S, et al. Serine phosphorylation of human P450c17 increases 17,20 -lyase activity; implications for adrenarche and the polycystic ovary syndrome. Proc Natl Acad Sci USA 1995;92:10,619–10,623.

35. Dunaif A, Book CB, Schenker E, Tang Z. Excessive insulin receptor serine phosphorylation in cultured fibroblasts and in skeletal muscle: a potential mechanism for insulin resistance in the polycystic ovary syndrome. J Clin Invest 1995;96:801–810.

36. Nestler JE, Jacubowicz DJ. Lean women with polycystic ovary syndrome respond to insulin reduction with decreases in ovarian P450c1 activity and serum androgens. J Clin Endocrinol Metab 1997;82:4075–4079.

37. Falcone T, Finegood DT, Fantus IG, Morris D. Androgen response to endogenous insulin secretion during the frequently sampled intravenous glucose tolerance test in normal and hyperandrogenic women. J Clin Endocrinol Metab 1990;71:1653–1657.

38. Toscano V, Bianchi P, Balducci R, et al. Lack of linear relationship between hyperinsulinaemia and hyperandrogenism. Clin Endocrinol (Oxf) 1992;36:197–202.

39. Poretsky L, Piper B. Insulin resistance, hypersecretion of LH, and a dual-defect hypothesis for the pathogenesis of polycystic ovary syndrome. Obstet Gynecol 1994;84:613–621.

40. Cara JF, Rosenfield RL. Insulin-like growth factor I and insulin potentiate luteinizing hormone-induced androgen synthesis. Endocrinology 1988;123:733–739.

41. Poretsky L, Clemons J, Bogovich K. Hyperinsulinemia and human chorionic gonadotropin synergistically promote the growth of ovarian follicular cysts in rats. Metabolism 1992;41:903–910.

42. Davoren JB, Kasson BG, Li CH, Hsueh AJ. Specific insulin-like growth factor (IGF)-I binding sites on rat granulosa cells: relation to IGF action. Endocrinology 1986;119:2155–2162.

43. Plymate SR, Matej LA, Jones RE, Friedl KE. Inhibition of sex hormone-binding globulin production in the human hepatoma (HepG2) cell line by insulin and prolactin. J Clin Endocrinol Metab 1988;67:460–464.

44. Nestler JE, Powers LP, Matt DW, et al. A direct effect of hyperinsulinemia on serum sex hormone-binding globulin levels in obese women with the polycystic ovary syndrome. J Clin Endocrinol Metab 1991;72:83–89.

45. Preziosi P, Barrett-Connor E, Papoz L, et al. Interrelation between plasma sex hormone-binding globulin and plasma insulin in healthy adult women: the Telecom study. J Clin Endocrinol Metab 1993;76:283–287.

46. Nestler JE. Editorial: Sex hormone-binding globulin: a marker for hyperinsulinemia and/or insulin resistance. J Clin Endocrinol Metab 1992;76:273–274.

47. Cleland WH, Mendelson CR, Simpson ER. Effects of aging and obesity on aromatase activity of human adipose cells. J Clin Endocrinol Metab 1985;60:174–177.

48. Mitwally MF, Casper RF. Use of an aromatase inhibitor for induction of ovulation in patients with an inadequate response to clomiphene citrate. Fertil Steril 2001;75:305–309.

49. Mu YM, Yanase T, Nishi Y, et al. Insulin sensitizer, troglitazone, directly inhibits aromatase activity in human ovarian granulosa cells. Biochem Biophys Res Commun 2000;271:710–713.

50. Vrbikova J, Hill M, Starka L, et al. The effects of long-term metformin treatment on adrenal and ovarian steroidogenesis in women with polycystic ovary syndrome. Eur J Endocrinol 2001;144: 619–628.

51. Gabrilove JL. The pathogenesis of the polycystic ovary syndrome: a hypothesis. Endocr Pract 2002;8:127–132.

52. Jakimiuk AJ, Weitsman SR, Brzechffa PR, et al. Aromatase mRNA expression in individual follicles from polycystic ovaries. Mol Hum Reprod 1998;4:1–8.

53. Erickson GF, Hsueh AJ, Quigley ME, et al. Functional studies of aromatase activity in human granulosa cells from normal and polycystic ovaries. J Clin Endocrinol Metab 1979;49:514–519.

54. Jones ME, Thoburn AW, Britt KL. Aromatase-deficient (ArKO) mice accumulate excess adipose tissue. J Steroid Biochem Mol Biol 2001;79:3–9.

55. MacGillivray MH, Morishima A, Conte F, et al. Pediatric endocrinology update: an overview. The essential roles of estrogens in pubertal growth, epiphyseal fusion and bone turnover: lessons from mutations in the genes for aromatase and estrogen receptor. Horm Res 1998;49:2–8.

56. Ahima RS, Flier JS. Leptin. In: DeGroot LJ, Jameson JL, Burger HG, et al, eds. Endocrinology, 4th ed. WB Saunders, Philadelphia, 2001, pp. 605–615.

57. Laughlin GA, Morales AJ, Yen SSC. Serum leptin levels in women with polycystic ovary syndrome: the role of insulin resistance/hyperinsulinemia. J Clin Endocrinol Metab 1997;82:1692–1696.

58. Mantzoros CS, Dunaif A, Flier JS. Leptin concentrations in the polycystic ovary syndrome. J Clin Endocrinol Metab 1997;82:1687–1697.

59. Carmina E, Ferin M, Gonzalez F, et al. Evidence that insulin and androgens may participate in the regulation of serum leptin levels in women. Fertil Steril 1999;72:926–931.

60. Pirwany IR, Fleming R, Sattar N, et al. Circulating leptin concentrations and ovarian function in polycystic ovary syndrome. Eur J Endocrinol 2001;145:289–294.

61. Spritzer PM, Poy M, Wiltgen D, et al. Leptin concentrations in hirsute women with polycystic ovary syndrome or idiopathic hirsutism: influence on LH and relationship with hormonal, metabolic, and anthropometrics measurements. Hum Reprod 2001;16(7):1340–1346.

62. Jessop DS, Dallman MF, Fleming D, et al. Resistance to glucocorticoid feedback in obesity. J Clin Endocrinol Metab 2001;86:4109–4114.

63. Strain GW, Zumoff B, Kream J, et al. Sex difference in the influence of obesity on the 24 hr mean plasma concentration of cortisol. Metabolism 1982;31:209–212.

64. Chin D, Shackleton C, Prasad VK: Increased 5 alpha-reductase and normal 11beta-hydroxysteroid dehydrogenase metabolism of C19 and C21 steroids in a young population with polycystic ovarian syndrome. J Pediatr Endocrinol Metab 2000;13:253–259.

65. Gennarelli G, Holte J, Stridsberg M, et al. Response of the pituitary-adrenal axis to hypoglycemic stress in women with the polycystic ovary syndrome. J Clin Endocrinol Metab 1999;84:76–81.

66. Guven M, Acbay O, Sultuybek G. Glucocorticoid receptors on mononuclear leukocytes in polycystic ovary syndrome. Int J Gynaecol Obstet 1998;63:33–37.

67. Masuzaki H, Paterson J, Shinyama H, et al. A transgenic model of visceral obesity and the metabolic syndrome. Science 2001;294:2166–2170.

68. Rask E, Walker BR, Soderberg S, et al. Tissue-specific changes in peripheral cortisol metabolism in obese women: increased adipose 11beta-hydroxysteroid dehydrogenase type 1 activity. J Clin Endocrinol Metab 2002;87:3330–3336.

69. Morton NM, Ramage L, Seckl JR. Down-regulation of adipose 11beta-hydroxysteroid dehydrogenase type-1 by high fat feeding in mice: a potential adaptive mechanism counteracting metabolic disease. Endocrinology 2004;145:2707–2712.

70. Kissebah AH, Vydelingum N, Murray R, et al. Relation of body fat distribution to metabolic complications of obesity. .J Clin Endocrinol Metab 1982;54:254–260.

71. Ross R, Freeman J, Hudson R, et al. Abdominal obesity, muscle composition, and insulin resistance in premenopausal women. J Clin Endocrinol Metab 2002;87:5044–5051.

72. Peiris AN, Struve MF, Kissebah AH. Relationship of body fat distribution to the metabolic clearance of insulin in premenopausal women. Int J Obesity 1987;11:581–589.

73. Dunaif A, Segal KR, Shelley DR, et al. Evidence for distinctive and intrinsic defects in insulin action in polycystic ovary syndrome. Diabetes 1992;41:1257–1266.

74. Svedberg J, Bjorntorp P, Smith U, et al. Free-fatty acid inhibition of insulin binding, degradation, and action in isolated rat hepatocytes. Diabetes 1990;39:570–574.

75. Boden G. Role of fatty acids in the pathogenesis of insulin resistance and NIDDM. Diabetes 1997;46:3–10.

76. Holte J, Bergh T, Berne C, et al. Serum lipoprotein lipid profile in women with the polycystic ovary syndrome: relation to anthropometric, endocrine and metabolic variables. Clin Endocrinol (Oxf) 1994;41:463–471.

77. Ek I, Arner P, Ryden M, et. al. A unique defect in the regulation of visceral fat cell lipolysis in the polycystic ovary syndrome as an early link to insulin resistance. Diabetes 2002;51:484–492.

78. Hotamisligil GS, Peraldi P, Budavari A. IRS-1-mediated inhibition of insulin receptor tyrosine kinase activity in TNF-alpha- and obesity-induced insulin resistance. Science 1996;271:665–668.

79. Escobar-Morreale HF, Calvo RM, Sancho J, et al. TNF-alpha and hyperandrogenism: a clinical, biochemical, and molecular genetic study. J Clin Endocrinol Metab 2001;86:3761–3767.

80. Dunaif A. Diabetes mellitus and polycystic ovary syndrome. In: Dunaif A, Given JR, Haseltine FP, Merriam GR, eds. Polycystic Ovary Syndrome. Blackwell Scientific, Boston, 1992, pp. 347–358.

81. Poretsky L, Cataldo N, Rosenwaks Z, et al. The insulin–related ovarian regulatory system in health and disease. Endocr Rev 1999;20:535–582.

82. Polderman KH, Gooren JG, Asscherman H. Induction of insulin resistance by androgens and estrogens. J Clin Endocrinol Metab 1994;79:265–271.

83. Dunaif A, Segal KR, Shelley DR, et al. Evidence for distinctive and intrinsic defects in insulin action in polycystic ovary syndrome. Diabetes 1992;41:1257–1266.

84. Lemieux S, Lewis GF, Ben-Chetrit A. Correction of hyperandrogenemia by laparoscopic ovarian cautery in women with polycystic ovarian syndrome is not accompanied by improved insulin sensitivity or lipid-lipoprotein levels. J Clin Endocrinol Metab 1999;84:4278–4282.

85. Dunaif A, Green G, Futterweit W. Suppression of hyperandrogenism does not improve peripheral or hepatic insulin resistance in the polycystic ovary syndrome. J Clin Endocrinol Metab 1990;70(3):699–704.

86. Ibanez L, Potau N, Marcos MV. Treatment of hirsutism, hyperandrogenism, oligomenorrhea, dyslipidemia, and hyperinsulinism in nonobese, adolescent girls: effect of flutamide. J Clin Endocrinol Metab 2000;85:3251–3255.

87. Ciaraldi TP, El-Roeiy A, Madar Z, et al. Cellular mechanisms of insulin resistance in polycystic ovary syndrome. J Clin Endocrinol Metab 1992;75:577–583.

88. Rosenbaum D, Haber RS, Dunaif A. Insulin resistance in polycystic ovary syndrome: decreased expression of GLUT-4 glucose transporters in adipocytes. Am J Physiol 1993;264:E197–E202.

89. Dunaif A. Hyperandrogenic anovulation (PCOS): a unique disorder of insulin action associated with an increased risk of non-insulin dependent diabetes mellitus. Am J Med 1995;98(S1A):33–39.

90. O'Meara NM, Blackman JD, Ehrmann DA, et al. Defects in β-cell function in functional ovarian hyperandrogenism. J Clin Endocrinol Metab 1993;76:1241–1247.

91. Flier JS, Minaker KL, Landsberg L, et al. Impaired *in vivo* insulin clearance in patients with severe target cell resistance to insulin. Diabetes 1982;31:132–135.

92. Flier JS, Kahn CR, Roth J, Bar RS. Antibodies that impair insulin receptor binding in an unusual diabetic syndrome with severe insulin resistance. Science 1975;190:63–65.

93. Barbieri R. Effects of insulin on ovarian steroidogenesis. In: Dunaif A, Givens JR, Haseltine F, Merriam GR, eds. The Polycystic Ovary Syndrome. Blackwell Scientific, Cambridge, MA, 1992, pp. 249–263.

94. el-Roeiy A, Chen X, Roberts VJ, et al. Expression of the genes encoding the insulin-like growth factors (IGF-I and II), the IGF and insulin receptors, and IGF-binding proteins 1–6 and the localization of their gene products in normal and polycystic ovary syndrome ovaries. J Clin Endocrinol Metab 1994;78:1488–1496.

95. Poretsky L, Glover B, Laumas V, et al. The effects of experimental hyperinsulinemia on steroid secretion, ovarian 125-I-insulin binding and ovarian 125-I-insulin-like growth factor I binding in the rat. Endocrinology 1988;122:581–585.

96. Willis D, Franks S. Insulin action in human granulosa cells from normal and polycystic ovaries is mediated by the insulin receptor and not the type-I insulin-like growth factor receptor. J Clin Endocrinol Metab 1995;80:3788–3790.

97. Willis D, Mason H, Gilling-Smith C, et al. Modulation by insulin of follicle-stimulating hormone and luteininzing hormone actions in human granulosa cells of normal and polycystic ovaries. J Clin Endocrinol Metab 1996;81:302–309.

98. Poretsky L, Seto-Young D, Shrestha A, et al. Phosphatidyl-inositol-3 kinase-independent insulin action pathway(s) in the human ovary. J Clin Endocrinol Metab 2001;86:3115–3119.

99. Seto-Young D, Zajac J, Lui HC, et al. The role of mitogen-activated protein kinase in insulin and insulin-like growth factor I (IGF-I) signaling cascades for progesterone and IGF-binding protein-1 production in human granulosa cells. J Clin Endocrinol Metab 2003;88:3385–3391.

100. Poretsky L, Grigorescu F, Seibel M, et al. Distribution and characterization of insulin and insulin-like growth factor I receptors in normal human ovary. J Clin Endocrinol Metab 1985;61:728–734.

101. Poretsky L, Bhargava G, Kalin MF, et al. Regulation of insulin receptors in the human ovary: in vitro studies. J Clin Endocrinol Metab 1988;67:774–778.
102. Suikkari AM, Koivisto VA, Rutanen EM, et al. Insulin regulates the serum levels of low molecular weight insulin-like growth factor-binding protein. J Clin Endocrinol Metab 1988;66:266–272.
103. Buyalos RP, Pekonen F, Halme JK, et al. The relationship between circulating androgens, obesity, and hyperinsulinemia on serum insulin-like growth factor binding protein-1 in the polycystic ovarian syndrome. Am J Obstet Gynecol 1995;172:932–939.
104. Giudice LC, Rosenfeld RG. Insulin-like growth factors and the ovary: an overview. In: Dunaif A, Givens JR, Haseltine F, Merriam GR, eds. The Polycystic Ovary Syndrome. Blackwell Scientific, Cambridge, MA, 1992, pp. 201–207.
105. Garcia-Rudaz MC. Amplified and orderly growth hormone secretion characterizes lean adolescents with polycystic ovary syndrome. Eur J Endocrinol 2002;147:207–216.
106. Morales AJ, Laughlin GA, Butzow T. Insulin, somatotropic, and luteinizing hormone axes in lean and obese women with polycystic ovary syndrome: common and distinct features. J Clin Endocrinol Metab 1996;81:2854–2864.
107. Gambineri A, Pelusi C, Vicennati V, et al. Obesity and the polycystic ovary syndrome. Int J Obes Relat Metab Disord 2002;26:883–896.
108. Veldhuis JD, Iranmanesh A, Ho KKY, Waters MJ, et al. Dual defects in pulsatile growth hormone secretion and clearance subserve the hyposomatropinism of obesity in man. J Clin Endocrinol Metab 1991;72:51–59.
109. Dahlgren E, Johansson S, Lindstedt G, et al: Women with polycystic ovary syndrome wedge resected in 1956 to 1965: a long-term follow up focusing on natural history and circulating hormones. Fertil Steril 1992;57:505–513.
110. Ehrmann DA, Barnes RB, Rosenfield RL, et al. Prevalence of imparied glucose tolerance and diabetes in women with polycystic ovary syndrome. Diabetes Care 1999;22:141–146.
111. Azziz R, Ehrmann D, Legro RS, et al. (PCOS/Troglitazone Study Group). Troglitazone improves ovulation and hirsutism in the polycystic ovary syndrome: a multicenter, double blind, placebo-controlled trial. J Clin Endocrinol Metab 2001;86:1626–1632.
112. Haakova L, Cibula D, Rezabek K, et al. Pregnancy outcome in women with PCOS and in control matched by age and weight. Hum Reprod 2003;18:1438–1441.
113. Vollenhoven B, Clark S, Kovacs G, et al. Prevalence of gestational diabetes in polycystic ovary syndrome patients pregnant after ovulation induction with gonadotropins. Aust N Z J Obstet Gynaecol 2000;40:54–58.
114. Mikola M, Hiilesmaa V, Halttunen M, et al. Obstetric outcome in women with polycystic ovarian syndrome. Hum Reprod 2001;16:226–229.
115. Radon PA, McMahon MJ, Meyer WR. Impaired glucose tolerance in pregnant women with polycystic ovary syndrome. Obstet Gynceol 1999;94:194–197.
116. Bjercke S, Dale PO, Tanbo T, et al. Impact of insulin resistance on pregnancy complications and outcome in women with polycystic ovary syndrome. Gynecol Obstet Invest 2002;54:94–98.
117. Expert panel on detection, evaluation, and treatment of high blood cholesterol in adults: executive summary of the third report of the National Cholesterol Education Program (NCEP) Expert Panel on detection, evaluation, and treatment of high blood cholesterol in adults (Adult Treatment Panel III). JAMA 2001;285:2486–2497.
118. Alberti KGMM, Zimmet PZ, the World Health Organization (WHO) Consultation. Definition, diagnosis, and classification of diabetes mellitus and its complications. Part I: diagnosis and classification of diabets mellitus: provisional report of a WHO consultation. Diabet Med 1998; 15:539–553.
119. American College of Endocrinology. Insulin resistance syndrome (position statement). Endocr Pract 2003;9:9–21.
120. Orio F Jr , Palomba S, Spinelli L, et al. The cardiovascular risk of young women with polycystic ovary syndrome: an observational, analytical, prospective case-control study. J Clin Endocrinol Metab 2004;89:3696–3701.
121. Zimmerman S, Phillips RA, Dunaif A, et al. Polycystic ovary syndrome: lack of hypertension despite profound insulin resistance. J Clin Endocrinol Metab 1992;75:508–513.
122. Talbott EO, Zborowski JV, Sutton-Tyrell K, et al. Cardiovascular risk in women with polycystic ovary syndrome. Obstet Gynecol Clin North Am 2001;28:111–133.
123. Amowitz LL, Sobel BE. Cardiovascular consequences of polycystic ovary syndrome. Endocrinol Metab Clin North Am 1999;28:439–458.

124. Legro RS, Kunselman AR, Dunaif A. Prevalence and predictors of dyslipidemia in women with polycystic ovary syndrome. Am J Med 2001;111:607–613.
125. Wild RA, Applebaum-Bowden D, Demers LM, et al. Lipoprotein lipids in women with androgen excess: independent associations with increased insulin and androgen. Clin Chem 1990;36:283–289.
126. Loverro G, Lorusso F, Mei L, et al. The plasma homocysteine levels are increased in polycystic ovary syndrome. Gynecol Obstet Invest 2002;53:157–162.
127. Schachter M, Raziel A, Friedler S, et al. Insulin resistance in patients with polycystic ovary syndrome is associated with elevated plasma homocysteine. Hum Reprod 2003;18:721–727.
128. Vgontzas AN, Legro RS, Bixler EO, et al. Polycystic ovary syndrome is associated with obstructive sleep apnea and daytime sleepiness: role of insulin resistance. J Clin Endocrinol Metab 2001;86:517–520.
129. Kiddy DS, Hamilton-Fairley D, Bush A, et al. Improvement in endocrine and ovarian function during dietary treatment of obese women with polycystic ovary syndrome. Clin Endocrinol 1992;36:105–111.
130. Anderson P, Seljeflot I, Abdelnoor M, et al. Increased insulin sensitivity and fibrinolytic capacity after dietary intervention in obese women with polycystic ovary syndrome. Metabolism 1995;44: 611–616.
131. Huber-Buchholz MM, Carey DGP, Norman RJ. Restoration of Reproductive potential by lifestyle modification in obese polycystic ovary syndrome: Role of insulin sensitivity and leutinizing hormones. J Clin Indocrinal Metab 1999;84:1470–1474.
132. De Leo V, Lanzetta D, D'Antona D, et al. Hormonal effects of flutamide in young women with polycystic ovary syndrome. J Clin Endocrinol Metab 1998;83:99–102.
133. Diamanti-Kandarakis E, Mitrakou A, Raptis S, et al. The effect of a pure antiandrogen receptor blocker, flutamide, on the lipid profile in the polycystic ovary syndrome. J Clin Endocrinol Metab 1998;83:2699–2705.
134. Moghetti P, Tosi F, Castello R, et al. The insulin resistance in women with hyperandrogenism is partially reversed by antiandrogen treatment: evidence that androgens impair insulin action in women. J Clin Endocrinol Metab 1996;81:952–960.
135. Falsetti L, Pasinetti E. Effects of long-term administration of an oral contraceptive containing ethinylestradiol and cyproterone acetate on lipid metabolism in women with polycystic ovary syndrome. Acta Obstet Gynecol Scand 1995;74:56–60.
136. Mastorakos G, Koliopouls C, Crestas G. Androgen and lipid profiles in adolescents with polycystic ovary syndrome who were treated with two forms of combined oral contraceptives. Fertil Steril 2002;77:919–927.
137. Guido M, Romualdi D, Guiliani M, et al. Drospirenone for the treatment of hirsute women with polycystic ovary syndrome: a clinical, endocrinological, metabolic pilot study. J Clin Endocrinol Metab 2004;89:2817–2823.
138. Kasdorf G, Kalkhoff RK. Prospective studies of insulin sensitivity in normal women receiving oral contraceptive agents. J Clin Endocrinol Metab 1988;66:846–852.
139. Cibula D, Fanta M, Hill M, Sindelka G, Skrha J, Zivny J. Insulin sensitivity in non-obese women with polycystic ovary syndrome during treatment with oral contraceptives containing low-androgenic progestin. Hum Reprod 2002;17:76–82.
140. Iuorno MJ, Nestler JE. Insulin lowering drugs in polycystic ovary syndrome. Obstet Gynecol Clin North Am 2001;28:153–164.
141. Ibanez L, Valls C, Ferrer A, et al. Sensitization to insulin induces ovulation in nonobese adolescents with anovulatory hyperandrogenism. J Clin Endocrinol Metab 2001;86:3595–3598.
142. Nestler JE, Jacubowicz DJ. Decreases in ovarian cytochrome p450c17-alpha activity and serum free testosterone after reduction of insulin secretion in polycystic ovary syndrome. N Engl J Med 1996; 335:617–623.
143. Gambineri A, Pelusi C, Genghini S, et al. Effect of flutamide and metformin administered alone or in combination in dieting obese women with polycystic ovary syndrome. Clin Endocrinol 2004; 60:241–249.
144. Ibanez L, de Zegher F. Low-dose combination of flutamide, metformin, and an oral contraceptive for non-obese young women with polycystic ovary syndrome. Hum Reprod 2003;18:57–60.
145. Bloomgarden ZT, Futterweit W, Poretsky L. Use of insulin-sensitizing agents in patients with polycystic ovary syndrome. Endocr Pract 2001;7:279–286.
146. Baillargeon JP, Jakubowicz DJ, Iuorno MJ, et al. Effects of metformin and rosiglitazone, alone and in combination, in non-obese women with polycystic ovary syndrome and normal indices of insulin sensitivity. Fertil Steril 2004;82:893–902.

147. Belli SH, Graffigna MN, Oneto A, et al. Effect of rosiglitazone on insulin resistance, growth factors, and reproductive disturbances in women with polycystic ovary syndrome. Fertil Steril 2004; 81:624–629.
148. Dereli D, Dereli T, Bayraktar F, et al. Endocrine and metabolic effects of nosiglitazone in non-obese women with polycystic ovary disease. Endocr J 2005;52:299–308.
149. Glueck CJ, Moreira A, Goldenberg N, et al. Pioglitazone and metformin in obese women with polycystic ovary syndrome not optimally responsive to metformin. Hum Reprod 2003;18:1618–1625.
150. Brettenthaler N, De Getyer C, Huber P, Keller U. Effect of the insulin sensitizer pioglitazone on insulin resistance, hypernadrogenism, and ovulatory dysfunction in women with polycystic ovary syndrome. J Clin Endocrinol Metab 2004;89:3835–3840.
151. Romualdi D, Guido M, Cioampelli M, et al. Selective effects of pioglitazone on insulin and androgen abnormailities in normo- and hyperinsulinaemic obese patients with polycystic ovary syndrome. Hum Reprod 2003;18:1210–1218.
152. Seto-Young D, Paliou M, Schlosser J, et al. Direct thiazolidinedione action in the human ovary insulin-independent and insulin-sensitizing effects on steroidogenesis and insulin-like growth factor binding protein-1 production. J Clin Endocrinal Metab 2005;90.
153. Baillargeon JP, Iuorno MJ, Jakubowicz DJ, et al. Metformin therapy increases insulin-stimulated release of D-chiro-inositol-containing inositolphosphoglycan mediator in women with polycystic ovary syndrome. J Clin Endocrinol Metab 2004;89:242–249.

16 Obesity and Type 2 Diabetes Mellitus in Childhood and Adolescence

Susann Blüher, MD and Wieland Kiess, MD

CONTENTS

INTRODUCTION

Obesity and type 2 diabetes mellitus used to be very rare in children and adolescents, but since the mid-1990s, an ever-increasing prevalence of obesity and diabetes in children has been observed. More important, both the prevalence and the degree of obesity in children and adolescents are significantly increasing in many populations around the world. For example, a dramatic increase in type 2 diabetes has been reported from investigators in Cincinnati, OH *(1)*. In Germany, more than 5000 youths meet the diagnostic criteria for type 2 diabetes *(2)*. The prevalence of type 2 diabetes mellitus is also very high in Australasia, depending on ethnicity and the degree of obesity. Currently, almost every fifth child is considered to be obese, and 25% of obese children present with impaired glucose tolerance (IGT). Childhood obesity is associated with substantial comorbidities and late sequelae, such as cardiovascular, orthopedic, and psychosocial problems, irrespective of whether obesity persists into adulthood. Thus, type 2 diabetes mellitus and obesity are currently regarded as two of the most challenging health issues facing young people *(3–7)*.

From: *Contemporary Diabetes: Obesity and Diabetes*
Edited by: C. S. Mantzoros © Humana Press Inc., Totowa, NJ

OBESITY IN CHILDHOOD AND ADOLESCENCE

Definition

Several factors influence the degree of body fat mass, such as ethnic background, gender, developmental stage, and age. The standard parameter to define obesity clinically is the body mass index ([BMI], weight in kilograms divided by the square of height in meters, or kg/m^2), which is easy to calculate and correlates significantly with direct measures of body fatness.

Overweight is defined as a BMI greater than the 90th but less than the 97th percentile corrected for age and gender. A child with a BMI above the 97th percentile corrected for age and gender is considered to be obese and should be referred to a pediatric endocrinologist for further diagnosis and treatment (8–12).

In addition, waist circumference, waist-to-hip ratio (to assess upper-body fat deposition), and skin fold thickness are also valuable measures to define obesity but are less extensively used in children and adolescents (9–13). Direct measurements of body fat content include dual-energy X-ray absorptiometry, hydrodensitometry, and bioimpedance, but these useful research tools are validated mainly for adult medicine and are currently used for scientific reasons (13).

Epidemiology

Childhood obesity has reached epidemic proportions in all industrialised countries. The prevalence is as high as 20–30% (8). A cross-sectional study performed in Leipzig, Germany involving more than 2500 children and adolescents between 7 and 18 yr of age revealed that 29% of the subjects were overweight (BMI between the 90th and 97th percentiles) and 16% were obese (BMI above the 97th centile). In another population-based study performed in the same geographic area, an incidence of obesity in children and adolescents of approx 12% was found (9,10). Interestingly, not only the prevalence but also the degree of obesity is increasing in children over time ([9,10]; unpublished data).

Genetic and Environmental Factors

Both genetic/endogenous and environmental/exogenous factors act in concert toward the development of increasing body fatness early in life (Table 1). Thus, a multifactorial etiopathogenesis seems to be responsible for the development of obesity in most patients. However, genetic studies including twin studies suggest that at least 50% of the tendency toward obesity is inherited (11,12). In addition, responsiveness to dietary intervention seems to be genetically determined (14–17).

Several monogenic causes of obesity have been recently identified. Genetic alterations of several genes, including the obgene (leptin) (18–22), the leptin-receptor (23), as well as the melanocortin-4 receptor (MC4-R) (24–27), have been shown to be associated with severe obesity that develops in childhood. The clinical characteristics of these syndromes, the most prevalent of which is currently owing to MC4-R mutations, accounting for up to 4–7% of severe obesity, are reported elsewhere (27).

A sedentary lifestyle, which includes lack of physical activity and excessive use of modern media, in particular, television viewing; and an overconsumption of carbohydrate-rich drinks and fat-rich diets are the most important risk factors for the development of obesity in childhood and adolescence (28–30). Nutrition and diet early in infancy is also thought to influence growth rate and body fatness beyond infancy. In summary, a model in which susceptibility to obesity is determined by genetic factors but the

Table 1
Factors Contributing to Development of Obesity
and Metabolic Syndrome

1. *Environmental/exogenous factors*
   - Increase in sedentary activities (e.g., television viewing)
   - Decrease in physical activity
   - Shift in diets rich in fast/prepackaged foods with high fat/calorie content
   - Loneliness and social isolation
   - Psychosocial/family problems
2. *Genetic/endogenous factors*
   Polymorphisms and/or mutations in any of the following genes:
   - Adrenergic receptors
   - Leptin
   - Leptin receptors (Ob-R)
   - MC4-R and MC3-R
   - Proopiomelanocortin
   - Melanocyte-concentrating hormone
   - Neuropeptide Y (NPY)
   - Prohormone convertase 1
   - SOCS-3 (possible)
   - Tumor necrosis factor-α (possible)
   - NPY receptors (possible)
   - Corticotropin-releasing hormone (possible)
   - Thyrotropin-releasing hormone (possible)
   - Urocortin (possible)
   - Orexin A and B (possible)
   - Serotonin (possible)
   - Galanin (possible)
3. *Genes x environment interactions*

environment determines individual phenotypic expression is currently widely supported and accepted *(12–14)*.

TYPE 2 DIABETES MELLITUS IN CHILDHOOD AND ADOLESCENCE

Definition and Pathogenesis

The World Health Organization and the American Diabetes Association have defined the diagnostic criteria for IGT and type 2 diabetes mellitus *(31)*. The use of simple algorithms helps to establish the clinical evaluation of the obese child (Fig. 1) *(31)*.

Caucasian teenagers from the United Kingdom *(32–34)*, Japanese youths *(35)*, and Indian adolescents *(36)* were the first children to be diagnosed with juvenile type 2 diabetes mellitus. Most of these individuals had a BMI above the 97th percentile at the time of diagnosis *(32–36)*. Currently, type 2 diabetes mellitus has been reported in obese children of virtually any ethnic background.

It is now well established that adipose tissue plays a role of major significance in the pathogenesis of type 2 diabetes. Adipocytes, more numerous and larger in obesity, synthesize and secrete an ever-expanding list of factors and signaling proteins (Tables 2 and 3). These factors are known to alter insulin secretion and insulin sensitivity and even cause insulin resistance under experimental and clinical conditions.

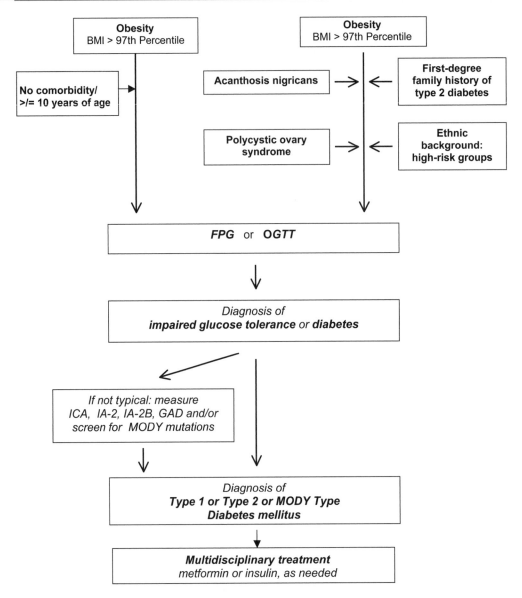

Fig. 1. Proposed algorithm to diagnose IGT and type 2 diabetes in obese children and adolescents FPG, fasting plasma glucose; ICA, islet cell antibodies; IA, islet antibodies; MODY, maturity onset diabetes of the young.

Epidemiology

The incidence of type 2 diabetes mellitus has increased significantly irrespective of ethnicity *(32)*. Children as young as 8 yr are now being diagnosed with the disease *(8,32,37–40)*.

The prevalence of overweight in childhood and adolescence is increasing at a tremendous pace. About 22 million children younger than age 5 are affected worldwide *(5,40)*. The prevalence of overweight among children ages 4–12 yr increased by 1998 to 21.8% in Hispanics, 21.5% in African Americans, and 12.3% in non-Hispanic whites *(41)*. Thus overweight prevalence has increased by more than 50% in the last 10 yr *(41)*.

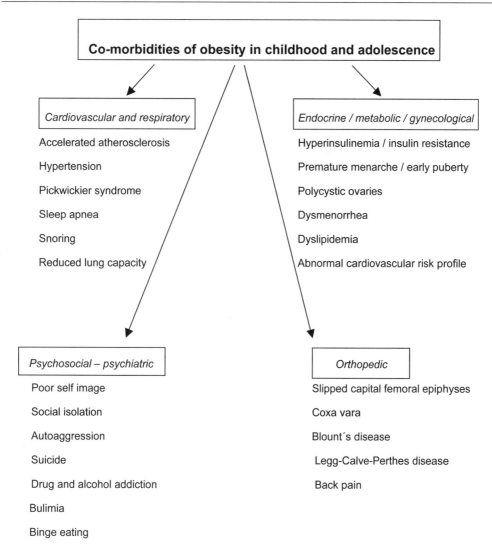

Fig. 2. Comorbidities of obesity in childhood and adolescence.

IGT was also found in lean and obese adolescents with polycystic ovary syndrome (PCOS) *(42,43)*.

Genetic and Environmental Factors

Family histories, ethnicity, and the concordance in monozygotic twins suggest that a genetic component plays a significant role in the development of type 2 diabetes. However, the striking increase in the number of individuals being affected over a short period of time points to exogenous factors and/or a combination of both genetic and environmental/exogenous factors acting in concert in the pathogenesis of type 2 diabetes *(3–8,35–37)*. In children with type 2 diabetes, pancreatic β- and α-cell dysfunction has been described, and insulin insensitivity seems to be an early predictor of the onset of the disease *(38)*.

Candidate genes that may be involved in the pathogenesis of type 2 diabetes mellitus are provided in Table 1. The genetics of diabetes is also covered in detail in Chapter 3.

Table 2
Factors Secreted from Adipose Tissue That May Play Important Role in Energy Homeostasis and Insulin Resistance

Metabolites	Signaling proteins	Molecules acting locally within adipose tissue
Fatty acids	Leptin	Cortisol (11β hydroxysteroid dehydrogenase activity)
Glycerol	Adipsin	
Acetate	Acylation-stimulating proteins	
	Plasminogen activator inhibitor-1	
	Interleukin-6, -8	
	Tumor necrosis factor-α	
	Adiponectin	
	Renin-angiotensinogen-angiotensin	
	Resistin	
	Prostaglandin(s)	

Table 3
Candidate Genes Putatively Implicated in Regulation of Glucose Homeostasis and Pathogenesis of Type 2 Diabetes[a]

Insulin signaling cascade	Tissue specific (insulin-sensitive) factors	Factors released from fat tissue
Insulin receptor	Glucose transporters	See Table 2
Insulin receptor substrates (IRS-1 to IRS-4)	(e.g., GLUT4)	
Enzymes (e.g., PI3kinase, tyrosine kinases, phosphatases, serine kinases)	Glycogen synthase	
	Enzymes (e.g., PEPCK)	
	Potassium channel	
Transcription factors	Sulfonylurea receptors	

[a]A complete discussion of these molecules can be found in specific reviews (75–77).

Genetic factors, such as several rare mutations, explain directly <5% of all cases of type 2 diabetes at present, and those factors are not yet as well defined as the role of human leukocyte antigen genes in the pathogenesis of type 1 diabetes.

Basal and postchallenge insulin levels are significantly higher in African American, Mexican American, and Pima Indian children compared with Caucasian children, suggesting that ethnic factors might play a role of major significance. These ethnic differences are independent of adiposity *per se,* which, by itself, is associated with greater insulin levels in all ethnic groups examined. African American children are more prone to develop type 2 diabetes given the same degree of adiposity, and Mexican American children may be more likely to develop syndrome X, owing to greater obesity-related hyperinsulinemia and dyslipidemia *(39,40).*

Changes in lifestyle, such as in specific eating patterns and the level of physical activity, might contribute to both the global epidemic of obesity and the increasing incidence of type 2 diabetes in the pediatric population (Table 1). Major components influencing this development are the number of meals eaten, availability of food, portion sizes, snacking and meal skipping as well as hours spent watching television *(41).*

SCREENING FOR AND CLINICAL FEATURES OF OBESITY AND TYPE 2 DIABETES MELLITUS

Clinical Presentations of Obesity and Type 2 Diabetes Mellitus and Their Comorbidities in Childhood and Adolescence (see Fig. 2)

The most important clinical features associated with juvenile obesity are hypertension, dyslipidemia, and psychosocial problems (9–11,44), predisposing for additional comorbidities such as cardiovascular disease in early adulthood (45). In addition, alcohol and illicit drug use seem to be associated with an earlier onset of type 2 diabetes mellitus (46).

It is crucial that blood pressure (BP) and lipid status monitoring be available to all obese children and, even more important, to children and adolescents with diabetes mellitus (38,39,45). Ambulatory BP monitoring is a helpful tool to investigate children and adolescents at an early stage of the disorder (45). In addition, orthopedic surgeons and pediatric psychiatrists should be involved as needed in the treatment of these patients.

Screening Procedures

In children with newly diagnosed type 2 diabetes mellitus, the disease counts for 5–45% of the cases of diabetes in different populations (47). It is advisable that obese children with a family history of type 2 diabetes be screened for the disease at a young age. Special care should be provided to obese African American, Native American, and Hispanic children.

Autoantibodies to IA-2 and GAD might be detected in children with type 2 diabetes mellitus, but also in patients with type 1 diabetes (48). Thus, although these antibodies are not specific for a special subtype of diabetes mellitus, screening involving measurement of autoantibodies might be advisable to define or rule out autoimmunity.

THERAPEUTIC APPROACH TOWARD OBESITY AND TYPE 2 DIABETES MELLITUS AND GOALS OF THERAPY: MULTIDISCIPLINARY TREATMENT OPTIONS

Because of the increasing prevalence of juvenile obesity as well as type 2 diabetes mellitus, it is imperative that effective treatment be developed and become widely available. Therapeutic strategies should be multidisciplinary and include psychological and family therapy interventions (49), lifestyle/behavior modification (50), exercise programs (51), and nutrition education (52,53). Optimal results are being achieved by comprehensive treatment protocols combining programs to reduce sedentary behaviors and include structured exercise as well as physical training (54,55).

Multidisciplinary treatment approaches are considered to be the most effective. The creaton of networks of primary care physicians, public health/medical schools, and medical institutions, specialists of pediatric and adolescent medicine, social workers, child psychologists, and dieticians, as well as sports educators should be achieved. Such networking concepts should be strongly supported by health insurance providers and government agencies. Using such approaches, some groups have reported high success rates and sufficient long-term weight reduction in relatively small groups of studied children (49–57).

Requirements Prior to Therapy

Empowerment and responsibility of the whole family toward achieving a solution of the problem i.e., the increasing prevalence of obesity and type 2 diabetes amongst our youngsters, are crucial for the successful management of body weight on a long-term basis. Prior to initiation of therapy, young patients and their families should obtain detailed information about the disease, its comorbidities, and available options for therapy. To evaluate the individual health risk and to plan for the optimal therapy, the patient should be examined carefully, and a detailed history should be obtained by a pediatric endocrinologist.

The history should focus on the following information:

- Family history (obesity, diabetes mellitus, hypertension, coronary artery disease).
- Weight and height curve.
- Level of physical activity.
- Diet.
- Social and occupational background.

The physical examination should include the following:

- Body weight, height, hip and waist circumference.
- BP (24-h profile if needed).
- Physical examination.
- Fasting blood glucose concentration, oral glucose tolerance test (OGTT).
- Total, high-density lipoprotein, and low-density lipoprotein cholesterol, triglycerides.
- Uric acid.
- Creatinine, electrolytes.
- Thyroid-stimulating hormone, thyroxine.
- Electrocardiogram.
- Sleep apnea screening.
- Abdominal ultrasound.
- Leptin, adiponectin, ghrelin, or other adipokines (only for scientific reasons in the context of ongoing studies).

Additional parameters might be necessary as needed, e.g., 24-h urine collection for free cortisol or a dexamethasone-suppression test if Cushing disease is suspected, or serum concentrations of gonadotropins if PCOS is suspected.

Whenever a specific syndrome, such as Prader-Willi syndrome, or a monogenetic form of obesity (i.e., mutations of MC4-R, leptin, leptin receptor) is suspected, molecular genetic screening should be considered.

Lifestyle and Behavior Modification

Obesity is an increasing problem in industrialized countries and is attributable, to an immense proportion, not only to individual lifestyle changes and habits, but also to general features in these countries. The level of physical activity has changed dramatically. Favorite leisure-time activities (not only of youngsters) now include playing video and computer games as well as watching television, rather than engaging in physical exercise or outdoor activities (56).

Nutrition is another important feature related to changes in lifestyle and the rise in the prevalence of obesity. "Junk food" is more easily available and affordable than a healthy diet to a growing number of individuals, depending on the time of year and country.

Thus, it is advisable that governments promote individual health and nutrition education as well as a healthy lifestyle of the entire community, including appropriate eating patterns and regular physical exercise, in order to stop the current epidemic of obesity in industrialized countries (56,57). Treatment of obesity as well as a cognitive awareness of a healthy lifestyle should start early in childhood, because certain lifestyle changes and patterns are more easily incorporated into adulthood if learned early in life (58).

Psychological, Group, and Family Therapy Interventions

To create an awareness of lifestyle changes, different strategies of psychotherapy have been used. The most important and most useful therapeutic approach has been reported to be family or cognitive behavioral therapy *(59)*.

Depending on the age of the obese child or adolescent and the social and/or family background, the most appropriate type of psychotherapy should be chosen. For preschoolers, group teaching seems to be a promising approach, because they normally accept groups formed from the outside. However, in older children, individual forms of therapy might be advisable, because they prefer to create their own groups. In general terms, family therapy is a helpful tool in early childhood but also with teenagers and adults, because the family of origin should always be involved in the treatment regimen. It is therefore advisable that treatment regimens should be adhered to by as many members of the family as possible.

In addition, not only changing eating as well as activity patterns within the family network is crucial for a successful and lasting therapy of obesity, but also the emotional and psychological support of family members. Family arrangements to meet the obese child's diet and exercise programs should be accompanied by encouragement, sensitive support, and appreciation by family members *(58,59)*.

Exercise and Physical Activity

Aerobic exercise has been reported to be the most suitable form of exercise for obese children and adolescents, and regular exercise aims at reducing body weight and comorbidiy and at correcting posture. Aerobic exercise not only increases cardiorespiratory capacity, but also utilizes fat metabolites during muscle work, which is facilitated by increased enzymatic activity of skeletal muscles *(60–62)*. In addition, an individual adapted to a higher level of dynamic, aerobic motor activity during growth may develop greater activity of specific enzymes, which metabolize and utilize fatty acids *(60)*.

Lean and obese subjects have different characteristic profiles in their enzymatic activity. In obese or obesity-prone subjects, the activity of fat-oxidizing enzymes in skeletal muscles is decreased. Moreover, smaller areas of type 1 and 2B muscle fibers are present in postobese vs nonobese individuals *(61)*. A key enzyme in the β-oxidation of fatty acids is known to be hydroxyacyl-coenzyme-A. This enzyme has been found to be significantly negatively correlated to the degree of adiposity *(62)*.

Because a reduction in body fat is best achieved by dynamic, aerobic exercise, exercise programs should be started with swimming, whenever possible. When some weight reduction and adaptation to increased physical activity have been achieved, exercise from lying down or sitting positions and the use of cycle ergometers are useful approaches as well *(62)*.

The degree of obesity and the social background show a significant variability. It is thus essential to consider the special features and needs of the particular obese child or adolescent prior to initiating an exercise program.

Nutritional Intervention

In the context of a multifactorial treatment approach for obesity, dietary intervention is a factor of considerable significance. Prior to initiating a nutritional intervention, a child's nutritional status should be evaluated, and several factors such as the age of the obese patient, comorbidities, and degree of obesity should be considered.

In general, overweight and moderate obesity in children and adolescents (BMI between the 90th and 97th percentiles) can be treated with a balanced low-calorie diet, in which energy intake is reduced by about 30%. The diet should provide approx 20% of energy from protein, 30–35% from fat, and 45–50% from carbohydrates, respectively (63).

When obesity is severe (i.e., the BMI is far above the 97th percentile) and comorbidities are already present, a very low-calorie diet (≤800 kcal/d) should be considered rather than a balanced low-calorie diet (63,64). In a very low-calorie diet, the calories provided per day should be partially balanced (i.e., 25% of energy derived from protein, 30% from fat, and 45% from carbohydrates). The protein-sparing modified fast or unbalanced very low-calorie diet is supposed to spare lean body mass while producing rapid weight loss (i.e., 66% of energy derived from protein, 24% from fat, 10% from carbohydrates). Children and adolescents with severe obesity are most widely treated with a protein-sparing modified fast (63,64).

All forms of low-calorie diets should be used very carefully in this age group of obese patients and only under strict medical supervision, because the weight loss can be rapid and remarkable. Thus, regular medical checkups are imperative when prescribing any form of diet to an obese child or adolescent.

Pharmacotherapy

In general, three main modes of action of antiobesity drugs can be distinguished:

1. Agents that influence *energy intake* via central or peripheral mechanisms: These substances either modify eating behavior or suppress appetite by acting on central neurons known to be involved in the regulation of energy homeostasis or to alter gastric emptying, causing malabsorption.
2. Substances that influence *energy storage,* by either decreasing lipid storage or increasing lipid oxidation in the fat tissue.
3. Drugs that regulate *energy output,* by acting via either central (i.e., on hypothalamic neuron populations known to be involved in energy homeostasis) or peripheral (skeletal muscle, brown and white adipose tissue) mechanisms to increase, among others, nonshivering thermogenesis (65–67).

Antiobesity drugs, including appetite suppressants and thermogenic drugs (i.e., epinephrine, caffeine, or β-adrenergic agonists), have not been approved for use in children and adolescents. Only very limited data from a few clinical trials are available about the use of digestive inhibitors such as lipase inhibitors and fat substitutes in children and adolescents. The only medication that has been extensively investigated as a therapeutic approach for both type 2 diabetes and obesity in children and adolescents is metformin (68,69).

At present, success rates and efficacy of the available treatment strategies for obesity in the pediatric population are very limited. Long-term treatment including pharmacotherapy might therefore be an important treatment option in extremely obese adolescents. However, antiobesity medications have not yet been studied with respect to efficacy, safety, and long-term effects in children and adolescents and are therefore not advisable for use in those patients at present (9,10,56,65–67).

IMPACT AND FUTURE DIRECTIONS

Obesity is the most common chronic disorder in the Western world (11–14). The financial and societal consequences of the emerging epidemic of obesity and type 2 diabetes are substantial and demand a prompt public health response. Approximately 60–85% of obese preschoolers will remain obese during adulthood, and comorbidities represent a major health burden in industrialized societies *(12,14)*.

The optimum BMI range associated with best longevity has been reported to be 23–25 kg/m^2 for Caucasians and 23–30 kg/m^2 for African Americans *(70)*. In the United States, the annual economic costs owing to medical expenses and lost income from obesity in adults amount to approx $70 billion. It is estimated that another $30 billion is spent on diet foods, products, and programs to lose weight *(70–72)*.

Thus, emphasis must be placed on preventive strategies. Prevention has to start very early in life and perhaps even before extrauterine life *(73,74)*. Good nutrition and modest exercise for pregnant women as well as monitoring of intrauterine growth of the child are mandatory, and breast feeding should be recommended *(74)*. Principles of good nutrition and physical activities should be taught at all ages. Parents and caretakers should ensure that children have easy access to healthy foods and should serve meals and snacks in a pleasant and positive environment to help children develop healthy food habits *(73)*.

All children and adolescents above the age of 10 with a BMI greater than the 97th percentile, defined as severe obesity, should undergo an OGTT as a screening for IGT or overt type 2 diabetes. Whenever treatment of obesity or type 2 diabetes is necessary, multidisciplinary teams should be formed, including a physician, a nutrition specialist, a psychologist, as well as care providers such as school nurses and teachers. Joint actions by physicians, health authorities, and government agencies using modern media are required for the implementation of nationwide prevention programs. These programs should consider cultural approaches and racial preferences with respect to food preparation and eating habits and should encourage increasing physical activity. In addition, the public should be made aware of both the epidemic of childhood obesity and its serious consequences, the most important of which is type 2 diabetes. Thus, one of the prime targets of public health intervention programs should be prevention and treatment of juvenile obesity and type 2 diabetes mellitus *(31–41)*.

CONCLUSIONS

Obesity is the most common chronic disorder in industrialized countries, and the number of obese children and adolescents is increasing significantly over time. Childhood obesity is associated with substantial comorbidities, such as type 2 diabetes mellitus. Its impact on individuals' lives and on health-care costs and economics is increasingly being recognized by physicians and the public alike.

Whereas diagnostic strategies are clear and straightforward, treatment often remains difficult and frustrating for the patient, the family, and the multidisciplinary team providing health care. As a result, much more attention should be given to prevention and the development of preventive strategies at all ages. Research on new and more effective treatment options is urgently needed. Finally, the public and politicians alike should become aware of the increasing health burden and economic dimensions of the epidemic of juvenile obesity and take appropriate action.

REFERENCES

1. Pinhas-Hamiel O, Dolan LM, Daniels SR. Increased incidence of non-insulin-dependent diabetes mellitus among adolescents. J Pediatr 1996;128:608–615.
2. Kiess W, Böttner A, Raile K, et al. Type 2 diabetes mellitus in children and adolescents—a review from a European perspective. Horm Res 2003;59(Suppl 1):77–84.

3. Arslanian SA. Type 2 diabetes mellitus in children: pathophysiology and risk factors. J Pediatr Endocrinol Metab 2000;13(Suppl 6):1385–1394.

4. American Diabetes Association. Type 2 diabetes in children and adolescents. Diabetes Care 2000;23:381–389.

5. Libman I, Arslanian S. Type 2 diabetes in childhood: the American perspective. Horm Res 2003; 56–63.

6. Brosnan CA, Upchruch S, Schreiner B. Type 2 diabetes in children and adolescents: an emerging disease. J Pediatr Health Care 2001;15:187–193.

7. Ortega-Rodriguez E, Levy-Marchal C, Tubiana N, Czernbichow P, Polak M. Emergence of type 2 diabetes in hospital based cohort of children with diabetes mellitus. Diabetes Metab 2001; 27:574–578.

8. Sinha R, Fisch G, Teague B, et al. Prevalence of impaired glucose tolerance among children and adolescents with marked obesity. N Engl J Med 2002;346:802–810.

9. Kiess W, Galler A, Reich A, et al. Clinical aspects of obesity in childhood and adolescence. Obes Rev 2001;2:29–36.

10. Kiess W, Böttner A. Obesity in the adolescent. Adolesc Med: 2002;13:181–190.

11. Kopelman PG. Obesity as a medical problem. Nature 2000; 404:635–643.

12. Ebbeling CB, Pawlak DB, Ludwig DS. Childhood obesity: public-health crisis, common sense cure. Lancet 2002;360:473–482.

13. Cole TJ, Bellizzi MC, Flegal KM, Dietz WH. Establishing a standard definition for child overweight and obesity worldwide: international survey. BMJ 2000;320:1240–1243.

14. Friedman JM. Obesity in the new millenium. Nature 2000;404:632–634.

15. Bouchard C. The causes of obesity: advances in molecular biology but stagnation on the genetic front. Diabetologia 1996;39:1532–1533.

16. Schwartz MW, Woods SC, Porte D, Seeley RJ, Baskin DG. Central nervous system control of food intake. Nature 2000;404:661–671.

17. Kennedy E, Powell R. Changing eating patterns of American children: a view from 1996. J Am Coll Nutr 1996;16:524–529.

18. Zhang Y, Proenca R, Maffei M, Barone M, Leopold L, Friedman JM. Positional cloning of the mouse obese gene and its human homologue. Nature 1994;372:425–432.

19. Montague CT, Farooqi IS, Whitehead JP, et al. Congenital leptin deficiency is associated with severe early-onset obesity in humans. Nature 1997;387:903–908.

20. Strobel A, Issad T, Camoin L, Ozata M, Strosberg AD. A leptin missense mutation associated with hypogonadism and morbid obesity. Nat Genet 1998;18:213–215.

21. Farooqi IS, Jebb SA, Langmack G, et al. Effects of recombinant leptin therapy in a child with congenital leptin deficiency. N Engl J Med 1999;341:879–884.

22. Farooqi IS, Matarese G, Lord GM, et al. Beneficial effects of leptin on obesity, T cell hyporesponsiveness, and neuroendocrine/metabolic dysfunction of human congenital leptin deficiency. J Clin Invest 2002;110:1093–1103.

23. Clement K, Vaisse C, Lahlou N, et al. A mutation in the human leptin receptor gene causes obesity and pituitary dysfunction. Nature 1998;392:398–401.

24. Huszar D, Lynch CA, Fairchild-Huntress V, Dunmore JH, Fang Q, Berkemeier LR. Targeted disruption of the melanocortin-4 receptor results in obesity in mice. Cell 1997;88:131–141.

25. Farooqi IS, Keogh JM, Yeo GS, Lank EJ, Cheetham T, O'Rahilly S. Clinical spectrum of obesity and mutations in the melanocortin 4 receptor gene. N Engl J Med 2003;348:1085–1095.

26. Farooqi IS, Yeo GS, Keogh JM, et al. Dominant and recessive inheritance of morbid obesity associated with melanocortin 4 receptor deficiency. J Clin Invest 2000;106:271–279.

27. Vaisse C, Clement K, Durand E, Hercberg S, Guy-Grand B, Froguel P. Melanocortin-4 receptor mutations are a frequent and heterogeneous cause of morbid obesity. J Clin Invest 2000;106(2): 253–262.

28. Robinson TN. Does television cause childhood obesity? JAMA 1998;279:959, 960.

29. Robinson TN. Television viewing and childhood obesity. Pediatr Clin North Am 2001;48:1017–1025.

30. Votruba SB, Horvitz MA, Schoeller DA. The role of exercise in the treatment of obesity. Nutrition 2000;16:179–188.

31. Report of the Expert Committee on the Diagnosis and Classification of Diabetes Mellitus. Diabetes Care 1997;20:1183–1197.

32. Rowell HA, Evans BJ, Quarry-Horn JL, Kerrigan JR. Type 2 diabetes mellitus in adolescents. Adolesc Med 2002;13:1–12.

33. Dyer O. First cases of type 2 diabetes found in white UK teenagers. BMJ 2002;324:506.

34. Drake AJ, Smith A, Betts PR, Crowne EC, Shiled JP. Type 2 diabetes in obese white children. Arch Dis Child 2002;86:207–208.
35. Ohara T, Kasuga M. Type 2 diabetes. Nippon Rinsho 2001;59(Suppl 8):223–230.
36. Narayan KM, Fagot-Campagna A, Imperatore G. Type 2 diabetes in children: a problem lurking for India? Indian Pediatr 2001;38:701–704.
37. Bourgeois MJ. Screening, diagnosis, and management of non-insulin dependent diabetes mellitus in adolescents. Tex Med 2002;98:47–50.
38. Beck J, Brandt EN Jr, Blackett P, Copeland K. Prevention and early detection of type 2 diabetes in children and adolescents. J Okla State Med Assoc 2001;94:355–361.
39. Anavian J, Brenner DJ, Fort P, Speiser PW. Profiles of obese children presenting for metabolic evaluation. J Pediatr Endocrinol Metab 2001;14:1145–1150.
40. Gower BA. Syndrome X in children: influence of ethnicity and visceral fat. Am J Hum Biol 1999;11:249–257.
41. Strauss RS, Pollack HA. Epidemic increase in childhood overweight, 1986–1998. JAMA 2001;286: 2845–2848.
42. Umpaichira W, Bastian W, Taha D, Banerji MA, AvRuskin TW, Castells S. C-peptide and glucagon profiles in minority children with type 2 diabetes. J Clin Endocrinol Metab 2001;86:1605–1609.
43. Palmert MR, Gordon CM, Kartashov AI, Legro RS, Emans SJ, Dunaif A. Screening for abnormal glucose tolerance in adolescents with polycystic ovary syndrome. J Clin Endocrinol Metab 2002;87:1017–1023.
44. Wabitsch M. Overweight and obesity in European children: definition and diagnostic procedures, risk factors and consequences for later health outcome. Eur J Pediatr 2000;159(Suppl 1):S8–S13.
45. Daniels SR. Cardiovascular disease risk factors and atherosclerosis in children and adolescents. Curr Atheroscl Rep 2001;3:479–485.
46. Johnson KH, Bazargan M, Cherpitel CJ. Alcohol, tobacco, and drug use and the onset of type 2 diabetes among inner-city minority patients. Am Board Fam Pract 2001;14:430–436.
47. Valente AM, Strong W, Sinaiko AR. Obesity and insulin resistance in young people. Am Heart J 2001;142:440–444.
48. Grasso YZ, Reddy SK, Rosenfeld CR, et al. Autoantibodies to IA-2 and GAD65 in patients with type 2 diabetes mellitus of varied duration: prevalence and correlation with clinical features. Endocr Pract 2001;7:339–345.
49. Steinberger J, Moran A, Hong CP, Jacobs DR Jr, Sinaiko AR. Adiposity in childhood predicts obesity and insulin resistance in young adulthood. J Pediatr 2001;138:453–454.
50. Birch LL, Krahnstoever Davison K. Family environmental factors influence the developing behavioral controls of food intake and childhood overweight. Pediatr Clin North Am 2001;48:893–907.
51. Epstein LH. Behavioral therapy in the treatment of pediatric obesity. Pediatr Clin North Am 2001;48:981–993.
52. Sothern MS. Exercise as a modality in the treatment of childhood obesity. Pediatr Clin North Am 2001;48:995–1015.
53. Nicklas TA, Baranowski T, Cullen KW, Berenson G. Eating patterns, dietary quality and obesity. J Am Coll Nutr 2001;20:599–608.
54. Ikeda JP, Mitchell RA. Dietary approaches to the treatment of the overweight pediatric patient. Pediatr Clin North Am 2001;48:955–968.
55. Flynn JT. What's new in pediatric hypertension? Curr Hypertens Rep 2001;3:503–510.
56. Poston WSC, Foreyt JP, Borrell L, Haddock CK. Challenges in obesity management. South Med J 1998;91:710–720.
57. Bray GA. Overweight is risking fate. J Clin Endocrinol Metab 1999;84:10–12.
58. Sothern MS, Loftin JM, Udall JN, et al. Inclusion of resistance exercise in a multidisciplinary outpatient treatment program for preadolescent obese children. Southern Med J 1999;92:585–592.
59. Flodmark CE, Lissau I. Psychotherapy. In: Burniat W, Cole T, Lissau I, Poskitt E, eds. Child and Adolescent Obesity. Cambridge University Press, 2002, pp. 282–307.
60. Parizkova J, Bunc V, Sprynarova S, Mackova E, Heller J. Body composition, aerobic power, ventilatory threshold, and food intake in different sports. Ann Sports Med 1987;3:171–177.
61. Raben A, Mygind E, Saltin B, Astrup A. Decreased activity of fat-oxidizing enzymes in muscle of obesity-prone subjects. Int J Obes 1997;21-2:S43.
62. Parizkova J, Maffeis C, Poskitt EME. Management through activity. In: Burniat W, Cole T, Lissau I, Poskitt E, eds. Child and Adolescent Obesity. Cambridge University Press, Cambridge, UK: 2002, pp. 282–307.
63. Wadden TA, Stunkard AJ, Brownell KD. Very low calorie diets: their efficacy, safety, and future. Ann Intern Med 1983;99:675–684.

64. Caroli M, Burniat W. Dietary management. In: Burniat W, Cole T, Lissau I, Poskitt E, eds. Child and Adolescent Obesity. Cambridge University Press, 2002, pp. 282–307.

65. Bray GA, Tartaglia LA. Medical strategies in the treatment of obesity. Nature 2000;404:672–677.

66. Molnar D, Malecka-Tendera E. Drug therapy. In: Burniat W, Cole T, Lissau I, Poskitt E, eds. Child and Adolescent Obesity. Cambridge University Press, 2002, pp. 345–354.

67. Finer N. Pharmacotherapy of obesity. Best Prac & Res Clin Endocrinol and Metab 2002;16:717–742.

68. Pasquali R, Gambineri A, Biscotti D, et al. Effect of long-term treatment with metformin added to hypocaloric diet on body composition, fat distribution, and androgen and insulin levels in abdominally obese women with and without polycystic ovary syndrome. J Clin Endocrinol Metab 2000;85:2767–2774.

69. Diabetes Prevention Program Research Group. Reduction in the incidence of type 2 diabetes with lifestyle intervention or metformin. N Engl J Med 2002;346:393–493.

70. Fontaine KR, Redden DT, Wang C, Westfall AO, Allison DB. Years of life lost due to obesity. JAMA 2003;289:187–193.

71. Fitzner K, Caputo N, Trendell W, French MV, Bondi MA, Jennings C. Recent tax changes may assist treatment of obesity. Manage Care Interface 2003;16:47–51.

72. Colditz GA. Economic costs of obesity and inactivity. Med Sci Sports Exerc 1999;31:663–667.

73. Koivisto Hursti UK. Factors influencing children's food choice. Ann Med 1999;31(Suppl 1):26–32.

74. Von Kries, Koletzko B, Sauerwald T, et al. Breast feeding and obesity: cross sectional study. BMJ 1999;319:147–150.

75. Kahn CR. Knockout mice challenge our concepts of glucose homeostasis and the pathogenesis of diabetes. Exp Diabesity Res 2003;4:169–182 (review).

76. Ueki K, Kondo T, Tseng YH, Kahn CR. Central role of suppressors of cytokine signaling proteins in hepatic steatosis, insulin resistance, and the metabolic syndrome in the mouse. Proc Natl Acad Sci USA 2004;13:10,422–10,427.

77. Flier JS. Obesity wars: molecular progress confronts an expanding epidemic [review]. Cell 2004;23:337–350.

17 Diabetic Retinopathy

Vassiliki Poulaki, MD, PhD and Joan W. Miller, MD

INTRODUCTION

Diabetes mellitus is the leading cause of blindness in people between the ages of 20 and 74 in the United States, and diabetic retinopathy (DR) will eventually affect most people with type 1 diabetes. Blindness is 25 times more common in patients with diabetes mellitus than in control subjects. In the Wisconsin Epidemiological Study of Diabetic Retinopathy (WESDR), 3.6% of patients with type 1 diabetes were legally blind (the majority owing to DR), whereas 1.6% of those with type 2 diabetes were legally blind (one-third owing to DR) *(1)*. DR began in type 1 diabetes 3–5 yr after diagnosis and in type 2 diabetes as early as 4–7 yr before the clinical diagnosis of diabetes. Almost all type 1 patients and 50–80% of type 2 patients were affected at 20 yr. Because the prevalence of type 2 diabetes mellitus is much higher in the general population, a larger proportion of severe proliferative diabetic retinopathy (PDR) cases are caused by type 2 diabetes mellitus. This chapter discusses the pathophysiology and current management, as well as novel emerging approaches for the treatment of DR.

Definition and Classification

DR is classified into two main groups: nonproliferative (mild, moderate, moderately severe, and severe) and proliferative (mild, moderate, and high risk) DR. Nonproliferative diabetic retinopathy (NPDR) is characterized by increased vascular permeability, dilation and tortuosity of the retinal veins, abnormal vascular communications between arterioles and venules, microaneurysms, intraretinal hemorrhages, and

From: *Contemporary Diabetes: Obesity and Diabetes*
Edited by: C. S. Mantzoros © Humana Press Inc., Totowa, NJ

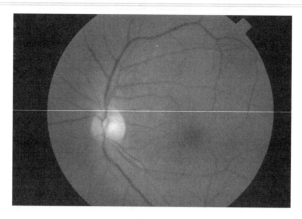

Fig. 1. Fundus appearance of normal retina. Disk margins are sharp, retinal vessels have normal caliber, and the macular area has a sharp reflex.

"cotton-wool" spots (areas of infarction in the nerve layer). Microvascular angiopathy results in exudation of plasma from breakdown of the blood–retinal barrier. Reabsorption of the fluid results in the deposition of protein and lipid exudates ("hard exudates"). PDR is marked by the formation of neovessels in the area of the optic disk (neovascularization of the optic disk [NVD]) or retinal neovascularization elsewhere (NVE). Fifty percent of type 1 and 10% of type 2 diabetics who have had DR for 15 yr will have PDR, whereas the prevalence is higher in type 2 patients who require insulin.

Prevalence and Incidence

Calculation of the prevalence of DR in the population, especially in early stages, is complicated by the type of physician making the diagnosis (general ophthalmologist vs retina specialist) and by the identification method (fundus photography vs opthalmoscopy). Grading of retinopathy in large clinical trials, such as the Early Treatment Diabetic Retinopathy Study (ETDRS) and the WESDR, uses the Airlie House classification *(2)*, with photographs covering seven standard fields of the retina. The reported prevalence of DR at diagnosis of type 1 diabetes mellitus is low (0–3%). Because type 2 diabetes mellitus can remain undiagnosed for years, DR is present in 6.7–30.2% of patients at diagnosis *(3)*. The prevalence of DR in type 1 and 2 diabetes is strongly correlated with duration of the disease. As many as 100% of patients with type 1 diabetes have been observed to develop some degree of retinopathy after 20–30 yr, with a peak incidence at about 10–15 yr after diagnosis *(3)*. Of type 2 patients 50–80%, are affected by 20 yr from diagnosis. Severe visual loss is owing to DR in 86% of patients with type 1 diabetes, but only 33% of older-onset groups, because other eye diseases increase with age *(4)*.

In the WESDR, the 4-yr incidence of any DR was 59% in patients with type 1 diabetes, 47.4% in type 2 patients treated with insulin, and 34.4% in type 2 patients not treated with insulin *(3,5)*. Among type 1 patients, 41.2% experienced progression of DR and 10.5% had progression to PDR during the 4-yr study. Progression of DR was seen in just over one-third (34%) of insulin-treated type 2 patients and 24.9% of noninsulin-treated type 2 patients. Progression to PDR was seen in 7.4 and 2.3% of these patients, respectively. In the three patient groups (type 1, insulin-treated type 2, and non-insulin-treated type 2), the incidence of legal blindness was found to be 1.5, 3.2, and 2.7%, respectively *(3,5)*. The 10-yr incidence of any DR or visual loss in patients enrolled in the WESDR was 89.3 and 9.2%, respectively, in type 1 diabetes; 79.2 and 32.8%, respectively, in insulin-treated type 2 diabetes; and 66.9 and 21.4%, respectively, in non-insulin-treated type 2 diabetes, respectively *(3,6)*. In these patients, those experiencing one or more steps of progression (on the Early Treatment of Diabetic Retinopathy Study [ETDRS] scale) after 4 yr were calculated to be 5.85 times more likely to develop PDR in the next 6 yr compared with those with no progression *(3)*.

PATHOPHYSIOLOGY OF DR

DR: A Disease of Vascular Remodeling and Uncontrolled Angiogenesis

The first ophthalmoscopically observed lesion is the formation of vascular microaneurysms (small outpouchings that stem from the retinal capillaries) and venular dilatation, although biochemical and cytokine perturbations have probably preexisted for years *(7)*. Thickening of the retinal basement membrane is thought by some investigators to be the earliest change in DR. Microvascular contractile cell (pericyte) death, followed by endothelial cell proliferation, may explain the formation of microaneurysms and may also lead to acellular capillaries, which tend to undergo occlusion, leading to retinal ischemia. "Cotton-wool" spots and soft exudates represent ischemic areas of the nerve-fiber retina layer. Acellular capillaries are also fragile and leaky, leading to blot hemorrhages and/or extravasation of fluid and retinal edema. These changes can still be asymptomatic, unless they affect the macula. Macular edema is an important cause of severe central vision loss. Reabsorbance of the fluid from the extracellular edema results in precipitation of lipids and protein, forming "hard exudates." Growth of new blood vessels in the retina in response to retinal hypoxia is the hallmark of PDR. New vessels may appear near the macula, directly affecting central vision. New vessels also rupture easily, leading to vitreous hemorrhage. In advanced PDR, fibrovascular tissue growing from the retina into the vitreous may result in traction and retinal detachment leading to blindness. New vessel proliferation can also occur on the surface of the iris and in the anterior chamber angle, the latter blocking the outflow path for aqueous humor in the eye, increasing the intraocular pressure and causing neovascular glaucoma. The significant advances in the field of angiogenesis have greatly increased the knowledge about the pathogenesis of the vascular lesions in DR and the regulation of retinal neovascularization.

DR: An Undiagnosed Chronic Inflammatory Disease

Over the past 15 yr, an increasing body of experimental and clinical evidence has suggested that a low-grade chronic, subclinical, inflammatory process takes place in the retinal microvasculature in the setting of DR and could be a major pathogenetic mechanism underlying its vascular pathology. This evidence has implications for understanding the pathophysiology of a major cause of blindness and may also shift the treatment paradigm for this condition by bringing anti-inflammatory therapies into the spotlight.

Within 1 wk of experimental diabetes in relevant animal models, retinal vascular endothelial growth factor (VEGF) levels increase *(8)* and serve to stimulate intercellular adhesion molecule-1 (ICAM-1) expression in the retinal vasculature, which promotes leukocyte binding to the diabetic retinal vasculature (leukostasis). Leukocytes then trigger a Fas/Fas ligand (FasL)-mediated endothelial cell death, and breakdown of the blood–retinal barrier *(9)*. These findings occur irrespectively of the method used to induce diabetes in the animal model (streptozotocin for pancreatic islet destruction or galactose-based diet that induces systemic hyperhexosemia or animals genetically prone to spontaneous diabetes development) and were confirmed in postmortem human retina tissue sections from diabetic subjects (10). Moreover, neutrophils from diabetic rats exhibit higher levels of surface β_2-integrin heterodimers LFA-1 (CD11a/CD18) and Mac-1 (CD11a/CD18) that serve as ICAM-1 receptors (11) and demonstrate enhanced superoxide radical production. Antibody-based neutralization of ICAM-1 and CD18 prevents leukocyte adhesion (12–14). Moreover, diabetic and galactosemic mice deficient for the leukocyte adhesion molecules CD18 and ICAM-1 show a marked and sustained suppression of retinal vascular leukocyte adhesion, endothelial cell injury and loss, blood–retinal barrier breakdown, pericyte death, acellular capillary formation, and neural cell death, compared with wild-type controls.

DR: Role of Apoptosis

Diabetic retinal leukostasis is temporally and spatially associated with retinal endothelial cell injury and death. Antibody-based neutralization of ICAM-1 and CD18 prevents retinal endothelial cell injury and death, presumably through its effect on leukocyte adhesion (14). Retinal endothelial cell and pericyte apoptosis is accelerated in human and experimental diabetes and precedes any histological evidence of retinopathy. This phenomenon can also be induced by experimental hyperhexosemia (galactosemia) (15). A cycle of accelerated death and cell renewal may contribute to vascular architectural changes and, on exhaustion of replicative life-span, to capillary occlusion (16). Retinal cells undergo apoptosis as well, resulting in reduction in thickness of the inner plexiform and inner nuclear and ganglion layers in diabetic rats (17). Apoptosis in the photoreceptor layer of diabetic models has also been reported (18).

A major mechanism of leukocyte-mediated induction of apoptosis is via the Fas pathway. Fas (also known as Apo1/CD95) is a transmembrane protein that belongs to the tumor necrosis factor receptor (TNFR) superfamily and is widely expressed throughout most tissues. On crosslinking by FasL (a member of the TNF family that is expressed in activated immune effector cells), Fas activates caspase-8 (19,20), which then triggers the downstream apoptotic caspase cascade. Retinal endothelial cells express Fas and caspase-8, but little FasL. High glucose concentrations increase their susceptibility to Fas-mediated apoptosis (21). Neutrophils from diabetic rats have increased FasL surface expression and can induce Fas/FasL-dependent endothelial cell apoptosis, vascular damage, and blood–retinal barrier breakdown (21).

Proinflammatory Mediators in DR: Role of Cyclooxygenase-2 and TNF-α

Additional support for the notion that DR has an inflammatory component comes from documentation of a role for traditional inflammatory mediators, such as prostaglandins and the enzyme responsible for their generation, cyclooxygenase-2 (COX-2). COX-2 expression is induced in human diabetic retinas and specific COX-2 (but not COX-1) inhibitors prevent neovascularization, whereas prostaglandin E2 induces VEGF and basic fibroblast growth factor mRNA expression and exacerbates neovascularization (22,23). Preclinical evidence suggests that specific COX-2 inhibitors (such as celecoxib and meloxicam), as well as high doses of aspirin, prevent diabetic retinal leukostasis and blood–retinal barrier breakdown in DR (24–26). High-dose aspirin (50 mg/[kg·d]) and high-dose meloxicam (a selective COX-2 inhibitor) (2.0 mg/[kg d]) reduce retinal ICAM-1 expression, leukostasis, and blood–retinal barrier breakdown in diabetic animal models, as well as TNF-α levels in the diabetic retina, suggesting a role for TNF-α in the pathopysiology of DR. This hypothesis is supported by the fact that the soluble TNF-α inhibitor (TNFR-Fc, etanercept) suppresses leukostasis in this model *(24)*.

The clinical significance of the aforementioned preclinical data remains controversial, because of the lack of supportive clinical evidence for a protective effect of aspirin on early DR. In the ETDRS, aspirin (650 mg/d) did not prevent the development of high-risk proliferative retinopathy and did not reduce the risk of visual loss. At the same time, it did not increase the risk of vitreous hemorrhage (suggesting that there are no ocular contraindications to aspirin when required for cardiovascular disease or other medical indications) *(27,28)*. However, in another double-blind, randomized, controlled clinical trial (the Dipyridamole Aspirin Microangiopathy of Diabetes [DAMAD] Study Group), a slightly higher aspirin dose (330 mg three times daily) significantly slowed the progression of early DR *(29)*. Taken together, these data suggest that conventional (650 mg/d) aspirin has no protective effect on early DR (and no complications), whereas higher doses (as high as 20–50 mg/[kg·d]) *(24,26)* have shown a protective effect in preclinical studies that still await conclusive support from clinical data.

Role of Platelets in DR

Platelets are operative in hemostasis; coagulation; thrombosis; and, notably, inflammatory responses. Platelet microthrombi, leading to capillary occlusion, are more prevalent in the diabetic retina of rats and humans. Boeri et al. *(30)* demonstrated a topographic association of microthromboses with apoptotic cells in the retinal vasculature. Platelet numbers are increased in the retina as early as after 2 wk of experimental diabetes. When neutralizing anti-FasL F(ab′)2 fragments given to inhibit endothelial cell death, retinal platelet numbers are reduced to nondiabetic levels. Within seconds of platelet activation, the inflammatory mediator CD40 ligand (CD40L, CD154), a transmembrane protein that belongs in the TNF-α family, is translocated to the cell surface. CD40L binds to CD40 on endothelial cells, triggering expression of the adhesion molecules ICAM-1 and vascular cell adhesion molecule-1, and chemokines such as interleukin-8 and monocyte chemoattractant protein-1. These proinflammatory molecules facilitate the extravasation of leukocytes at sites of vascular injury. In addition, platelets contain preformed VEGF, TNF-α, and platelet-derived growth factor (PDGF), which can be released on platelet activation. Taken together, these data indicate that in addition to their hemostatic role, platelets can participate in inflammation and may release growth factors affecting the vasculature. Insulin can significantly stimulate plasminogen activator inhibitor-1 activity in endothelial cells, potentially precipitating thrombogenesis *(31)*. Platelet microthrombi and capillary occlusion can also lead to focal ischemia and hypoxia that will lead to VEGF expression and neovascularization.

Role of VEGF in DR

VEGF SIGNALING SYSTEM

VEGF, also known as vascular permeability factor, is an endothelial cell mitogen and motogen *(32)* that promotes the formation of new vessels. VEGF is also a powerful permeability factor. On a molar basis, it is 50,000 times more potent than histamine. It exists in five different isoforms of 121, 145, 165, 189, and 206 amino acids, which are derived from alternatively spliced mRNAs, of which $VEGF_{165}$ is the predominant molecular species. It binds two high-affinity receptors, the 180-kDa fms-like tyrosine kinase (Flt-1, also known as VEGFR1) and the 200-kDa kinase insert domain-containing receptor (KDR), also known as fetal liver kinase (flk) or VEGFR2,

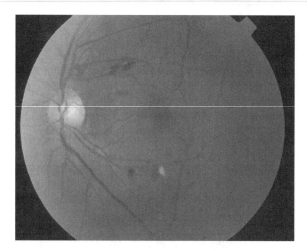

Fig. 2. NPDR. Flame-shaped, dot-blot retinal hemorrhages and "cotton-wool" spots are shown.

but KDR transduces the signals for endothelial proliferation and chemotaxis *(33,34)*. VEGF participates in the pathogenesis and progression of a wide range of angiogenesis-dependent diseases, including cancer *(32,35)*, certain inflammatory disorders *(32,35)*, and DR.

VEGF: A KEY MEDIATOR IN DR

In the eye, VEGF mediates normal retinal vascular development, as well as pathological neovascularization of the cornea, iris, retina, and choroid. Abundant evidence implicates VEGF in both preproliferative and proliferative DR *(36–43)*. VEGF mRNA and protein expression is present in retinal pigment epithelial cells, pericytes, astrocytes, glia, and endothelial cells *(44)* and VEGF levels are tightly correlated temporally and spatially with PDR. Intravitreal injections of VEGF in primates produces vascular pathology that recapitulates human DR: vessel dilation, tortuosity, microaneurysm-like formations, leukostasis, blood–retinal barrier breakdown, and neovascularization *(45)*. Intraocular VEGF levels are increased in diabetic patients with blood–retinal barrier breakdown and neovascularization *(36,41,46–48)*. Increased expression of VEGF-R2 has also been reported in diabetic retinas *(49)*. Interestingly, patients who did not develop any evidence of DR even after long-standing diabetes were found to have a deficiency in the hypoxic induction of VEGF in peripheral blood monocytes *(50)*. Specific inhibition of VEGF suppresses retinal ICAM-1–level upregulation, leukostasis, and blood–retinal barrier breakdown in animal models *(38,42,51,52)*. Therefore, regulation of VEGF expression conceivably could be both a mediator for converging local and systemic stimuli modulating vessel pathophysiology in DR, and a target for therapeutic intervention.

REGULATION OF VEGF EXPRESSION IN DR

VEGF expression can be induced by many factors associated with DR, including tissue hypoxia, hyperglycemia, advanced glycation end products (AGEs), reactive oxygen intermediates (ROIs), inflammatory mediators, insulin growth factor-1 (IGF-I), and insulin.

Hypoxia. For some types of neovascularization, including PDR, tissue ischemia and hypoxia is a very potent inducer of VEGF gene expression. Retinal VEGF expression temporally and spatially correlates with neovascularization in PDR *(53)*. Hypoxic retinal pericytes and retinal pigment epithelial cells stimulate retinal endothelial cell growth in a VEGF-dependent manner *(54)*. Hypoxia stimulates VEGF mRNA expression mainly via the inducible helix-loop-helix (bHLH)-PAS transcription factor hypoxia-inducible factor-1α (HIF-1α), which heterodimerizes with the constitutively present bHLH Per/ARNT/Sim (PAS) protein ARNT (HIF-1β) *(55–58)*, and binds to consensus and ancillary hypoxia-response elements in the VEGF promoter. In addition, hypoxia may increase the stability of VEGF mRNA *(59,60)*.

Hyperglycemia. Hyperglycemia has been implicated in VEGF stimulation via several pathways. Glucose toxicity can directly affect endothelial cell and pericyte function and viability, resulting in distorted retinal microvascular blood flow; hypoxia; and, thus, stimulation of VEGF expression. Hyperglycemia can also impair autoregulation of retinal blood flow, causing increased shear stress on the retinal blood vessels, injury, and subsequent production of VEGF *(61)*. Furthermore, hyperglycemia may induce VEGF gene expression directly via intracellular signaling pathways such as the aldose reductase pathway and the protein kinase C (PKC) pathway *(62,63)*, and via the formation of AGEs and ROIs *(64,65)*.

Advanced Glycation End Products. AGEs increase VEGF mRNA in vitro in cultured human retinal pigment epithelial (RPE) and bovine vascular smooth muscle cell levels and in vivo in the ganglion, inner nuclear, and RPE cell layers of the rat retina. Use of an anti-VEGF antibody blocked the capillary endothelial cell proliferation induced by the conditioned media of AGE-treated cells *(66)*. Albumin-AGE stimulates VEGF mRNA and protein expression in RPE cells through an extracellular signal-regulated kinase (ERK) dependent pathway that also involves an increase in accumulation of the HIF-1α protein and activation of its DNA-binding activity *(67)*. Thus, AGEs may participate in the pathogenesis of DR through their ability to increase retinal VEGF gene expression *(66)*.

Reactive Oxygen Intermediates. Superoxide and H_2O_2 rapidly stimulated VEGF mRNA levels in human RPE cells in vitro, largely through increases in VEGF mRNA stability. Reoxygenation of human RPE cells in vitro and ocular reperfusion in vivo increased retinal VEGF mRNA levels *(68)*. H_2O_2 increases macrophage VEGF through an oxidant induction of VEGF promoter *(69)*. ROIs also accelerate AGE-stimulated VEGF expression *(70)*. Attempts to use antioxidants to lower VEGF expression have been successful in animal models, with resulting improvement in vascular pathology *(71–73)*, but clinical proof in human trials is still lacking.

Prostaglandins. The role of prostaglandins in VEGF expression and the preclinical studies using COX-2 inhibitors are reported under Proinflammatory Mediators in DR.

Insulin-like Growth Factor-1. IGF-1 potently stimulates VEGF expression in the diabetic retina: vitreous IGF-1 levels correlate with the presence and severity of ischemia-associated diabetic retinal neovascularization *(74)*; intravitreal IGF-1 injection dose dependently causes retinal neovascularization and microangiopathy *(75)*; reduction in serum IGF-1 levels inhibits retinal neovascularization in an ischemic murine model *(76)*; exogenous recombinant IGF-1 exacerbated DR when administered to patients with diabetes (in an attempt to suppress growth hormone [GH] secretion and reverse insulin resistance) *(77,78)*; conversely, pituitary ablation acutely improved visual acuity and suppressed PDR, suggesting that decreases in GH and IGF-1 underlie this phenomenon *(79,80)*; and PDR is rare in dwarfs who are deficient in GH and IGF-1 *(81)*. Finally, mice with a vascular endothelial cell-specific knockout (KO) of the IGF-1 receptor are less susceptible to hypoxia-induced retinal neovascularization as compared with controls *(82)*.

In vitro, IGF-1 potently stimulates VEGF expression in RPE cells and in vivo has an additive effect with hypoxia *(83)*. Intravitreous administration of IGF-1 increased retinal Akt, c-Jun kinase (JNK), HIF-1α, nuclear factor-κB (NF-κB), and AP-1 activity, and VEGF levels. IGF-1 stimulated VEGF promoter activity in vitro, mainly via HIF-1α, and secondarily via NF-κB and activator protein (AP)-1, as demonstrated by deletional mapping of the VEGF promoter and by electrophoretic mobility shift assays (EMSA) *(84)*. Systemic inhibition of IGF-1 signaling with a receptor-neutralizing antibody, or with inhibitors of phosphatidylinositol-3-kinase (PI-3K), JNK, or Akt, suppressed retinal Akt, JNK, HIF-1α, NF-κB, and AP-1 activity; VEGF expression; as well as ICAM-1 levels, leukostasis, and blood–retinal barrier breakdown in a diabetic animal model *(84)*.

These findings, in addition to providing clinically important conclusions about the pathophysiology of DR, propose targets for pharmacological intervention to preserve vision in patients with diabetes. Compounds that inhibit the activity of the IGF-1 receptor or its downstream intracellular signaling pathways (e.g., inhibitors of PI-3K or Akt) may be novel therapeutic agents for this disease. Geldanamycin (the prototypic member of the family of ansamycin antibiotics that inhibit the hsp90 molecular chaperone, leading to depletion of several kinases, including Akt) lowered Akt and JNK enzymatic activity, VEGF levels, and vascular leakage in a rodent model of DR *(84)*. Geldanamycin analogs are currently undergoing clinical evaluation as inhibitors of growth factor-induced signaling in neoplastic diseases and have demonstrated a favorable pharmacological profile *(85)*. These compounds, as well as other inhibitors of the IGF-1 receptor or its downstream effectors, such as Akt, NF-κB, and AP-1, represent potential novel pharmacological agents for the treatment of DR.

Insulin. Acute, intensive insulin therapy transiently worsens DR and is known epidemiologically as an independent risk factor. Insulin stimulates growth of microvascular endothelial cells by upregulating VEGF mRNA. A neutralizing antibody against VEGF can completely suppress insulin-induced endothelial cell proliferation. The angiogenic effects of insulin are additive with those of hypoxia *(31)*. Mice with a vascular endothelial cell-specific KO of the insulin receptor are less susceptible to hypoxia-induced retinal neovascularization and demonstrate a blunted rise in VEGF, endothelial nitric oxide synthase (eNOS), and endothelin-1 (ET-1) *(82)*. Acute, intensive insulin therapy markedly increases VEGF mRNA and protein levels in the retinae of diabetic rats, by activating HIF-1α via a pathway that involves p38 mitogen-activated protein kinase (MAPK) and PI-3K, but not p42/p44 MAPK or PKC *(86)*. Blood–retinal barrier breakdown is markedly increased with acute, intensive insulin therapy but can be reversed by treating diabetic animals with a VEGFR–Fc fusion-soluble protein *(86)*.

WHAT ARE THE DOWNSTREAM TARGETS OF VEGF IN DR?

As mentioned previously, VEGF is primarily a mitogen for endothelial cells and drives endothelial cell proliferation and neovascularization in DR. A MAPK-dependent pathway of proliferation has been described *(87)*. VEGF may also promote endothelial cell migration and vascular permeability *(88)*. The resulting vessel leakiness promotes interstitial edema and worsens hypoxia, further stimulating VEGF production. VEGF stimulates the expression of eNOS, and the resulting nitric oxide (NO) production promotes ICAM-1 expression and leukocyte adhesion *(89)*.

VEGF also provides endothelial cells with a cytoprotective, antiapoptotic stimulus through Flk-1/KDR-mediated phosphorylation/activation of Akt *(90–93)*. Because Akt can stimulate VEGF expression, the latter may be part of an autocrine loop through which VEGF stimulates its own gene expression. Another loop may involve STAT3, because VEGF can activate STAT3 signaling in retinal microvascular endothelial cells via a VEGFR2/STAT3 complex that induces STAT3 tyrosine phosphorylation, nuclear translocation, and stimulation of VEGF expression *(94,95)*.

RISK FACTORS

Most of the studies that identified risk factors for the progression of DR involved patients with type 1 diabetes mellitus. Duration of diabetes mellitus, prior development of high-risk PDR, impaired visual acuity at baseline, high HbA1c levels, history of diabetic neuropathy, lower hematocrit, elevated triglycerides, lower serum albumin, mild to moderate nonproliferative retinopathy, and younger age (or type 1 diabetes) are all predictors for a worse outcome *(96)*.

Duration of Diabetes Mellitus

In the WESDR, the prevalence of any retinopathy among young type 1 patients was 25% at 5 yr and reached 80% at 15 yr, whereas the prevalence of PDR increased from 0% at 3 yr to 25% at 15 yr. The 4-yr incidence of retinopathy also increased with increasing duration of the disease, from 0% the first 5 yr to 28% after 14 yr. In the Pittsburgh Epidemiology of Diabetes Complications Study (PEDCS), patients between 18 and 30 yr of age with type 1 diabetes mellitus and PDR had longer duration of diabetes in relation to patients without retinopathy. The effect of the duration of the disease to the development and progression of DR is variable after 20 yr.

Hyperglycemia

In the Diabetes Control and Complications Trial (DCCT), progressive retinopathy was uncommon in patients with HbA1c values below 7%. In the WESDR, type 1 patients with higher levels of HbA1c and diabetes mellitus of <10 yr of duration were 1.5 times as likely to have any retinopathy compared with those with lower levels. Among older-onset patients, those with the highest HbA1c levels were 2.5 times more likely to develop retinopathy than those with lower levels. In the PEDCS, type 1 patients with retinopathy had higher levels of HbA1c than those without retinopathy whereas no such association was found in older ages. In parallel, in several trials of type 2 diabetes mellitus, a significantly higher risk of developing DR and progressing to PDR was associated with higher blood glucose levels, whereas there was a continuous relationship between the glycemia and the risk of microvascular disease.

In several randomized studies, institution of tight glycemic control with intensive insulin therapy resulted in "early worsening," but with a long-term delay in the progression of DR (see Insulin). It is also known that once DR reaches a certain stage, its progression becomes irreversible, even with adequate glycemic and blood pressure (BP) control ("retinopathic momentum") *(3)*.

Proteinuria and Renal Disease

Even after controlling confounding factors such as HbA1c levels, presenting age and duration of the disease, and BP, proteinuria is associated with a higher prevalence of DR and development of PDR. An association of proteinuria with background DR was found in the PEDCS in the 18 to 29-yr age group. The association was observed in type 1 patients mainly and in some studies in type 2 patients as well.

Blood Pressure

BP is a controversially discussed risk factor for the progression of DR. The UK Prospective Diabetes Study (UKPDS) showed that tight pressure control with an angiotensin-converting enzyme (ACE) inhibitor or a β-blocker reduced the risk of vision loss and progression of retinopathy, as well as mortality, from diabetes *(97)*. However, the Appropriate Blood Pressure Control in Diabetes trial (ABCD) showed that intensive BP control offers no benefit regarding to the progression of retinopathy compared with moderate control *(98)*. It seems that in young patients with type 1 diabetes mellitus, diastolic blood pressure (DBP) but not systolic blood pressure (SBP) was predictive of progression of DR, whereas both systolic and DBPs were associated with PDR. Among older-onset patients or type 2 patients, neither SBP nor DBP is associated with the progression of DR, whereas DBP <70 mmHg is a protective factor in patients with long-standing diabetes. Because hypertension is a known risk factor for heart and central nervous system (CNS) morbidity, it should be treated vigorously regardless of its effect on DR.

Pregnancy

Whereas pregnant diabetic patients without retinopathy do not experience progression of retinoplasty during pregnancy, in patients with established PDR, pregnancy is associated with progression *(99)*.

Genetic Factors

Siblings of affected patients tend to have significantly higher risk of severe DR *(100,101)*, and several studies have shown a difference in the frequency of DR among ethnic populations *(102)*. Areas in chromosomes 3 and 9 influence retinopathy and nephropathy, although a specific region dedicated for DR has not been identified *(103)*. Genes of the major histocompability complex, in particular HLA-DQ, contribute to the risk of type 1 diabetes mellitus, depending on the ethnicity of the population studied. This region is linked to the susceptibility of DR in both type 1 *(104,105)* and 2 diabetes mellitus patients *(106)*, although larger samples of adult populations are required. Other genes proposed to be linked to DR susceptibility are the aldose reductase gene (AR2) *(107–109)*, GLUT1 *(110,111)*, a number of genes involved in cellular communication and extracellular matrix homeostasis (APOE *[112]*, PAI-1 *[113]*, TNF-α *[114]*, neuropeptide Y *[115]*, G protein β3-subunit *[116]*, β3-adrenergic receptor gene *[117]*, Paroxonase 1 *[118]*, collagen IV *[119]*, and α2β integrin *[120]*), ETs (ET-1,ET-2,ET-3) *(121)*, and NOSs (NOS 1, NOS 2A, NOS 3) *(122)*, but the role of many of these candidate genes is still controversial. Lack of association with a genetic risk of DR was reported for the ACE gene *(123)*.

Sex, race, age at examination, genetic predisposition, age at diagnosis, body weight, socioeconomic status, and tobacco and alcohol use are controversial risk factors and are generally not believed to constitute risk factors for the development or progression of DR.

SCREENING

Examination by an Ophthalmologist

The diabetic patient's eye care should be a collaborative effort between the ophthalmologist and the primary care physician. It is very important for the primary care provider to know when to refer the patient for ophthalmological consultation. The early and treatable stages of DR are asymptomatic; therefore, regular checkups are essential. It is crucial to identify patients who have high risk characteristics (pregnancy, chronic hyperglycemia, hypertension, renal disease, hyperlipidemia, and cardiovascular autonomic neuropathy; see under Risk Factors). Patients with these conditions require careful medical evaluation and follow-up for the progression of DR.

Patients must be warned about the eye-threatening complications of diabetes mellitus. DR encompasses a wide spectrum of manifestations from mild to profound vision loss, and early screening and appropriate treatment determine prognosis. Patients with type 1 diabetes should be examined 3–5 yr after the disease's onset or during puberty and then yearly thereafter (unless findings requiring urgent care occur before). The examination includes a history of visual symptoms, a visual acuity measurement, measurement of intraocular pressure and a dilated fundus examination. Patients with type 2 diabetes should be examined at the time of diagnosis and then yearly thereafter. Pregnant diabetic patients should be examined prior to pregnancy for counseling, early in the first trimester, each trimester or more frequently as indicated, and then 6 wk postpartum. This does not apply for patients who develop gestational diabetes, because they are at no increased risk of developing retinopathy.

In general, patients with macular edema, severe background DR or PDR should be followed by an experienced ophthalmologist or a retina specialist, and patients with low visual potential should also be evaluated by a low-vision specialist for visual rehabilitation.

Diagnosis of DR

Diagnosis of DR can be established by fundoscopy, which reveals the characteristic lesions of NPDR (cotton wool spots, soft and hard exudates) or neovessels in PDR, which occur within the optic disc or elsewhere in the posterior pole within 45° of the disc. Fundus fluorescein angiography (FA) can be used to evaluate NVE, although not routinely; NVE can be best detected by a thorough fundus examination, with binocular indirect ophthalmoscopy combined with biomicroscopy using a lens or fundus. Optical coherence tomography (OCT) (used to measure the thickness of the retinal structures and the progression of macular edema by the interference pattern of a pair of near-infrared beams sent from a diode through the pupil of the eye as it passes through the vitreous, retina, and choroids [124,125]) can be used to detect and follow the progression of macular edema. New and experimental diagnostic methods include laser Doppler flowmetry (which measures retinal blood flow by quantifying the Doppler shifts of a laser beam that is projected to a column of moving erythrocytes [126]), scanning laser ophthalmoscopy (which measures the movement of a fixed fluorescent point along a vessel and, therefore, quantifies the movement of a plasma column in the photographic field), contrast-enhanced magnetic resonance imaging (MRI), which uses iv injection of gadolinium-diethylenetriamine pentaacetic acid to assess vascular leakage and compares in sensitivity to regular FA [127], and functional MRI (which indirectly assesses retinal oxygenation by measuring the change in retinal oxygenation when a patient breathes air with varying concentrations of oxygen [100 and 95%]). The latter method is so sensitive that it detects changes in oxygenation in areas of a few hundred micrometers (128).

COMPLICATIONS OF DR AND CLINICAL MECHANISM OF VISION LOSS

Macular Disease

As mentioned, macular edema results from the breakdown of the blood–retinal barrier that occurs early in DR and can result in vision loss in both NPDR and PDR. Additionally, central vision can be endangered by various insults to the macula: nonperfusion of parafoveal capillaries, traction of the macula (from fibrovascular proliferation) with or without detachment, intra- or preretinal hemorrhage, or retinal holes.

Vitreous and Preretinal Hemorrhage

Hemorrhage from neovessels can be confined to the vitreous face (the most anterior portion of the vitreous), where it and is usually easily cleared, or to the vitreous cavity, where it and usually requires months to be absorbed. Neovessels can bleed from Valsava maneuvers or from avulsion of retinal vessels from vitreous or fibrovascular membrane traction.

Vitreous Traction and Fibrovascular Proliferation

During the course of neovessel formation, fibrous tissue accompanies the new vessels and contracts over time, resulting in vitreous detachment and traction retinal detachment that can vary in severity and extent. Fibrovascular tissue can develop in the macular region and lead to distortion of the macula that can significantly reduce visual acuity.

Rubeosis

Retinal ischemia, long-standing retinal detachment, and fibrovascular proliferation can cause iris neovascularization (rubeosis), which consists of a fine vascular network within the iris that can cross the scleral spur of the angle and block the outflow path for aqueous humor, causing neovascular glaucoma, a condition difficult to treat that can lead to a painful eye with rapidly progressing visual loss.

Involutional PDR

The end result of DR is the involutional stage, characterized by a variable visual outcome; complete vitreous detachment, usually with retinal detachment; optic disc pallor; attenuated arterioles; and rarely microaneurysms, hemorrhages, and pigmentary RPE changes. Macular edema, ischemia or detachment, or optic nerve disease can account for the observed visual loss.

PREVENTION

Glycemic Control

The most effective approach for primary prevention of DR, as well as for delaying of the rate of progression, is intensive glycemic control. In the DCCT, tight glucose control reduced the risk of development and progression of DR and other complications of type 1 diabetes mellitus, despite an insulin-induced "early worsening" of DR *(129)*. Owing to the large long-term risk reduction with intensive treatment, outcomes in intensively treated patients who had early worsening were similar to or more favorable than outcomes in conventionally treated patients who had no early worsening. The most important risk factors for early worsening were higher HbA1c level, particularly if retinopathy

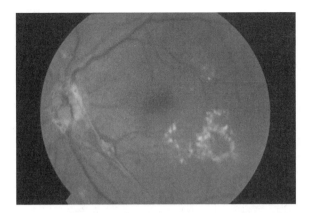

Fig. 3. Clinically significant macular edema. Circinate exudates are seen around the macula with the characteristic yellowish appearance deep to the retinal vessels. An area of fibrovascular traction is shown near the optic disk.

was at or past the moderate nonproliferative stage. In patients whose retinopathy is already approaching the high-risk stage, it may be prudent to delay the initiation of intensive treatment until prophylactic photocoagulation can be completed, particularly if HbA1c is high. The reduction in the risk of DR resulting from prior intensive therapy in patients with type 1 diabetes persists for at least 4 yr, despite increasing hyperglycemia after the end of intensive therapy *(130)*. Intensive therapy was most effective when initiated early in the course of type 1 diabetes mellitus *(131)*. Therefore, patients with type 1 diabetes mellitus have to aim for levels of HbA1c close to the nondiabetic range *(132)*.

BP Control

Hypertension, and particularly diastolic hypertension, is a likely risk factor for the development and progression of DR *(133)*; the UKPDS showed that tight control of BP with an ACE inhibitor or a β-blocker reduced significantly the deterioration of visual function in diabetic patients. However, the EUCLID study *(134)* investigated the effect of ACE inhibitors in normotensive diabetic adults and suggested that this drug class may have BP-independent effects on the progression of DR, and there is an ongoing larger study to investigate the effects of ACE inhibitors. Short-term losartan treatment of type 2 patients with macular edema and hard exudates (diabetic maculopathy) does not seem to have a beneficial effect, although long-term studies are required *(135)*. Because hypertension is a known risk factor for heart and CNS morbidity, it should be treated vigorously regardless of its effect on DR.

Lipid Control

Elevated serum lipids, particularly increased cholesterol levels, are associated with the presence of retinal hard exudates in macular edema in patients with type 1 diabetes mellitus *(136)*. Severe hard exudates can lead to subretinal fibrosis and visual deterioration. For more on clinical studies using lipid-lowering agents, see under Lipid-Lowering Agents.

Follow-Up

Equally important as tight glycemic control are regular, comprehensive eye examinations for all individuals with diabetes mellitus. Most diabetic eye disease can be

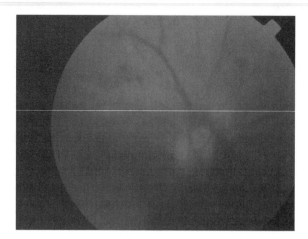

Fig. 4. Severe PDR. An area of vitreous hemorrhage is shown inferiorly. In addition, areas of scattered retinal hemorrhages are present.

successfully treated if detected early. Routine, nondilated eye examinations by the primary care provider or diabetes specialist are *inadequate* to detect diabetic eye diseases properly. The treatment of diabetic eye diseases requires an ophthalmologist experienced in these disorders.

The controversy regarding the effect of antiplatelet agents was discussed earlier (see under Proinflammatory Mediators in DR).

TREATMENT OF DR

Conventional Management

The current therapeutic options available for the treatment of DR, such as laser photocoagulation and vitrectomy, do not completely prevent progression. Scattered laser photocoagulation is used in the treatment of PDR and involves the placement of 200–1600 argon blue-green or krypton red laser burns on the midperipheral retina in two or more sessions. Focal photocoagulation is used for the treatment of diabetic macular edema and involves the focal placement of argon green laser burns on capillaries and microaneurysms that appear leaky during FA between 500 and 3000 μm from the center of the macula. Eyes complicated with nonclearing vitreous hemorrhage precluding the view to the back or eyes with traction retinal detachment involving the fovea, combined traction-rhegmatogenous retinal detachment, or epiretinal membrane formation can benefit from vitrectomy.

Three multicenter, randomized, controlled clinical trials sponsored by the National Eye Institute (NEI) investigated the role of scattered laser photocoagulation and vitrectomy surgery on the management of DR. The Diabetic Retinopathy Study (DRS) showed a reduction with laser photocoagulation treatment in neovascularization and vision loss in patients with severe NPDR or PDR that persisted for 5 yr. Although the DRS showed that there is a moderate risk of visual acuity reduction from the laser treatment, this outweighed by far the benefits for eyes with high-risk PDR *(137)*. The complications of laser photocoagulation can present in the immediate postoperative period or long term and include macular edema or burn, choroidal or retinal detachment, pain during treatment, increased intraocular pressure, and corneal abrasions that can lead to permanent visual loss or disability.

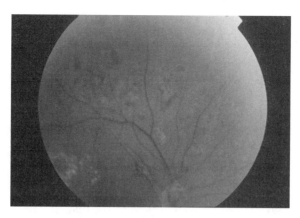

Fig. 5. Fundus appearance after laser scatter photocoagulation. Pigmented atrophic scars were generated in the retinal periphery.

Laser treatment is not recommended in mild to moderate NPDR. The Early Treatment Diabetic Retinopathy Study showed that treatment with photocoagulation is not beneficial for eyes with mild or moderate NPDR until high-risk characteristics are observed, but it is beneficial for the treatment of clinically significant macular edema *(138,139)*. It identified three factors that were predictive of progression: venous beading, intraretinal microvascular abnormalities, and hemorrhages/microaneurysms. It also showed that aspirin did not affect the course of the retinopathy in patients with mild or moderate NPDR *(27,28)*. On the contrary, the DAMAD study assessed higher doses of aspirin and dipyridamole and concluded that aspirin may have a protective role against the progression of retinopathy in NPDR *(29)* (see also Proinflammatory Mediators in DR).

The Diabetic Retinopathy Vitrectomy Study (DRVS) showed that vitrectomy surgery is efficacious in the management of type 1 diabetes mellitus patients with nonclearing vitreous hemorrhage and/or active fibrovascular proliferation *(140)*. With subsequent substantial improvements in technique and instrumentation, surgeons currently intervene with vitrectomy for a broader range of indications. High-risk PDR requires initial scatter laser photocoagulation treatment (because the greatest threat to vision is traction retinal detachment, especially involving the macula, rather than vitreous hemorrhage), or focal photocoagulation if clinically significant macular edema (CSME) is present. Patients with type 1 diabetes may benefit from vitrectomy earlier than those with type 2 diabetes. Complications from vitrectomy include corneal injury, cataract formation, postoperative hemorrhage with ghost cell glaucoma, iris and angle neovascularization, and anterior hyaloidal fibrovascular proliferation.

Patients without DR are not at increased risk of progression after cataract surgery *(141)*, but those with substantial DR may suffer worsening *(142)*. Eyes with active PDR and cataract are better treated with combined cataract removal and pars plana vitrectomy with intraoperative endolaser. The use of oral or local nonsteroidal anti-inflammatory drugs and close follow-up postoperatively is advised in patients with diabetes because of the high incidence of macular edema.

Attempts to treat diabetic macula edema with pars plana vitrectomy with internal limiting membrane peeling gave mixed results. Currently, intravitreal steroid injections are preferable for this indication [see under Intravitreal Steroids (Triamcinolone)].

Emerging and Experimental Treatments

Even with laser treatment available, DR remains one of the primary causes of vision loss, leading to the increased need for new treatments. Pharmacological therapy that improves the metabolic control or prevents the biochemical sequela of hyperglycemia, such as aldose reductase inhibitors (ARIs), AGE, or PKC inhibitors, could be an alternative as a stand-alone treatment or in combination with laser therapy. Neovascularization in PDR can be targeted with inhibitors of growth factors that are responsible for angiogenesis, such as IGF-1 and VEGF, or inhibitors of integrins (a-v, b-3), intracellular signal transduction cascades (MAPK, PKC), or intravitreous steroids.

INTRAVITREAL STEROIDS (TRIAMCINOLONE)

Corticosteroids have been traditionally used for many years for the treatment of intraocular inflammation and to suppress blood–retinal barrier breakdown and fluid extravasation into the retinal tissue. Based on the above clinical observations (*see* "DR: An Undiagnosed Chronic Inflammatory Disease"), Machamer suggested that intravitreal application of a crystalline form of cortisone that creates a vitreal "depot" of the drug could be used to suppress the intraocular inflammation and cellular proliferation that characterizes aggressive vitreoretinopathies *(143,144)*. Intravitreal injection of triamcinolone acetonide improved visual acuity in diabetes mellitus patients with clinically significant diffuse macular edema who had received no prior treatment *(145)* and even in patients in whom prior laser photocoagulation had failed *(146)*. Intravitreal triamcinolone induced regression of iris neovascularization in a small series of 14 patients and can be used as an adjuvant therapy for neovascular glaucoma *(147)*. Intravitreal triamcinolone is also used as an adjuvant treatment in PDR after vitrectomy to reduce intraocular inflammation *(148)*, although its use to reduce the risk of pseudophakic macular edema after cataract surgery remains controversial *(149)*. It should be noted that the formulation of triamcinolone currently used is not manufactured specifically for intravitreal use. An NEI-sponsored trial is under way to investigate a new preservative-free formulation of triamcinolone.

ANTIHYPERTENSIVES: ACE INHIBITORS

In the EUCLID study, lisinopril delayed the progression of DR in nonhypertensive patients with type 1 diabetes mellitus and no nephropathy *(134)*. A decrease in SBP by 30 mmHg against placebo was enough to decrease the risk of DR progression by 50% and the progression to PDR by 80%. However, the presence of other confounding factors and the fact that DR was not one of the primary end points of the EUCLID study raised concerns. The ABCD *(98)* and Heart Outcomes Prevention Evaluation *(150)* studies, which included DR as one of their primary end points, did not support the EUCLID conclusion that ACE inhibitors might be beneficial. Short-term losartan treatment of type 2 patients with macular edema and hard exudates (diabetic maculopthy) does not seem to have a beneficial effect, although long-term studies are required *(135)*.

LIPID-LOWERING AGENTS

Deregulated lipid metabolism contributes to the microvascular alterations in DR by activating the coagulation-fibrinolysis system, inducing endothelial injury and subsequent death, and increasing vascular permeability. HMG-CoA reductase inhibitors are potential therapeutic candidates for DR partly owing to their strong lipid effects. Oral administration of lipid-lowering agents such as atorvastatin or simvastatin in type 1 diabetes mellitus patients with dyslipidemia reduces the severity of hard exudates and lipid migration *(151–153)*. Although these data are based on short-term studies and the need for long-term studies is obvious before clinical guidelines can be established, it is generally agreed that aggressive management of diabetic dyslipidemia would benefit both macrovascular and microvascular diabetic disease.

ALDOSE REDUCTASE INHIBITORS

Early trials involving the ARIs sorbinil and polarnestat were complicated by serious side effects and failed to demonstrate a favorable effect on DR *(154,155)*. Newer compounds have shown promising results in preclinical studies. ARIs such as WAY-121,509 prevented galactose-induced cataract formation and retinal microvascular abnormalities in diabetic dogs *(156)*. ARI-509 and aminoguanidine prevent or delay DR and VEGF upregulation *(157)*. Epalrestat (Kinedak) was found to prevent the galactose-induced loss of corneal barrier function *(158)*, whereas SG-210 *(159)*, which is currently in clinical trials in Japan and the United States, reduces the formation of cataract.

AGE INHIBITORS

Aminoguanidine was one of the original AGE inhibitors. The clinical trial that was designed to determine the effectiveness of aminoguanidine in humans was prematurely stopped owing to financial reasons *(160)*. Preliminary results from a phase III trial involving aminoguanidine show a beneficial effect in the progression of DR but its use is associated with mild anemia *(161)*. Two AGE inhibitors, pimagedine and the crosslink breaker ALT-711, have shown a favorable pharmacokinetic profile in preclinical trials and have demonstrated a reduction in the severity of AGE-related pathologies *(162)*. ALT-711 reduced blood pressure in patients with diabetes *(162)*. Administration of pimagedine in patients with type 1 diabetes demonstrated a reduction in the progression of DR *(161)*.

PKC INHIBITORS

PKC activation results in a variety of metabolic and cellular abnormalities, such as increased expression of connective-tissue proteins, growth factors, and mediators that contribute to the basement membrane thickening and decrease in retinal blood flow characteristics of DR microangiopathy. Among the PKC isoforms, PKCβ is preferentially activated in DR and is a crucial element of the VEGF signaling cascade that mediates ocular neovascularization and macular edema. Oral administration of LY333531 (ruboxistaurin; Eli Lilly), a specific PKCβ inhibitor, in diabetes mellitus patients with minimal or no retinopathy had a dose-dependent normalizing effect on retinal blood flow without significant side effects *(163)*. However, the Protein Kinase C β-Inhibitor Diabetic Retinopathy Study (PKC-DRS) failed to demonstrate a significant impact of ruboxistaurin on the progression of DR *(164,165)*. A subgroup analysis indicated a slower progression of diabetic macular edema in patients treated with the highest dose of ruboxistaurin, compared to placebo, which was thought to warrant further investigation. Oral administration of another inhibitor, PKC412, at doses of 100 mg/d in diabetes mellitus patients with macular edema reduced significantly retinal thickening and improved visual acuity without significant side effects *(166,167)*.

ANTIOXIDANTS

Glucose-stimulated production of free radicals is associated with microvascular damage in diabetes, and normalization of this production has been shown to halt vascular endothelial damage through a variety of pathways *(168)*. High-dose vitamin E therapy has normalized retinal blood flow in patients with diabetes without affecting glycemic control *(169,170)*. Further clinical trials are needed to determine the dose and long-term effectiveness of antioxidants in DR and macular edema.

ANTITHROMBOTIC AGENTS AND COX-2 INHIBITORS

The combination of decreased antithrombotic function of the endothelium and platelet activation leads to a prothrombotic state and retinal ischemia in diabetes mellitus. Although the ETDRS concluded that aspirin treatment did not affect the development and progression of DR, the DAMAD study showed that aspirin alone in higher doses or in combination with dipyridamole delayed the progression of DR *(29)* (*see* also under Proinflammatory Mediators in DR). Because higher doses of aspirin can have troublesome side effects, such as increased risk of bleeding and gastrointestinal ulcers, when given long-term in patients with diabetes, an active search for equally efficient alternatives was undertaken. COX-2 inhibitors suppress DR progression in various animal models *(24)*. The COX-2 inhibitor rofecoxib is currently undergoing a small-scale clinical trial in patients with diabetic macular edema. The TIMAD study showed that ticlopidine, a IIa/IIIb inhibitor, delayed the formation of microaneurysms *(171)*. Defibrotide, a compound with profibrinolytic effects, was shown to improve visual acuity and other ophthalmological parameters of retinal function in a small-scale trial with type 1 diabetes mellitus patients *(172)*.

ENDOTHELINS: NO

ETs, especially ET-1 and ET-3, have vasocontrictive properties, whereas prostacyclin and NO induce vasodilation. Alteration of this delicate balance between vasoconstriction and vasodilation in diabetes mellitus with increased ET expression and a deficit in prostacyclin and NO correlates with the progression of DR. Inhibition of ETs or facilitation of prostacyclin or NO action can be used as a therapeutic target in DR. Although ET receptor inhibitors have shown favorable pharmacokinetic profiles and beneficial effects in experimental DR models, they have not been used in large-scale controlled trials yet. Another vasoactive drug that increases NO production and potentiates its effects is calcium dobesilate (doxium), which reduced the blood hyperviscosity, intraocular pressure, blood–retinal barrier breakdown, and retinal hemorrhages and improved the visual fields of patients with DR *(173,174)*.

ANTIANGIOGENIC THERAPY

Although an angiogenesis inhibitor is not yet approved for use in DR, more than 30 antiangiogenic agents are currently in clinical trials. Owing to its pivotal role in DR, VEGF signaling has been the target of many preclinical and ongoing clinical studies using agents such as neutralizing monoclonal antibodies *(175)*, VEGFR–Fc fusion soluble protein *(86)*, receptor tyrosine kinase inhibitors *(176)* (SU5416 *[177]*, SU6668 *[178]*, ZD6474 *[179]*, CP-547,632 *[180,181]*, PTK787, and ZD4190 *[182]*), or ribozymes (angiozyme *[183]*). EYE001 (macugen) is a pegylated antisense RNA oligonucleotide that binds to VEGF165, preventing its action (aptamer) *(184)*. Phase I trials with macugen have established the systemic safety of a single intravitreous injection, and noncontrolled II/III trials showed encouraging preliminary results in exudative age-related macular degeneration *(184)*. Additionally, there are various other agents that downregulate VEGF expression in experimental models of DR, such as ACE inhibitors and pentoxifylline. Pentoxifyllin is well tolerated, increases ocular blood flow in healthy volunteers and almost normalized choroidal blood flow in a study of patients with NPDR *(185,186)*, and it decreases erythrocyte friability, fibrinogen levels, and microvascular complications *(187)*.

Other promising approaches involve various proteins with antiangiogenic properties (angiostatin and endostatin *[188,189]*, platelet factor-4 *[190]*, and the Tie-angiopoietin system *[191]*), inhibitors of matrix metalloproteinases (BB-3644 *[192]*, AG3340 *[193,194]*, metastat *[195]*, neovastat *[196,197]*, CGS-27023A *[198]*, Bay-129566), inhibitors of PDGF (SU101 *[199]*), and inhibitors of integrins responsible for the interaction of the endothelial cell with the extracellular matrix (EMD121974 *[200]*, Vitaxin *[201]*). Peroxisome proliferator-activated receptor γ agonists have antiangiogenic activity, in addition to their effect on blood glucose levels *[207,203]*. Levels of pigment epithelium-derived factor (PEDF) in the aqueous humor are decreased in DR *(198,204,205)* and exogenous PEDF administration has reduced retinal neovascularization in various animal models of ocular disease *(206)*. A dose-escalation phase I clinical trial of adenovirally mediated PEDF is currently ongoing in patients with advanced neovascular age-related macular degeneration (AMD) *(207)* that will identify the maximum tolerated dose and activity of adenovirally encoded PEDF, which can lead to a similar study for DR.

SOMATOSTATIN ANALOGS

Octreotide has been shown to retard the progression of DR in patients with severe NPDR or early non-high-risk PDR and reduce the number of vitreous hemorrhages, while preserving visual acuity in a small-scale trial *(208,209)*. A small trial of the GH inhibitor pegvisomant in patients with non-high-risk PDR failed to demonstrate a significant effect and induce reduction of neovascularization *(210)*. Clinical trials with long-acting somatostatin analogs are currently in progress and they constitute a promising treatment for patients who fail panretinal photocoagulation.

GENE THERAPY

Intraocular in vivo gene delivery has been proposed to treat DR by delivering "suicide genes" to specifically target abnormally proliferating fibroblasts and RPE cells using a retroviral vector (herpes simplex virus) to deliver the gene thymidine kinase in the target cells and, therefore, make them susceptible to the cytotoxic effects of ganciclovir *(211)*. This method has been used in various experimental models with success even when the viral transduction efficiency is low *(211,212)*. VEGF expression can be targeted with antisense or ribozyme gene therapy. Another proposed approach that could be useful in cases of retinal detachment would be to prevent the death of photoreceptors and retinal cells via the intravitreal injection of neuroprotective growth factors such as brain-derived neurotrophic factor *(213)*. Neovascularization can also be targeted with the forced expression of antiangiogenic molecules such as angiostatin or endostatin in RPE cells *(212)*. Although there is significant excitement about the envisioned uses of gene therapy, there is justified skepticism regarding unique challenges on the translational application of this proposed therapy.

CONCLUSIONS

DR is a major cause of vision loss in Western societies. Tight glycemic control is the mainstay of current medical management. Appropriate surgical therapy with photocoagulation or vitrectomy can delay progression and preserve vision. Recent advances in the knowledge of the pathophysiology of DR and elucidation of its inflammatory and angiogenic mechanisms have identified numerous therapeutic targets and herald an era of very active clinical research for new, effective, and safe targeted therapies.

REFERENCES

1. Klein R, Klein BE, Moss SE. Visual impairment in diabetes. Ophthalmology 1984;91(1):1–9.
2. Klein BE, Davis MD, Segal P, et al. Diabetic retinopathy: assessment of severity and progression. Ophthalmology 1984;91(1):10–17.
3. Williams R, Airey M, Baxter H, Forrester J, Kennedy-Martin T, Girach A. Epidemiology of diabetic retinopathy and macular oedema: a systematic review. Eye 2004;18:963–983.
4. Klein R, Klein BE, Moss SE, DeMets DL, Kaufman I, Voss PS. Prevalence of diabetes mellitus in southern Wisconsin. Am J Epidemiol 1984;119(1):54–61.
5. Klein R, Klein BE, Moss SE. The Wisconsin epidemiologic study of diabetic retinopathy: an update. Aust N Z J Ophthalmol 1990;18(1):19–22.
6. Klein R, Klein BE, Moss SE. Relation of glycemic control to diabetic microvascular complications in diabetes mellitus. Ann Intern Med 1996;124(1 Pt 2):90–96.
7. Klein R, Klein BEK. Diabetic eye disease. Lancet 1997;350(9072):197–204.
8. Miller JW, Adamis AP, Shima DT, et al. Vascular endothelial growth factor/vascular permeability factor is temporally and spatially correlated with ocular angiogenesis in a primate model. Am J Pathol 1994;145(3):574–584.
9. Joussen AM, Poulaki V, Mitsiades N, et al. Suppression of Fas-FasL-induced endothelial cell apoptosis prevents diabetic blood–retinal barrier breakdown in a model of streptozotocin-induced diabetes. FASEB J 2003;17(1):76–78.
10. McLeod DS, Lefer DJ, Merges C, Lutty GA. Enhanced expression of intracellular adhesion molecule-1 and P-selectin in the diabetic human retina and choroid. Am J Pathol 1995;147(3):642–653.
11. Barouch FC, Miyamoto K, Allport JR, et al. Integrin-mediated neutrophil adhesion and retinal leukostasis in diabetes. Invest Ophthalmol Vis Sci 2000;41(5):1153–1158.
12. Miyamoto K, Khosrof S, Bursell SE, et al. Prevention of leukostasis and vascular leakage in streptozotocin-induced diabetic retinopathy via intercellular adhesion molecule-1 inhibition. Proc Nat Acad Sci USA 1999;96(19):10,836–10,841.
13. Miyamoto K, Khosrof S, Bursell S-E, et al. Vascular endothelial growth factor (VEGF)–induced retinal vascular permeability is mediated by intercellular adhesion molecule-1 (ICAM-1). Am J Pathol 2000;156(5):1733–1739.
14. Joussen AM, Murata T, Tsujikawa A, Kirchhof B, Bursell SE, Adamis AP. Leukocyte-mediated endothelial cell injury and death in the diabetic retina. Am J Pathol 2001;158(1):147–152.
15. Kern TS, Engerman RL. A mouse model of diabetic retinopathy. Arch Ophthalmol 1996;114(8):986–990.
16. Mizutani M, Kern TS, Lorenzi M. Accelerated death of retinal microvascular cells in human and experimental diabetic retinopathy. J Clin Invest 1996;97(12):2883–2890.
17. Barber AJ, Lieth E, Khin SA, Antonetti DA, Buchanan AG, Gardner TW. Neural apoptosis in the retina during experimental and human diabetes: early onset and effect of insulin. J Clin Invest 1998;102(4):783–791.
18. Park SH, Park JW, Park SJ, et al. Apoptotic death of photoreceptors in the streptozotocin-induced diabetic rat retina. Diabetologia 2003;46(9):1260–1268.
19. Muzio M, Stockwell BR, Stennicke HR, Salvesen GS, Dixit VM. An induced proximity model for caspase-8 activation. J Biol Chem 1998;273(5):2926–2930.
20. Salvesen GS, Dixit VM. Caspase activation: the induced-proximity model. Proc Natl Acad Sci USA 1999;96(20):10,964–10,967.
21. Joussen AM, Poulaki V, Mitsiades N, et al. Suppression of Fas-FasL-induced endothelial cell apoptosis prevents diabetic blood–retinal barrier breakdown in a model of streptozotocin-induced diabetes. FASEB J 2003;17(1):76–78.
22. Cheng T, Cao W, Wen R, Steinberg RH, LaVail MM. Prostaglandin E2 induces vascular endothelial growth factor and basic fibroblast growth factor mRNA expression in cultured rat Muller cells. Invest Ophthalmol Vis Sci 1998;39(3):581–591.

23. Sennlaub F, Valamanesh F, Vazquez-Tello A, et al. Cyclooxygenase-2 in human and experimental ischemic proliferative retinopathy. Circulation 2003;108(2):198–204.

24. Joussen AM, Poulaki V, Mitsiades N, et al. Nonsteroidal anti-inflammatory drugs prevent early diabetic retinopathy via TNF-alpha suppression. FASEB J 2002;16(3):438–440.

25. Ayalasomayajula SP, Kompella UB. Celecoxib, a selective cyclooxygenase-2 inhibitor, inhibits retinal vascular endothelial growth factor expression and vascular leakage in a streptozotocin-induced diabetic rat model. Eur J Pharmacol 2003;458(3):283–289.

26. Kern TS, Engerman RL. Pharmacological inhibition of diabetic retinopathy: aminoguanidine and aspirin. Diabetes 2001;50(7):1636–1642.

27. Early Treatment Diabetic Retinopathy Study Research Group. Effects of aspirin treatment on diabetic retinopathy. ETDRS report number 8. Ophthalmology 1991;98(5 Suppl):757–765.

28. Chew EY, Klein ML, Murphy RP, Remaley NA, Ferris FL 3rd. Effects of aspirin on vitreous/preretinal hemorrhage in patients with diabetes mellitus. Early Treatment Diabetic Retinopathy Study report no. 20. Arch Ophthalmol 1995;113(1):52–55.

29. The DAMAD Study Group. Effect of aspirin alone and aspirin plus dipyridamole in early diabetic retinopathy: A multicenter randomized controlled clinical trial. Diabetes 1989;38(4):491–498.

30. Boeri D, Maiello M, Lorenzi M. Increased prevalence of microthromboses in retinal capillaries of diabetic individuals. Diabetes 2001;50(6):1432–1439.

31. Yamagishi S, Kawakami T, Fujimori H, et al. Insulin stimulates the growth and tube formation of human microvascular endothelial cells through autocrine vascular endothelial growth factor. Microvasc Res 1999;57(3):329–339.

32. Folkman J. Tumor angiogenesis. In: Bast RC, Kufe DW, Pollock RE, et al, eds. Cancer Medicine. B.C. Decker Hamilton, Ontario, 2000, pp. 132–152.

33. Senger DR, Galli SJ, Dvorak AM, Perruzzi CA, Harvey VS, Dvorak HF. Tumor cells secrete a vascular permeability factor that promotes accumulation of ascites fluid. Science 1983;219(4587): 983–985.

34. Ferrara N, Houck K, Jakeman L, Leung DW. Molecular and biological properties of the vascular endothelial growth factor family of proteins. Endocr Rev 1992;13(1):18–32.

35. Folkman J. Seminars in Medicine of the Beth Israel Hospital, Boston: clinical applications of research on angiogenesis. N Engl J Med 1995;333(26):1757–1763.

36. Aiello LP, Avery RL, Arrigg PG, et al. Vascular endothelial growth factor in ocular fluid of patients with diabetic retinopathy and other retinal disorders. N Engl J Med 1994;331(22):1480–1487.

37. Aiello LP, Wong JS. Role of vascular endothelial growth factor in diabetic vascular complications. Kidney Int Suppl 2000;77:S113–S119.

38. Qaum T, Xu Q, Joussen AM, et al. VEGF-initiated blood–retinal barrier breakdown in early diabetes. Invest Ophthalmol Vis Sci 2001;42(10):2408–2413.

39. Miller JW, Adamis AP, Shima DT, et al. Vascular endothelial growth factor/vascular permeability factor is temporally and spatially correlated with ocular angiogenesis in a primate model. Am J Pathol 1994;145(3):574–584.

40. Tolentino MJ, Miller JW, Gragoudas ES, Chatzistefanou K, Ferrara N, Adamis AP. Vascular endothelial growth factor is sufficient to produce iris neovascularization and neovascular glaucoma in a nonhuman primate. Arch Ophthalmol 1996;114(8):964–970.

41. Adamis AP, Miller JW, Bernal MT, et al. Increased vascular endothelial growth factor levels in the vitreous of eyes with proliferative diabetic retinopathy. Am J Ophthalmol 1994;118(4):445–450.

42. Adamis AP, Shima DT, Tolentino MJ, et al. Inhibition of vascular endothelial growth factor prevents retinal ischemia-associated iris neovascularization in a nonhuman primate. Arch Ophthalmol 1996;114(1):66–71.

43. Joussen AM, Poulaki V, Qin W, et al. Retinal vascular endothelial growth factor induces intercellular adhesion molecule-1 and endothelial nitric oxide synthase expression and initiates early diabetic retinal leukocyte adhesion in vivo. Am J Pathol 2002;160(2):501–509.

44. Caldwell RB, Bartoli M, Behzadian MA, et al. Vascular endothelial growth factor and diabetic retinopathy: pathophysiological mechanisms and treatment perspectives. Diabetes Metab Res Rev 2003;19(6):442–455.

45. Adamis AP, Shima DT, Tolentino MJ, et al. Inhibition of vascular endothelial growth factor prevents retinal ischemia-associated iris neovascularization in a nonhuman primate. Arch Ophthalmol 1996;114(1):66–71.

46. Aiello LP, Avery RL, Arrigg PG, et al. Vascular endothelial growth factor in ocular fluid of patients with diabetic retinopathy and other retinal disorders. N Engl J Med 1994;331(22):1480–1487.

47. Malecaze F, Clamens S, Simorre-Pinatel V, et al. Detection of vascular endothelial growth factor messenger RNA and vascular endothelial growth factor-like activity in proliferative diabetic retinopathy. Arch Ophthalmol 1994;112(11):1476–1482.

48. Murata T, Ishibashi T, Khalil A, Hata Y, Yoshikawa H, Inomata H. Vascular endothelial growth factor plays a role in hyperpermeability of diabetic retinal vessels. Ophthalmic Res 1995;27(1):48–52.

49. Gilbert RE, Vranes D, Berka JL, et al. Vascular endothelial growth factor and its receptors in control and diabetic rat eyes. Lab Invest 1998;78(8):1017–1027.

50. Marsh S, Nakhoul FM, Skorecki K, et al. Hypoxic induction of vascular endothelial growth factor is markedly decreased in diabetic individuals who do not develop retinopathy. Diabetes Care 2000;23(9):1375–1380.

51. Aiello LP, Pierce EA, Foley ED, et al. Suppression of retinal neovascularization in vivo by inhibition of vascular endothelial growth factor (VEGF) using soluble VEGF-receptor chimeric proteins. Proc Natl Acad Sci USA 1995;92(23):10,457–10,461.

52. Aiello LP, Pierce EA, Foley ED, et al. Suppression of retinal neovascularization in vivo by inhibition of vascular endothelial growth factor (VEGF) using soluble VEGF-receptor chimeric proteins. Proc Natl Acad Sci USA 1995;92(23):10,457–10,461.

53. Pe'er J, Shweiki D, Itin A, Hemo I, Gnessin H, Keshet E. Hypoxia-induced expression of vascular endothelial growth factor by retinal cells is a common factor in neovascularizing ocular diseases. Lab Invest 1995;72(6):638–645.

54. Aiello LP, Northrup JM, Keyt BA, Takagi H, Iwamoto MA. Hypoxic regulation of vascular endothelial growth factor in retinal cells. Arch Ophthalmol 1995;113(12):1538–1544.

55. Pollenz RS, Sullivan HR, Holmes J, Necela B, Peterson RE. Isolation and expression of cDNAs from rainbow trout (Oncorhynchus mykiss) that encode two novel basic helix-loop-Helix/PER-ARNT-SIM (bHLH/PAS) proteins with distinct functions in the presence of the aryl hydrocarbon receptor: evidence for alternative mRNA splicing and dominant negative activity in the bHLH/PAS family. J Biol Chem 1996;271(48):30,886–30,896.

56. Jiang BH, Semenza GL, Bauer C, Marti HH. Hypoxia-inducible factor 1 levels vary exponentially over a physiologically relevant range of O2 tension. Am J Physiol 1996;271(4 Pt 1):C1172–C1180.

57. Wang GL, Jiang BH, Rue EA, Semenza GL. Hypoxia-inducible factor 1 is a basic-helix-loop-helix-PAS heterodimer regulated by cellular O_2 tension. Proc Natl Acad Sci USA 1995;92(12):5510–5514.

58. Wang GL, Semenza GL. Purification and characterization of hypoxia-inducible factor 1. J Biol Chem 1995;270(3):1230–1237.

59. Levy AP, Levy NS, Goldberg MA. Hypoxia-inducible protein binding to vascular endothelial growth factor mRNA and its modulation by the von Hippel–Lindau protein. J Biol Chem 1996;271(41): 25,492–25,497.

60. Levy AP, Levy NS, Goldberg MA. Post-transcriptional regulation of vascular endothelial growth factor by hypoxia. J Biol Chem 1996;271(5):2746–2753.

61. Gan L, Miocic M, Doroudi R, Selin-Sjogren L, Jern S. Distinct regulation of vascular endothelial growth factor in intact human conduit vessels exposed to laminar fluid shear stress and pressure. Biochem Biophys Res Commun 2000;272(2):490–496.

62. Williams B, Gallacher B, Patel H, Orme C. Glucose-induced protein kinase C activation regulates vascular permeability factor mRNA expression and peptide production by human vascular smooth muscle cells in vitro. Diabetes 1997;46(9):1497–1503.

63. Aiello LP, Bursell SE, Clermont A, et al. Vascular endothelial growth factor–induced retinal permeability is mediated by protein kinase C in vivo and suppressed by an orally effective beta-isoform-selective inhibitor. Diabetes 1997;46(9):1473–1480.

64. Ellis EA, Guberski DL, Somogyi-Mann M, Grant MB. Increased H2O2, vascular endothelial growth factor and receptors in the retina of the BBZ/Wor diabetic rat. Free Radic Biol Med 2000; 28(1):91–101.

65. El-Remessy AB, Behzadian MA, Abou-Mohamed G, Franklin T, Caldwell RW, Caldwell RB. Experimental diabetes causes breakdown of the blood–retina barrier by a mechanism involving tyrosine nitration and increases in expression of vascular endothelial growth factor and urokinase plasminogen activator receptor. Am J Pathol 2003;162(6):1995–2004.

66. Lu M, Kuroki M, Amano S, et al. Advanced glycation end products increase retinal vascular endothelial growth factor expression. J Clin Invest 1998;101(6):1219–1224.

67. Treins C, Giorgetti-Peraldi S, Murdaca J, Van Obberghen E. Regulation of vascular endothelial growth factor expression by advanced glycation end products. J Biol Chem 2001;276(47):43,836–43,841.

68. Kuroki M, Voest EE, Amano S, et al. Reactive oxygen intermediates increase vascular endothelial growth factor expression in vitro and in vivo. J Clin Invest 1996;98(7):1667–1675.

69. Cho M, Hunt TK, Hussain MZ. Hydrogen peroxide stimulates macrophage vascular endothelial growth factor release. Am J Physiol Heart Circ Physiol 2001;280(5):H2357–H2363.

70. Urata Y, Yamaguchi M, Higashiyama Y, et al. Reactive oxygen species accelerate production of vascular endothelial growth factor by advanced glycation end products in RAW264.7 mouse macrophages. Free Radic Biol Med 2002;32(8):688–701.

71. Obrosova IG, Minchenko AG, Marinescu V, et al. Antioxidants attenuate early up regulation of retinal vascular endothelial growth factor in streptozotocin-diabetic rats. Diabetologia 2001;44(9):1102–1110.

72. Rota R, Chiavaroli C, Garay RP, Hannaert P. Reduction of retinal albumin leakage by the antioxidant calcium dobesilate in streptozotocin-diabetic rats. Eur J Pharmacol 2004;495(2–3):217–224.

73. Kowluru RA, Kern TS, Engerman RL, Armstrong D. Abnormalities of retinal metabolism in diabetes or experimental galactosemia. III. Effects of antioxidants. Diabetes 1996;45(9):1233–1237.

74. Meyer-Schwickerath R, Pfeiffer A, Blum WF, et al. Vitreous levels of the insulin-like growth factors I and II, and the insulin-like growth factor binding proteins 2 and 3, increase in neovascular eye disease: studies in nondiabetic and diabetic subjects. J Clin Invest 1993;92(6):2620–2625.

75. Danis RP, Bingaman DP. Insulin-like growth factor-1 retinal microangiopathy in the pig eye. Ophthalmology 1997;104(10):1661–1669.

76. Smith LE, Kopchick JJ, Chen W, et al. Essential role of growth hormone in ischemia-induced retinal neovascularization. Science 1997;276(5319):1706–1709.

77. Simpson HL, Umpleby AM, Russell-Jones DL. Insulin-like growth factor-I and diabetes: a review. Growth Horm IGF Res 1998;8(2):83–95.

78. Jeffcoate W. Can growth hormone therapy cause diabetes? Lancet 2000;355(9204):589, 590.

79. Poulsen JE. Diabetes and anterior pituitary insufficiency: final course and postmortem study of a diabetic patient with Sheehan's syndrome. Diabetes 1966;15(2):73–77.

80. Luft R, Notter G. Preliminary results from treatment of juvenile diabetics with progressive vascular complications and neuropathy by implantation of the hypophysis with radioactive yttrium. Acta Isotopica 1964;4(4):387–398.

81. Merimee TJ. A follow-up study of vascular disease in growth-hormone-deficient dwarfs with diabetes. N Engl J Med 1978;298(22):1217–1222.

82. Kondo T, Vicent D, Suzuma K, et al. Knockout of insulin and IGF-1 receptors on vascular endothelial cells protects against retinal neovascularization. J Clin Invest 2003;111(12):1835–1842.

83. Punglia RS, Lu M, Hsu J, et al. Regulation of vascular endothelial growth factor expression by insulin-like growth factor I. Diabetes 1997;46(10):1619–1626.

84. Poulaki V, Joussen AM, Mitsiades N, Mitsiades CS, Iliaki EF, Adamis AP. Insulin-like growth factor-I plays a pathogenetic role in diabetic retinopathy. Am J Pathol 2004;165(2):457–469.

85. Workman P, Maloney A. HSP90 as a new therapeutic target for cancer therapy: the story unfolds. Expert Opin Biol Ther 2002;2(1):3–24.

86. Poulaki V, Qin W, Joussen AM, et al. Acute intensive insulin therapy exacerbates diabetic blood–retinal barrier breakdown via hypoxia-inducible factor-1alpha and VEGF. J Clin Invest 2002;109(6):805–815.

87. Murata M, Kador PF, Sato S. Vascular endothelial growth factor (VEGF) enhances the expression of receptors and activates mitogen-activated protein (MAP) kinase of dog retinal capillary endothelial cells. J Ocul Pharmacol Ther 2000;16(4):383–391.

88. Antonetti DA, Barber AJ, Khin S, Lieth E, Tarbell JM, Gardner TW. Vascular permeability in experimental diabetes is associated with reduced endothelial occludin content: vascular endothelial growth factor decreases occludin in retinal endothelial cells. Penn State Retina Research Group. Diabetes 1998;47(12):1953–1959.

89. Joussen AM, Poulaki V, Qin W, et al. Retinal vascular endothelial growth factor induces intercellular adhesion molecule-1 and endothelial nitric oxide synthase expression and initiates early diabetic retinal leukocyte adhesion in vivo. Am J Pathol 2002;160(2):501–509.

90. Gerber HP, McMurtrey A, Kowalski J, et al. Vascular endothelial growth factor regulates endothelial cell survival through the phosphatidylinositol 3′-kinase/Akt signal transduction pathway: requirement for Flk-1/KDR activation. J Biol Chem 1998;273(46):30,336–30,343.

91. Fujio Y, Walsh K. Akt mediates cytoprotection of endothelial cells by vascular endothelial growth factor in an anchorage-dependent manner. J Biol Chem 1999;274(23):16,349–16,354.

92. Suhara T, Mano T, Oliveira BE, Walsh K. Phosphatidylinositol 3-kinase/Akt signaling controls endothelial cell sensitivity to Fas-mediated apoptosis via regulation of FLICE-inhibitory protein (FLIP). Circ Res 2001;89(1):13–19.

93. Tran J, Master Z, Yu JL, Rak J, Dumont DJ, Kerbel RS. A role for survivin in chemoresistance of endothelial cells mediated by VEGF. Proc Natl Acad Sci USA 2002;99(7):4349–4354.

94. Bartoli M, Platt D, Lemtalsi T, et al. VEGF differentially activates STAT3 in microvascular endothelial cells. FASEB J 2003;17(11):1562–1564.

95. Yahata Y, Shirakata Y, Tokumaru S, et al. Nuclear translocation of phosphorylated STAT3 is essential for vascular endothelial growth factor–induced human dermal microvascular endothelial cell migration and tube formation. J Biol Chem 2003;278(41):40,026–40,031.

96. Davis MD, Fisher MR, Gangnon RE, et al. Risk factors for high-risk proliferative diabetic retinopathy and severe visual loss: Early Treatment Diabetic Retinopathy Study Report #18. Invest Ophthalmol Vis Sci 1998;39(2):233–352.

97. UK Prospective Diabetes Study Group. Tight blood pressure control and risk of macrovascular and microvascular complications in type 2 diabetes: UKPDS 38. BMJ 1998;317(7160):703–713.

98. Estacio RO, Jeffers BW, Gifford N, Schrier RW. Effect of blood pressure control on diabetic microvascular complications in patients with hypertension and type 2 diabetes. Diabetes Care 2000;23 (Suppl 2):B54–B64.

99. Cassar J, Kohner EM, Hamilton AM, Gordon H, Joplin GF. Diabetic retinopathy and pregnancy. Diabetologia 1978;15(2):105–111.

100. The Diabetes Control and Complications Trial Research Group. Clustering of long-term complications in families with diabetes in the diabetes control and complications trial. Diabetes 1997;46(11):1829–1839.

101. Leslie RD, Pyke DA. Diabetic retinopathy in identical twins. Diabetes 1982;31(1):19–21.

102. Guillausseau PJ, Tielmans D, Virally-Monod M, Assayag M. Diabetes: from phenotypes to genotypes. Diabetes Metab 1997;23(Suppl 2):14–21.

103. Imperatore G, Hanson RL, Pettitt DJ, Kobes S, Bennett PH, Knowler WC. Sib-pair linkage analysis for susceptibility genes for microvascular complications among Pima Indians with type 2 diabetes. Pima Diabetes Genes Group. Diabetes 1998;47(5):821–830.

104. Falck AA, Knip JM, Ilonen JS, Laatikainen LT. Genetic markers in early diabetic retinopathy of adolescents with type 1 diabetes. J Diabetes Complications 1997;11(4):203–207.

105. Serrano-Rios M, Regueiro JR, Severino R, Lopez-Larrea C, Arnaiz-Villena A. HLA antigens in insulin dependent and non-insulin dependent Spanish diabetic patients. Diabetes Metab 1983;9(2):116–120.

106. Hawrami K, Mohan R, Mohan V, Hitman GA. A genetic study of retinopathy in south Indian type 2 (non-insulin-dependent) diabetic patients. Diabetologia 1991;34(6):441–444.

107. Patel A, Hibberd ML, Millward BA, Demaine AG. Chromosome 7q35 and susceptibility to diabetic microvascular complications. J Diabetes Complications 1996;10(2):62–67.

108. Chistiakov DA, Turakulov RI, Girashko NM, et al. [Polymorphism of the dinucleotide repeat inside the aldose reductase gene in normal states and in patients with insulin-dependent diabetes mellitus with vascular complications]. Mol Biol (Mosk) 1997;31(5):778–783.

109. Demaine A, Cross D, Millward A. Polymorphisms of the aldose reductase gene and susceptibility to retinopathy in type 1 diabetes mellitus. Invest Ophthalmol Vis Sci 2000;41(13):4064–4068.

110. Hodgkinson AD, Millward BA, Demaine AG. Polymorphisms of the glucose transporter (GLUT1) gene are associated with diabetic nephropathy. Kidney Int 2001;59(3):985–989.

111. Liu ZH, Guan TJ, Chen ZH, Li LS. Glucose transporter (GLUT1) allele (XbaI-) associated with nephropathy in non-insulin-dependent diabetes mellitus. Kidney Int 1999;55(5):1843–1848.

112. Tarnow L, Stehouwer CD, Emeis JJ, et al. Plasminogen activator inhibitor-1 and apolipoprotein E gene polymorphisms and diabetic angiopathy. Nephrol Dial Transplant 2000;15(5):625–630.

113. Nagi DK, McCormack LJ, Mohamed-Ali V, Yudkin JS, Knowler WC, Grant PJ. Diabetic retinopathy, promoter (4G/5G) polymorphism of PAI-1 gene, and PAI-1 activity in Pima Indians with type 2 diabetes. Diabetes Care 1997;20(8):1304–1309.

114. Hawrami K, Hitman GA, Rema M, et al. An association in non-insulin-dependent diabetes mellitus subjects between susceptibility to retinopathy and tumor necrosis factor polymorphism. Hum Immunol 1996;46(1):49–54.

115. Niskanen L, Voutilainen-Kaunisto R, Terasvirta M, et al. Leucine 7 to proline 7 polymorphism in the neuropeptide y gene is associated with retinopathy in type 2 diabetes. Exp Clin Endocrinol Diabetes 2000;108(3):235,236.

116. Shcherbak NS, Schwartz EI. The C825T polymorphism in the G-protein beta3 subunit gene and diabetic complications in IDDM patients. J Hum Genet 2001;46(4):188–191.

117. Vendrell J, Gutierrez C, Broch M, Fernandez-Real JM, Aguilar C, Richart C. Beta 3-adrenoreceptor gene polymorphism and leptin: lack of relationship in type 2 diabetic patients. Clin Endocrinol (Oxf) 1998;49(5):679–683.

118. Mackness B, Durrington PN, Abuashia B, Boulton AJ, Mackness MI. Low paraoxonase activity in type II diabetes mellitus complicated by retinopathy. Clin Sci (Lond) 2000;98(3):355–363.

119. Chen JW, Hansen PM, Tarnow L, Hellgren A, Deckert T, Pociot F. Genetic variation of a collagen IV alpha 1-chain gene polymorphism in Danish insulin-dependent diabetes mellitus (IDDM) patients: lack of association to nephropathy and proliferative retinopathy. Diabet Med 1997;14(2):143–147.

120. Matsubara Y, Murata M, Maruyama T, et al. Association between diabetic retinopathy and genetic variations in alpha2beta1 integrin, a platelet receptor for collagen. Blood 2000;95(5):1560–1564.

121. Warpeha KM, Ah-Fat F, Harding S, et al. Dinucleotide repeat polymorphisms in EDN1 and NOS3 are not associated with severe diabetic retinopathy in type 1 or type 2 diabetes. Eye 1999;13(Pt 2): 174–178.

122. Warpeha KM, Chakravarthy U. Molecular genetics of microvascular disease in diabetic retinopathy. Eye 2003;17(3):305–311.

123. Tarnow L, Cambien F, Rossing P, et al. Lack of relationship between an insertion/deletion polymorphism in the angiotensin I-converting enzyme gene and diabetic nephropathy and proliferative retinopathy in IDDM patients. Diabetes 1995;44(5):489–494.

124. Huang D, Swanson EA, Lin CP, et al. Optical coherence tomography. Science 1991;254(5035): 1178–1181.

125. Drexler W, Morgner U, Ghanta RK, Kartner FX, Schuman JS, Fujimoto JG. Ultrahigh-resolution ophthalmic optical coherence tomography. Nat Med 2001;7(4):502–507.

126. Grunwald JE, Riva CE, Sinclair SH, Brucker AJ, Petrig BL. Laser Doppler velocimetry study of retinal circulation in diabetes mellitus. Arch Ophthalmol 1986;104(7):991–996.

127. Wilson CA, Fleckenstein JL, Berkowitz BA, Green ME. Preretinal neovascularization in diabetic retinopathy: a preliminary investigation using contrast-enhanced magnetic resonance imaging. J Diabetes Complications 1992;6(4):223–229.

128. Berkowitz BA. Adult and newborn rat inner retinal oxygenation during carbogen and 100% oxygen breathing: comparison using magnetic resonance imaging delta Po2 mapping. Invest Ophthalmol Vis Sci 1996;37(10):2089–2098.

129. The relationship of glycemic exposure (HbA1c) to the risk of development and progression of retinopathy in the diabetes control and complications trial. Diabetes 1995;44(8):968–983.

130. The Diabetes Control and Complications Trial/Epidemiology of Diabetes Interventions and Complications Research Group. Retinopathy and nephropathy in patients with type 1 diabetes four years after a trial of intensive therapy. N Engl J Med 2000;342(6):381–389.

131. Diabetes Control and Complications Trial Research Group. Progression of retinopathy with intensive versus conventional treatment in the Diabetes Control and Complications Trial. Ophthalmology 1995;102(4):647–661.

132. The effect of intensive diabetes treatment on the progression of diabetic retinopathy in insulin-dependent diabetes mellitus: the Diabetes Control and Complications Trial. Arch Ophthalmol 1995;113(1):36–51.

133. Klein R, Klein BE, Moss SE, Cruickshanks KJ. The Wisconsin Epidemiologic Study of Diabetic Retinopathy: XVII. The 14-year incidence and progression of diabetic retinopathy and associated risk factors in type 1 diabetes [see comment]. Ophthalmology 1998;105(10):1801–1815.

134. Chaturvedi N, Sjolie AK, Stephenson JM, et al. Effect of lisinopril on progression of retinopathy in normotensive people with type 1 diabetes. The EUCLID Study Group. EURODIAB Controlled Trial of Lisinopril in Insulin-Dependent Diabetes Mellitus [see comment]. Lancet 1998;351(9095):28–31.

135. Knudsen ST, Bek T, Poulsen PL, Hove MN, Rehling M, Mogensen CE. Effects of losartan on diabetic maculopathy in type 2 diabetic patients: a randomized, double-masked study. J Intern Med 2003;254(2):147–158.

136. Klein BE, Moss SE, Klein R, Surawicz TS. The Wisconsin Epidemiologic Study of Diabetic Retinopathy. XIII. Relationship of serum cholesterol to retinopathy and hard exudate. Ophthalmology 1991;98(8):1261–1265.

137. Fine SL, Patz A. Ten years after the Diabetic Retinopathy Study. Ophthalmology 1987;94(7):739, 740.

138. Early Treatment Diabetic Retinopathy Study Research Group. Early photocoagulation for diabetic retinopathy. ETDRS report number 9. Ophthalmology 1991;98(5 Suppl):766–785.

139. Early Treatment Diabetic Retinopathy Study research group. Photocoagulation for diabetic macular edema. Early Treatment Diabetic Retinopathy Study report number 1. Arch Ophthalmol 1985; 103(12):1796–1806.

140. Arrigg PG, Cavallerano J. The role of vitrectomy for diabetic retinopathy. J Am Optom Assoc 1998;69(11):733–740.

141. Squirrell D, Bhola R, Bush J, Winder S, Talbot JF. A prospective, case controlled study of the natural history of diabetic retinopathy and maculopathy after uncomplicated phacoemulsification cataract surgery in patients with type 2 diabetes. Br J Ophthalmol 2002;86(5):565–571.

142. Borrillo JL, Mittra RA, Dev S, et al. Retinopathy progression and visual outcomes after phacoemulsification in patients with diabetes mellitus. Trans Am Ophthalmol Soc 1999;97:435–445; discussion 45–49.

143. Machemer R. Proliferative vitreoretinopathy (PVR): a personal account of its pathogenesis and treatment. Proctor lecture. Invest Ophthalmol Vis Sci 1988;29(12):1771–1783.

144. Machemer R, Sugita G, Tano Y. Treatment of intraocular proliferations with intravitreal steroids. Trans Am Ophthalmol Soc 1979;77:171–180.

145. Jonas JB, Kreissig I, Sofker A, Degenring RF. Intravitreal injection of triamcinolone for diffuse diabetic macular edema. Arch Ophthalmol 2003;121(1):57–61.

146. Martidis A, Duker JS, Greenberg PB, et al. Intravitreal triamcinolone for refractory diabetic macular edema. Ophthalmology 2002;109(5):920–927.

147. Jonas JB, Hayler JK, Sofker A, Panda-Jonas S. Regression of neovascular iris vessels by intravitreal injection of crystalline cortisone. J Glaucoma 2001;10(4):284–287.

148. Chalam KV, Malkani S, Shah VA. Intravitreal dexamethasone effectively reduces postoperative inflammation after vitreoretinal surgery. Ophthalmic Surg Lasers Imaging 2003;34(3):188–192.

149. Singal N, Hopkins J. Pseudophakic cystoid macular edema: ketorolac alone vs. ketorolac plus prednisolone. Can J Ophthalmol 2004;39(3):245–250.

150. Yusuf S, Sleight P, Pogue J, Bosch J, Davies R, Dagenais G. Effects of an angiotensin-converting-enzyme inhibitor, ramipril, on cardiovascular events in high-risk patients. The Heart Outcomes Prevention Evaluation Study Investigators. N Engl J Med 2000;342(3):145–153.

151. Gupta A, Gupta V, Thapar S, Bhansali A. Lipid-lowering drug atorvastatin as an adjunct in the management of diabetic macular edema. Am J Ophthalmol 2004;137(4):675–682.

152. Sen K, Misra A, Kumar A, Pandey RM. Simvastatin retards progression of retinopathy in diabetic patients with hypercholesterolemia. Diabetes Res Clin Pract 2002;56(1):1–11.

153. Misra A, Vikram NK, Kumar A. Diabetic maculopathy and lipid-lowering therapy. Eye 2004;18(1):107–108.

154. Sorbinil Retinopathy Trial Research Group. A randomized trial of sorbinil, an aldose reductase inhibitor, in diabetic retinopathy. Arch Ophthalmol 1990;108(9):1234–1244.

155. Arauz-Pacheco C, Ramirez LC, Pruneda L, Sanborn GE, Rosenstock J, Raskin P. The effect of the aldose reductase inhibitor, ponalrestat, on the progression of diabetic retinopathy. J Diabetes Complications 1992;6(2):131–137.

156. Robinson WG Jr, Laver NM, Jacot JL, et al. Diabetic-like retinopathy ameliorated with the aldose reductase inhibitor WAY-121,509. Invest Ophthalmol Vis Sci 1996;37(6):1149–1156.

157. Frank RN, Amin R, Kennedy A, Hohman TC. An aldose reductase inhibitor and aminoguanidine prevent vascular endothelial growth factor expression in rats with long-term galactosemia. Arch Ophthalmol 1997;115(8):1036–1047.

158. Kubo E, Mori K, Kobayashi T, et al. Effect of aldose reductase inhibitor on corneal epithelial barrier function in galactose-fed dogs. J Ocul Pharmacol Ther 1998;14(2):181–190.

159. Horie S, Nagai H, Yuuki T, et al. Effect of SG-210, a novel aldose reductase inhibitor, on impaired polyol pathway in rats received diabetic manipulations. J Diabetes Complications 1998;12(3):163–169.

160. No authors listed. A curious stopping rule from Hoechst Marion Roussel. Lancet 1997; 350(9072):155.

161. Bolton WK, Cattran DC, Williams ME, et al. Randomized trial of an inhibitor of formation of advanced glycation end products in diabetic nephropathy. Am J Nephrol 2004;24(1):32–40.

162. Vasan S, Foiles PG, Founds HW. Therapeutic potential of AGE inhibitors and breakers of AGE protein cross-links. Expert Opin Investig Drugs 2001;10(11):1977–1987.

163. Aiello LP. The potential role of PKC beta in diabetic retinopathy and macular edema. Surv Ophthalmol 2002;47(Suppl 2):S263–S269.

164. Davis M, Atello L, Milton R, Sheetz M, Arora V, Vignati L. Diabetic retinopathy and macular edema progression rates in recent placebo-controlled clinical trials. Diabetes 2003;52(Suppl 1):A200.

165. Milton R, Aiello L, Davis M, Sheetz M, Arora V, Vignati L. Initial results of the Protein Kinase C b Inhibitor Diabetic Retinopathy Study (PKC-DRS). Diabetes 2003;52(Suppl 1):A127.

166. Campochiaro PA. Reduction of diabetic macular edema by oral administration of the kinase inhibitor PKC412. Invest Ophthalmol Vis Sci 2004;45(3):922–931.

167. Donnelly R, Idris I, Forrester JV. Protein kinase C inhibition and diabetic retinopathy: a shot in the dark at translational research. Br J Ophthalmol 2004;88(1):145–151.

168. Nishikawa T, Edelstein D, Du XL, et al. Normalizing mitochondrial superoxide production blocks three pathways of hyperglycaemic damage. Nature 2000;404(6779):787–790.

169. Bursell SE, Cavallerano JD, Cavallerano AA, et al. Stereo nonmydriatic digital-video color retinal imaging compared with Early Treatment Diabetic Retinopathy Study seven standard field 35-mm stereo color photos for determining level of diabetic retinopathy. Ophthalmology 2001;108(3): 572–585.

170. Bursell SE, Clermont AC, Aiello LP, et al. High-dose vitamin E supplementation normalizes retinal blood flow and creatinine clearance in patients with type 1 diabetes. Diabetes Care 1999;22(8): 1245–1251.

171. The TIMAD Study Group. Ticlopidine treatment reduces the progression of nonproliferative diabetic retinopathy. Arch Ophthalmol 1990;108(11):1577–1583.

172. Vingolo EM, De Mattia G, Giusti C, Forte R, Laurenti O, Pannarale MR. Treatment of nonproliferative diabetic retinopathy with Defibrotide in noninsulin-dependent diabetes mellitus: a pilot study. Acta Ophthalmol Scand 1999;77(3):315–320.

173. Leite EB, Mota MC, de Abreu JR, Cunha-Vaz JG. Effect of calcium dobesilate on the blood–retinal barrier in early diabetic retinopathy. Int Ophthalmol 1990;14(2):81–88.

174. Berthet P, Farine JC, Barras JP. Calcium dobesilate: pharmacological profile related to its use in diabetic retinopathy. Int J Clin Pract 1999;53(8):631–636.

175. Ferrara N, Hillan KJ, Gerber HP, Novotny W. Discovery and development of bevacizumab, an anti-VEGF antibody for treating cancer. Nat Rev Drug Discov 2004;3(5):391–400.

176. Rosen LS. Clinical experience with angiogenesis signaling inhibitors: focus on vascular endothelial growth factor (VEGF) blockers. Cancer Control 2002;9(Suppl 2):36–44.

177. Giles FJ, Cooper MA, Silverman L, et al. Phase II study of SU5416—a small-molecule, vascular endothelial growth factor tyrosine-kinase receptor inhibitor—in patients with refractory myeloproliferative diseases. Cancer 2003;97(8):1920–1928.

178. Hoekman K. SU6668, a multitargeted angiogenesis inhibitor. Cancer J 2001;7(Suppl 3):S134–S138.

179. Bates D. ZD-6474. AstraZeneca. Curr Opin Investig Drugs 2003;4(12):1468–1472.

180. Fong TA, Shawver LK, Sun L, et al. SU5416 is a potent and selective inhibitor of the vascular endothelial growth factor receptor (Flk-1/KDR) that inhibits tyrosine kinase catalysis, tumor vascularization, and growth of multiple tumor types. Cancer Res 1999;59(1):99–106.

181. Sridhar SS, Shepherd FA. Targeting angiogenesis: a review of angiogenesis inhibitors in the treatment of lung cancer. Lung Cancer 2003;42(Suppl 1):S81–S91.

182. Shepherd FA, Sridhar SS. Angiogenesis inhibitors under study for the treatment of lung cancer. Lung Cancer 2003;41(Suppl 1):S63–S72.

183. Rosen LS. Inhibitors of the vascular endothelial growth factor receptor. Hematol Oncol Clin North Am 2002;16(5):1173–1187.

184. Eyetech Study Groups. Preclinical and phase 1A clinical evaluation of an anti-VEGF pegylated aptamer (EYE001) for the treatment of exudative age-related macular degeneration. Retina 2002; 22(2):143–152.

185. Sebag J, Tang M, Brown S, Sadun AA, Charles MA. Effects of pentoxifylline on choroidal blood flow in nonproliferative diabetic retinopathy. Angiology 1994;45(6):429–433.

186. Sonkin PL, Kelly LW, Sinclair SH, Hatchell DL. Pentoxifylline increases retinal capillary blood flow velocity in patients with diabetes. Arch Ophthalmol 1993;111(12):1647–1652.

187. Ferrari E, Fioravanti M, Patti AL, Viola C, Solerte SB. Effects of long-term treatment (4 years) with pentoxifylline on haemorheological changes and vascular complications in diabetic patients. Pharmatherapeutica 1987;5(1):26–39.

188. Folkman J. Role of angiogenesis in tumor growth and metastasis. Semin Oncol 2002;29(6 Suppl 16):15–18.

189. Curran WJ. New chemotherapeutic agents: update of major chemoradiation trials in solid tumors. Oncology 2002;63(Suppl 2):29–38.

190. Belman N, Bonnem EM, Harvey HA, Lipton A. Phase I trial of recombinant platelet factor 4 (rPF4) in patients with advanced colorectal carcinoma. Invest N Drugs 1996;14(4):387–389.

191. Laird AD, Cherrington JM. Small molecule tyrosine kinase inhibitors: clinical development of anti-cancer agents. Expert Opin Investig Drugs 2003;12(1):51–64.

192. Wall L, Talbot DC, Bradbury P, Jodrell DI. A phase I and pharmacological study of the matrix metalloproteinase inhibitor BB-3644 in patients with solid tumours. Br J Cancer 2004;90(4):800–804.

193. Hidalgo M, Eckhardt SG. Development of matrix metalloproteinase inhibitors in cancer therapy. J Natl Cancer Inst 2001;93(3):178–193.

194. Santos O, McDermott CD, Daniels RG, Appelt K. Rodent pharmacokinetic and anti-tumor efficacy studies with a series of synthetic inhibitors of matrix metalloproteinases. Clin Exp Metastasis 1997;15(5):499–508.

195. Seftor RE, Seftor EA, De Larco JE, et al. Chemically modified tetracyclines inhibit human melanoma cell invasion and metastasis. Clin Exp Metastasis 1998;16(3):217–225.

196. Falardeau P, Champagne P, Poyet P, Hariton C, Dupont E. Neovastat, a naturally occurring multi-functional antiangiogenic drug, in phase III clinical trials. Semin Oncol 2001;28(6):620–625.

197. Gingras D, Boivin D, Deckers C, Gendron S, Barthomeuf C, Beliveau R. Neovastat—a novel antiangiogenic drug for cancer therapy. Anticancer Drugs 2003;14(2):91–96.

198. Ogata N, Nishikawa M, Nishimura T, Mitsuma Y, Matsumura M. Unbalanced vitreous levels of pigment epithelium-derived factor and vascular endothelial growth factor in diabetic retinopathy. Am J Ophthalmol 2002;134(3):348–353.

199. George D. Platelet-derived growth factor receptors: a therapeutic target in solid tumors. Semin Oncol 2001;28(5 Suppl 17):27–33.

200. Eskens FA, Dumez H, Hoekstra R, et al. Phase I and pharmacokinetic study of continuous twice weekly intravenous administration of Cilengitide (EMD 121974), a novel inhibitor of the integrins alphavbeta3 and alphavbeta5 in patients with advanced solid tumours. Eur J Cancer 2003;39(7):917–926.

201. Posey JA, Khazaeli MB, DelGrosso A, et al. A pilot trial of Vitaxin, a humanized anti-vitronectin receptor (anti alpha v beta 3) antibody in patients with metastatic cancer. Cancer Biother Radiopharm 2001;16(2):125–132.

202. Panigrahy D, Shen LQ, Kieran MW, Kaipainen A. Therapeutic potential of thiazolidinediones as anticancer agents. Expert Opin Investig Drugs 2003;12(12):1925–1937.

203. Margeli A, Kouraklis G, Theocharis S. Peroxisome proliferator activated receptor-gamma (PPAR-gamma) ligands and angiogenesis. Angiogenesis 2003;6(3):165–169.

204. Ogata N, Tombran-Tink J, Nishikawa M, et al. Pigment epithelium-derived factor in the vitreous is low in diabetic retinopathy and high in rhegmatogenous retinal detachment. Am J Ophthalmol 2001;132(3):378–382.

205. Boehm BO, Lang G, Feldmann B, et al. Proliferative diabetic retinopathy is associated with a low level of the natural ocular anti-angiogenic agent pigment epithelium-derived factor (PEDF) in aqueous humor. a pilot study. Horm Metab Res 2003;35(6):382–386.

206. Stellmach V, Crawford SE, Zhou W, Bouck N. Prevention of ischemia-induced retinopathy by the natural ocular antiangiogenic agent pigment epithelium-derived factor. Proc Natl Acad Sci USA 2001;98(5):2593–2597.

207. Rasmussen H, Chu KW, Campochiaro P, et al. Clinical protocol: an open-label, phase I, single administration, dose-escalation study of ADGVPEDF.11D (ADPEDF) in neovascular age-related macular degeneration (AMD). Hum Gene Ther 2001;12(16):2029–2032.

208. Grant MB, Caballero S. Somatostatin analogues as drug therapies for retinopathies. Drugs Today (Barc) 2002;38(11):783–791.

209. Boehm BO, Lang GK, Jehle PM, Feldman B, Lang GE. Octreotide reduces vitreous hemorrhage and loss of visual acuity risk in patients with high-risk proliferative diabetic retinopathy. Horm Metab Res 2001;33(5):300–306.

210. Growth Hormone Antagonist for Proliferative Diabetic Retinopathy Study Group. The effect of a growth hormone receptor antagonist drug on proliferative diabetic retinopathy. Ophthalmology 2001;108(12):2266–2272.

211. Kimura H, Sakamoto T, Cardillo JA, et al. Retrovirus-mediated suicide gene transduction in the vitreous cavity of the eye: feasibility in prevention of proliferative vitreoretinopathy. Hum Gene Ther 1996;7(7):799–808.

212. Lai CC, Wu WC, Chen SL, et al. Suppression of choroidal neovascularization by adeno-associated virus vector expressing angiostatin. Invest Ophthalmol Vis Sci 2001;42(10):2401–2407.

213. Lewis GP, Linberg KA, Geller SF, Guerin CJ, Fisher SK. Effects of the neurotrophin brain-derived neurotrophic factor in an experimental model of retinal detachment. Invest Ophthalmol Vis Sci 1999;40(7):1530–1544.

18 Obesity and Renal Disease

Ayman Geneidy, MD *and Richard Solomon,* MD

INTRODUCTION

With the increasing prevalence of obesity and its impact on metabolic and cardiovascular diseases, more attention is now being focused on the relationship between obesity and renal function. It is now recognized that obesity enhances the progression of renal function deterioration to end-stage renal disease (ESRD) in subjects with known preexisting renal disease. In addition, obesity is associated with a well-described glomerulopathy called focal segmental glomerulosclerosis (FSGS). Finally, and most important, through its close association with type 2 diabetes and hypertension, the two most important causes of ESRD in the United States *(1)*, obesity is now felt to be a major risk factor for the development of chronic kidney disease.

PREVALENCE OF RENAL DISEASE IN OBESITY

Obese individuals are often found to have asymptomatic microalbuminuria and proteinuria. Some individuals, however, present with nephrotic-range proteinuria, with or without edema, and on renal biopsy have FSGS. Whether these presentations represent different ends of the same spectrum or different diseases is unknown. Sleep apnea, often present in the obese, is also associated with similar glomerular lesions *(2,3)*. Data on the epidemiology of renal dysfunction among the obese population are sparse. Several reports have described a higher incidence of microalbuminuria among obese subjects both with and without hypertension *(4,5)*. In a subanalysis of a large population study, microalbuminuria was noted in 9.5% of lean nondiabetic, nonhypertensive males compared with 18.3% in overweight (body mass index [BMI] = 25–29.9 kg/m^2) and 29.3% in obese (BMI > 30 kg/m^2) subjects. In women, the values were 6.6, 9.2, and 16%, respectively *(6)*. Liese et al. *(7)* described a consistent association of microalbuminuria with measures of adiposity in nondiabetic men and women. Hypertension and central adiposity were the two strongest correlates of microalbuminuria.

From: *Contemporary Diabetes: Obesity and Diabetes*
Edited by: C. S. Mantzoros © Humana Press Inc., Totowa, NJ

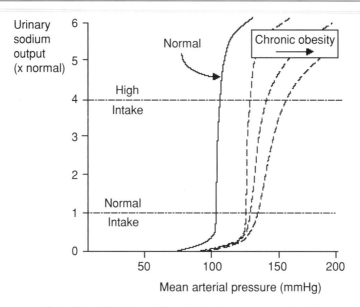

Fig. 1. The presence of obesity shifts the relationship between mean arterial pressure and urinary sodium excretion to the right. Thus, for any level of sodium excretion, a higher mean arterial pressure is required.

Although obesity-associated FSGS is an infrequent finding among the obese population, its frequency was recently noted to have increased 10-fold among native kidney biopsies, from 0.2% in 1986–1990 to 2.0% in 1996–2000 *(8)*.

PATHOPHYSIOLOGICAL BASIS OF KIDNEY DYSFUNCTION IN OBESITY

Several hemodynamic and hormonal abnormalities contribute to renal dysfunction in obese individuals. Hypertension is very prevalent in the obese and plays a role in the pathogenesis of renal dysfunction. However, nonhemodynamic renal effects of various hormonal factors also play a role in contributing to renal dysfunction in the obese.

Hypertension in Obesity

One of the hallmarks of the hemodynamic changes in obesity is extracellular fluid volume expansion resulting from sodium retention *(9)*. A number of mechanisms may contribute to this sodium retention. These mechanisms (*see* below) result in a shift of the normal pressure–natriuresis curve to the right (Fig. 1). This means that obese subjects require higher than normal arterial pressure to bring sodium excretion into balance with sodium intake *(10)*. The main mechanisms thought to be responsible for this shift in the pressure–natriuresis curve include increased sympathetic nervous system (SNS) activity, activation of the renin–angiotensin system (RAS), hyperinsulinemia, and physical compression of the kidneys by visceral obesity *(11,12)*.

SYMPATHETIC ACTIVATION

Obesity increases SNS activity in many tissues, including skeletal muscles, adipose tissue, and kidneys *(13)*. Increased SNS activity, especially in the kidneys, plays a major role in raising arterial pressure in obesity. In the setting of increased renal sympathetic tone, renal sodium excretion is reduced as a result of renal vasoconstriction and decreased glomerular filtration of sodium and by a direct tubular effect to increase sodium reabsorption. Activation of the SNS is also associated with hyperinsulinemia, hyperleptinemia, and hyperangiotensinemia (see below). As a reflection of SNS activation, the use of adrenergic blocking agents resulted in greater reduction in blood pressure (BP) in obese than lean hypertensive subjects (14). Renal denervation significantly reduced sodium retention and hypertension in obese dogs (15). This suggests that in obesity the effect of SNS activation on BP is mediated through the kidney and sodium reabsorption.

LEPTIN

Serum leptin levels have been shown to be directly related to body adiposity (16). Acute iv administration of leptin increased sympathetic activity in the kidneys, adrenals, and adipose tissue (17). On the other hand, human leptin was shown to promote natriuresis in rats (18) and to induce vasorelaxant effects through endothelial nitric oxide (NO) production (19,20). Thus, acutely, administration of leptin seems to have little effect on BP. However, chronic infusion of leptin to raise blood levels to those found in the obese raised BP in rats despite hypophagia and weight loss (21,22). This was associated with a decrease in renal blood flow and a shift in the pressure–natriuresis curve to the right (18). This effect was further enhanced when NO synthesis was inhibited (23), as may occur in obese or diabetic subjects with endothelial dysfunction. Since obesity is associated with resistance to the metabolic and anorexic actions of leptin, the preservation of leptin's other actions can only be explained by the presence of "selective leptin resistance." This concept has been suggested in several recent studies (24,25).

HYPERINSULINEMIA

The role of insulin in promoting sodium reabsorption in humans is still unclear, despite extensive experimental studies in animals. The clinical phenomenon of "refeeding edema" is often cited as an example of insulin's ability to induce sodium retention in humans. Insulin resistance and hyperinsulinemia correlate with BP in obese subjects. In addition, studies of acute insulin infusion suggested that hyperinsulinemia raises BP by increasing sodium reabsorption directly, enhancing sympathetic activity (26), and increasing the secretion of aldosterone in response to angiotensin II (Ang II) (27). On the other hand, neither acute nor chronic insulin infusion has been shown to cause a shift in the pressure–natriuresis relationship in humans and dogs (28).

It may be that another stimulus for sodium retention is necessary to "unmask" the direct effect of insulin on renal tubular function. In this regard, hyperglycemia has been cited as a possible additional factor. Increased filtration of glucose enhances sodium reabsorption in the proximal tubule (via the sodium-glucose cotransporter). As long as the amount of filtered glucose does not exceed the ability of the tubular reabsorptive process for glucose and result in an osmotic diuresis, enhanced proximal sodium reabsorption will occur. This shifts the amount of sodium that is excreted at any level of BP (shifts the pressure–natriuresis curve to the right).

One additional consequence of increased proximal sodium reabsorption that may be relevant to obesity-induced renal dysfunction is that it decreases delivery of sodium to more distal sites (such as the macula densa) and stimulates the tubuloglomerular feedback loop TGF. Activation of the tubuloglomerular feedback loop results in afferent arteriolar vasodilation leading to an increase in glomerular hydrostatic pressure and hyperfiltration. This is often cited as a mechanism for the early hyperfiltration in diabetes, and a similar pathogenesis may be operative in obesity-induced hyperfiltration *(29)*. Hyperfiltration reflects the transmission of more systemic pressure into the glomerulus (glomerular hypertension). The effects of systemic hypertension on vessels throughout the body are well appreciated. A similar pathophysiology applies to glomerular hypertension.

In animal models, improvement in hyperinsulinemia reverses many of these hemodynamic abnormalities. For example, treatment with troglitazone in heminephrectomized Wistar fatty rats markedly reduced serum insulin levels with resultant improvement in proteinuria *(30)*.

RENIN–ANGIOTENSIN SYSTEM

Despite volume expansion and sodium retention, obesity is associated with activation of the RAS *(31)*. Adipose tissue, besides its other endocrine functions, contains all elements of the RAS *(32)*. It is speculated that adipose-derived Ang II could be a potential mediator of obesity-related glomerular and systemic hypertension *(33)*. Finally, activation of the SNS (as noted earlier) may also increase renal renin production and circulating Ang II, contributing to systemic hypertension.

Nonhemodynamic Mechanisms

LEPTIN

Accumulating data suggest a potential role for leptin in the progression of chronic kidney disease. Leptin stimulated the proliferation of cultured glomerular endothelial cells. Transforming growth factor-β (TGF-β) is a profibrotic cytokine that is implicated in the progressive fibrosis that occurs with any renal injury. Leptin was shown to enhance TGF-β1 mRNA expression and type IV collagen secretion by these glomerular endothelial cells *(34)*.

The db/db mouse, a model for type 2 diabetes and morbid obesity, has leptin resistance and high circulating leptin levels (>80 ng/mL). These mice have been shown to develop glomerular hypertrophy, mesangial expansion, proteinuria, and eventually renal insufficiency *(35)*. Although leptin failed to stimulate TGF-β1 synthesis, it increased TGF-β type II receptor expression and type I collagen secretion in db/db mouse mesangial cells *(36)*. Thus, activation of this paracrine TGF-β system by leptin may contribute to extracellular matrix deposition, glomerulosclerosis, and proteinuria *(37)*. Interestingly, ob/ob mice, which are leptin deficient but phenotypically morbidly obese, rarely develop renal disease *(38)*.

ANG II

Ang II is also widely believed to contribute to target organ damage by directly causing vascular hypertrophy and increasing collagen formation in various tissues including mesangial cells *(39)*. The role of blockade of the RAS in patients with and without diabetes has firmly established the importance of this system on the progression of renal function loss. Evidence from animal *(40)* and human *(41)* studies of the beneficial renal effects of RAS blockade argues that the hemodynamic actions of Ang II are one of the main mechanisms in moderating renal injury. Nevertheless, nonhemodynamic mechanisms are probably important. Blockade of the RAS system with angiotensin receptor blockers alters the expression of key proteins in the slit diaphragm between renal podocytes. The slit diaphragm is the final barrier to movement of protein and albumin into the urine. Restoration of the normal components of this slit diaphragm by inhibition of Ang II may account for the antiproteinuric effects of such treatments. Proteinuria and albuminuria are both markers for renal disease and also pathogenic factors contributing to progressive loss of renal function. The finding of microalbuminuria in up to 30% of obese individuals may reflect both the hemodynamic effects of Ang II and these more specific tissue effects.

HYPERINSULINEMIA

Insulin has been shown to stimulate mesangial cell hypertrophy and excess mesangial matrix production in in vitro and in vivo animal models resulting in glomerulosclerosis *(42,43)*. Whether insulin contributes to glomerulosclerosis in humans is unknown.

OBESITY-INDUCED LIPOTOXICITY

Lipotoxicity refers to the array of disorders caused by overaccumulation of lipids in nonadipose tissues with subsequent steatosis, lipoapoptosis, and toxicity secondary to fatty acid non-β oxidation *(44)*. There is clear evidence that increased accumulation of lipids has deleterious effects on various organs such as the heart *(45)*, and on pancreatic β-cells *(29)*, but the role of renal lipotoxicity is still unclear. However, indirect evidence for such a disorder comes from experimental animal studies showing that obesity is associated with marked accumulation of fatty tissue, especially in the renal sinuses *(46)*. In addition, it has been observed that lipid peroxidation biomarkers are markedly elevated in glomeruli and renal microvessels in type 2 diabetes. Lipid-lowering agents (e.g., 3-hydroxy-3-methyl-glutaryl-CoA reductase inhibitors) reduce proteinuria and the rate of progression of kidney disease in patients with hypercholesterolemia and proteinuria *(47)*.

POTENTIAL ROLE OF INFLAMMATORY CYTOKINES DERIVED FROM EXCESS ADIPOSITY

A low-grade inflammatory state is described in obesity and is thought to result from increased adipocyte production of inflammatory cytokines (adipokines) such as tumor necrosis factor-α, interleukin-6, and C-reactive protein *(48)*. Whether such inflammation has any role in glomerular and interstitial fibrosis associated with obesity is still unclear. Studies examining the time course of renal interstitial fibrosis in Zucker obese rats suggest that inflammation cannot explain the initial onset of renal interstitial fibrosis that occurs in obese Zucker rats but may aggravate it once it begins *(49)*. Peroxisome proliferator-activated receptor γ (PPARγ) agonists have been found to reduce plasma levels of various adipokines and to improve endothelial function as well as glucose regulation *(48)*. Similarly, the PPARγ agonist rosiglitazone was effective in reducing the proteinuria and glomerular and tubular kidney damage in obese Zucker rats. In this model, the PPARγ agonist exerted superior renal protection compared with angiotensin-converting enzyme (ACE) inhibitor therapy *(50)*.

RENAL FUNCTIONAL AND STRUCTURAL CONSEQUENCES OF OBESITY

Hyperfiltration and Micro/Macroalbuminuria

The combined effect of sympathetic activation and volume expansion gives a classic hyperdynamic circulatory state characterized by increased cardiac output, heart rate, mean arterial pressure, and renal blood flow *(51,52)*.

As noted, more systemic pressure is transmitted to the glomerulus *(52)* as a result of afferent arteriolar vasodilation. The latter occurs in obesity because of increased proximal sodium reabsorption resulting from activation of the SNS and RAS and possibly the effect of increased availability of glucose. A consequence of increased proximal reabsorption is decreased distal delivery of sodium to the macula densa. This activates the tubuloglomerular feedback loop, resulting in afferent arteriolar vasodilation *(51)*.

Hyperfiltration, a hallmark of obesity-related kidney disease, reflects the increased glomerular hydrostatic pressure *(53)*. The early glomerular hyperfiltration in obesity is often as great as that observed in uncontrolled type 1 diabetes *(54)*. Such hyperfiltration stresses the wall of the glomerulus and causes the appearance of microalbuminuria or proteinuria even before there are major structural changes *(55,56)*. For example, in their dog model for human obesity, Henegar et al. *(57)* showed that dogs fed a high-fat diet for 7–9 wk or 24 wk developed hypertension and had an increased glomerular filtration rate (GFR) (145% of baseline) and renal plasma flow. Renal histopathology revealed an expansion of Bowman's capsule, increased cell proliferation in the glomerulus, thickening of the mesangial matrix and Bowman's capsule basement membrane, plus increased glomerular TGF-β expression.

Over the long term, the effects of glomerular hyperfiltration and arterial hypertension—especially if combined with metabolic and profibrotic effects of hyperleptinemia, hyperinsulinemia and hyperglycemia—could result in glomerular structural changes, glomerulosclerosis, and eventually nephron loss, resulting in a decrease in GFR *(57,58)*.

Obesity-Related Glomerulopathy

Nephrotic-range proteinuria was first reported as a complication of massive obesity in 1974. The renal histological picture was identical to that of FSGS *(59)*. FSGS is a common cause of nephrotic syndrome in adults and steroid-resistant nephrotic syndrome in children. A form of this condition called "collapsing FSGS" also occurs in human immunodeficiency virus-associated nephropathy and is associated with rapid loss of renal function. The pathogenesis is unknown. Since 1974, several case reports have described this syndrome *(2,60–62)*. In 2001, two different centers reported on a series of patients and described the clinical and pathological features of the obesity-related disease compared to cases of idiopathic FSGS (I-FSGS) *(8,63)*.

The patients were mostly Caucasians, with a male-to-female ratio of 2:1 in obese-FSGS, whereas it was 1:1 in I-FSGS. Mean age at time of biopsy diagnosis was significantly older (46 yr) in obese-FSGS compared with I-FSGS patients (32 yr). A large percentage (40–60%) of patients with obesity-related FSGS had submorbid obesity (BMI = 30–40 kg/m^2), whereas those with I-FSGS were lean (average BMI = 25 kg/m^2). Half of the obese patients were hypertensive at the time of biopsy diagnosis, a significantly higher percentage compared with that of the I-FSGS group. Mild renal insufficiency was also present in the obese, with a mean serum creatinine of 1.5 mg/dL at the time of biopsy. An important clinical distinction was noted: Although nearly half of the patients had nephrotic-range proteinuria, most had no clinical evidence of nephrotic syndrome, including the absence of edema, and normal serum albumin and total serum protein. This is in marked contrast to what is typically seen in adult nephrotic syndrome. FSGS and glomerulomegaly were present in 80% of cases, whereas 20% of biopsies had glomerulomegaly alone. "Diabetoid" changes were also noted, such as mild focal mesangial sclerosis or focal glomerular and tubular basement membrane thickening.

An inconsistent course was noted in the two studies. In the study by Praga et al. *(63)* (smaller number but longer follow-up), 33% of cases progressed to ESRD requiring dialysis. The use of ACE inhibitors was common and initially resulted in some decrease in the level of proteinuria, but at the end of 1 yr of follow-up, proteinuria had returned to the same level as at baseline. The loss of antiproteinuric effect of ACE inhibitors coincided with an increase in body weight at follow-up. The risk of progressive loss of renal function correlated with baseline creatinine and creatinine clearance.

By contrast, in the study by Kambham et al. *(8)* (larger number of patients but shorter follow-up), only 3.4% progressed to ESRD. The use of ACE inhibitors was associated with a decline in the amount of proteinuria. Five patients were able to lose weight by 10–36% of their original weight. Those patients exhibited a reduction in proteinuria by at least 50% and in one case by 75%. Predictors of poor outcome were the initial serum creatinine and severity of proteinuria.

Adelman et al. *(64)* described seven African American adolescents with severe obesity (average BMI = 46) who presented with proteinuria and had typical biopsy findings of glomerular hypertrophy, FSGS, increased mesangial matrix, and relative foot process preservation. One patient had dramatically reduced proteinuria with weight reduction, and one 15-yr-old patient developed ESRD. Although ACE inhibitors reduced proteinuria in three patients, the long-term benefit remained unclear.

Note that the development of proteinuria, the amount of proteinuria, and the response of proteinuria to various therapies are all considered powerful determinants of the rate of progression of renal disease. Proteinuria not only is a marker of renal dysfunction; it also plays a pathogenic role in producing progressive fibrosis in the interstitium of the kidney and glomerulosclerosis. The uptake of filtered proteins by cells of the proximal tubule results in the generation of cytokines resulting in an inflammatory milieu in the surrounding renal parenchyma. This adds to the burden of glomerulosclerosis and dropout of nephrons. The amount of proteinuria correlates with the rate of loss of renal function. For every gram of urinary protein excreted per day, the risk of end-stage kidney disease increases fivefold *(65)*. The percentage reduction of proteinuria by pharmacological therapies correlates with a reduction in the risk of developing end-stage kidney disease or a doubling of serum creatinine. Indeed, there is recent evidence that the renoprotective effect of angiotensin receptor blockers is totally explained by their ability to reduce proteinuria *(66)*.

Obesity as a Risk Factor for Progression of Preexisting Chronic Kidney Disease

Whereas most patients reported with obesity-related glomerulopathy have had no other underlying condition, some reports suggest that obesity may be an additive risk factor in patients with preexisting conditions such as reduced renal mass or chronic nephritis.

UNILATERAL NEPHRECTOMY

Praga et al. *(67)* studied 73 patients who had undergone unilateral nephrectomy. On follow-up, 72% of patients had normal renal function, whereas the remaining 28% had proteinuria, averaging 3.4 g/d, of whom over half also had renal insufficiency. Proteinuria was related directly to BMI. The group with proteinuria had a significantly higher BMI. Among 14 patients with a BMI >30 kg/m^2, 92% developed proteinuria or renal insufficiency, whereas among 59 patients with a BMI <30 kg/m^2, only 12% developed such complications. This observation suggests that obesity is a risk factor for new-onset proteinuria and the development of chronic renal insufficiency when renal function is reduced anatomically.

Immunoglobulin A Nephropathy

Bonnet et al. *(68)* examined excess body weight as a risk factor for disease progression in 162 patients with primary immunoglobulin A nephropathy. Overweight patients (BMI = 42.5 kg/m^2) had more proteinuria, arterial hypertension, and more advanced biopsy findings than those without excess weight. When followed for a mean of 46 mo after initial biopsy, overweight patients had a worse survival curve than those who were not overweight. BMI was an independent risk factor along with hypertension and initial biopsy score.

Diabetic/Hypertensive Nephrosclerosis

In the United Kingdom Prospective Diabetes Study, the risk of microalbuminuria increased with increased BP, hemoglobin A$_{1c}$, triglycerides, and non-Caucasian ethnicity. However, it was also shown that each 0.1 unit increase in waist-to-hip ratio was associated with a further 15% increase in risk *(69)*. In addition, BMI was associated with an increased risk of chronic kidney disease *(70)*. However, the relation appeared to be limited to morbid obesity (BMI $\geq$ 35 kg/m^2) and was felt to be largely mediated by diabetes and hypertension because adjustment for these conditions significantly decreased the relative risk.

Obesity and Renal Cell Cancer

Obesity has been associated with an increased risk of renal cell cancer. Bergstrom et al. *(71)* reviewed 22 studies from 1966 to 1998 examining body weight in relation to kidney cancer and found that increased BMI was strongly associated with an increased risk among both men and women. Chow et al. *(72)* examined the health records of 363,000 Swedish men entering the study at an average age of 44 yr and followed these subjects for an average of 16 yr. Higher BMI and elevated BP independently increased the risk of renal cancer. Compared with men in the lowest three-eighths of the cohort for BMI, those in the middle three-eighths had a 30–60% greater risk of renal cancer and those in the highest two-eighths had nearly double the risk.

MANAGEMENT

Impact of Weight Reduction

Weight management is considered the most beneficial strategy for controlling BP in obese hypertensive patients. It is also believed to be a key tool in the management of proteinuria and glomerulosclerosis of obesity. Furthermore, it ameliorates associated cardiovascular risk factors such as hyperlipidemia and insulin resistance. Weight management can be achieved by calorie restriction through diet, increased physical activity, or pharmacological and surgical interventions.

Diet

Morales et al. *(73)* investigated the effect of weight loss (through a low-calorie normoprotein diet) in 30 overweight patients (BMI > 27) with chronic proteinuric nephropathies of different etiologies. Over the course of 5 mo, a significant decrease in body weight and BMI was associated with a significant reduction in the amount of proteinuria compared to baseline and to a non-weight-losing control group. There was a significant positive correlation between the amount of weight loss and the extent of proteinuria reduction. Although changes in renal function did not differ significantly between the groups, there was a trend toward worsening in the control group whereas renal function remained stable in the diet group. There is also strong evidence for the beneficial effect of weight reduction on BP control *(74–76)*. There is a dose response relation between the degree of weight loss and the reduction in BP *(77)* independent of sodium intake *(78)*.

Many consider obesity a sodium-sensitive form of hypertension (*see* above). Sodium restriction was shown to reduce BP modestly in obese individuals *(77)*. This was further reinforced recently in a trial in obese postmenopausal women *(79)* in whom modest sodium restriction resulted in a dramatic reduction in systolic BP ($\approx$16 mmHg).

SURGERY

Obesity surgery has gained increasing popularity as a therapy for severe forms of obesity. Little information is available on the impact of such surgery on renal function and/or long-term BP control. Among subjects with severe obesity (BMI = 48 ± 2.4 kg/m^2) and no overt renal disease, weight reduction at 1 yr after gastroplasty resulted in a significant reduction in obesity-related hyperfiltration, microalbuminuria, BP and renal plasma flow *(80)*. Another study among 40 morbidly obese patients found that a reduction in BMI from 52.3 to 34.4 kg/m^2 through vertical band gastroplasty significantly improved control of hypertension at 27 mo of follow-up. Hypertension disappeared or improved in 86% of patients *(81)*. However, the long-term effect of surgery-induced weight loss on BP might not be as impressive. The Swedish Obese Subjects study, the largest study on obesity surgery and its effect on obesity-related comorbidities, demonstrated no effect of significant weight reduction on the development of hypertension at 8 yr of follow-up *(82)*.

Pharmacological Interventions to Correct Hyperfiltration and Retard Progression of Chronic Kidney Disease in Obesity

Prevention and treatment of obesity-associated renal disease should be aimed at normalizing glomerular hydrostatic pressure, as well as systemic arterial pressure. Adequate control of BP may be as effective or even more effective than adequate control of plasma glucose in obese patients with type 2 diabetes in preventing the development of serious kidney disease *(83)*. The RAS is generally regarded as playing a pathogenetic role in the development of progressive renal insufficiency. Both hemodynamic and nonhemodynamic effects play a role. ACE inhibitors and angiotensin receptor antagonists have been studied in large prospective randomized clinical trials in which their efficacy in renal protection was established *(84)*. Although these studies did not prospectively stratify the populations on the basis of weight, post hoc subgroup analysis indicated similar benefits in obese compared with nonobese patients.

The use of diuretics is invariably necessary to control BP in obese subjects with or without diabetes. As previously noted, volume expansion secondary to sodium retention contributes importantly to the hypertension of obesity. The use of diuretics should always be accompanied by sodium restriction for effective antihypertensive efficacy.

Recently, the selective aldosterone antagonist Eplerenone was also shown to attenuate glomerular hyperfiltration, sodium retention, and hypertension associated with chronic dietary-induced obesity in dogs *(85)*. This effect was dependent on the BP-lowering effect of Eplerenone. Similarly, PPARγ agonists have been shown to have a renoprotective effect in obese diabetic rats *(50)* as well as retard development of obesity-related hypertension in Sprague-Dawley hypertensive rats *(50,86)*. These effects were thought to be related to both an insulin-sensitizing action and a possible direct renal action.

REFERENCES

1. USRDS: the United States Renal Data System. Am J Kidney Dis 2003;42(6)(Suppl 5):1–230.
2. Jennette JC, Charles L, Grubb W. Glomerulomegaly and focal segmental glomerulosclerosis associated with obesity and sleep-apnea syndrome. Am J Kidney Dis 1987;10(6):470–472.
3. Bailey RR, Lynn KL, Burry AF, Drennan C. Proteinuria, glomerulomegaly and focal glomerulosclerosis in a grossly obese man with obstructive sleep apnea syndrome. Aust N Z J Med 1989;19(5):473, 474.
4. Valensi P, Assayag M, Busby M, Paries J, Lormeau B, Attali JR. Microalbuminuria in obese patients with or without hypertension. Int J Obes Relat Metab Disord 1996;20(6):574–579.
5. Ribstein J, du Callar G, Mimran A. Combined renal effects of overweight and hypertension. Hypertension 1995;26(4):610–615.
6. Hillege HL, Janssen WM, Bak AA, et al. Microalbuminuria is common, also in a nondiabetic, nonhypertensive population, and an independent indicator of cardiovascular risk factors and cardiovascular morbidity. J Intern Med 2001;249(6):519–526.
7. Liese AD, Hense HW, Doring A, Stieber J, Keil U. Microalbuminuria, central adiposity and hypertension in the non-diabetic urban population of the MONICA Augsburg survey 1994/95. J Hum Hypertens 2001;15(11):799–804.
8. Kambham N, Markowitz GS, Valeri AM, Lin J, D'Agati VD. Obesity-related glomerulopathy: an emerging epidemic. Kidney Int 2001;59(4):1498–1509.
9. Hall JE, Kuo JJ, da Silva AA, de Paula RB, Liu J, Tallam L. Obesity-associated hypertension and kidney disease. Curr Opin Nephrol Hypertens 2003;12(2):195–200.
10. Hall JE. The kidney, hypertension, and obesity. Hypertension 2003;41(3 Pt 2):625–633.
11. Bloomfield GL, Sugerman HJ, Blocher CR, Gehr TW, Sica DA. Chronically increased intra-abdominal pressure produces systemic hypertension in dogs. Int J Obes Relat Metab Disord 2000;24(7):819–824.
12. Hall JE, Brands MW, Henegar JR. Mechanisms of hypertension and kidney disease in obesity. Ann NY Acad Sci 1999;892:91–107.
13. Esler M, Rumantir M, Wiesner G, Kaye D, Hastings J, Lambert G. Sympathetic nervous system and insulin resistance: from obesity to diabetes. Am J Hypertens 2001;14(11 Pt 2):304S–309S.
14. Wofford MR, Anderson DC Jr, Brown CA, Jones DW, Miller ME, Hall JE. Antihypertensive effect of alpha- and beta-adrenergic blockade in obese and lean hypertensive subjects. Am J Hypertens 2001;14(7 Pt 1):694–698.
15. Kassab S, Kato T, Wilkins FC, Chen R, Hall JE, Granger JP. Renal denervation attenuates the sodium retention and hypertension associated with obesity. Hypertension 1995;25(4 Pt 2):893–897.
16. Considine RV, Sinha MK, Heiman ML, et al. Serum immunoreactive-leptin concentrations in normal-weight and obese humans. N Engl J Med 1996;334(5):292–295.
17. Haynes WG, Sivitz WI, Morgan DA, Walsh SA, Mark AL. Sympathetic and cardiorenal actions of leptin. Hypertension 1997;30(3 Pt 2):619–623.
18. Jackson EK, Li P. Human leptin has natriuretic activity in the rat. Am J Physiol 1997;272(3 Pt 2): 333–338.
19. Lembo G, Vecchione C, Fratta L, et al. Leptin induces direct vasodilation through distinct endothelial mechanisms. Diabetes 2000;49(2):293–297.
20. Vecchione C, Maffei A, Colella S, et al. Leptin effect on endothelial nitric oxide is mediated through Akt-endothelial nitric oxide synthase phosphorylation pathway. Diabetes 2002;51(1):168–173.
21. Shek EW, Brands MW, Hall JE. Chronic leptin infusion increases arterial pressure. Hypertension 1998;31(1 Pt 2):409–414.
22. Aizawa-Abe M, Ogawa Y, Masuzaki H, et al. Pathophysiological role of leptin in obesity-related hypertension. J Clin Invest 2000;105(9):1243–1252.
23. Kuo JJ, Jones OB, Hall JE. Inhibition of NO synthesis enhances chronic cardiovascular and renal actions of leptin. Hypertension 2001;37(2 Pt 2):670–676.
24. Correia ML, Haynes WG, Rahmouni K, Morgan DA, Sivitz WI, Mark AL. The concept of selective leptin resistance: evidence from agouti yellow obese mice. Diabetes 2002;51(2):439–442.
25. Rahmouni K, Haynes WG, Morgan DA, Mark AL. Selective resistance to central neural administration of leptin in agouti obese mice. Hypertension 2002;39(2 Pt 2):486–490.
26. Emdin M, Gastaldelli A, Muscelli E, et al. Hyperinsulinemia and autonomic nervous system dysfunction in obesity: effects of weight loss. Circulation 2001;103(4):513–519.
27. Rocchini AP. Obesity hypertension, salt sensitivity and insulin resistance. Nutr Metab Cardiovasc Dis 2000;10(5):287–294.
28. Hall JE. Hyperinsulinemia: a link between obesity and hypertension? Kidney Int 1993;43(6):1402–1417.

29. Shimabukuro M, Zhou YT, Levi M, Unger RH. Fatty acid–induced beta cell apoptosis: a link between obesity and diabetes. Proc Natl Acad Sci USA 1998;95(5):2498–2502.

30. Fujiwara K, Hayashi K, Ozawa Y, Tokuyama H, Nakamura A, Saruta T. Renal protective effect of troglitazone in Wistar fatty rats. Metabolism 2000;49(10):1361–1364.

31. Hall JE, Brands MW, Dixon WN, Smith MJ Jr. Obesity-induced hypertension: renal function and systemic hemodynamics. Hypertension 1993;22(3):292–299.

32. Engeli S, Sharma AM. The renin-angiotensin system and natriuretic peptides in obesity-associated hypertension. J Mol Med 2001;79(1):21–29.

33. Massiera F, Bloch-Faure M, Ceiler D, et al. Adipose angiotensinogen is involved in adipose tissue growth and blood pressure regulation. FASEB J 2001;15(14):2727–2729.

34. Wolf G, Hamann A, Han DC, et al. Leptin stimulates proliferation and TGF-beta expression in renal glomerular endothelial cells: potential role in glomerulosclerosis [see comments]. Kidney Int 1999;56(3):860–872.

35. Ziyadeh FN, Hoffman BB, Han DC, et al. Long-term prevention of renal insufficiency, excess matrix gene expression, and glomerular mesangial matrix expansion by treatment with monoclonal anti-transforming growth factor-beta antibody in db/db diabetic mice. Proc Natl Acad Sci USA 2000; 97(14):8015–8020.

36. Han DC, Isono M, Chen S, et al. Leptin stimulates type I collagen production in db/db mesangial cells: glucose uptake and TGF-beta type II receptor expression. Kidney Int 2001;59(4):1315–1323.

37. Ballermann BJ. A role for leptin in glomerulosclerosis? Kidney Int 1999;56(3):1154, 1155.

38. Wolf G, Chen S, Han DC, Ziyadeh FN. Leptin and renal disease. Am J Kidney Dis 2002;39(1):1–11.

39. Border WA, Noble NA. Interactions of transforming growth factor-beta and angiotensin II in renal fibrosis. Hypertension 1998;31(1 Pt 2):181–188.

40. Griffin KA, Abu-Amarah I, Picken M, Bidani AK. Renoprotection by ACE inhibition or aldosterone blockade is blood pressure-dependent. Hypertension 2003;41(2):201–206.

41. Kurtz TW. False claims of blood pressure-independent protection by blockade of the renin angiotensin aldosterone system? Hypertension 2003;41(2):193–196.

42. Anderson PW, Zhang XY, Tian J, et al. Insulin and angiotensin II are additive in stimulating TGF-beta 1 and matrix mRNAs in mesangial cells. Kidney Int 1996;50(3):745–753.

43. Abrass CK, Spicer D, Raugi GJ. Induction of nodular sclerosis by insulin in rat mesangial cells in vitro: studies of collagen. Kidney Int 1995;47(1):25–37.

44. Unger RH. Lipotoxic diseases. Annu Rev Med 2002;53:319–336.

45. Zhou Y-T, Grayborn P, Karim A, et al. Lipotoxic heart disease in obese rats:implications for human obesity. Proc Natl Acad Sci USA 2000;97:1784–1789.

46. Dwyer TM, Mizelle HL, Cockrell K, Buhner P. Renal sinus lipomatosis and body composition in hypertensive, obese rabbits. Int J Obes Relat Metab Disord 1995;19(12):869–874.

47. Keane WF. The role of lipids in renal disease: future challenges. Kidney Int Suppl 2000;75:S27–S31.

48. Lyon CJ, Law RE, Hsueh WA. Minireview: adiposity, inflammation, and atherogenesis. Endocrinology 2003;144(6):2195–2200.

49. Lavaud S, Poirier B, Mandet C, et al. Inflammation is probably not a prerequisite for renal interstitial fibrosis in normoglycemic obese rats. Am J Physiol Renal Physiol 2001;280(4):683–694.

50. Baylis C, Atzpodien EA, Freshour G, Engels K. Peroxisome proliferator-activated receptor [gamma] agonist provides superior renal protection versus angiotensin-converting enzyme inhibition in a rat model of type 2 diabetes with obesity. J Pharmacol Exp Ther 2003;307(3):854–860.

51. Dobrian AD, Davies MJ, Prewitt RL, Lauterio TJ. Development of hypertension in a rat model of diet-induced obesity. Hypertension 2000;35(4):1009–1015.

52. Messerli FH, Christie B, DeCarvalho JG, et al. Obesity and essential hypertension: hemodynamics, intravascular volume, sodium excretion, and plasma renin activity. Arch Intern Med 1981;141(1):81–85.

53. Chagnac A, Weinstein T, Korzets A, Ramadan E, Hirsch J, Gafter U. Glomerular hemodynamics in severe obesity. Am J Physiol Renal Physiol 2000;278(5):F817–F822.

54. Hall JE, Crook ED, Jones DW, Wofford MR, Dubbert PM. Mechanisms of obesity-associated cardiovascular and renal disease. Am J Med Sci 2002;324(3):127–137.

55. Wesson DE, Kurtzman NA, Frommer JP. Massive obesity and nephrotic proteinuria with a normal renal biopsy. Nephron 1985;40(2):235–237.

56. Metcalf P, Baker J, Scott A, Wild C, Scragg R, Dryson E. Albuminuria in people at least 40 years old: effect of obesity, hypertension, and hyperlipidemia. Clin Chem 1992;38(9):1802–1808.

57. Henegar JR, Bigler SA, Henegar LK, Tyagi SC, Hall JE. Functional and structural changes in the kidney in the early stages of obesity. J Am Soc Nephrol 2001;12(6):1211–1217.

58. de Jong PE, Verhave JC, Pinto-Sietsma SJ, Hillege HL. Obesity and target organ damage: the kidney. Int J Obes Relat Metab Disord 2002;26(Suppl 4):21–24.

59. Weisinger JR, Kempson RL, Eldridge FL, Swenson RS. The nephrotic syndrome: a complication of massive obesity. Ann Intern Med 1974;81(4):440–447.

60. Praga M, Morales E, Herrero JC, et al. Absence of hypoalbuminemia despite massive proteinuria in focal segmental glomerulosclerosis secondary to hyperfiltration. Am J Kidney Dis 1999;33(1):52–58.

61. Kasiske BL, Crosson JT. Renal disease in patients with massive obesity. Arch Intern Med 1986; 146(6):1105–1109.

62. Kasiske BL, Napier J. Glomerular sclerosis in patients with massive obesity. Am J Nephrol 1985; 5(1):45–50.

63. Praga M, Hernandez E, Morales E, et al. Clinical features and long-term outcome of obesity-associated focal segmental glomerulosclerosis. Nephrol Dial Transplant 2001;16(9):1790–1798.

64. Adelman RD, Restaino IG, Alon US, Blowey DL. Proteinuria and focal segmental glomerulosclerosis in severely obese adolescents. J Pediatr 2001;138(4):481–485.

65. Jafar TH, Stark PC, Schmid CH, et al. Proteinuria as a modifiable risk factor for the progression of non-diabetic renal disease. Kidney Int 2001;60(3):1131–1140.

66. Zhang Z, Shahimtar S, Keane WF, et al. Importance of baseline distribution of proteinuria in renal outcome trials: lessons from the reduction of endpoints in NIDDM with the angiotensin II antagonist (RENAAL) study. J Am Soc Nephrol 2005;16:1775–1780.

67. Praga M, Hernandez E, Herrero JC, et al. Influence of obesity on the appearance of proteinuria and renal insufficiency after unilateral nephrectomy. Kidney Int 2000;58(5):2111–2118.

68. Bonnet F, Deprele C, Sassolas A, et al. Excessive body weight as a new independent risk factor for clinical and pathological progression in primary IgA nephritis. Am J Kidney Dis 2001;37(4):720–727.

69. Adler AI, Stevens RJ, Manley SE, Bilous RW, Cull CA, Holman RR. Development and progression of nephropathy in type 2 diabetes: the United Kingdom Prospective Diabetes Study (UKPDS 64). Kidney Int 2003;63(1):225–232.

70. Stengel B, Tarver-Carr ME, Powe NR, Eberhardt MS, Brancati FL. Lifestyle factors, obesity and the risk of chronic kidney disease. Epidemiology 2003;14(4):479–487.

71. Bergstrom A, Hsieh CC, Lindblad P, Lu CM, Cook NR, Wolk A. Obesity and renal cell cancer—a quantitative review. Br J Cancer 2001;85(7):984–990.

72. Chow WH, Gridley G, Fraumeni JF Jr, Jarvholm B. Obesity, hypertension, and the risk of kidney cancer in men. N Engl J Med 2000;343(18):1305–1311.

73. Morales E, Valero MA, Leon M, Hernandez E, Praga M. Beneficial effects of weight loss in overweight patients with chronic proteinuric nephropathies. Am J Kidney Dis 2003;41(2):319–327.

74. Krebs JD, Evans S, Cooney L, et al. Changes in risk factors for cardiovascular disease with body fat loss in obese women. Diabetes Obes Metab 2002;4(6):379–387.

75. Metz JA, Stern JS, Kris-Etherton P, et al. A randomized trial of improved weight loss with a prepared meal plan in overweight and obese patients: impact on cardiovascular risk reduction. Arch Intern Med 2000;160(14):2150–2158.

76. Sjostrom CD, Peltonen M, Wedel H, Sjostrom L. Differentiated long-term effects of intentional weight loss on diabetes and hypertension. Hypertension 2000;36(1):20–25.

77. Stevens VJ, Obarzanek E, Cook NR, et al. Long-term weight loss and changes in blood pressure: results of the Trials of Hypertension Prevention, phase II. Ann Intern Med 2001;134(1):1–11.

78. Fagerberg B, Andersson OK, Isaksson B, Bjorntorp P. Blood pressure control during weight reduction in obese hypertensive men: separate effects of sodium and energy restriction. Br Med J (Clin Res Ed) 1984;288(6410):11–14.

79. Seals DR, Tanaka H, Clevenger CM, et al. Blood pressure reductions with exercise and sodium restriction in postmenopausal women with elevated systolic pressure: role of arterial stiffness. J Am Coll Cardiol 2001;38(2):506–513.

80. Chagnac A, Weinstein T, Herman M, Hirsh J, Gafter U, Ori Y. The effects of weight loss on renal function in patients with severe obesity. J Am Soc Nephrol 2003;14(6):1480–1486.

81. Haciyanli M, Erkan N, Bora S, Gulay H. Vertical banded gastroplasty in the Aegean region of Turkey. Obes Surg 2001;11(4):482–486.

82. Torgerson JS, Sjostrom L. The Swedish Obese Subjects (SOS) study—rationale and results. Int J Obes Relat Metab Disord 2001;25(Suppl 1):S2–S4.

83. Sowers JR, Haffner S. Treatment of cardiovascular and renal risk factors in the diabetic hypertensive. Hypertension 2002;40(6):781–788.

84. Brenner BM, Cooper ME, de Zeeuw D, et al. Effects of losartan on renal and cardiovascular outcomes in patients with type 2 diabetes and nephropathy. N Engl J Med 2001;345(12):861–869.
85. de Paula RB, da Silva AA, Hall JE. Aldosterone antagonism attenuates obesity-induced hypertension and glomerular hyperfiltration. Hypertension 2004;43(1):41–47.
86. Dobrian AD, Schriver SD, Khraibi AA, Prewitt RL. Pioglitazone prevents hypertension and reduces oxidative stress in diet-induced obesity. Hypertension 2004;43(1):48–56.

19 Diabetic Peripheral Neuropathy

Rachel Nardin, MD and Roy Freeman, MD

CONTENTS

INTRODUCTION

Diabetic peripheral neuropathy is the most prevalent peripheral neuropathy in the Western world. It has been reported to affect nearly 50% of people with diabetes *(1,2)*. It is responsible for a significant proportion of the mortality and morbidity that accompany diabetes and ranks third in lifetime expenditures associated with diabetic complications *(3)*. Diabetic peripheral neuropathy was until recently thought to be a late complication of diabetes; however, there is growing evidence that neuropathy may be associated with glucose intolerance and may even be the presenting symptom of diabetes *(4–6)*. Diabetes affects the peripheral nervous system in at least four distinctive patterns *(see* Table 1). Chronic, distal sensory-motor polyneuropathy, referred to as diabetic neuropathy, is the most common. However, there are acute forms of diabetic neuropathy and various focal syndromes.

CHRONIC DIABETIC POLYNEUROPATHY

Epidemiology

Chronic diabetic polyneuropathy is the most common of the diabetic neuropathies. Epidemiological studies suggest that the prevalence of diabetic polyneuropathy ranges from 5 to 93% among patients with diabetes. The wide range is related to the population under study and to the diagnostic criteria, especially whether neuropathy is defined as symptomatic or presymptomatic. In a large population-based epidemiological study, Pirart *(1)* followed a cohort of 4400 patients from 1947 to 1978 and found evidence of neuropathy using clinical criteria in 7.5% of patients at the time of diagnosis. The

From: *Contemporary Diabetes: Obesity and Diabetes*
Edited by: C. S. Mantzoros © Humana Press Inc., Totowa, NJ

Table 1
Classification of Diabetic Neuropathies

Chronic diabetic polyneuropathy
   Mixed sensory-motor-autonomic
   Variants
      Predominantly sensory
         Small-fiber sensory polyneuropathy
         Large-fiber sensory polyneuropathy
      Autonomic polyneuropathy
      Polyneuropathy with prominent demyelination
Acute diabetic polyneuropathy
   Acute painful diabetic neuropathy (with worsening diabetic control)
   Insulin neuritis (with improved control)
Proximal diabetic neuropathy (diabetic amyotrophy)
Diabetic radiculopathies and mononeuropathies
   Multisegmental truncal radiculoneuropathy
   Limb mononeuropathies
      Resulting from diabetes
      Focal compression neuropathies
   Cranial neuropathies

prevalence of neuropathy increased to 50% after 25 yr of follow-up. More recently, in a controlled, longitudinal study of 132 patients with type 2 diabetes, Partanen et al. *(7)* documented the progression of polyneuropathy. The prevalence of nerve conduction abnormalities in the legs and feet increased from 8.3% at baseline to 16.7% after 5 yr and to 41.9% after 10 yr *(7)*. Polyneuropathy is associated with older age, other microvascular complications, duration of diabetes, height, background, proliferative retinopathy, and smoking *(8)*. Lipid abnormalities such as elevated fasting triglycerides and abnormal high-density lipoprotein levels are associated with diabetic peripheral neuropathy in some *(8,9)* but not all *(10)* studies. There is some evidence that obesity may be a risk factor for polyneuropathy in patients with diabetes. This may be indirect, such as via the adverse effect of obesity on lipid profiles or other risk factors; however there may be an independent effect of obesity as well. Controlling for other known risk factors, Straub et al. found that obese patients with noninsulin-dependent diabetes mellitus had worse scores on a neuropathy assessment and an autonomic function test than lean patients *(11)*.

Clinical Features

Chronic diabetic polyneuropathy is a slowly progressive, distal, axonal polyneuropathy without distinguishing features. Both large and small myelinated and unmyelinated nerve fibers are affected; however, diabetic polyneuropathy usually presents clinically as a sensory or a sensory > motor polyneuropathy. In cases in which only sensory symptoms and signs are clinically apparent, electrophysiological testing will often reveal motor involvement. Overt autonomic symptoms are rare until the neuropathy is advanced, but subclinical autonomic involvement is common. Typically, numbness and paresthesias begin in the toes and gradually and insidiously ascend to involve the feet and lower legs. Because the distal portions of longer nerves are affected first, the feet and lower legs are involved before the hands, producing the typical "stocking and glove" pattern of sensory deficit. Neuropathic pain in the feet is a common accompaniment.

Mild distal weakness of the lower extremities usually follows sensory symptoms and signs, but significant weakness and atrophy are present only in advanced polyneuropathy. In most cases ankle reflexes are lost, but more diffuse areflexia occurs only in advanced cases. The symptoms of diabetic polyneuropathy are typically more severe at night. In some cases, there is preferential involvement of a particular group of fibers, leading to variant presentations, which are discussed next.

PREDOMINANTLY SENSORY POLYNEUROPATHY

The most common subgroup of diabetic polyneuropathy is characterized by selective small-fiber involvement. Features characteristic of a small-fiber peripheral neuropathy include burning pain, paresthesias and dysesthesias, and deficits in pain and temperature perception, with relative sparing of proprioception and reflexes. There is often dysautonomia owing to coexistent involvement of autonomic fibers. Foot ulceration and Charcot joints can occur with any type of generalized polyneuropathy, although there is a predisposition to these complications with small-fiber polyneuropathy because of the background insensitivity to pain. Impaired proprioception and atrophy of intrinsic foot muscles, with consequent maldistribution of weight bearing, disturbed sweating, impaired capillary blood flow caused by autonomic neuropathy, and noninflammatory edema, further increase the predisposition to ulceration *(12–15)*.

A smaller number of patients have a variant involving predominantly large sensory fibers. Here, there is early loss of position and vibration perception sense, manifested as impaired balance, and widespread loss of deep tendon reflexes. Diabetes is not believed to cause a selective motor neuropathy. When a patient with diabetes has significant weakness, diagnostic considerations include proximal diabetic neuropathy, acquired demyelinating polyneuropathy, anterior horn cell loss from recurring treatment-induced hypoglycemia, and coincidental motor neuronopathy.

AUTONOMIC POLYNEUROPATHY

A small number of patients have a predominantly autonomic diabetic polyneuropathy. This variant occurs disproportionately in young patients with type 1 diabetes. Classic symptoms include gastroparesis; constipation or diabetic diarrhea; incomplete bladder emptying; impotence; resting tachycardia; orthostatic hypotension; and sudomotor dysfunction, including gustatory sweating and hyper- or anhidrosis. Autonomic neuropathy may be associated with hypoglycemic unawareness. Usually there is a coexisting sensory polyneuropathy *(16)*. If the duration of diabetes is less than expected for the severity of autonomic dysfunction, amyloidosis and other causes of dysautonomia must be considered.

POLYNEUROPATHY WITH PROMINENT DEMYELINATION

Segmental demyelination is not usually a feature of diabetic polyneuropathy. However, several investigators have drawn attention to the association between chronic inflammatory demyelinating polyradiculoneuropathy (CIDP) and diabetes *(17–19)*. The typical presentation of CIDP appears similar in those with and without diabetes and includes numbness and paresthesias of the feet and hands, symmetrical proximal and distal weakness, and global hypo- or areflexia. Primary demyelination and conduction block are seen on nerve conduction studies and demyelination on nerve biopsy. The clinical progression is characteristically more rapid than chronic diabetic polyneuropathy and weakness is often more prominent. The distinction is important to make because CIDP often responds to immunomodulatory treatment *(17–20)*.

Table 2
Possible Pathogenic Mechanisms in Diabetic Polyneuropathy

Direct glucose neurotoxicity
Metabolic derangements
   Polyol pathway activation
   Reduced N^+/K^+ ATPase
   Abnormal glycation and glycosylation of proteins
   Slowed axonal transport
   Reactive oxygen species formation
   PKC activation
   Abnormal lipid metabolism
Microvascular abnormalities
   Decreased prostaglandins
   Decreased nerve blood flow
   Endoneurial ischemia
NGF deficiency
Autoimmune-mediated neurotoxicity

PATHOGENESIS

The pathophysiological basis of chronic diabetic polyneuropathy remains uncertain, and it is likely that multiple interacting factors play a role. The strongest evidence that polyneuropathy is owing to hyperglycemia, rather than other primary pathogenic factors in diabetes, comes from the success of glycemic treatment in preventing polyneuropathy *(21)*. There are a large number of potential mechanisms by which chronic hyperglycemia could lead to neuropathy (Table 2).

Elevated blood glucose may be directly toxic to the nerves; intravenous infusions of glucose have been shown to increase neuropathic pain *(22)*. Hyperglycemia may also injure nerves by a number of indirect mechanisms. Hyperglycemia causes activation of the polyol pathway, leading to the conversion of glucose into sorbitol by aldose reductase. The accumulation of the organic osmolyte sorbitol leads to compensatory depletion of other intercellular osmolytes such as myoinositol and taurine, which, in turn, leads to reduced Na^+/K^+ adenosine triphosphatase (ATPase) activity *(23)*.

The polyol pathway also generates fructose, which, together with several other compounds, such as glucose, glucose-6-phosphate, and galactose, stimulates nonenzymatic glycation, another metabolic effect of hyperglycemia. In this process, reducing sugars form reversible glycosylation products with proteins, some of which rearrange to form irreversible advanced glycosylation end products (AGEs). These AGEs can crosslink proteins, including neurofilaments and basement membrane components *(24)*.

The vascular abnormalities observed in patients with diabetic polyneuropathy include basement membrane thickening, endothelial hyperplasia, endothelial dysfunction, increased expression of endothelin, and alterations in vascular endothelial growth factor expression *(25,26)*. Pathological studies of proximal and distal segments of nerve in diabetic polyneuropathy have shown multifocal fiber loss along the length of the nerves, suggesting ischemia as a pathogenetic contributor *(27)*.

Vascular and metabolic mechanisms likely interact; hyperglycemia has been shown to have a number of deleterious effects on blood vessels. For example, the polyol pathway has been shown to consume nicotinamide adenine dinucleotide phosphate, reducing its availability for nitric oxide (NO) synthase; reduced bioavailability of NO can cause nerve ischemia in animal models of diabetes. Vessel wall matrix proteins may be affected by nonenzymatic glycation. Hyperglycemia can lead to increased oxidative stress with production of superoxides and NO. These substances can interact, leading to protein nitration or nitrosylation, lipid peroxidation, DNA damage, and endothelial and neuronal cell death. Superoxides also lead to activation of protein kinase C (PKC), which induces vasoconstriction and reduces neuronal blood flow (28,29). Hyperglycemia may also cause polyadenosine diphosphate ribosylation depletion of adenosine triphosphate resulting in cell necrosis and activation of genes involved in endothelial cell damage (30,31).

Additional mechanisms may play a role in the pathogenesis of diabetic neuropathy as well. Nerve growth factors (NGFs) are suppressed in diabetes (32). Immunological mechanisms are suggested by the circulating antineuronal antibodies found in some patients with diabetes and the inflammatory cells observed in the nerves of diabetic patients with neuropathy (33).

The recent finding that neuropathy can be seen with impaired glucose tolerance (IGT) as well as frank diabetes suggests that nerve injury from hyperglycemia may lie on a continuum and that prolonged exposure to high levels of glucose may not be necessary. Recent studies have shown that approx 35% of patients with idiopathic neuropathy have IGT, an incidence much greater than that seen in historical control subjects without neuropathy (6,34).

Reduced intraepidermal nerve fiber density on skin biopsy is found in subjects with neuropathy associated with both IGT and diabetes (35). Sumner et al. (36) showed that the neuropathy associated with IGT is less severe (based on electrophysiological measurements and intraepidermal nerve fiber densities) than that seen with diabetes, suggesting progressive injury to nerves with worsening glucose dysmetabolism.

The results of the Diabetes Control and Complications Trial (DCCT) showing that intensive insulin therapy instituted before development of retinopathy or albuminuria can reduce the appearance of neuropathy significantly compared with conventional insulin therapy also supports that early impaired glycemic control is toxic to the nerves (37). IGT is part of the syndrome of insulin resistance, which also includes obesity, hyperlipidemia, and increased risk of large-vessel atherosclerotic disease. Whether or not other markers of this syndrome, such as hyperlipidemia, are increased in patients with polyneuropathy is unclear, with the published evidence conflicting (38,39). Whether other pathophysiological pathways of nerve injury beyond those associated with hyperglycemia itself are involved in the neuropathy associated with IGT has still not been elucidated.

DIAGNOSIS AND EVALUATION OF NEUROPATHY

History and Examination

For the patient with known diabetes, a diagnosis of diabetic polyneuropathy can often be made on clinical grounds alone when the history and examination are typical. It is our practice to consider other causes of polyneuropathy before assuming diabetes as the cause. It is necessary to ask about any exposure to neurotoxins, and whether there is a history of other systemic disorders; including uremia; a possible dietary deficiency; or a family history of neuropathy. Clues that a patient's neuropathy may not be from diabetes alone include non-length-dependent sensory loss; stepwise, multifocal nerve involvement; weakness without sensory loss; bulbar or proximal weakness without advanced distal weakness; neuropathy of a severity beyond that expected for the patient's degree of diabetes; and disproportionate loss of reflexes suggesting demyelination.

Conversely, diabetes and IGT should be looked for in all patients with a newly diagnosed axonal polyneuropathy. The 2-h glucose tolerance test is recommended as a screen for IGT in patients with neuropathy given the insensitivity of the hemoglobin A1C as a screening test and the data showing that use of IFG underestimates the prevalence of impaired glucose regulation in population studies (4).

Although a careful sensory examination is usually adequate to assess sensory loss in the patient with suspected polyneuropathy, there are quantitative measures of sensory function that can be useful when more objective evidence of sensory deficit will help in the diagnosis or in following an individual patient. These include the assessment of touch perception with calibrated filaments and the use of calibrated vibrating rods. Various standardized scales incorporating elements of the history and physical examination are available to aid in the diagnosis and staging of polyneuropathy; these include the Neuropathy Impairment Score (2), the Michigan Neuropathy Screening Instrument, and the Michigan Diabetic Neuropathy Score (40).

Quantitative Sensory Testing

Quantitative sensory testing (QST) is now available in many clinical settings and allows determination of the absolute sensory threshold to various stimulus modalities (41,42). QST may be helpful in screening for mild neuropathy in which there are few symptoms or signs. It also provides objective assessment of small-fiber sensory function; this class of fibers is inaccessible to evaluation with standard nerve conduction studies. QST abnormalities correlate well with the presence of neuropathy in diabetic populations (2) and in individual patients.

Electrophysiological Testing

Nerve conduction studies and electromyography are not always necessary in patients with a history and physical examination consistent with diabetic polyneuropathy. These are useful in excluding other causes of a patient's symptoms, such as differentiating polyneuropathy from lumbosacral polyradiculopathy in a diabetic patient with severe degenerative spine disease. They are also useful in differentiating a demyelinating polyneuropathy from the predominantly axonal neuropathy of diabetes; demyelinating neuropathy should be suspected in patients with proximal weakness, global areflexia in the absence of severe weakness, and weakness in the absence of muscle atrophy. These studies can also be helpful in diagnosing superimposed compressive neuropathies in patients with underlying polyneuropathy, such as in sorting out whether intermittent hand numbness is owing to polyneuropathy or a superimposed carpal tunnel syndrome (43).

Autonomic Testing

Autonomic testing can be used to confirm a clinical suspicion of autonomic neuropathy. Autonomic testing consists of a variety of techniques for assessing the small myelinated and unmyelinated fibers of the sympathetic and parasympathetic autonomic nervous systems. The most commonly used techniques involve measures of cardiovascular influences on heart rate and blood pressure (BP). These include the Valsalva maneuver, heart rate response to deep breathing, heart rate response to standing up, BP response to standing up, and BP response to sustained handgrip. Sudomotor sympathetic function can be evaluated with the quantitative sudomotor axon reflex test, sweat imprint quantitation, thermoregulatory sweat testing, and the sympathetic skin response. Skin vasoconstrictor reflexes are produced by various maneuvers, such as Valsalva, and the resultant change in microvascular skin flow can be measured with laser Doppler flowmetry (16,44). Abnormalities on tests of autonomic function are correlated with the duration of diabetes and severity of polyneuropathy (45).

Nerve Biopsy and Skin Biopsy

Standard sural nerve biopsy is not necessary in the routine evaluation of the patient with suspected diabetic polyneuropathy. It is useful primarily in variant presentations of neuropathy in diabetics to exclude an alternative cause such as vasculitis or amyloidosis. Nerve biopsies in diabetic polyneuropathy show loss of both large- and small-caliber axons. Endoneurial capillaries are thickened and microvascular occlusions can be seen. Segmental demyelination is a rare finding (25,46).

Skin biopsy for intraepidermal nerve fiber (IENF) density analysis is a relatively new technique. It provides information about the loss of both myelinated and unmyelinated nerve fibers and can be uniquely helpful in demonstrating axon loss in pure small-fiber polyneuropathies for which routine nerve conduction studies are normal (47). IENF density in skin biopsies from distal leg sites has been shown to correlate with the densities of sural nerve total myelinated, small myelinated, and large myelinated fibers in patients with neuropathy (48).

MANAGEMENT OF CHRONIC DIABETIC POLYNEUROPATHY

Treatment of Hyperglycemia

Management of diabetic neuropathy begins with treatment of hyperglycemia. There is unequivocal evidence, based on multicenter, randomized, controlled trials, supporting strict control of blood glucose levels in patients with or without diabetic neuropathy (21,49–54). In a groundbreaking study, the DCCT unquestionably established the necessity of meticulous control of hyperglycemia. Intensive therapy significantly reduced the development of confirmed clinical neuropathy by 64% in the combined cohorts after 5 yr of follow-up; five percent of the intensive therapy group developed a confirmed clinical neuropathy compared with 13% of the conventional therapy group. The prevalence of nerve conduction abnormalities was reduced by 44%; twenty-six percent of the intensive treatment group developed abnormal nerve conductions compared with 46% of the conventional treatment group (21,37,55).

There are also data supporting the benefits of meticulous control of hyperglycemia in type 2 diabetes. A similar, although smaller, trial was conducted in Kumamoto, Japan. One hundred ten Japanese patients with type 2 diabetes were randomly assigned to receive multiple or conventional insulin injections. After 6 yr, the intensively treated cohort showed significant improvement in nerve conduction velocities, whereas the conventionally treated group showed significant deterioration in the median nerve conduction velocities and vibration threshold (50). Intensive glycemic control slows the development of autonomic neuropathy, as well (54).

Pancreatic transplantation in humans and animal models of diabetes restores the euglycemic state and obviates the need for exogenous insulin. Results from several centers have consistently reported that pancreatic transplantation in patients with well-established diabetes improves nerve conduction velocities, small- and large-fiber sensory thresholds, and measures of somatosensory and autonomic function (56–62).

Treatment of Metabolic Abnormalities

Based on the understanding of the pathogenesis of diabetic peripheral neuropathy, a number of different agents from diverse chemical classes have entered clinical trials. Although some of these agents have shown promise in clinical trials, none is approved for clinical use.

Aldose reductase inhibitors have been extensively studied, because they prevent activation of the polyol pathway. Large multicenter studies of several agents have shown some improvements in autonomic function or nerve conduction velocity slowing, but did not show a clinically meaningful effect.

Despite early data that recombinant human NGF might improve neuropathy, a larger phase III trial was not able to confirm a beneficial effect (63). Trials of dietary supplementation with myoinositol, evening primrose oil, thiamine, vitamin B$_{12}$, and pantothenic acid have been disappointing. Treatment with γ-linoleic acid has been shown to improve nerve conduction studies, but trials to show a clinically meaningful benefit have not been performed (64,65). Clinical studies of several antioxidants have shown promise. A randomized study of α-lipoic acid given intravenously for 3 wk showed improvement in neuropathic symptoms and a meta-analysis of α-lipoic acid used over 3 wk suggested benefit (66,67). A large multi-center trial with this agent is currently in progress. Although a small study of vitamin E supplementation showed improvement in nerve conduction study parameters (68), there are no convincing clinical trials providing evidence for the efficacy of supplementation with vitamin E, vitamin C, or other antioxidants in diabetic polyneuropathy.

Symptomatic Treatment of Pain

Pain is one of the more distressing and difficult to manage symptoms of diabetic neuropathy. Patients with diabetes experience spontaneous and stimulus-evoked pain. Hyperalgesia and allodynia are frequently present by history and on examination. The pathophysiological basis for the pain of diabetic neuropathy has not been established. Several investigators have attempted to define the structural basis of painful diabetic polyneuropathy. Morphological abnormalities that have been associated with neuropathic pain include axonal sprouting, acute axonal degeneration, active degeneration of myelinated fibers, and disproportionate loss of large-caliber nerve fibers. Recent controlled studies, however, have failed to support these associations consistently (69,70).

Treatment of pain requires attempts at strict control of blood glucose levels, because there is evidence that hyperglycemia may reduce the pain threshold (22,71). A variety of agents from diverse pharmacological classes have been used to treat neuropathic pain (72). These include tricyclic antidepressants (73,74), serotonin and norepinephrine uptake inhibitors (75), first (76) and second-generation anticonvulsants (77–80), and opioids (81,82). Table 3 provides some commonly used medications and dosing regimens. Because the pain of diabetic neuropathy is characteristically worse at night, regular dosing of medication in the evening may reduce analgesic requirements at night and improve sleep.

Symptomatic Treatment of Autonomic Dysfunction

Orthostatic hypotension can be treated in a stepwise fashion, depending on severity, with a high-salt diet and compression stockings, the use of 9-α-fluorohydrocortisone

Table 3
Medications for Neuropathic Pain

Agent	Initial dose	Dose increment	Usual effective dose
Antidepressants			
Tricyclics	10–25 mg every night	10–25 mg/wk	25–150 mg/d
Venlafaxine	37.5 mg every day	75 mg every wk	75–150 mg twice daily
Duloxetine	20 mg twice daily	20 mg every wk	60 mg/d
Paroxetine	10 mg every day	10 mg every 3 wk	20–60 mg/d
Anticonvulsants			
Gabapentin	100–300 mg every night	300 mg every 3–5 d	300–1800 mg three times daily
Pregabalin	75 mg twice daily	150 mg every wk	50–100 mg three times daily
Carbamazepine	100 mg twice daily	200 mg every 1–2 wk	200–400 mg three times daily
Lamotrigine	25 mg every day	25–50 mg every wk	100–200 mg twice daily
Topiramate	25 mg twice daily	50 mg every wk	100–200 mg twice daily
Analgesics			
Tramadol	50 mg every day	50 mg every day	50–100 mg four times daily
Oxycodone CR	10 mg every day	10 mg every wk	20–40 mg twice daily
Other agents			
Mexilitene	150 mg every day	150 mg every wk	150–300 mg three times daily
Capsaicin cream	0.075% four times daily	None needed	0.075% four times daily
5% Lidocaine patch	Maximum of 3 patches every day	None needed	Maximum of 3 patches every day

(0.1–0.5 mg daily) to expand intravascular volume, and the use of the peripherally acting α-agonist midodrine (2.5–10 mg three times a day). These therapies carry a risk of inducing supine hypertension, so patients should sleep with the head of the bed elevated 15–30°.

Treatment of gastroparesis involves optimizing blood glucose control, which improves gastric motility. Patients should eat multiple small meals per day. Prokinetic agents used to treat diabetic gastropathy include metoclopramide (10 mg orally 30 min before meals), domperidone (10–20 mg four times a day), erythromycin (250 mg three times a day, and levosulpiride (25 mg three times daily) (16).

Treatments for impotence owing to autonomic neuropathy include sildenafil (50 mg), a phosphodiesterase inhibitor that enhances blood flow to the corpora cavernosae with sexual stimulation. Tadalafil (20 mg) (83) and vardenafil (20 mg) (84) are also effective in >60% of diabetic patients with erectile dysfunction. Other therapies include the injection of vasoactive substances such as papaverine, and the use of mechanical vacuum devices or penile constricting rings.

Patients with a neurogenic bladder owing to a diabetic autonomic neuropathy should be taught to initiate micturition with a Credé maneuver every 4 h. Parasympathomimetic agonists such as bethanechol (10–30 mg three times a day) are sometimes helpful. Intermittent self-catheterization can also be used.

Gustatory sweating may respond to anticholinergic agents (85) and to injections of botulinum toxin type A (86).

ACUTE DIABETIC POLYNEUROPATHY

Patients with diabetes may develop an acute, rapidly progressive, painful polyneuropathy associated with weight loss *(87)*. In this condition, there is a sudden appearance of severe burning pain in the extremities, combined with deep aching pain in proximal muscles; jabs of pain radiating from the feet to the legs; and striking hypersensitivity or allodynia of the extremities and trunk to touch, clothing, or bed sheets that is often likened to sunburn. Neuropathic pain and cutaneous hypersensitivity overshadow sensory loss, which may be minor on examination. Patients with this condition may appear ill and acutely overwhelmed by pain, distinguishing them from patients who are newly aware of chronic polyneuropathy. Acute diabetic polyneuropathy occurs after a change in glycemic control and is given different names, depending on the triggering event.

One form, sometimes called "insulin neuritis," appears for the first time coincident with improved glycemic control owing to treatment with insulin or oral hypoglycemic agents, or to weight loss *(88–90)*. Although the cause is unknown, one hypothesis is that the normalization of blood sugar after prolonged hyperglycemia could result in energy deprivation in nerves that had shifted to anaerobic metabolism in a glucose-rich environment.

A second form, called acute painful diabetic neuropathy or diabetic neuropathic cachexia, is associated with poor diabetic control. It is seen primarily in men with poorly controlled type 2 diabetes and is associated with anorexia and unintentional weight loss *(91)*. It is distinct from the phenomenon of widespread paresthesias of the extremities and trunk, referred to as hyperglycemic neuropathy, that occasionally occur in patients with newly diagnosed or poorly controlled diabetes. These symptoms of hyperglycemic neuropathy are rapidly corrected with the institution of normoglycemia *(92)*. This is in contrast to the course of both forms of acute diabetic polyneuropathy, in which improvement occurs slowly over months, perhaps as axonal regrowth occurs. Although pain improves, an underlying polyneuropathy remains.

PROXIMAL DIABETIC NEUROPATHY

Proximal diabetic neuropathy, also called proximal motor neuropathy, diabetic polyradiculopathy *(93)*, diabetic amyotrophy, and diabetic lumbosacral radiculoplexus neuropathy *(94)*, is much less common than chronic diabetic polyneuropathy, with a prevalence estimated at 0.8%. It is more common in men than women and typically occurs with a peak incidence in the sixth decade in patients with type 2 diabetes, usually after a period of poorly controlled hyperglycemia *(95)*. Anorexia and substantial weight loss usually occur before or during the syndrome. Blood glucose may normalize after weight loss, which can confuse the picture.

The clinical picture is one of acute or subacute thigh and back pain, usually severe, followed within weeks by weakness and atrophy of lower-extremity muscles. The iliopsoas, quadriceps, and thigh adductors are usually involved. Distal muscles may also be weak, particularly peroneal-innervated muscles, but proximal muscles are always more affected than distal. Mild sensory loss or hyperesthesia may be seen over the anterior thigh in about half of patients *(96,97)*. The knee jerk is nearly always reduced or absent on the affected side, whereas ankle jerks may be preserved unless compromised by a coexistent distal polyneuropathy. Symptoms usually begin unilaterally, but the opposite extremity can be affected within weeks to months *(94)*. Recurrent episodes are uncommon *(93,97)*.

The symptoms may have a monophasic or stepwise progression *(98–100)*. The progression of weakness most often occurs in two phases, with a rapid phase associated with pain followed by a slower phase that progresses over weeks or months *(95)*. On occasion, patients can develop a similar disorder affecting the proximal upper extremity.

The diagnosis of proximal diabetic neuropathy rests on the typical clinical presentation. Electrophysiological studies can be helpful in demonstrating an axonal radiculoplexopathy and in excluding an alternative cause of proximal weakness, such as CIDP, polymyositis, or motor neuron disease. Evidence of a distal polyneuropathy is found in the majority of patients as well *(93,101)*. A lesion of the lumbar nerve roots should be excluded by magnetic resonance imaging (MRI) of the lumbar spine. Imaging of the pelvis and lumbosacral plexus should be done in patients with a history suggesting a risk of an alternative cause, such as anticoagulation or a history of cancer. Cerebrospinal fluid protein is usually elevated *(101)*. Serum creatine kinase can be mildly elevated as seen in other denervating disorders.

Recent studies have emphasized the likelihood that proximal diabetic neuropathy has an inflammatory basis *(96,102)*, which has led to the use of immune-modulating therapies. Intravenous immunoglobulins, plasmapheresis, and oral and iv corticosteroids have all been used in open-label uncontrolled studies *(101–103)*. If immunotherapy is used, it makes theoretical sense to institute it early, during the period of presumed active inflammation. Because of reports that patients who regain lost weight improve faster than those who remain cachectic, patients should be encouraged to regain weight until they have recovered, even if this requires more intensive glucose therapy. The pain of proximal diabetic neuropathy can be severe and often requires treatment with narcotic analgesics. Assessment of the effects of treatments in uncontrolled trials is confounded by the fact that the natural history of the disease is one of a phase of progression followed by improvement. One study suggests a mean time to the start of recovery of 3 mo, with a variance of 1–12 mo *(97)*. Pain improves first, followed by gradual return of strength over a period of 6–18 mo *(93,104,105)*. Improvement in strength occurs in a majority of patients but is often incomplete and significant weakness can persist *(101)*.

DIABETIC RADICULOPATHIES AND MONONEUROPATHIES

With the exception of secondary compressive mononeuropathies, the mononeuropathies and radiculopathies associated with diabetes tend to be acute or subacute in onset, often associated with pain. Like proximal diabetic neuropathy, they occur in middle or later life, often associated with recent weight loss, and can be the presenting feature of diabetes. They tend to spontaneously improve over 6–12 mo. These features have suggested an ischemic and possibly an inflammatory etiology.

Truncal Radiculoneuropathy

Truncal radiculoneuropathy is also called thoracic polyradiculopathy, truncal neuropathy, or diabetic thoracoabdominal neuropathy. It usually occurs in middle-aged patients and often in those who have relatively mild diabetes *(106)*. It is characterized by the onset of pain, cutaneous hypersensitivity, sensory loss, and sometimes weakness in the distribution of one or more somatic nerves or roots *(107,108)*. Onset of pain is usually acute, and the pain may be located in the back, chest, or abdomen, causing confusion with medical conditions such as myocardial ischemia and acute appendicitis.

The character of the pain is usually deep and aching with some elements of superficial sharp or burning pain. Focal muscle weakness affecting the abdominal wall may simulate a hernia. Symptoms commonly appear during an episode of changing diabetic control and are often associated with weight loss; occasionally, the disorder occurs simultaneously with proximal diabetic neuropathy (108). The diagnosis of diabetic truncal radiculoneuropathy is generally a clinical one, although most patients have abnormalities on electromyography consistent with a multisegmental disorder at the nerve roots, proximal intercostal and abdominal nerves, or both that can confirm the disorder (108,109). The symptoms usually progress over days to weeks. Remission of pain typically occurs within 4–12 mo, although cutaneous sensory loss may persist. The role of immunotherapies in this disorder is uncertain.

Limb Mononeuropathies

There are rare cases of acute, painful mononeuropathy in diabetes, likely on the basis of focal nerve infarction (110). Isolated femoral neuropathy, which was once thought to be a diabetic mononeuropathy, is now largely felt to be a variant of proximal diabetic neuropathy. Most diabetic mononeuropathies are the result of local nerve entrapment or compression. Patients with diabetes are considered more susceptible to focal compression neuropathies, which are clinically and electrophysiologically similar to those that develop in the absence of diabetes (111).

Carpal tunnel syndrome caused by median-nerve entrapment in the wrist is particularly common among people with diabetes. Retrospective and population studies have shown an increased incidence of carpal tunnel syndrome in patients with diabetes (2,111,112). Dyck et al. (2) found asymptomatic median neuropathies at the wrist in 32% of patients with diabetes and symptomatic median neuropathies at the wrist in 9%. Obesity may be an independent risk factor for carpal tunnel syndrome as well (113). The diagnosis of carpal tunnel syndrome is best made with nerve conduction studies, although the diagnostic challenges are greater in those with underlying polyneuropathy. The treatment of carpal tunnel syndrome is the same for patients with and without diabetes and consists of neutral wrist splinting for early cases. Steroid injections into the carpal tunnel may provide temporary relief from symptoms but lead to increased hyperglycemia and should be used with caution. Once there is evidence of axon loss from median-nerve compression, consideration should be given to surgical decompression. It is important to remember that if there is underlying polyneuropathy, decompression may not relieve acral numbness entirely.

Ulnar mononeuropathy also occurs with greater frequency in diabetes, found in about 2% of patients, and is probably related to the position of the nerve at the elbow that renders it vulnerable to chronic trauma (2). Symptoms usually appear insidiously. There is usually progressive weakness and atrophy in ulnar-innervated hand muscles. Although some patients have sensory symptoms in the ring and small fingers, there may be no associated pain or numbness. The hand weakness from ulnar neuropathy needs to be differentiated from the distal weakness from polyneuropathy, in which median-innervated thenar muscles are also involved. Electrophysiological studies can be helpful in the diagnosis. Treatment is the same as in patients without diabetes, consisting of conservative measures early with elbow padding and splinting, and surgical decompression for more severe cases.

Other mononeuropathies are rare in diabetes and may occur coincidentally. Peroneal mononeuropathy typically produces sudden painless foot drop usually owing to compression of the nerve at the fibular head. Lateral femoral cutaneous neuropathy, or meralgia paresthetica, occurs in approx 1% of patients with diabetes, although obesity may be an alternative explanation in this population *(2)*. Phrenic neuropathy resulting in diaphragmatic paralysis may occur rarely in patients with diabetes *(114)*.

Cranial Mononeuropathies

The most common of diabetic cranial neuropathies affects the third and sixth cranial nerves *(115,116)*, and the fourth cranial nerve is rarely affected alone *(115)*. Unilateral oculomotor neuropathies are of sudden onset and are usually painful, with onset of diplopia progressing to complete ophthalmoplegia over several days. In cases of third-nerve involvement, there may be complete ptosis but the pupil is typically spared. Sparing of the pupil may be a consequence of the relative sparing of the peripherally located pupillomotor fibers from the effects of nerve ischemia; however, pupillary sparing can be seen in up to 20% of patients with third-nerve compression from a mass lesion *(117)*. Although typical cases of painful, acute-onset oculomotor neuropathy in patients with diabetes over age 50 can be observed without imaging, brain MRI is indicated in cases with progression after 1 wk, in cases with lack of improvement in 8 wk, or in any case of a third-nerve palsy in which there is either pupillary involvement or pupillary sparing in the absence of a complete third-nerve palsy. MRI imaging is most useful in excluding an alternative cause such as a mass lesion in the orbital fissure or cavernous sinus, cerebral aneurysm, or focal midbrain infarction *(118)*. There is no specific treatment for these ocular mononeuropathies. The prognosis is excellent, with data suggesting complete or partial recovery in 72% over 1 to 2 mo *(119,120)*.

Facial paralysis owing to seventh-nerve palsy may occur with increased frequency in patients with diabetes *(121)*. The incidence of diabetes in typical Bell's palsy is 6–10%, and facial palsy is more common in older patients with diabetes *(122,123)*. Pecket and Schattner *(123)* found a disturbance of taste in 14% of patients with Bell's palsy and diabetes compared with 83% of those without diabetes; this suggests that the lesion in patients with diabetes is usually distal to the chorda tympani. Other features are similar to those of Bell's palsy without diabetes, consisting of acute onset of facial weakness associated with pain and sometimes hyperacusis progressing over several days. Patients with incomplete facial weakness usually recover fully over weeks to month; those with complete facial paralysis have slower and less complete recovery. The prognosis for recovery may be worse than in patients without diabetes *(124)*.

REFERENCES

1. Pirart J. Diabetes mellitus and its degenerative complications: a prospective study of 4,400 patients observed between 1947 and 1973 (3rd and last part) [in French]. Diabetes Metab 1977;3(4):245–256.
2. Dyck PJ, Kratz KM, Karnes JL, et al. The prevalence by staged severity of various types of diabetic neuropathy, retinopathy, and nephropathy in a population-based cohort: the Rochester Diabetic Neuropathy Study [published erratum appears in Neurology 1993;43(11):2345]. Neurology 1993;43(4):817–824.
3. Caro JJ, Ward AJ, O'Brien JA. Lifetime costs of complications resulting from type 2 diabetes in the US Diabetes Care 2002;25(3):476–481.
4. Russell JW, Feldman EL. Impaired glucose tolerance—does it cause neuropathy? Muscle Nerve 2001;24(9):1109–1112.
5. Singleton JR, Smith AG, Bromberg MB. Increased prevalence of impaired glucose tolerance in patients with painful sensory neuropathy. Diabetes Care 2001;24(8):1448–1453.
6. Novella SP, Inzucchi SE, Goldstein JM. The frequency of undiagnosed diabetes and impaired glucose tolerance in patients with idiopathic sensory neuropathy. Muscle Nerve 2001;24(9):1229–1231.

7. Partanen J, Niskanen L, Lehtinen J, et al. Natural history of peripheral neuropathy in patients with non- insulin-dependent diabetes mellitus. N Engl J Med 1995;333(2):89–94.

8. Tesfaye S, Stevens LK, Stephenson JM, et al. Prevalence of diabetic peripheral neuropathy and its relation to glycaemic control and potential risk factors: the EURODIAB IDDM Complications Study. Diabetologia 1996;39(11):1377–1384.

9. Maser RE, Steenkiste AR, Dorman JS, et al. Epidemiological correlates of diabetic neuropathy: report from Pittsburgh Epidemiology of Diabetes Complications Study. Diabetes 1989;38(11): 1456–1461.

10. Dyck PJ, Davies JL, Wilson DM, et al. Risk factors for severity of diabetic polyneuropathy: intensive longitudinal assessment of the Rochester Diabetic Neuropathy Study cohort. Diabetes Care 1999;22(9):1479–1486.

11. Straub RH, Thum M, Hollerbach C, et al. Impact of obesity on neuropathic late complications in NIDDM. Diabetes Care 1994;17(11):1290–1294.

12. Edmonds ME. The diabetic foot: pathophysiology and treatment. Clin Endocrinol Metab 1986;15:889–916.

13. Boulton AJ. The pathogenesis of diabetic foot problems: an overview [review]. Diabet Med 1996;13(Suppl 1):S12–S16.

14. Reiber GE. The epidemiology of diabetic foot problems. Diabet Med 1996;13(Suppl 1):S6–S11.

15. Reiber GE, Vileikyte L, Boyko EJ, et al. Causal pathways for incident lower-extremity ulcers in patients with diabetes from two settings. Diabetes Care 1999;22(1):157–162.

16. Vinik AI, Maser RE, Mitchell BD, Freeman R. Diabetic autonomic neuropathy. Diabetes Care 2003;26(5):1553–1579.

17. Stewart JD, McKelvey R, Durcan L, et al. Chronic inflammatory demyelinating polyneuropathy (CIDP) in diabetics. J Neurol Sci 1996;142(1–2):59–64.

18. Gorson KC, Ropper AH, Adelman LS, Weinberg DH. Influence of diabetes mellitus on chronic inflammatory demyelinating polyneuropathy. Muscle Nerve 2000;23(1):37–43.

19. Haq RU, Pendlebury WW, Fries TJ, Tandan R. Chronic inflammatory demyelinating polyradiculoneuropathy in diabetic patients. Muscle Nerve 2003;27(4):465–470.

20. Sharma KR, Cross J, Farronay O, et al. Demyelinating neuropathy in diabetes mellitus. Arch Neurol 2002;59(5):758–765.

21. Anonymous. The effect of intensive treatment of diabetes on the development and progression of long-term complications in insulin-dependent diabetes mellitus. The Diabetes Control and Complications Trial Research Group [see comments]. N Engl J Med 1993;329:977–986.

22. Morley GK, Mooradian AD, Levine AS, Morley JE. Mechanism of pain in diabetic peripheral neuropathy. Effect of glucose on pain perception in humans. Am J Med 1984;77(1):79–82.

23. Greene DA, Lattimer SA, Sima AA. Sorbitol phosphinositides, and sodium-potassium ATPase in pathogenesis of diabetic complications. N Engl J Med 1978;316:599–606.

24. Brownlee M. Glycation products and the pathogenesis of diabetic complications. Diabetes Care 1992;15(12):1835–1843.

25. Dyck PJ, Giannini C. Pathologic alterations in the diabetic neuropathies of humans: a review [see comments]. J Neuropathol Exp Neurol 1996;55(12):1181–1193.

26. Sheetz MJ, King GL. Molecular understanding of hyperglycemia's adverse effects for diabetic complications. JAMA 2002;288(20):2579–2588.

27. Dyck PJ, Karnes JL, O'Brien P, et al. The spatial distribution of fiber loss in diabetic polyneuropathy suggests ischemia. Ann Neurol 1986;19:440–449.

28. Low PA, Nickander KK, Tritschler HJ. The roles of oxidative stress and antioxidant treatment in experimental diabetic neuropathy. Diabetes 1997;46(Suppl 2):S38–S42.

29. Feldman EL. Oxidative stress and diabetic neuropathy: a new understanding of an old problem. J Clin Invest 2003;111(4):431–433.

30. Du X, Matsumura T, Edelstein D, et al. Inhibition of GAPDH activity by poly(ADP-ribose) polymerase activates three major pathways of hyperglycemic damage in endothelial cells. J Clin Invest 2003;112(7):1049–1057.

31. Obrosova IG, Li F, Abatan OI, et al. Role of poly(ADP-ribose) polymerase activation in diabetic neuropathy. Diabetes 2004;53(3):711–720.

32. Leinninger GM, Vincent AM, Feldman EL. The role of growth factors in diabetic peripheral neuropathy. J Peripher Nerv Syst 2004;9(1):26–53.

33. Younger DS, Rosoklija G, Hays AP, et al. Diabetic peripheral neuropathy: a clinicopathologic and immunohistochemical analysis of sural nerve biopsies. Muscle Nerve 1996;19(6):722–727.

34. Singleton JR, Smith AG, Bromberg MB. Painful sensory polyneuropathy associated with impaired glucose tolerance. Muscle Nerve 2001;24(9):1225–1228.

35. Smith AG, Ramachandran P, Tripp S, Singleton JR. Epidermal nerve innervation in impaired glucose tolerance and diabetes-associated neuropathy. Neurology 2001;57(9):1701–1704.

36. Sumner CJ, Sheth S, Griffin JW, et al. The spectrum of neuropathy in diabetes and impaired glucose tolerance. Neurology 2003;60(1):108–111.

37. Anonymous. The effect of intensive diabetes therapy on the development and progression of neuropathy. The Diabetes Control and Complications Trial Research Group. Ann Intern Med 1995;122(8):561–568.

38. Periquet MI, Novak V, Collins MP, et al. Painful sensory neuropathy: prospective evaluation using skin biopsy [see comments]. Neurology 1999;53(8):1641–1647.

39. Jeppesen U, Gaist D, Smith T, Sindrup SH. Statins and peripheral neuropathy. Eur J Clin Pharmacol 1999;54(11):835–838.

40. Feldman EL, Stevens MJ, Thomas PK, et al. A practical two-step quantitative clinical and electrophysiological assessment for the diagnosis and staging of diabetic neuropathy. Diabetes Care 1994;17(11):1281–1289.

41. Gruener G, Dyck PJ. Quantitative sensory testing: methodology, applications, and future directions [review]. J Clin Neurophysiol 1994;11(6):568–583.

42. Stewart JD, Freeman R. Quantitative sensory testing. In: Brown WF, Bolton CF, Aminoff MJ, eds. Neuromuscular Function and Disease. WB Saunders, Philadelphia, 2002, pp. 131–144.

43. Freeman R. The peripheral nervous system and diabetes. In: Kahn CR, Weir GC, King GL, eds. Joslin's Diabetes Mellitus. Lippincott Williams & Wilkins, Philadelphia, 2002.

44. Ewing DJ, Martyn CN, Young RJ, Clarke BF. The value of cardiovascular autonomic function tests: 10 yr experience in diabetes. Diabetes Care 1985;8:491–498.

45. Ziegler D, Dannehl K, Muhlen H, et al. Prevalence of cardiovascular autonomic dysfunction assessed by spectral analysis, vector analysis, and standard tests of heart rate variation and blood pressure responses at various stages of diabetic neuropathy. Diabet Med 1992;9(9):806–814.

46. Sima AA, Brown MB, Prashar A, et al. The reproducibility and sensitivity of sural nerve morphometry in the assessment of diabetic peripheral polyneuropathy. Diabetologia 1992;35(6):560–569.

47. McArthur JC, Stocks EA, Hauer P, et al. Epidermal nerve fiber density: normative reference range and diagnostic efficiency [see comments]. Arch Neurol 1998;55(12):1513–1520.

48. Herrmann DN, Griffin JW, Hauer P, et al. Epidermal nerve fiber density and sural nerve morphometry in peripheral neuropathies. Neurology 1999;53(8):1634–1640.

49. Anonymous. The effect of intensive diabetes therapy on measures of autonomic nervous system function in the Diabetes Control and Complications Trial (DCCT). Diabetologia 1998;41(4):416–423.

50. Ohkubo Y, Kishikawa H, Araki E, et al. Intensive insulin therapy prevents the progression of diabetic microvascular complications in Japanese patients with non-insulin- dependent diabetes mellitus: a randomized prospective 6-yr study [see comments]. Diabetes Res Clin Pract 1995;28(2):103–117.

51. Reichard P, Britz A, Carlsson P, et al. Metabolic control and complications over 3 yr in patients with insulin dependent diabetes (IDDM): the Stockholm Diabetes Intervention Study (SDIS). J Intern Med 1990;228(5):511–517.

52. Reichard P, Berglund B, Britz A, et al. Intensified conventional insulin treatment retards the microvascular complications of insulin-dependent diabetes mellitus (IDDM): the Stockholm Diabetes Intervention Study (SDIS) after 5 yr. J Intern Med 1991;230:101–108.

53. Reichard P, Nilsson BY, Rosenqvist U. The effect of long-term intensified insulin treatment on the development of microvascular complications of diabetes mellitus [see comments]. N Engl J Med 1993;329(5):304–309.

54. Gaede P, Vedel P, Parving HH, Pedersen O. Intensified multifactorial intervention in patients with type 2 diabetes mellitus and microalbuminuria: the Steno type 2 randomised study [see comments]. Lancet 1999;353(9153):617–622.

55. Anonymous. Effect of intensive diabetes treatment on nerve conduction in the Diabetes Control and Complications Trial. Ann Neurol 1995;38(6):869–880.

56. Kennedy WR, Navarro X, Goetz FC, et al. Effects of pancreatic transplantation on diabetic neuropathy [see comments]. N Engl J Med 1990;322:1031–1037.

57. Navarro X, Kennedy WR, Loewenson RB, Sutherland DE. Influence of pancreas transplantation on cardiorespiratory reflexes, nerve conduction, and mortality in diabetes mellitus. Diabetes 1990;39:802–806.

58. Navarro X, Sutherland DE, Kennedy WR. Long-term effects of pancreatic transplantation on diabetic neuropathy [see comments]. Ann Neurol 1997;42(5):727–736.

59. Nusser J, Scheuer R, Abendroth D, et al. Effect of pancreatic and/or renal transplantation on diabetic autonomic neuropathy. Diabetologia 1991;34(Suppl 1):S118–S120.

60. Solders G, Wilczek H, Gunnarsson R, et al. Effects of combined pancreatic and renal transplantation on diabetic neuropathy: a two-yr follow-up study. Lancet 1987;2:1232–1235.

61. Solders G, Tyden G, Persson A, Groth CG. Improvement in diabetic neuropathy 4 yr after successful pancreatic and renal transplantation. Diabetologia 1991;34(Suppl 1):S125–S127.

62. Trojaborg W, Smith T, Jakobsen J, Rasmussen K. Effect of pancreas and kidney transplantation on the neuropathic profile in insulin-dependent diabetics with end-stage nephropathy. Acta Neurol Scand 1994;90(1):5–9.

63. Apfel SC, Schwartz S, Adornato BT, et al. Efficacy and safety of recombinant human nerve growth factor in patients with diabetic polyneuropathy: a randomized controlled trial. JAMA 2000;284(17): 2215–2221.

64. Jamal GA, Carmichael H. The effect of gamma-linolenic acid on human diabetic peripheral neuropathy: a double-blind placebo-controlled trial. Diabet Med 1990;7(4):319–323.

65. Keen H, Payan J, Allawi J, et al. Treatment of diabetic neuropathy with gamma-linolenic acid. The gamma- Linolenic Acid Multicenter Trial Group [see comments]. Diabetes Care 1993; 16(1):8–15.

66. Ametov AS, Barinov A, Dyck PJ, et al. The sensory symptoms of diabetic polyneuropathy are improved with alpha-lipoic acid: the SYDNEY trial. Diabetes Care 2003;26(3):770–776.

67. Ziegler D, Nowak H, Kempler P, et al. Treatment of symptomatic diabetic polyneuropathy with the antioxidant alpha-lipoic acid: a meta-analysis. Diabet Med 2004;21(2):114–121.

68. Tutuncu NB, Bayraktar M, Varli K. Reversal of defective nerve conduction with vitamin E supplementation in type 2 diabetes: a preliminary study. Diabetes Care 1998;21(11):1915–1918.

69. Llewelyn JG, Gilbey SG, Thomas PK, et al. Sural nerve morphometry in diabetic autonomic and painful sensory neuropathy: a clinicopathological study. Brain 1991;114:867–892.

70. Malik RA. The pathology of human diabetic neuropathy. Diabetes 1997;46(Suppl 2):S50–S53.

71. Oyibo SO, Prasad YD, Jackson NJ, et al. The relationship between blood glucose excursions and painful diabetic peripheral neuropathy: a pilot study. Diabet Med 2002;19(10):870–873.

72. Sindrup SH, Jensen TS. Pharmacologic treatment of pain in polyneuropathy. Neurology 2000;55(7): 915–920.

73. Max MB, Lynch SA, Muir J, et al. Effects of desipramine, amitriptyline, and fluoxetine on pain in diabetic neuropathy. N Engl J Med 1992;326(19):1250–1256.

74. Sindrup SH, Gram LF, Brosen K, Eshoj O, Mogensen EF. The selective serotonin reuptake inhibitor paroxetine is effective in the treatment of diabetic neuropathy symptoms. Pain 1990;42:135–144.

75. Sindrup SH, Bach FW, Madsen C, et al. Venlafaxine versus imipramine in painful polyneuropathy: a randomized, controlled trial. Neurology 2003;60(8):1284–1289.

76. Saudek CD, Werns S, Reidenberg MM. Phenytoin in the treatment of diabetic symmetrical polyneuropathy. Clin Pharmacol Ther 1977;22(2):196–199.

77. Backonja M, Beydoun A, Edwards KR, et al. Gabapentin for the symptomatic treatment of painful neuropathy in patients with diabetes mellitus: a randomized controlled trial [see comments]. JAMA 1998;280(21):1831–1836.

78. Rosenstock J, Tuchman M, LaMoreaux L, Sharma U. Pregabalin for the treatment of painful diabetic peripheral neuropathy: a double-blind, placebo-controlled trial. Pain 2004;110(3):628–638.

79. McCleane GJ. Lamotrigine in the management of neuropathic pain: a review of the literature. Clin J Pain 2000;16(4):321–326.

80. Eisenberg E, Lurie Y, Braker C, et al. Lamotrigine reduces painful diabetic neuropathy: a randomized, controlled study. Neurology 2001;57(3):505–509.

81. Harati Y, Gooch C, Swenson M, et al. Maintenance of the long-term effectiveness of tramadol in treatment of the pain of diabetic neuropathy. J Diabetes Complications 2000;14(2):65–70.

82. Gimbel JS, Richards P, Portenoy RK. Controlled-release oxycodone for pain in diabetic neuropathy: a randomized controlled trial. Neurology 2003;60(6):927–934.

83. Saenz de Tejada I, Anglin G, Knight JR, Emmick JT. Effects of tadalafil on erectile dysfunction in men with diabetes. Diabetes Care 2002;25(12):2159–2164.

84. Goldstein I, Young JM, Fischer J, et al. Vardenafil, a new phosphodiesterase type 5 inhibitor, in the treatment of erectile dysfunction in men with diabetes: a multicenter double-blind placebo-controlled fixed-dose study. Diabetes Care 2003;26(3):777–783.

85. Shaw JE, Abbott CA, Tindle K, et al. A randomised controlled trial of topical glycopyrrolate, the first specific treatment for diabetic gustatory sweating. Diabetologia 1997;40(3):299–301.

86. Restivo DA, Lanza S, Patti F, et al. Improvement of diabetic autonomic gustatory sweating by botulinum toxin type A. Neurology 2002;59(12):1971–1973.

87. Archer AG, Watkins PJ, Thomas PK, et al. The natural history of acute painful neuropathy in diabetes mellitus. J Neurol Neurosurg Psychiatry 1983;46(6):491–499.

88. Caravati CM. Insulin neuritis: a case report. Va Med Monthly 1933;59:745, 746.

89. Ellenberg M. Diabetic neuropathy precipitating after institution of diabetic control. Am J Med Sci 1958;236:466.

90. Llewelyn JG, Thomas PK, Fonseca V, et al. Acute painful diabetic neuropathy precipitated by strict glycemic control. Acta Neuropathol (Berl) 1986;72:157–163.

91. Said G, Goulon-Goeau C, Slama G, Tchobroutsky G. Severe early-onset polyneuropathy in insulin-dependent diabetes mellitus. A clinical and pathological study. N Engl J Med 1992;326:1257–1263.

92. Thomas PK. Diabetic neuropathy: mechanisms and future treatment options. J Neurol Neurosurg Psychiatry 1999;67(3):277–279.

93. Bastron JA, Thomas JE. Diabetic polyradiculopathy: clinical and electromyographic findings in 105 patients. Mayo Clin Proc 1981;56(12):725–732.

94. Dyck PJ, Norell JE, Dyck PJ. Microvasculitis and ischemia in diabetic lumbosacral radiculoplexus neuropathy. Neurology 1999;53(9):2113–2121.

95. Barohn RJ, Sahenk Z, Warmolts JR, Mendell JR. The Bruns-Garland syndrome (diabetic amyotrophy). Revisited 100 yr later. Arch Neurol 1991;48(11):1130–1135.

96. Said G, Elgrably F, Lacroix C, et al. Painful proximal diabetic neuropathy: inflammatory nerve lesions and spontaneous favorable outcome. Ann Neurol 1997;41(6):762–770.

97. Coppack SW, Watkins PJ. The natural history of diabetic femoral neuropathy [see comments]. Q J Med 1991;79(288):307–313.

98. Chokroverty S. Proximal nerve dysfunction in diabetic proximal amyotrophy: electrophysiology and electron microscopy. Arch Neurol 1982;39(7):403–407.

99. Chokroverty S. AAEE case report 13: diabetic amyotrophy. Muscle Nerve 1987;10(8):679–684.

100. Chokroverty S, Sander HW. AAEM case report 13: diabetic amyotrophy [published erratum appears in Muscle Nerve 1996;19(12):1655]. Muscle Nerve 1996;19(8):939–945.

101. Pascoe MK, Low PA, Windebank AJ, Litchy WJ. Subacute diabetic proximal neuropathy. Mayo Clin Proc 1997;72(12):1123–1132.

102. Said G, Goulon-Goeau C, Lacroix C, Moulonguet A. Nerve biopsy findings in different patterns of proximal diabetic neuropathy. Ann Neurol 1994;35(5):559–569.

103. Krendel DA, Costigan DA, Hopkins LC. Successful treatment of neuropathies in patients with diabetes mellitus [see comments]. Arch Neurol 1995;52(11):1053–1061.

104. Hamilton CR Jr, Dobson HL, Marshall J. Diabetic amyotrophy: clinical and electronmicroscopic studies in six patients. Am J Med Sci 1968;256(2):81–90.

105. Casey EB, Harrison MJ. Diabetic amyotrophy: a follow-up study. BMJ 1972;1(801):656–659.

106. Lauria G, McArthur JC, Hauer PE, et al. Neuropathological alterations in diabetic truncal neuropathy: evaluation by skin biopsy. J Neurol Neurosurg Psychiatry 1998;65(5):762–766.

107. Stewart JD. Diabetic truncal neuropathy: topography of the sensory deficit. Ann Neurol 1989;25(3):233–238.

108. Sun SF, Streib EW. Diabetic thoracoabdominal neuropathy: clinical and electrodiagnostic features. Ann Neurol 1981;9(1):75–79.

109. Kikta DG, Breuer AC, Wilbourn AJ. Thoracic root pain in diabetes: the spectrum of clinical and electromyographic findings. Ann Neurol 1982;11(1):80–85.

110. Fraser DM, Campbell IW, Ewing DJ, Clarke BF. Mononeuropathy in diabetes mellitus. Diabetes 1979;28:96–101.

111. Mulder DW, Lambert EH, Bastron JA, Sprague RG. The neuropathies associated with diabetes mellitus: a clinical and electromyographic study of 103 unselected diabetic patients. Neurology 1961;11(4)(Pt 1):275–284.

112. Albers JW, Brown MB, Sima AA, Greene DA. Frequency of median mononeuropathy in patients with mild diabetic neuropathy in the early diabetes intervention trial (EDIT). Tolrestat Study Group for Edit (Early Diabetes Intervention Trial). Muscle Nerve 1996;19(2):140–146.

113. Nathan PA, Keniston RC, Myers LD, Meadows KD. Obesity as a risk factor for slowing of sensory conduction of the median nerve in industry: a cross-sectional and longitudinal study involving 429 workers. J Occup Med 1992;34(4):379–383.

114. de Carvalho MA, Matias T, Evangelista T, et al. Bilateral phrenic nerve neuropathy in a diabetic patient. Eur J Neurol 1996;3:481–482.

115. Zorrilla E, Kozak GP. Ophthalmoplegia in diabetes mellitus. Arch Intern Med 1967;67:968–976.
116. Ross AT. Recurrent cranial nerve palsies in diabetes mellitus. Neurology 1962;12:180–185.
117. Jacobson DM. Relative pupil-sparing third nerve palsy: etiology and clinical variables predictive of a mass. Neurology 2001;56(6):797, 798.
118. Breen LA, Hopf HC, Farris BK, Gutmann L. Pupil-sparing oculomotor nerve palsy due to midbrain infarction [see comments]. Arch Neurol 1991;48(1):105, 106.
119. Richards BW, Jones FR Jr, Younge BR. Causes and prognosis in 4,278 cases of paralysis of the oculomotor, trochlear, and abducens cranial nerves. Am J Ophthalmol 1992;113(5):489–496.
120. Goldstein JE, Cogan DG. Diabetic ophthalmoplegia with special reference to the pupil. Arch Ophthalmol 1960;64:592–600.
121. Korczyn AD. Bell's palsy and diabetes mellitus. Lancet 1971;1(7690):108, 109.
122. Aminoff MJ, Miller AL. The prevalence of diabetes mellitus in patients with Bell's palsy. Acta Neurol Scand 1972;48(3):381–384.
123. Pecket P, Schattner A. Concurrent Bell's palsy and diabetes mellitus: a diabetic mononeuropathy? J Neurol Neurosurg Psychiatry 1982;45(7):652–655.
124. Adour KK, Wingerd J. Idiopathic facial paralysis (Bell's palsy): factors affecting severity and outcome in 446 patients. Neurology 1974;24(12):1112–1116.

20 The Diabetic Foot

Thanh L. Dinh, DPM
and Aristidis Veves, MD, MSc, DSc

Contents

INTRODUCTION

Foot pathology remains the leading diabetic complication requiring hospitalization *(1)*. Because the incidence of diabetes in the general population is expected to rise, the prevalence of diabetic foot complications will follow. The resulting cost to society can be measured in direct costs attributed to treatment, as well as indirect costs in lost productivity. The total cost of diabetic foot complications in the United States has been estimated to approach $4 billion annually, as extrapolated from the costs of ulcer care and amputations *(2)*. However the costs are measured, diabetic foot problems represent a major public health challenge of growing proportions.

The prevalence of secondary complications of diabetes, such as diabetic foot complications, appears to be associated with risk factors such as duration of diabetes and obesity *(3)*. The role of obesity in the development and prolongation of diabetic foot complications can be described as an indirect pathway. It has been presumed that increases in body weight result in increased peak plantar pressures in the foot. Because plantar peak pressures are a major risk factor for the development of foot ulcers, obesity was thought to increase the development of foot ulcerations as well as negatively impact their timely resolution.

However, there is currently conflicting evidence on the role of obesity in peak plantar foot pressures. One study found that an increase in body weight directly resulted in an increase in peak plantar pressures of the foot *(4)*. Another study found that although body mass is correlated with peak plantar pressures, the functional relationship between the two variables was weak. Instead, body mass accounted for <14% of the variance in peak plantar pressure observed *(5)*. Further studies investigating the role of obesity on peak plantar pressures and the development of foot ulcerations will assist in clarifying this debate.

From: *Contemporary Diabetes: Obesity and Diabetes*
Edited by: C. S. Mantzoros © Humana Press Inc., Totowa, NJ

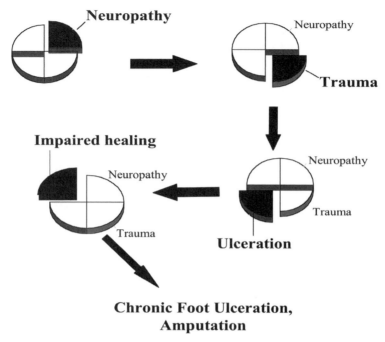

Fig. 1. Pathway to foot ulceration. Sensory neuropathy, associated with pain insensitivity, is the first component of the pathway. However, the development of ulceration also requires the existence of trauma, usually related to the plantar tissue stress and injury that results from the development of high foot pressures during walking. The presence of the third component, impaired wound healing, owing to reduced blood flow in the ulcer area and aberrant expression of growth factors and cytokines, prevents wound closure and leads to the development of chronic ulceration and, in some cases, amputation. (Modified from ref. *10*.)

DIABETIC FOOT ULCERATION

Etiology

PATHWAY TO FOOT ULCERATION

Major risk factors for the development of diabetic foot ulcers include peripheral neuropathy, high foot pressures, and impaired wound healing. It is important to note that these risk factors do not act independently to produce foot ulceration. Instead, a combination of risk factors acts to trigger the pathway leading to ulceration. A critical triad of neuropathy, minor foot trauma, and foot deformity was found in >63% of foot ulcers in one study *(6)*.

As shown in Fig. 1, in the vast majority of diabetic foot ulceration, the first major component is the development of sensory neuropathy that results in pain insensitivity component *(7)*. The next step is the development of trauma, usually related to the high foot pressures that develop under the foot while walking. Finally, impaired wound healing, related to reduced blood supply at the wound area and abnormal expression of growth factors and other cytokines that are involved in the healing process, results in the body's inability to repair the trauma. It is usually the combination of these three major components that lead to the development of chronic ulceration and, in some cases, amputation of the lower extremity.

PERIPHERAL SENSORY NEUROPATHY

Reported in approx 30–50% of all patients with diabetes, peripheral sensory neuropathy has been found to be the most common and sensitive predictor for foot ulceration in such patients *(8,9)*. In a study that specifically examined casual pathways of diabetic foot ulceration, the presence of neuropathy was reported in 78% of feet with ulcers *(6)*.

The presence of peripheral sensory neuropathy initiates a series of events that eventually result in foot ulceration. With an inability to detect the pain signals that warn of impending tissue trauma, the insensate foot is exposed to increased pressures that hasten tissue damage, leading to ulceration. The propagation of this vicious cycle, of increased forces coupled with impaired protective sensation, causes the ulcer to worsen.

AUTONOMIC AND MOTOR NEUROPATHY

Autonomic neuropathy is a common finding in patients with long-standing diabetes. In the lower extremity, autonomic neuropathy can cause arteriovenous shunting, resulting in a vasodilatory condition in the small arteries *(10)*. Abnormalities in autonomic neuropathy are also responsible for decreased activity of the sweat glands of the feet. These changes in the diabetic foot can result in skin that is prone to dryness and fissuring, predisposing the patient to the risk of infection *(11)*.

Motor neuropathy in the foot causes weakness and wasting of the small intrinsic muscles, classically termed the intrinsic minus foot. This leads to muscular imbalance with a characteristic clawing of the toes and plantar flexion of the metatarsal heads. The prominences at the plantar metatarsal head level and the digital level serve as areas of focal pressures with possible irritation from footwear. Coupled with sensory neuropathy, these prominences are susceptible to increased forces with subsequent ulceration.

PEAK PLANTAR PRESSURES

Diabetic ulcers can occur on any part of the foot but are clinically observed most frequently on the plantar surfaces. The predilection of diabetic foot ulcers to the plantar surfaces is related to the trauma that develops in these areas as the result of increased peak plantar pressures during walking *(12)*.

The development of high foot pressures starts in the early stages of diabetic neuropathy, even in the subclinical phase of the disease. One of the first steps is the transfer of high peak pressures from the heel area to the forefoot area, in the absence of any clinically detectable neuropathy. As a result, the pressures under certain areas of the diabetic foot can be considerably high and lead to tissue injury even after walking not very long distances. In the presence of sensory neuropathy, the patient is unaware of the first warning symptoms of this injury, such as pain, and continues to walk until tissue integrity is compromised and foot ulceration occurs.

LIMITED JOINT MOBILITY

Restriction of joint mobility is well documented in diabetes and is related mainly to collagen glycosylation that results in thickening of the periarticular structures such as tendons, ligaments, and joint capsules *(13,14)*. At the foot level, the subtalar and metatarsalphalangeal joints are most commonly involved. Involvement of the subtalar joint seems critical because it impairs the ability of the foot to adapt to the ground surface and absorb the shock that develops when the heel makes contact with the ground during walking. Subsequently, high foot pressures develop, mainly in the forefoot area, and are believed to contribute further to the development of foot ulceration *(15–17)*.

Collagen glycosylation is also implicated in decreasing the resiliency of the Achilles tendon in patients with diabetes *(18)*. Decreased motion of the Achilles tendon creates an equinus deformity with a further shift of plantar forces to the forefoot region that results in increased plantar pressures under the metatarsal area *(19)*. Surgical lengthening of the Achilles tendon has been found to effectively distribute plantar pressures more uniformly, thus decreasing the peak forces at the metatarsal region *(20)*.

PERIPHERAL VASCULAR DISEASE

Peripheral vascular disease (PVD) on average is identified in 30% of foot ulcers *(6)*. It is important to note that ischemia in itself is not a risk factor for the development of a foot ulcer. Instead, ischemia complicates and slows wound healing, as a result of insufficient blood flow. PVD in diabetes is characterized by impairment at both the microcirculation and macrocirculation level. Macrocirculatory disease in the patient with diabetes is identical to the atherosclerotic changes found in individuals without diabetes, whereas microcirculatory disease is unique to the patient with diabetes.

Recent investigation into the microcirculation of the diabetic foot has revealed significant structural and functional changes that may contribute to the impaired wound healing observed in diabetic foot ulcers. Impairment of the diabetic foot at the level of the microcirculation has been coined a "functional ischemia," owing to its inability to vasodilate under conditions of stress. This functional ischemia may be a possible mechanism for the nonhealing observed in diabetic foot ulcers.

IMPAIRED WOUND HEALING

An understanding of the faulty wound healing in the diabetic foot ulcer is essential in providing appropriate treatment. The normal wound healing process entails a complex interplay among connective-tissue formation, cellular activity, and growth factor activation. All three of these physiological processes are altered in the diabetic state and contribute to the poor healing of diabetic foot ulcers.

The normal inflammatory stage of wound repair involves an orchestrated interaction of resident cells such as epithelial cells, fibroblasts, dendritic cells, and endothelial cells with biochemical activity *(21)*. In addition to these resident cells, platelets, neutrophils, T-cells, natural killer cells, and macrophages are recruited to the wound site. These cells migrate to the injury site to mediate the inflammation, coagulation, and angiogenesis processes occurring in the wound-healing process.

Instead of progressing through the normal stages of wound healing, it is now clear that diabetic ulcers are "stuck" in the inflammatory phase of the wound-healing process. During this delay, there is a cessation of epidermal growth and migration over the wound surface *(22,23)*. Analysis of fluid from these chronic wounds has demonstrated elevated levels of matrix metalloproteinases directly resulting in increased proteolytic activity and inactivation of the growth factors necessary for proper wound healing. Additionally, these chronic wounds have been found to exhibit deficiencies in growth factors and cytokines along with elevated levels of inhibitory proteases. Therefore, impaired wound healing is manifested in aberrant protein synthesis, cellular activity, and growth factor secretion.

Growth factors influence the wound-healing process through inhibitory or stimulatory effects on the local wound environment. Growth factors such as growth platelet-derived growth factor (PDGF), basic fibroblast growth factor, and vascular endothelial growth factor have all been found in wound fluid. These growth factors are known to be integral in the chemotaxis, migration, stimulation, and proliferation of cells and matrix substances necessary for wound healing. Therefore, the altered secretion or absence of these growth factors in diabetic foot ulcers can potentially impair wound healing. Recent investigation of the role that these growth factors play in wound healing appears to support this hypothesis *(24)*.

Treatment Principles

The best means of treating diabetic foot ulcerations appears to be prevention through screening for those individuals at high risk and patient education regarding early warning signs of ulceration and infection. Primary care physicians should refer patients with diabetes with evidence of loss of protective sensation (easily performed with the Semmes-Weinstein monofilament) to a podiatric specialist for routine evaluation.

In the event that an ulceration is present, the cornerstones of treatment for full-thickness ulcers should consist of adequate debridement, off-loading of pressure, treatment of infection, and local wound care. In addition to these basic tenets of diabetic ulcer treatment, greater understanding of the pathophysiology of wound healing has led to advanced wound care products demonstrating promise in accelerating wound healing.

DEBRIDEMENT

Debridement allows removal of all nonviable tissue and greater visual assessment of the wound base as well as promotes the release of growth factors. The goal of wound debridement should be the complete removal of all necrotic, dysvascular, and nonviable tissue in order to achieve a red, granular wound bed. In the event that ischemia is suspected, aggressive debridement should be delayed until vascular examination and revascularization are achieved.

Debridement can be performed in a variety of methods. Sharp technique for removal of necrotic tissue is considered the "gold standard" for debridement of diabetic foot ulcers *(25)*. Using sharp instruments such as a scalpel blade, all nonviable tissue can be removed until a healthy bleeding ulcer bed is produced with saucerization of the wound edges. This procedure can be performed in the office setting; however, if debridement is extensive or sensation to the foot intact, sharp debridement should be carried out in an operating room under appropriate anesthesia and sterility.

PRESSURE OFF-LOADING

As discussed previously, ulcerations occur in high-pressure areas of the insensate foot; therefore, reduction of pressures is essential to healing. A number of methods are employed for the reduction of foot pressures, with varying success rates. The most popular methods include the use of total-contact casting, half shoes, short leg walkers, and felted-foam dressings.

Total-contact casting has been considered the most effective means of off-loading diabetic foot ulcers as measured by wound-healing rate *(26)*. Described by Paul Brand, total-contact casting involves the use of a well-molded minimally padded plaster cast to distribute pressures evenly to the entire limb. It allows patient mobility during treatment and has been found to help control edema, linked to impairment of healing *(27)*. The main advantage and likely effectiveness of total-contact casting, however, is the forced patient compliance owing to the inability to remove the apparatus. Disadvantages include the considerable skill and time required for application, the possibility of secondary skin lesions as the result of cast irritation, and the inability to assess the wound daily.

Because of the significant disadvantages associated with the total-contact cast, few clinicians use that particular off-loading technique. Instead, commercially available off-the-shelf devices such as the half shoe and short leg walker are more commonly used. Both of these devices are relatively inexpensive, easy to use, and readily accepted by the patient. However, pressure reduction is significantly less compared to total contact casting, and patient compliance cannot be ensured owing to the removable nature of the devices (28).

Felted-foam dressings are accommodative off-loading devices fashioned from a felt-foam pad with an aperture corresponding to the ulceration for customized pressure relief. The pad is generally attached by tape or rubber cement directly to the patient's skin, preventing migration of the pad and ensuring a degree of patient compliance. Wound care and wound assessment can be performed through the aperture portion of the pad. The felted foam is often used in conjunction with a surgical shoe or half shoe and must be changed every 10–14 d to ensure integrity of the dressing. Felted-foam dressings in combination with a surgical shoe or half shoe were found to be more effective in pressure reduction when compared to a short leg walker or a half shoe alone (29).

TREATMENT OF INFECTION

A diabetic foot ulcer can serve as a portal of entry for bacteria, with subsequent infection. Diagnosis of infection is primarily based on clinical appearance, relying on clinical signs such as erythema, edema, pain, tenderness, and warmth. The severity of an infection can range from a superficial cellulitis to a deep abscess or necrotizing fasciitis with systemic toxicity. Note that clinically uninfected ulcers should not be cultured, because the organisms recovered will consist only of colonizing flora.

Radiographic imaging of the infected foot can demonstrate increased density and thickening of the sc fat along with blurring of the usually visible fat planes. The presence of osseous changes such as periosteal reaction, cortical bone destruction, and focal osteopenia may suggest a diagnosis of osteomyelitis. However, these changes become evident only after osteomyelitis has been present for 10–14 d and require up to 50% bone loss before becoming recognizable (30). When a diagnosis of osteomyelitis is in doubt, advanced imaging techniques such as magnetic resonance imaging (MRI) and computed tomography (CT), which are more sensitive compared to radiographs, may aid in accurate diagnosis.

Treatment of infection involves debridement of all necrotic tissue and drainage of purulent collections along with antibiotic therapy. Selection of antibiotic should take into account the likely causative organisms while considering the potential toxicity of the agents. In the diabetic foot, the bacteria most likely responsible for nonlimb-threatening infections are staphylococcus and streptococci, while limb-threatening infections are generally the consequence of a polymicrobial infection (31).

Empiric selection of antibiotic should be based on the suspected bacterial pathogens along with modifications to address anticipated resistant pathogens that may have been selected during prior hospitalizations. Selection of antibiotic should minimize toxicity and be cost-effective. Broad-spectrum antimicrobial therapy should be begun empirically with reassessment following the results of culture and sensitivities. Treatment regimens should then be simplified based on the culture data.

The duration of antimicrobial therapy for severe soft-tissue infections of the foot is based on response to the antibiotics and wound care. Two weeks of therapy is the usual guideline; however, recalcitrant infections may require longer courses. Even if the ulcer has not fully healed, antibiotics can be discontinued when evidence of infection has resolved. Continuation of antibiotics beyond this duration has not demonstrated any effect on wound healing *(32,33)*.

WOUND CARE

The effective use of dressings is essential to ensure optimal management of diabetic foot ulcers. In recent years, the concept of a clean, moist wound-healing environment has been widely accepted. Benefits to this approach include prevention of tissue dehydration and cell death, acceleration of angiogenesis, and facilitation of the interaction of growth factors with the target cells *(34)*. Additionally, patients have reported less discomfort with moist wound dressings. A multitude of wound care products are available on the market that promote moist wound healing; however, wet-to-dry normal saline gauze remains the standard of care of the majority of diabetic foot ulcers.

ADVANCED WOUND CARE PRODUCTS

Advanced wound care products have been developed in response to an improved understanding of the impaired wound healing integral in the diabetic foot ulcer. Pathophysiological defects such as decreased growth factor production and cellular inactivity have led to the development of products that address these deficiencies. Products in this category include recombinant PDGF and biological skin substitutes.

Recombinant human PDGF-BB (rhPDGF-BB) (becaplermin) is the only growth factor to date approved by the US Food and Drug Administration for the treatment of diabetic foot ulcers. Levels of PDGF have been shown to be lower in chronic wounds *(35)*. Administered topically to the ulcer daily, becaplermin gel both increased the incidence of complete wound closure and decreased the time to achieve complete wound healing *(36)*. Becaplermin is believed to enhance wound healing through the expression of PDGF-BB by macrophages, endothelial cells, and platelets. PDGF-BB is known to be a potent mitogen and chemotactic agent for connective tissue and stromal cells and may act to increase wound vascularization by stimulating endothelial cell proliferation, movement, and tube formation.

Biological skin substitutes, also known as living skin equivalents (LSEs), are produced from neonatal fibroblasts and keratinocytes using tissue-engineering technology. Available in epidermal, dermal, and composite (epidermal and dermal) forms, LSEs offer distinct advantages over traditional skin grafting: LSEs are noninvasive, do not require anesthesia, can be performed in an outpatient setting, and avoid potential donor site complications such as infection and scarring *(37)*. Furthermore, more rapid wound coverage of chronic diabetic foot ulcers with the use of LSEs can provide both social and economic advantages by reducing the number of office visits and hospital stays and preventing serious wound complications that often lead to amputation.

Two LSEs currently approved for use in diabetic foot ulcers are Dermagraft (Advanced Tissue Sciences, La Jolla, CA) and Apligraf (Organogenesis, Canton, MA, distributed by Novartis, East Hanover, NJ). Dermagraft consists of neonatal dermal fibroblasts cultured in vitro onto a bioabsorbable polygalactin mesh, producing a living, metabolically active tissue containing the normal dermal matrix proteins and cytokines. Dermagraft has been shown to incorporate quickly into the wound with good vascularization and no adverse side effects *(38,39)*. In a prospective randomized multicenter study, Dermagraft-treated ulcers were associated with more complete and rapid healing with the added benefit of a reduction in ulcer recurrence rate compared to conventional therapy *(40)*.

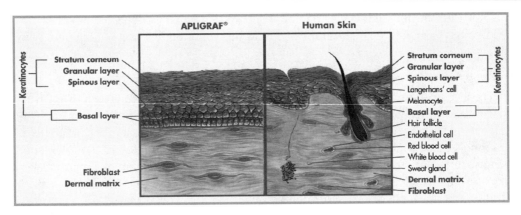

Fig. 2. Histological comparison of Apligraf and human skin.

Apligraf is considered a composite graft, containing both epidermal and dermal components. The outer layer consists of allergenic human keratinocytes constructed with an inner dermal layer consisting of human fibroblasts on type 1 collagen dispersed in a protein matrix. Although Apligraf histologically resembles human skin, it does not contain structures such as blood vessels, hair follicles, or sweat glands (Fig. 2). Interestingly, Apligraf acts like human skin, producing all the cytokines and growth factors produced by normal skin during the wound-healing process *(41)*. In diabetic foot ulcers, Apligraf was shown to statistically significantly increase wound healing rate as well as decrease the median time to complete wound closure *(42,43)*.

Although the precise mechanism of action of Dermagraft and Apligraf is not completely understood, it is believed that improved wound healing is a result of filling the wound with extracellular matrix proteins and with the subsequent induction and expression of growth factors and cytokines necessary for wound healing. Additionally, the matrix components may further facilitate the recruitment of cells to the wound, improving wound repair.

CHARCOT NEUROARTHROPATHY

Charcot neuroarthropathy is a noninfectious progression of joint destruction characterized by pathological fractures and joint dislocations. Described initially in 1868 by J. M. Charcot *(44)*, Charcot joint destruction can occur in a number of disease states that manifest peripheral neuropathy such as leprosy, tertiary syphilis, chronic alcoholism, and spina bifida *(45)*. However, with the increase in the prevalence of diabetes, diabetes mellitus is now the leading cause of Charcot neuroarthropathy.

Etiology

The exact etiology of Charcot neuroarthropathy remains unclear. There are two leading theories: the neurotraumatic theory and the neurovascular theory. The neurotraumatic theory proposes that repeated microtrauma on neuropathic joints results in eventual joint destruction *(46)*. In this theory, repetitive minor stresses on insensate joints produces intracapsular effusions, ligamentous laxity, and joint instability. With continued use of the foot, degeneration of the joints continues, often resulting in severe joint dislocation and deformity.

By contrast, the neurovascular theory hypothesizes that hyperemia owing to autonomic neuropathy results in excessive bone resorption resulting in weakening of the bone *(47)*.

The hyperemic bone resorption thus allows increased risk of pathological fractures with joint dislocation and destruction evident in Charcot joints. This theory corresponds to the clinical observation that Charcot neuroarthropathy occurs most commonly in patients with palpable pedal pulses (48). In actuality, the process of Charcot neuroarthropathy is likely owing to a combination of both the neurovascular and neurotraumatic theories.

Clinical Findings

Regardless of the etiology, the Charcot foot usually presents as a warm, nonpainful swelling of the foot. More often than not, there is no evidence of an open wound. Therefore, an infectious process can be excluded based on the lack of a portal of entry. Occasionally, patients may describe a precedent history of minor trauma; however, this is frequently so trivial that the patient is unable to recall the incident.

Initial evaluation of Charcot neuroarthropathy requires a thorough clinical and radiographic examination of the foot. Clinical examination often reveals a warm, edematous foot with crepitus with joint range of motion. Most commonly, pain is absent or significantly less than expected from the clinical presentation. Radiographic findings demonstrate osseous debris and fragmentation with mild to frank joint subluxation. The most common site affected in the foot is the tarsometatarsal joint (49). The extent of fragmentation and joint destruction is variable and most often related to the particular joints affected and the degree of ambulation prior to diagnosis. Advanced imaging techniques such as CT scans and MRIs are rarely necessary to make a diagnosis of Charcot joint and, instead, may be more useful in preoperative surgical planning in certain cases.

There are three identifiable clinical phases of Charcot neuroarthropathy: acute, coalescence, and remodeling. The acute phase is characterized by clinical findings of edema, erythema, localized warmth, and joint crepitus with range-of-motion examination. The coalescence phase begins when skin temperature normalizes and joint crepitus diminishes. With a period of duration lasting from months to years, the remodeling phase is characterized by joint stabilization and remodeling. Unfortunately, resolution of Charcot neuroarthropathy can result in a deformed foot with obvious bony prominences susceptible to ulceration (45).

Treatment Principles

The treatment of choice for acute Charcot foot is complete immobilization and non-weight bearing. Immobilization can be achieved with casts, splints, or braces and non-weight bearing aided with the use of crutches, walkers, or wheelchairs. Failure to immobilize the foot adequately may result in further fragmentation of bone with progression of the joint deformity, resulting in a foot with a rocker-bottom deformity (Fig. 3). The ultimate goal of immobilization therapy is to allow the foot to coalesce in a shape that will allow eventual ambulation.

Immobilization and non-weight bearing should continue until the acute phase of Charcot has ended and the coalescence phase commenced. The recommended duration of immobilization varies from 8 wk (50) to 3–6 mo (51). The decision to discontinue immobilization and begin weight bearing may be best made by clinical parameters such as increased warmth and edema, rather than an arbitrary time period. Resolution of both edema and warmth are good indicators of progression to the coalescence stage; therefore, immobilization and weight bearing may be safely discontinued. Serial radiographs may also aid in the decision-making process. Evidence of osseous consolidation, union of fractures, and reduction in soft-tissue edema are radiographic indications that coalescence has begun.

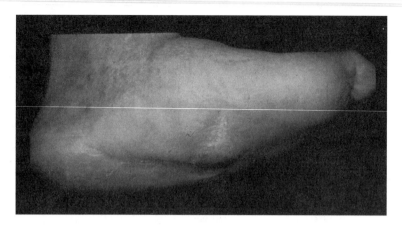

Fig. 3. Photograph of a Charcot foot with rocker-bottom deformity.

Once weight bearing is deemed safe, return to ambulation should be performed in a gradual manner. Typically, weight bearing is begun allowing only 15–20 lb of weight on the affected limb, with 10-lb increments added on a weekly basis. Should symptoms of the acute phase such as edema, erythema, and warmth appear, immobilization and non-weight bearing should be resumed until resolution of these symptoms occurs.

In recent years, increased attention has been given to surgical reconstruction of the severely deformed Charcot foot. In cases in which immobilization and non-weight bearing have failed to prevent extensive joint dislocation, a rocker-bottom type of foot with osseous prominences can be the end result. This type of foot is not amenable to ambulation and is highly susceptible to ulceration. Therefore, arthrodesis of the involved joints may provide a stable platform for ambulation in addition to preventing future ulcerations. However, patients undergoing joint fusions will require extended periods of immobilization and non-weight bearing postoperatively and, therefore, should be screened carefully.

CONCLUSIONS

Diabetic foot ulcerations represent a significant and growing health problem. Although obesity has not been conclusively demonstrated to be a risk factor in the development of diabetic foot ulcerations, there is some evidence that its presence may hinder the timely resolution of these ulcers. With a greater understanding of the risk factors and pathophysiological processes involved, new treatments are continually evolving.

There is no question that the growth of diabetes in the United States is reaching epidemic proportions. This appears to be related to the observed trend in obesity. As the incidence of diabetes rises, the rate of secondary complications such as diabetic foot ulcerations will follow. Therefore, addressing the trend in obesity may be the best means of preventing diabetic foot complications.

REFERENCES

1. Gibbons G, Eliopolos G. Infection of the diabetic foot. In: Kozak G, Hoar CJ, Rowbotham J, Wheelock F, Gibbons G, Campbell DR, eds. Management of Diabetic Foot Problems. Saunders, Philadelphia, 1984, pp. 97–102.
2. Harrington C, Zagari MJ, Corea J, Klitenic J. A cost analysis of diabetic lower-extremity ulcers. Diabetes Care 2002;25:630–631.

3. Shera AS, Jawad F, Maqsood A, Jamal S, Azfar M, Ahmed U. Prevalence of chronic complications and associated factors in type 2 diabetes. J Pak Med Assoc 2004;54(2):54–59.

4. Vela SA, Lavery LA, Armstrong DG, Anaim AA. The effect of increased weight on peak pressures: implications for obesity and diabetic foot pathology. J Foot Ankle Surg 1998;37:416–420.

5. Cavanagh PR, Sims DS Jr, Sanders LJ. Body mass is a poor predictor of peak plantar pressure in diabetic men. Diabetes Care 1991;14(8):750–755.

6. Reiber GE, Vileikyte L, Boyko EJ, et al. Causal pathways for incident lower-extremity ulcers in patients with diabetes from two settings. Diabetes Care 1999;22:157–162.

7. Pecoraro RE, Reiber GE, Burgess EM. Pathways to diabetic limb amputation: basis for prevention. Diabetes Care 1990;13:513–521.

8. Young MJ, Breddy JL, Veves A, Boulton AJM. The prediction of diaetic neuropathic foot ulceration using vibration perception thresholds: a prospective study. Diabetes Care 1994;17:557–560.

9. Adler AI, Boyko EJ, Ahroni JH, Stensel V, Forsberg RC, Smith DG. Risk factors for diabetic peripheral sensory neuropathy: results of the Seattle prospective diabetic foot study. Diabetes Care 1997;96:223–228.

10. Ward JD, Simms JM, Knight G, Boulton AJM, Sandler DA. Venous distension in the diabetic neuropathic foot. J R Soc Med 1983;76:1011–1014.

11. Tegner R. The effect of skin temperature on vibratory sensitivity in polyneuropathy. J Neurol Neurosurg Psychiatry 1985;48:176–178.

12. Boulton AJ, Hardisty CA, Betts RP, et al. Dynamic foot pressure and other studies as diagnostic and management aids in diabetic neuropathy. Diabetes Care 1983;1:26–33.

13. Kumar S, Fernando DJ, Veves A, Knowles EA, Young MJ, Boulton AJ. Semmes-Weinstein monofilaments: a simple, effective and inexpensive screening device for identifying diabetic patients at risk of foot ulceration. Diabetes Res Clin Pract 1991;13:63–67.

14. Stokes IA, Furis IB, Hutton WC. The neuropathic ulcer and loads on the foot in diabetic patients. Acta Orthop Scand 1975;46:839–847.

15. Ctercteko G, Dhanendran M, Hutton WC, et al. Vertical forces acting on the feet of diabetic patients with neuropathic ulceration. Br J Surg 1981;68:608–614.

16. Veves A, Fernando DJ, Walewski P, et al. A study of plantar pressures in a diabetic clinic population. Foot 1991;2:89–92.

17. Fernando DJ, Masson EA, Veves A, Boulton AJ. Relationship of limited joint mobility to abnormal foot pressures and diabetic foot ulceration. Diabetes Care 1991;14(1):8–11.

18. Grant WP, Sullivan R, Soenshine DE, et al. Electron microscopic investigation of the effects of diabetes mellitus on the Achilles tendon. J Foot Ankle Surg 1997;36:272–278.

19. Vlassara H, Brownlee M, Cerami A. Nonenzymatic glycosylation: rose in the pathogenesis of diabetic complications. Clin Chem 1986;32:B37–B41.

20. Armstrong DG, Stacpoole-Shea S, Nguyen HC, Harkless LB. Lengthening of the Achilles tendon in diabetic patients who are at high risk for ulceration of the foot. J Bone Joint Surg 1999;81A:535–538.

21. Schilling JA. Wound healing. Physiol Rev 1968;48:374–423.

22. Jude EB, Boulton AJ, Ferguson MW, Appleton I. The role of nitric oxide synthase isoforms and arginase in the pathogenesis of diabetic foot ulcers: possible modulatory effects by transforming growth factor beta 1. Diabetologia 1999;42:748–757.

23. Loots MA, Lamme EN, Zeegelaar J, Mekkes JR, Bos JD, Middelkoop E. Differences in cellular infiltrate and extracellular matrix of chronic diabetic and venous ulcers versus acute wounds. J Invest Dermatol 1998;111:850–857.

24. Cooper DM, Yu EZ, Hennesey P, et al. Determination of endogenous cytokines in chronic wounds. Ann Surg 1994;219:688–692.

25. Clark RAF. Mechanisms of cutaneous wound repair. In: (Fitzpatrick TB, Eisen AZ, Wolff K, Freedberg IM, Austin KF, eds.), Dermatology in General Medicine. McGraw-Hill, New York, 1993, pp. 473–483.

26. Armstrong DG, Nguyen HC, Lavery LA, et al. Offloading the diabetic foot wound: a randomized clinical trial. Diabetes Care 2001;24:1019–1022.

27. Mueller MJ, Diamond JE, Sinacore DR, et al. Total contact casting in treatment of diabetic plantar ulcers. Diabetes Care 1989;12:364–387.

28. Lavery LA, Vela SA, Lavery DC, et al. Reducing dynamic foot pressures in high-risk diabetics with foot ulcerations: a comparison of treatments. Diabetes Care 1996;19:818–821.

29. Birke JA, Fred B, Krieger LA, Sliman K. The effectiveness of an accommodative dressing in offloading pressure over areas of previous metatarsal head ulceration. Wounds 2003;15:33–39.

30. Bonakdar-Pour A, Gaines VD. The radiology of osteomyelitis. Orthop Clin North Am 1983;14:21–37.

31. Lipsky BA, Pecoraro RE, Wheat LJ. The diabetic foot: soft tissue and bone infection. Infect Dis Clin North Am 1990;4:409–432.

32. Lipsky BA, Pecoraro RE, Larson SA, Hanley ME, Ahroni JH. Outpatient management of uncomplicated lower-extremity infections in diabetic patients. Arch Intern Med 1990;150:790–797.

33. Jones EW, Edwards R, Finch R, Jaffcoate WJ. A microbiologic study of diabetic foot lesions. Diabet Med 1984;2:213–215.

34. Field FK, Kerstein MD. Overview of wound healing in a moist environment. Am J Surg 1994; 167(1A):2S–6S.

35. Cooper DM, Yu EZ, Hennesey P, et al. Determination of endogenous cytokines in chronic wounds. Ann Surg 1994;219:688–692.

36. Wieman TJ, Smiell JM, Su Y. Efficacy and safety of a topical gel formulation of recombinant human platelet-derived growth factor-BB (Becaplermin) in patients with chronic neuropathic diabetic ulcers. Diabetes Care 1998;21:822–827.

37. Muhart M, McFalls S, Kirsner RS, et al. Behavior of tissue-engineered skin. Arch Dermatol 1999;135:913–918.

38. Hansbrough JF, Dore C, Hansbrough WB: Clinical trials of a living dermal tissue replacement placed beneath meshed, split-thickness skin grafts on excised burn wounds. J Burn Care Rehabil 1992;13:519–529.

39. Cooper ML, Hansbrough JF, Spielvogel RL, et al. In vivo optimization of a living dermal substitute employing cultured human fibroblasts on a biodegradable polyglycolic acid or polyglactin mesh. Biomaterials 1991;12:243–248.

40. Gentzkow GD, Iwasaki SD, Hershon KS, et al. Use of Dermagraft, a cultured human dermis, to treat diabetic foot ulcers. Diabetes Care 1996;19:350–354.

41. Eaglstein WH, Iriondo M, Laszio K. A composite skin substitute (Graftskin) for surgical wounds: a clinical experience. Dermatol Surg 1995;21:839–843.

42. Brem H, Balledux J, Bloom T, Kerstein M, Hollier L. Healing of diabetic foot ulcers and pressure ulcers with human skin equivalent. Arch Surg 2000;135:627–634.

43. Veves A, Falanga V, Armstrong DG, Sabolinski ML. Graftskin, a human skin equivalent, is effective in the management of noninfected neuropathic diabetic foot ulcers. Diabetes Care 2001;24:290–295.

44. Charcot JM. Sur quelques arthropathies qui paraissent dependre d'une lesion du cerveau ou de la moelle epiniere. Arch Physiol Norm Pathol 1868;1:161–178.

45. Sanders LJ, Frykberg RG. Diabetic neuropathic osteoarthropathy: Charcot Foot. In: (Frykberg RG, ed.). The High Risk Foot in Diabetes Mellitus. Churchill Livingstone, New York, 1991, pp. 297–338.

46. Delano PJ. The pathogenesis of Charcot's joint. AJR 1946;(56)2:189–200.

47. Edmonds ME, Roberts VC, Watkins PJ. Blood flow in the diabetic neuropathic foot. Diabetologia 1982;22:9–15.

48. Edelman SV, Kosofsky EM, Paul RA, et al. Neuro-osteoarthropathy (Charcot's joint) in diabetes mellitus following revascularization surgery: three case reports and a review of the literature. Arch Intern Med 1987;147:1504–1508.

49. Sinha S, Munichoodappa C, Kozak GP. Neuroarthropathy (Charcot joints) in diabetes mellitus: clinical study of 101 cases. Medicine 1972;52:191–210.

50. Giurini JM, Chrzan JS, Gibbons GW, Habershaw GH. Charcot's disease in diabetic patients. Postgrad Med 1991;89:163–169.

51. Frykberg RG. Charcot changes in the diabetic foot. In: Veves A, Giurini JM, LoGerfo FW, eds. The Diabetic Foot. Humana, Totowa, NJ, 2002, pp. 221–246.

21 Erectile Dysfunction

Kenneth J. Snow, MD

CONTENTS

DEFINITION AND EPIDEMIOLOGY

Erectile dysfunction (ED) is defined as the consistent or recurrent inability to attain and/or maintain a penile erection sufficient for sexual performance and is a common sexual dysfunction especially among men with diabetes *(1)*. Sexual dysfunctions can include problems with libido, erectile function, and ejaculation. Although previously the term *impotence* was used interchangeably for all aspects of sexual dysfunction, this vague term led to confusion. Thus, in 1992, a National Institutes of Health consensus conference recommended that the term *erectile dysfunction* be used to describe problems relating to penile erections *(2)*.

Kinsey's initial data in 1948 revealed an incidence of ED of less than 2% in men under age 40 but 27% by age 70 *(3)*. Subsequent studies revealed that this percentage has increased, and ED is now recognized as a significant health problem for many men. The Massachusetts Male Aging Study (MMAS) found some degree of ED in 52% of the nearly 1300 men ages 40–70 studied *(4)*. Several risk factors have clearly been associated with ED. The most significant factor is aging. Men over age 70 have a six-fold increase in the risk of ED. Medical conditions associated with endothelial dysfunction have also been shown to increase the likelihood of ED. Diabetes mellitus, hypertension, hyperlipidemia, and coronary artery disease are known to increase the likelihood of having ED *(4,5)*. Braunsteins, *(6)*, in a review on ED, found that the prevalence of ED in men with diabetes varied from 27.5 to 75% in various studies. As the age of the men in the studies increased, the incidence increased, with up to 95% of men with diabetes over the age of 70 having some degree of dysfunction, whereas only 20% of those under the age of 30 had ED. In addition, blood glucose control in men with diabetes has also been shown to be inversely associated with the presence of ED *(7)*. By contrast, exercise, which is known to improve endothelial cell dysfunction, was shown in the MMAS to decrease the likelihood of developing ED *(8)*.

From: *Contemporary Diabetes: Obesity and Diabetes*
Edited by: C. S. Mantzoros © Humana Press Inc., Totowa, NJ

PATHOPHYSIOLOGY

Normal Erections

Although both an adequate blood supply and neural function are necessary for erections, the key factor to normal erections is adequate intrapenile blood flow. The penis has two elongated shafts, the corpora cavernosa, which comprise multiple sacs surrounded by smooth muscle. The flaccid resting state of the penis is the result of contraction of penile smooth muscle. This state is mediated through α-adrenergic stimulation, as well as other compounds such as prostaglandin $F_{2\alpha}$ ($PGF_{2\alpha}$) and endothelins *(9,10)*. In the presence of sexual stimulation, cholinergic fibers in the central nervous system (CNS) release acetylcholine, which partially blocks the adrenergic fibers. The major substance formed from the stimulation of the nonadrenergic noncholinergic (NANC) nerve fibers is nitric oxide (NO), which is produced through the action of NO synthase. NO is also released from vascular endothelial cells in the corpus cavernosum.

NO leads to stimulation of guanylyl cyclase, which converts guanosine 5′-triphosphate (GTP) into cyclic guanosine 5′-monophosphate (cGMP). cGMP then stimulates protein kinase C, which causes a decrease in intracellular calcium, which then leads to vasodilation. As the smooth muscle of the corpus cavernosa relaxes, the corporal sacs dilate and fill with blood. This filling leads to an increased intracavernosal pressure. The dilated sacs cause the corpora cavernosa to expand and press against the tunica albuginea, an elastic membrane surrounding the corpora. This expansion then compresses the veins that drain the corpora against the tunica albuginea. This compression decreases the drainage of blood from the corpora, maintaining intracavernosal pressure. After ejaculation, phosphodiesterase type 5 (PDE5), present in penile smooth muscle, metabolizes cGMP to 5′ GMP. Intracellular calcium increases, leading to contraction of the corpora smooth muscle, and detumescence ensues. Any process that decreases the production or release of NO or that causes endothelial dysfunction and inhibits adequate vasodilation will adversely affect erectile dysfunction (Fig. 1).

Normal Changes in Aging

Some men seeking help for ED may be experiencing normal changes that are seen in the aging male; Table 1 provides these changes. As men age they have a decreased ability to experience spontaneous erections from fantasy or visual stimulation, and more direct genital stimulation is required. In addition, loss of focus occurs more easily, so sexual activity needs to be attempted in a quiet place with minimum distractions when a man is well rested.

Penile sensation also decreases with age. Premature ejaculation is less common, but retarded ejaculation or anejaculation is more likely. This may lead to fatigue and detumescence without orgasm. The refractory period, the time from ejaculation to the next penile erection, lengthens with age and may be 30 min at age 20 but 2 d at age 70 *(11)*.

Pathophysiology of ED

The major chemical mediator of smooth muscle relaxation in the corpora cavernosum is NO, which is produced by both the nonadrenergic noncholinergic nerve fibers and endothelial cells. NO vasodilation has been shown to be impaired in patients with diabetes. Both neuropathy and vasculopathy are common complications in patients with diabetes. Studies have shown a decrease in acetylcholine synthesis in men with diabetes, which would hinder the ability of penile smooth muscle to relax. This decrease is associated with the duration of diabetes *(12)*. In addition, autonomic-mediated relaxation of corporal smooth muscle is impaired in diabetes *(13)*.

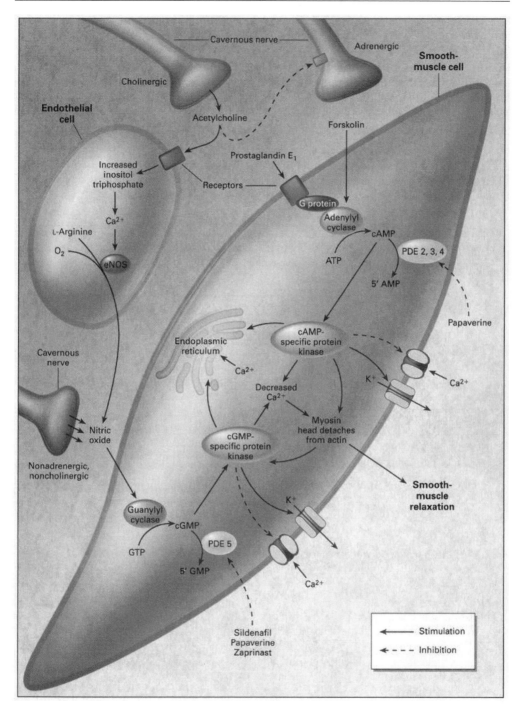

Fig. 1. Any process that decreases the production or release of nitric oxide or that causes endothelial dysfunction and inhibits adequate vasodilation will adversely affect erectile dysfunction. eNOS, endothelial nitric oxide synthase; ATP, adenosine triphosphate. (Copyright © 2000, Massachusetts Medical Society.)

Vascular impairment in diabetes will lead to ED from large-vessel disease but, more important, from problems with intrapenile blood flow. Decreased penile blood flow into the lacuna spaces will cause ED *(14)*.

Table 1
Sexual Changes in Aging Men

Decreased ability to have spontaneous erections
Increased need for foreplay
Decreased penile sensitivity
    Decreased premature ejaculation
    Increased retarded ejaculation
Increased length of refractory period
Increased episodes of detumescence without orgasm
Increased likelihood of loss of erection with loss of focus

Table 2
Commonly Used Drugs That Affect Sexual Function (16)

CNS acting
    Antidepressants (including tricyclics and SSRIs)
    Antipsychotics
    Tranquilizers
    Anorexiants
Cardiovascular
    Digoxin
    Older antihypertensives (reserpine, guanethidine, hydralazine)
    β-Blockers (especially propranolol, metoprolol, penbutolol, pindolol, timolol)
    Certain α-blockers (clonidine, guanfacine, prazosin)
    α- and β-Blockers (labetalol)
    α-Methyldopa
    Thiazide diuretics
    Spironolactone
    Calcium channel blockers (fairly low risk)
Allergy related
    Corticosteroids
    Theophylline
    Bronchodilators
Antifungals
    Fluconazole, ketoconazole, itraconazole
Recreational
    Marijuana
    Alcohol
Miscellaneous
    Metoclopramide, flutamide, clofibrate, gemfibrozil
Nonprescription
    Antihistamines (chlorpheniramine, diphenhydramine, chlotrimeton)
    Decongestants
    Cimetidine

One other issue in the pathophysiology of ED may be the presence of hypogonadism. Primary hypogonadism has been shown to increase the likelihood of ED, and correction of hypogonadism improves ED (15). Mild central hypogonadism is frequently seen in patients with diabetes and/or obesity. Whether mild decreases in testosterone significantly contribute to ED or not has not definitively been shown.

Many medications can affect various aspects of sexual function including libido, erectile function, and ejaculation. Table 2 provides some of the more commonly used

Table 3
Evaluation of the Patient With ED

History
    Duration
    Onset
    Progression
    Social setting
    Duration and control of diabetes
    Diabetes complications
    Other medical conditions
    Medications (prescription and nonprescription)
Physical examination
    BP
    Cardiovascular examination
    Neurological examination
    Breast examination
    Genital examination
Diagnostic tests
    A1C, lipids, creatinine, liver function, hemoglobin, testosterone

medications, especially in men with diabetes. Because of the frequency of hypertension in patients with diabetes, antihypertensives are commonly prescribed. Although many of the older medications, such as reserpine and propranolol, had a high rate of sexual side effects, newer agents such as angiotensin-converting enzyme inhibitors are less likely to contribute significantly to ED.

Many over-the-counter drugs such as pseudoephedrine and certain antihistamines such as diphenhydramine and chlorpheniramine are also known to contribute to ED. Other agents, such as metaclopramide, for the treatment of diabetic gastroparesis, may elevate prolactin (PRL) levels. Finally, many centrally acting drugs may inhibit sexual function by their direct actions on the CNS (as seen with selective serotonin reuptake inhibitors [SSRIs]) or by production of PRL (as seen with tricyclic antidepressants).

DIAGNOSTIC EVALUATION

Table 3 summarizes the evaluation of a patient with ED. The components involved are taking the patient's history, performing a physical examination, and doing diagnostic testing. In addition, measuring nocturnal penile activity and using surveys may be helpful.

History

When evaluating a patient with ED, the health care provider must take a careful, detailed history with emphasis on the sexual history. The first issue is to understand what type of sexual health problem the patient has. Although ED is a common sexual complaint, other issues such as concerns about ejaculation or issues regarding libido must be identified. Important features in ED include the duration of the problem, whether it presented suddenly or gradually, whether it has progressed, and whether it has any relation to other events in the patient's life.

These features provide information to help differentiate an organic cause from a psychogenic one. The presence of morning erections suggests a psychogenic component to the ED, but their absence does not prove the presence of an organic cause because morning erections decrease in frequency as men age. Prior to 1960, most men with ED were evaluated by physicians at psychiatric clinics, and in most men the problem was attributed to psychological causes. More recently, it has been recognized that the most common etiology for ED is an organic cause *(17)*, but men with diabetes are not exempt from having performance anxiety and relationship problems.

Because poor blood glycemic control increases the likelihood of ED, one must ascertain the patient's glycemic control as well as the presence of diabetic complications. Concomitant medical illnesses should be identified, with particular attention paid to other diseases associated with endothelial cell dysfunction such as hypertension, hyperlipidemia, and vascular disease. Because, men with ED, and especially those with obesity and glucose intolerance or diabetes, are more likely to have any of these conditions, all patients presenting with ED should be screened for these conditions.

The use of all medications, including prescription drugs, over-the-counter drugs, and nutritional supplements, should be identified and the relationship between starting these therapies and the development of ED assessed.

Physical Examination

The physical examination includes the measurement of blood pressure (BP), and a detailed cardiovascular and neurological examination. A breast and genital exam must be performed, with particular attention paid to evidence of normal virilization and any anatomic changes such as Peyronie disease.

Laboratory Testing

For the diabetic patient, laboratory testing should assess glycemic control by measuring a hemoglobin A1c value. The presence of nephropathy, a common complication of diabetes, is assessed with a creatinine measurement. Other common comorbid conditions such as hyperlipidemia, liver disease, or anemia, should be assessed by measuring a lipid profile, liver function tests, and a hemoglobin test. An initial testosterone determination should be considered, especially if the patient has any complaints consistent with testosterone deficiency, such as decreased libido.

Other Testing

Further diagnostic testing usually is not necessary. However, if the differentiation between organic and psychogenic ED is difficult to determine, measuring nocturnal penile activity may be beneficial. Assessment of the vascular status can be achieved with duplex ultrasound to monitor cavernosal artery pressure after the intracavernosal injection of papaverine or PGE_1. The greater the number of risk factors for arterial insufficiency, such as aortoiliac disease, history of tobacco abuse, and hypertension, the greater the chance that intrapenile blood flow will be decreased *(18)*.

Survey Tools

Several survey tools are now available to assess the severity of ED. Two of the most widely used are the International Index of Erectile Function (IIEF) *(19)* and the Sexual Encounter Profile (SEP). The IIEF is a validated tool that can be used to assess sexual function. The erectile function domain questions, questions 1–5 and 15 of the IIEF, address the ability to attain and maintain erections (Table 4, part A). Scoring ranges from 5 to 30, with lower scores reflecting a greater degree of ED (Table 4, part A). The SEP is composed of seven diary questions that allow patients to record results after a sexual encounter. Questions 2 and 3 are of greatest interest in assessing erectile function (Table 4, part B).

Table 4
Survey Tools to Assess ED

A. IIEF—EF Domain Questions

Over the past 4 wk

1. How often were you able to get an erection during sexual activity?
   0 = No sexual activity
   1 = Almost never/never
   2 = A few times (much less than half the time)
   3 = Sometimes (about half the time)
   4 = Most times (much more than half the time)
   5 = Almost always/always
2. When you had erections with sexual stimulation, how often were your erections hard enough to be able to penetrate your partner?
   0 = No sexual activity
   1 = Almost never/never
   2 = A few times (much less than half the time)
   3 = Sometimes (about half the time)
   4 = Most times (much more than half the time)
   5 = Almost always/always
3. When you attempted sexual intercourse, how often were you able to enter your partner?
   0 = Did not attempt intercourse
   1 = Almost never/never
   2 = A few times (much less than half the time)
   3 = Sometimes (about half the time)
   4 = Most times (much more than half the time)
   5 = Almost always/always
4. During intercourse, how often were you able to maintain your erection after penetration?
   0 = Did not attempt intercourse
   1 = Almost never/never
   2 = A few times (much less than half the time)
   3 = Sometimes (about half the time)
   4 = Most times (much more than half the time)
   5 = Almost always/always
5. During intercourse, how difficult was it to maintain your erection to completion?
   0 = Did not attempt intercourse
   1 = Extremely difficult
   2 = Very difficult
   3 = Difficult
   4 = Slightly difficult
   5 = Not difficult
6. How would you rate your confidence that you could get and keep an erection?
   1 = Very low
   2 = Low
   3 = Moderate
   4 = High
   5 = Very high

(Continued)

Table 4 *(Continued)*

Score	Severity of ED
26–30	Normal
22–25	Mild
17–21	Mild to moderate
11–16	Moderate
5–10	Severe

B. SEP Questions

SEP 2: Were you able to insert your penis into your partner's vagina?
    —Yes   —No
SEP 3: Did your erection last long enough for you to have successful intercourse?
    —Yes   —No

TREATMENT

While proceeding with therapy for ED, it is helpful to consider improving those factors that can be improved and may be contributing to the ED. These factors include optimizing glycemic control with avoidance of hypoglycemia. If the patient is taking a drug that is known to affect erectile function, one must consider changing the medication if possible to an agent less likely to be a problem. Even if the agent is not completely responsible for the ED, it may be contributing along with other factors and, thus, may adversely affect the degree of benefit achieved with therapy.

If appropriate, a qualified therapist should be part of the health care team. Performance anxiety or relationship issues may need to be addressed. At times, problems with decreased libido may point to an underlying conflict within the relationship that has to be evaluated, and some couples have to be taught about the need for more foreplay with aging.

Patients with primary gonadal failure need testosterone replacement therapy. Apart from causing libido and erectile problems, testosterone deficiency may cause lethargy, depression, anemia, muscle weakness, and osteoporosis. Men with diabetes often have secondary hypogonadism. These patients may also be treated with testosterone, although the benefit of this therapy is far less clear.

Oral Therapies for ED

Sildenafil (Viagra) was first released in 1998 and quickly revolutionized the treatment of ED. During sexual stimulation, NO is released from NANC nerves and from endothelial cells in the corpus cavernosum, which activate guanylyl cyclase, causing an increase in the level of cGMP. As previously discussed, this increase in cGMP causes a decrease in intracellular calcium, which in turn, leads to relaxation in smooth muscle and results in vasodilation of the corpus cavernosum. PDE5 degrades cGMP. Sildenafil works by inhibiting PDE5, causing an increase in cGMP (Fig. 1).

Sildenafil is available in 25-, 50-, and 100-mg strengths. The starting dose is 50 mg, with the option of titrating up to 100 mg for those who do not achieve an adequate response. The option to titrate down to 25 mg is available for those who have side effects at 50 mg. Typically, men with diabetes are less likely to respond to any PDE5 inhibitor and should be encouraged to utilize the 100-mg dose if an optimal response is not achieved with the 50-mg dose. The drug is absorbed with a maximal concentration reached at about 1 h. Therefore, patients should be advised to take the drug about 1 h prior to intercourse. Studies have shown that for half of all users, the onset of an adequate erection may occur within 20 min after taking the drug *(20)*. The half-life of the drug is about 4 h and, thus, patients will note decreasing efficacy beyond 4 h.

Sildenafil is very specific for the PDE5 isotype although it does crossreact with PDE6, an isoform found in the retina. This crossreactivity can lead to changes in blue-green color discrimination or the presence of a blue-green halo around objects. Since this effect is caused by the binding of the sildenafil to PDE6, the effect resolves as the drug is metabolized over a few hours.

The most common side effects from the drug include headache (16%), flushing (10%), dyspepsia (7%), and nasal congestion (4%) *(21)*. These side effects are related to the distribution of PDE5 in other tissues. There has not been any evidence that the drug causes cardiovascular events. Initially, there was a concern of an increased risk of cardiovascular events. This increased risk has been shown to be related to patients who have preexisting cardiovascular disease and are at high risk of a cardiovascular event when participating in any new form of exercise.

Vardenafil (Levitra) was approved for use in the United States in August 2003. This agent also works by inhibiting PDE5. The drug is available in 2.5-, 5-, 10-, and 20-mg strengths, with a typical starting dose of 10 mg. The dose can be increased to 20 mg if an adequate response is not obtained. Lower starting doses are appropriate for patients receiving antifungal or antiretroviral therapy. The drug reaches a maximal concentration in about 60 min, with a half-life of about 4 to 5 h. As with sildenafil, patients should be advised to take this agent approx 1 h before intercourse. The drug has been shown to facilitate erections as rapidly as 16 min *(22)*. It has minimal binding to PDE6, so, unlike sildenafil, blue-green color changes have not been observed with this agent. Common side effects include headache (15%), flushing (11%), rhinitis (9%), and dyspepsia (4%), related to the distribution of PDE5 in other tissues *(23)*.

Tadalafil (Cialis) was approved for use in the United States in November 2003. The third PDE5 inhibitor on the market, it is available in 5-, 10-, and 20-mg strengths, with a starting dose of 10 mg. The time to peak concentration and the half-life of this agent are dramatically different from those seen with sildenafil or vardenafil. Peak concentration is reached at 2 h (0.5–6 h) and the half-life of the drug is 24 h. Instead of taking this agent on demand, patients should be advised that once it reaches a peak concentration, the agent will provide benefit for the next 24 h *(24)*.

Tadalafil also has minimal PDE6 binding, so blue-green color changes have not been reported. The drug does inhibit PDE11 with an affinity about one-fifth that of PDE5. PDE11 is present in skeletal muscle, and this inhibition may account for the lower-back pain reported to occur in some patients (6%) the day following use. PDE11 exists in many other tissues including the testes, prostate, and kidneys, but no clinical significance has been attributed to PDE11 inhibition in these tissues. Side effects are similar to those of the other two agents because of the distribution of PDE5 in other tissues. These include headache (15%), dyspepsia (10%), nasal congestion (3%), and flushing (3%) *(24)*. Finally, because of the development of symptomatic hypotension in otherwise healthy volunteers taking PDE5 inhibitors and nitrate-based vasodilators concomitantly, the use of a PDE5 inhibitor is contraindicated in any patient taking a nitrate-containing agent *(21,23,24)*.

Postmarketing studies did reveal an interaction between sildenafil and α-blockers. These agents were found to have a greater effect on lowering BP in the presence of sildenafil, whereas a similar effect was not seen with other antihypertensives. The recommendation is to use 25 mg of sildenafil when combining with an α-blocker or 50 or 100 mg of sildenafil if the dose is separated from the use of the α-blocker by 4 h *(21)*. When healthy volunteers took 20 mg of vardenafil with 10 mg of terazosin, 25% were found to have a drop in systolic BP to <85 mmHg. Thus, vardenafil is contraindicated for use with α-blockers *(23)*. When 20 mg of tadalafil was administered with 0.4 mg of tamsulosin, an α-blocker with less antihypertensive effect, no significant decrease in BP was noted. As such, there is no contraindication to the use of tadalafil with tamsulosin *(24)*. Further studies are needed to determine whether the same antihypertensive effect is seen with vardenafil in lower doses and in combination with tamsulosin.

All three PDE5 inhibitors have been shown to be effective in patients regardless of the severity or the etiology of the ED, including diabetes. The response to the agent, however, is related to the severity of the ED, with a lower likelihood of an appropriate response or a less satisfactory response in those with more severe ED *(21,23,24)*. Response to therapy can be assessed by either a change in the IIEF score or changes to SEP 2 or SEP 3. In addition, a simple Global Assessment Question (GAQ) (i.e., "Has the treatment you have been taking during the past 4 wk improved your erections?") that is answered "yes" or "no" provides a valid simple assessment. The problem with the GAQ is that the degree of the response is not taken into account and even minimal responses may be considered as a "yes." As such, the response rate to the GAQ tends to be higher than to SEP 2 or SEP 3 and may not reflect a degree of response that is satisfactory to the patient.

In general, IIEF improvements of 8–10 points have been seen after treatment of patients with ED with a PDE5 inhibitor. SEP 2 and SEP 3 positive response rates of 80 and 65%, respectively, and GAQ positive response rates of 90% have been reported *(21,23,24)*. Factors such as age of the study population, concomitant medical conditions, and the severity of the ED will have a significant impact on the results, but to date no good study has shown a significant difference in the response rate from one agent to the next.

Apomorphine (Uprima) is a dopamine receptor agonist that treats erectile function by increasing the hypothalamic signal that causes erections. Although this agent was approved by the European Union in 2001, the US Food and Drug Administration (FDA) issued a nonapprovable letter for the drug in August 2003 and approval is not currently being pursued. In Europe, the drug is available in 2- and 3-mg doses and is administered sublingually. The mean onset of action is 20 min. Studies have shown that the effectiveness of the drug is significantly less than that of the PDE5 inhibitors. The most common side effects of this agent are yawning, nausea, dizziness, and somnolence, occurring in 5–8% of patients *(25)*.

Yohimbine is an α2-adrenergic blocker derived from the bark of the Yohimbe tree in Africa. Studies have not shown a significant benefit especially in patients with organic ED. Available without prescription, the usual starting dose is 5.4 mg three times a day. Side effects include hypertension, nervousness, tremor, tachycardia, and urinary retention, related to its action as an α-blocker *(26)*.

Injectable Therapy

In 1983, Brindley demonstrated that injecting papavarine, a vasodilator, into the corpus cavernosa will cause an erection *(27)*. The use of papaverine was complicated by a high incidence of penile fibrosis, which was decreased when phentolamine was added. Since then, mixtures of papaverine and phentolamine (bimix) have been used. The addition of PGE_1 (trimix) has been shown to improve effectiveness even further. Success rates in excess of 80% are commonly reported (28).

The most common side effects include pain on injection and the formation of painless fibrotic nodules in 1.5–60% of patients. This variability may be related to how the nodules are identified, the frequency of use, and the duration of therapy (29). Priapism is a rare but known complication and will usually occur initially before an optimal dose is identified or if the patient injects a dose in excess of the prescribed amount. In addition to being quite painful, priapism can lead to intracorporeal damage if not treated appropriately.

Despite widespread use, neither bimix nor trimix have FDA approval for use in treating ED. The FDA approved the first intracavernosal injection treatment in 1995. This therapy utilizes alprostadil (Caverject, Edex), which is a synthetic compound identical to PGE_1. Alprostadil increases intracellular cyclic adenosine monophosphate (cAMP), leading to vasodilation. Doses range from 2.5 to 20 µg. Studies have reported that >80% of men achieve erections adequate for sexual activity with the use of this therapy (30), but follow-up studies have shown that half of patients who had an adequate response to therapy were not using the therapy after 1 yr (31,32).

Transurethral Therapy

In addition to the injectable form, alprostadil has been formulated into a urethral suppository (MUSE). This format allows absorption across the urethral mucosa, avoiding the need for intracavernosal injections, but significantly higher doses are required. MUSE is available in 125-, 250-, 500-, and 1000-µg doses. Success rates as high as 65% have been reported (33). The most common side effects include penile and peroneal burning (30%), although it is usually not severe enough to lead to discontinuation of the drug.

Vacuum Assistance Devices

Vacuum devices for erections have been widely available for use in the United States for the past 30 yr. These devices consist of a plastic tube that is placed over the penis. As air is pumped out of the tube, a vacuum is created, which draws venous blood into the penis. An erection is thus obtained. It is maintained by using a rubber constriction ring that fits over the base of the penis.

Erections that are adequate for intercourse have been reported in >75% of men using these devices. A firm erection with no drug interactions and the absence of a cost for each use are the major attractions for this therapy. The major disadvantage of this treatment is the mechanical nature of the process. A unique side effect is a lack of tumescence proximal to the constriction band, which can lead to a "hinge" effect of the penis. In addition, decreased ejaculation and mild bruising can occur (34).

Constriction Rings

Patients who are still able to attain an adequate erection but find difficulty in maintaining it do not necessarily need therapies that improve erectile quality. This early detumescence or venous leakage can be treated with just a constriction device. Various products are now available.

Table 5
Costs of Therapy

Agent	Available strengths	Retail cost per use ($)[a]
PDE5 inhibitors		
Sildenafil	25, 50, 100 mg	9.10–9.40
Tadalafil	5, 10, 20 mg	9.00
Vardenafil	2.5, 5, 10, 20 mg	8.80–9.00
Injection therapy		
Bimix or trimix	[b]	[b]
Alprostadil		
Caverject	10, 20 µg	24.02–32.91
Edex	5, 10, 20, 40 µg	15.57–35.00
Urethral suppository	125, 250, 500, 1000 µg	19.78–23.94
Vacuum pump	NA[c]	0[d]

[a]Based on pricing from www.drugstore.com.
[b]The dose is customized and the final cost is greatly affected by the cost of mixing.
[c]NA, not applicable.
[d]There is no cost per use with a vacuum assistance device; however, there is the onetime initial cost of acquisition.

Penile Implants

Predating pharmacological therapy, penile implants have been a highly successful form of therapy for ED. As newer therapies have been developed, the percentage of men treated with this form of therapy has decreased. This therapy is an option for those men who have failed other options for therapy or with anatomic changes that make success with other forms of therapy impossible. There are two basic types: the semi-rigid rod and the inflatable rod. The latter has more hardware that is placed in the penis, scrotum, and suprapubic area, thus increasing the risk of mechanical failure and/or infection. The earlier models had a higher rate of mechanical failure, but this has decreased over time. Satisfaction rates among men with diabetes and their partners vary, depending on the study, but are often quite high *(35)*. Although dramatically improved, the major concerns continue to be infections and mechanical failure.

COSTS OF TREATMENT

The costs of these various treatments are quite variable and may influence compliance with a particular form of therapy. Therefore, one should take into account the cost per use and the expected number of uses per month. Table 5 provides the costs of the various therapies. Insurance coverage is highly variable, with some plans having restrictions on the choices of therapy or on the number of treatments per month. Others offer no coverage of therapy.

REFERENCES

1. Meuleman E, Broderick G, Meng Tan H. Clinical evaluation and the doctor–patient dialogue. In: Jardin A, Wagner G, Khoury S, Giuliano F, Padma-Nathan H, Rosen R, eds. Erectile Dysfunction. Plymbridge Distributors, Plymouth, UK, 2000, pp. 115–138.
2. NIH Consensus Development Panel on Impotence. Impotence. JAMA 1993;270:83–90.

3. Kinsey AC, Pomeroy WB, Martin CE. Sexual Behavior in the Human Male. WB Saunders, Philadelphia, 1998, pp. 235–238.
4. Feldman HA, Goldstein I, Hatzichristou DG, Krane RJ, McKinlay JB. Impotence and its medical and psychosocial correlates: results of the Massachusetts Male Aging Study. J Urol 1994;151:54–61.
5. Morillo LE, Diaz J, Estevez E, et al. Prevalence of erectile dysfunction in Columbia, Ecuador, and Venezuela: a population-based study (DENSA). Int J Impot Res 2002;14(Suppl. 2):S10–S18.
6. GD Braunstein. Impotence in diabetic men. Mt Sinai J Med 1987;54:236–240.
7. Romeo JH, Seftel AD, Madhun ZT, Aron DC. Sexual function in men with diabetes type 2: association with glycemic control. J Urol 2000;163:788–791.
8. Derby CA, Araujo AB, Johannes CB, Feldman HA, McKinlay JB. Measurement of erectile dysfunction in population-based studies: the use of a single question self-assessment in the Massachusetts Male Aging Study. Int J Impot Res 2000;12:197–204.
9. Italiano G, Calabro A, Spini S, Ragazzi E, Pagano F. Functional response of cavernosal tissue to distension. Urol Res 1998;26:39–44.
10. Gondre M, Christ GJ. Endothelin-1-induced alterations in phenylephrine-induced contractile responses are largely additive in physiologically diverse rabbit vasculature. J Pharmacol Exp Ther 1998;286:635–642.
11. Masters WH, Johnson VE. Sex after sixty-five. Reflections 1977;12:31–43.
12. Blanco R, Saenz de Tejada I, Goldstein I, Krane RJ, Wotiz HH, Cohen RA. Dysfunctional penile cholinergic nerves in diabetic impotent men. J Urol 1990;144:278–280.
13. Saenz de Tejada I, Goldstein I, Azadzoi K, Krane RJ, Cohen RA. Impaired neurogenic and endothelium-mediated relaxation of penile smooth muscle from diabetic men with impotence. N Engl J Med 1989;320:1025–1030.
14. Breza J, Aboseif SR, Orvis BR, Lue TF, Tanagho EA. Detailed anatomy of penile neurovascular structures: surgical significance. J Urol 1989;141:437–443.
15. Davidson JM, Camargo CA, Smith ER. Effects of androgen on sexual behavior in hypogonadal men. J Clin Endocrinol Metab 1979;48:955–958.
16. Drugs that cause sexual dysfunction: An update. Med Lett 1992;34:73–74.
17. Lue, TF. Erectile dysfunction. N Engl J Med 2000;342:1802–1813.
18. Wang CJ, Shen SY, Wu CC, Huang CH, Chiang CP. Penile blood flow study in diabetic impotence. Urol Int 1993;50:209–212.
19. Rosen RC, Riley A, Wagner G, Osterloh IH, Kirkpatrick J, Mishra A. The international index of erectile function (IIEF): a multidimensional scale for assessment of erectile dysfunction. Urology 1997;49:822–830.
20. Padma-Nathan H, Stecher VJ, Sweeney M, Orazem J, Tseng LJ, Deriesthal H. Minimal time to successful intercourse after sildenafil citrate: results of a randomized, double-blind, placebo-controlled trial. Urology 2003;62:400–403.
21. Sildenafil package insert. Pfizer. September 2002.
22. Hellstrom WJ. Vardenafil: a new approach to the treatment of erectile dysfunction. Curr Urol Rep 2003;4:479–487.
23. Levitra package insert. Bayer Pharmaceuticals. August 2003.
24. Cialis package insert. Lilly ICOS. November 2003.
25. Dula E, Bukofzer S, Perdok R, George M, for the apomorphine SL Study Group. Double-blind, crossover comparison of 3 mg apomorphine SL with placebo and with 4 mg apomorphine SL in male erectile function. Eur Urol 2001;39:558–564.
26. Mann K, Klingler T, Noe S, Roschke J, Muller S, Benkert O. Effects of yohimbine on sexual experiences and nocturnal penile tumescence and rigidity in erectile dysfunction. Arch Sex Behav 1996;25:1–16.
27. Brindley GS. Cavernosal alpha-blockade: a new technique for investigating and treating erectile impotence. Br J Psychiatry 1983;143:332–337.
28. Zorgniotti AW, Lefleur RS. Auto-injection of the corpus cavernosum with a vasoactive drug combination for vasculogenic impotence. J Urol 1985;133:39–41.
29. Krane, Goldstein I, Saenz de Tejada I. Impotence. N Engl J Med 1989;321:1648–1659.
30. Linet OI, Ogrinc FG. Efficacy and safety of intracavernosal alprostadil in men with erectile dysfunction. The Alprostadil Study Group. N Engl J Med 1996;334:873–877.
31. Weiss JN, Badlani GH, Ravalli R, Brettschneider N. Reasons for high drop-out rate with self-injection therapy for impotence. Int J Impot Res 1994;6:171–174.
32. Gupta R, Kirschen J, Barrow RC 2nd, Eid JF. Predictors of success and risk factors for attrition in the use of intracavernous injection. J Urol 1997;157:1681–1686.

33. Padma-Nathan Hellstrom WJ, Kaiser FE, Labasky RF, et al. Treatment of men with erectile dysfunction with transurethral alprostadil. Medicated Urethral System for Erection (MUSE) Study Group. N Engl J Med 1997;336:1–7.

34. Nadig PW, Ware JC, Blumoff R. Noninvasive device to produce and maintain an erection-like state. Urology 1986;27:126–131.

35. Lewis R. Surgery for Erectile Dysfunction. In: Walsh PC, Retik AB, Vaughan ED, Wein AJ, eds. Campbell's Urology, 7th ed. WB Saunders, Philadelphia, 1998, pp. 1215–1226.

22 Infections in Diabetes Mellitus

Sotirios Tsiodras, MD, Iosif Kelesidis, MD,
Christos S. Mantzoros, MD, DSc,
and Adolf W. Karchmer, MD

INTRODUCTION

Infections constitute the most common cause of diabetic ketoacidosis and uncontrolled diabetes but diabetes also predisposes to the development of serious infections *(1,2)*. The risk of infection and consequent hospitalization is higher in individuals with diabetes than in those without diabetes *(3)*, and some infections, such as rhinocerebral mucormycosis and emphysematous pyelonephritis, occur almost exclusively in patients with diabetes *(4)*. Individuals with diabetes mellitus might be at higher risk of moderate or severe infection-related morbidity and mortality, with almost a double risk of death related to an infection *(3)*. This propensity for infection is attributed to effects of the metabolic dysregulation not only on immune function *(5–8)* but also on the nervous and circulatory systems leading to disruption of the natural barriers to infection *(9)*. For example, neuropathic and ischemic ulcers in patients with diabetes provide portals of entry for microorganisms, and neuropathic urinary bladder dysfunction predisposes to urinary tract infections (UTIs) *(5,6,9)*.

In this chapter we summarize current knowledge on clinical infections seen in patients with diabetes.

COMMON INFECTIONS IN PATIENTS WITH DIABETES (Table 1)

Microorganisms Strongly Associated With Infections in Diabetes

Gram-positive bacteria most commonly encountered in diabetics are *Staphylococcus* spp., *Streptococcus* group B spp., *Pneumonococcus*, and *Enterococcus* spp. Although *S. aureus* infections have been suggested to be more common among patients with diabetes, it is difficult to estimate any proportional risk of such infections among these patients

From: *Contemporary Diabetes: Obesity and Diabetes*
Edited by: C. S. Mantzoros © Humana Press Inc., Totowa, NJ

Table 1
Common Infections in Diabetes

Respiratory tract infections	Urinary tract infections	Skin and soft-tissue infections	Other infections
Lower respiratory tract infection	Asymptomatic bacteriuria	Cellulitis	Zygomycosis rhinocerebral mucormycosis
	Acute pyelonephritis	Necrotizing fasciitis	
	Renal abscess	Pyomyositis	
	Emphysematous pyelonephritis, pyelitis, cystitis	Diabetic foot infections	Malignant necrotizing external otitis
		Osteomyelitis	
	Fungal cystitis	Candida skin infections	Emphysematous cholecystitis
		Dermatophytosis	Periodontitis

(10), and a study of *S. aureus* bacteremia found no difference in mortality between patients with diabetes and those without (11). By contrast, patients with diabetes seem to be at particularly high risk of infection with *Streptococccus* group B. For example, in a group of nonpregnant adults with group B streptococcal bacteremia, the prevalence of diabetes was found to be 27.5% (12). Gram-negative bacteria, most commonly *Escherichia coli, Klebsiella* spp., and *Pseudomonas aeruginosa,* frequently colonize and infect patients with diabetes. A disproportionately high incidence (30–60%) of diabetes has been reported in several series of patients with *Klebsiella* spp. infections, including bacteremia (13) and endophthalmitis (14), and diabetes has also been identified as a risk factor for infection with *Salmonella enteritidis (15).* Other microorganisms commonly seen in association with diabetes include anaerobes, *Mycobacterium tuberculosis, Candida* spp., and the Zygomycetes. Data on infections seen in subjects with diabetes and associated with these microorganisms are discussed in detail next.

Respiratory Tract Infections

Whether diabetes is an independent risk factor for the incidence of common upper or lower respiratory tract infections remains uncertain (16–19). It is widely accepted, however, that patients with underlying comorbidities such as diabetes, have more severe respiratory tract infections (20). Diabetes may be associated with functional lung abnormalities leading to decreased defense mechanisms against respiratory tract infections (16,21), and individuals with diabetes may also have altered host defenses and/or underlying abnormalities that predispose to increased morbidity and mortality (22–24). In the largest meta-analysis of community-acquired pneumonia to date, the odds ratio for death associated with diabetes mellitus was only 1.3 (18). Respiratory tract infections owing to certain microorganisms, such as *S. aureus,* Gram-negative organisms (e.g., *Klebsiella*), and *My. Tuberculosis*, may occur in patients with diabetes with increased frequency (16). Reduction of pulmonary ciliary clearance by influenza, together with the high incidence of nasal carriage of *S. aureus* among patients with diabetes, leads to an increased incidence of staphylococcal pneumonia in patients with diabetes. Although diabetes is a risk factor for bacteremia in patients with pneumococcal pneumonia, it remains unknown whether pneumococcal pneumonia in patients with diabetes is associated with increased mortality (20). Pulmonary tuberculosis has also been reported to occur more frequently among patients with diabetes than in the general population and to follow a more aggressive course in patients with poorly controlled diabetes (25).

Fungal infections (coccidioidomycosis, aspergillosis, and mucormycosis) may be seen more frequently in patients with diabetes *(16)*.

Pneumonia in patients with diabetes presents with typical clinical signs, fever and cough, and chest X-ray remains the main diagnostic tool. Although the widely used Patient Outcome Research Team (PORT) predictive scoring system does not include diabetes *per se (26)*, serum glucose values >250 convey an extra 10 points in calculation of the score *(26)*. The choice of initial antimicrobial treatment for community-acquired pneumonia in patients with diabetes should be based on standard recommendations and use of the PORT score, but standard regimens should be modified if clinical or epidemiological considerations suggest less common pathogens. Similarly, nosocomial pneumonia in patients with diabetes should be treated in concert with published guidelines and with particular attention to the etiological agents common to the patients' setting, while specific efforts should be made to recover the causative organism in individual patients.

Patients with diabetes have a normal response to pneumococcal vaccination, but although vaccination is recommended *(16)*, the benefit is likely restricted to the prevention of extrapulmonary complications, rather than of pneumonia *per se*. Thus, current recommendations are that all patients with diabetes receive annual influenza immunization *(27)*.

Urinary Tract Infections

Pathogenesis and Etiology of Asymptomatic Bacteriuria and/or UTI in Patients With Diabetes

UTIs rank among the top 10 concurrent or complicating illnesses occurring in patients with diabetes *(28–30)*. Evidence from epidemiological studies suggests that bacteriuria and UTI are more common in women with diabetes than among those without diabetes *(29,31,32)*. Anatomic and functional abnormalities of the urinary tract, recurrent vaginitis, poor glycemic control, long duration of diabetes, and the presence of microangiopathy have all been proposed as risk factors for UTI in diabetes *(33,34)*. Anatomic and/or functional abnormalities of the urinary tract, particularly bladder dysfunction, are also more frequent among men and women with diabetes and increase the likelihood of infection from urinary tract instrumentation *(29,35,36)*.

Although polymorphonuclear (PMN) leukocyte dysfunction has been suggested to contribute to increased risk of UTI in patients with diabetes, in certain studies, PMN leukocyte function has not been found to differ significantly between diabetic women with or without bacteriuria and/or between these women and nondiabetic control subjects *(37)*. Decreased antibacterial capacity of urine and increased adherence of bacteria to uroepithelial cells from patients with diabetes *(37)*, as well as altered baseline levels of cytokines (e.g., interleukin-6 [IL-6] and IL-8) in serum and urine from patients with diabetes *(38,39)*, have also been proposed to contribute, but more studies are necessary to better define immune dysfunction in diabetes and its potential effect on UTIs.

The organism most commonly causing UTI in patients with diabetes is *E. coli*, albeit at a significantly lower percentage when compared to age-matched nondiabetic patients with both nosocomial and community-acquired UTI *(40)*. Several series have shown a significant contribution by *Klebsiella* spp. especially among patients with uncommon, severe forms of UTI, such as emphysematous pyelonephritis (see Emphysematous

Pyelonephritis) *(41,42)*. *Acinetobacter* spp., group B streptococcus, and other unusual causes of UTI are more frequently reported among patients with diabetes mellitus *(43,44)*.

ASYMPTOMATIC BACTERIURIA

When compared with women without diabetes, those women with diabetes experience two to four times increased frequency of asymptomatic bacteriuria *(39,45,46)*. Although asymptomatic bacteriuria occurs in 4 to 5% of women with anatomically normal urinary tracts and is significantly associated with subsequent UTI, it is not associated with other adverse health outcomes in nonpregnant women with normal urinary tracts *(47)*. A prospective, randomized, double-blind, placebo-controlled trial has demonstrated that treatment of asymptomatic bacteriuria in women with diabetes does not reduce the chance of having one episode of symptomatic UTI, the time to the first symptomatic episode of UTI, the rate of symptomatic UTI, the rate of pyelonephritis, or the rate of hospitalization for UTI. Thus, diabetes itself is not a reason to screen women for asymptomatic bacteriuria nor to treat women for this finding *(48–50)*, and there is a consensus that asymptomatic bacteriuria should not be treated *(49,51–53)*.

ACUTE PYELONEPHRITIS

The incidence of acute pyelonephritis is higher in patients with diabetes compared with control subjects, and, more important, its complications may be substantially more significant. The upper urogenital tract is involved in up to 80% of UTIs in patients with diabetes, and these patients are also hospitalized more frequently *(54–56)*. The clinical presentation of acute pyelonephritis is similar to that in nondiabetic patients (fever, lumbar pain) except that bilateral infection is more common. *E. coli*, *Proteus* spp. and *Klebsiella* spp. are most commonly isolated, and bacteremia is four times more likely to originate from the urinary tract in patients with diabetes than in control subjects. Moreover, patients with diabetes and bacteremia are twice as likely to develop acute renal failure *(56)*. In fact, there is an increased risk, approximately threefold, of enterobacterial bacteremia in persons with diabetes vs those without, and this is, in large measure, driven by UTI *(57)*. Hematogenous spread to distant sites, including the eye *(58,59)* bone, vertebral joints *(60)*, and lungs, has been reported. Other complications of pyelonephritis in patients with diabetes include the development of acute papillary necrosis, perinephric and intrarenal abscesses, emphysematous pyelonephritis (discussed subsequently), and xanthogranulomatous pyelonephritis *(1,2)*.

THERAPY

Empiric therapy of community-acquired acute UTI in patients with diabetes can be initiated orally with trimethoprim/sulfamethoxazole (TMP/SMZ) or a fluoroquinolone, although in many regions of the United States resistance rates to TMP/SMZ among Gram-negative uropathogens exceed 15%. When a patient is septic, or unable to tolerate oral therapy, treatment with parenteral antibiotics is necessary. Fluoroquinolones, broad-spectrum β-lactams (carbapenems and cephalosporins), and aminoglycosides can be used contingent on anticipated susceptibility of the uropathogens. In diabetic patients with preexisting renal dysfunction, potential nephrotoxicity of aminoglycosides makes these less desirable therapeutic agents. Empirical therapy should be revised when the results of urine and blood cultures are available. If a patient does not improve in 4 to 5 d, obstruction, papillary necrosis, perinephric or renal abscess, or emphysematous pyelonephritis should be considered and the diagnosis pursued using ultrasound or computed tomography (CT).

PAPILLARY NECROSIS

Papillary necrosis is the consequence of renal damage owing to ischemia and infection. Although diabetes is the most common underlying condition associated with this, analgesic abuse sickle hemoglobinopathy should also be considered. Papillary necrosis is suspected when diabetic patients with pyelonephritis do not respond to antibiotic therapy or when they develop renal failure. Symptoms include persistent flank and abdominal pain accompanied by fever *(61)*. The diagnosis is usually established by imaging studies such as retrograde pyelography *(62)*. Therapy consists of relief of obstruction and effective iv antibiotics.

PERINEPHRIC AND INTRARENAL ABSCESSES

Perinephric and intrarenal abscesses are an infrequent but important complication of acute pyelonephritis. In one series of patients with perinephric abscess, 36% had diabetes *(63)*. *E. coli* and other enterobacterial organisms are typical bacteria causing acute pyelonephritis, but when renal infection is a consequence of bacteremia, *S. aureus* is the likely cause. Fever that persists for more than 4 d after the initiation of appropriate antibiotic therapy is the most useful clinical finding differentiating patients with a perinephric abscess from those with uncomplicated pyelonephritis. The diagnosis is established by ultrasonography or CT scan. Effective therapy requires percutaneous or surgical drainage and systemic antibiotics.

EMPHYSEMATOUS PYELONEPHRITIS

Emphysematous pyelonephritis, a condition that occurs most commonly in diabetic patients, is a rare, acute, life-threatening necrotizing renal and perirenal infection caused by gas-forming uropathogens *(64–67)*. It results from an interaction among gas-forming bacteria, impaired tissue perfusion, high tissue glucose, and a defective immune response. Fermentation of glucose with carbon dioxide production by the organisms has been proposed as the cause of gas in the tissues *(68)*.

Similar to acute pyelonephritis, emphysematous pyelonephritis occurs more commonly in women than men. High levels of glycosylated hemoglobin or high levels of blood sugar are usually noted in affected patients. Alcoholism, malnourishment, renal calculi, or diabetic ketoacidosis is often present *(66,69)*. Rare cases have been reported in nondiabetic persons who have anatomic abnormalities of the urinary tract, ureteral obstruction, renal failure, or immunosuppression as predisposing factors *(68,70,71)*. *E. coli* is the predominant pathogen, followed by *Klebsiella* spp., as well as *Proteus* spp., *Pseudomonas* spp., and *Streptococcus* spp. Mixed culture results are observed in 10% of patients. Rarely organisms such as *Clostridium* and *Candida* species have also been isolated *(66)*. Bacteremia is usually observed.

Patients with emphysematous pyelonephritis are typically very ill, with high fever, abdominal or flank pain, nausea and vomiting, dyspnea, acute renal impairment, altered sensorium, and shock. Crepitus over the flank area may occur in advanced cases. Pneumaturia is uncommon unless emphysematous cystitis is present. Most cases are unilateral, but in 10% of cases, the condition is bilateral and associated with high mortality *(72,73)*.

A high index of suspicion is important for diagnosing emphysematous pyelonephritis. Patients suspected of having this entity should be stabilized with iv fluids and antibiotics before performing imaging studies of the urogenital tract, which often reveal gas in the renal parenchyma and potentially in the collecting system and perinephric tissues. Renal ultrasonography is useful, but the CT scan is currently considered the definitive diagnostic imaging study *(66)*. A four-stage clinicoradiological classification scheme has been proposed based on the extent of tissue containing gas to assess prognosis and to guide management *(65)*.

Aggressive treatment is essential. Intensive care to allow fluid restoration, initiation of systemic antibiotics, cardiorespiratory stabilization, and control of diabetes is required immediately; surgical therapy can be subsequently undertaken. Nephrectomy was the treatment of choice in most patients in the past and appears to be associated with reduced mortality when compared with less aggressive surgery in early stages *(67,74–76)*. However, more recent reports suggest that less aggressive strategies such as systemic antibiotic therapy alone or together with alleviation of any obstruction (either by percutaneous drainage or by stent placement) may suffice *(77–80)*. Specifically, cases with less extensive tissue involvement (i.e., emphysematous pyelonephritis class 1 and 2) may be managed effectively by percutaneous drainage and antibiotics. Even with more extensive tissue involvement (class 3 and 4), percutaneous drainage and systemic antibiotic therapy may be used initially if renal failure, septic shock, and coagulopathy are not present. However, when these features are noted, nephrectomy yields better results *(65)*. Definitive treatment for stones may be deferred until later *(77–80)*. With therapy mortality remains high *(65)*, and when treatment includes nephrectomy mortality rates reach 15–20% *(68,71)*, but untreated, the disease is uniformly fatal.

EMPHYSEMATOUS PYELITIS

Emphysematous pyelitis is characterized by gas solely in the renal collecting system and is strongly associated with underlying obstruction of the urinary tract. Presenting symptoms are similar to those noted in noncomplicated pyelonephritis: fever, nausea, vomiting, and abdominal pain. On a plain radiograph, gas outlines the renal pelvis. Therapy with antibiotics alone can be effective and successful if obstruction either is not present or is relieved promptly *(79)*.

EMPHYSEMATOUS CYSTITIS

Emphysematous cystisis may accompany emphysematous pyelitis or emphysematous pyelonephritis and can cause pneumaturia and hematuria. Other causes of air in the urinary bladder should also be considered in the differential diagnosis, however, including cysteocolic or cysteovaginal fistula.

FUNGAL CYSTITIS

Diabetes mellitus is a common predisposing factor for UTIs caused by yeast, particularly *Candida* species. Infection ranges from bladder colonization and clinical cystitis to severe upper tract disease, including emphysematous cystitis *(81)*, and renal or perinephric abscess *(82,83)*. Treatment of upper UTIs, with or without dissemination, requires systemic therapy. Imaging should be used to evaluate for obstructing "fungal balls" (a mass arising from a group of organisms), which requires removal and relief of obstruction when detected. Occasionally, patients with diabetes have such extensive fungal pyelonephritis and parenchymal abscess that nephrectomy is required for cure. The appropriate treatment of candida colonization or infection confined to the bladder remains controversial. Although spontaneous resolution of funguria occurs often *(84)*, if an indwelling catheter is present, it should ideally be removed. Removal of an indwelling catheter, control of hyperglycemia, and discontinuation of antibiotics will result in spontaneous resolution of bladder colonization/infection in many patients and should be part of any attempted treatment *(85,86)*. Other treatment options include bladder irrigation with amphotericin B, a single dose of iv amphotericin B, or oral fluconazole *(84,87)*. In a placebo-controlled trial of fluconazole treatment of candiduria, candidas were eliminated from the urine at the end of therapy in 50% of patients receiving fluconazole vs 29% of those receiving placebo. However, cultures performed at 2 wk after treatment in patients remaining hospitalized showed similar rates of candiduria in the two study groups *(88)*. Although patients receiving amphotericin B bladder irrigation may have higher rates of eradication a few days after the beginning of therapy than those receiving oral fluconazole, cure rates are similar 1 mo after the beginning of therapy *(85)*. When treatment is considered necessary, fluconazole may be preferred because of its ease of administration and relative absence of toxicity; however, increasing resistance to fluconazole among yeast may limit its utility.

Skin and Soft-Tissue Infections

Skin and soft-tissue infections occur commonly in patients with diabetes and can be life-threatening *(89)*.

CELLULITIS

Cellulitis in diabetics is usually caused by the same organisms as in healthy hosts: group A streptococci and *S. aureus (90,91)*. Cellulitis caused by group B streptococci, which may be complicated by bacteremia, is more common in patients with diabetes than in individuals without diabetes. Tender, edematous erythematous skin lesions are usually noted to merge gradually with adjacent uninvolved skin. Group A streptococcal cellulitis is classically associated with the presence of lymphangitis. The portal of entry for infection varies widely and ranges from imperceptible breaks in skin to neuropathic ulcerations.

Aspiration of fluid or biopsy from the leading edge of the erythematous lesion for culture is usually not necessary. However, if the causative organism must be identified, a biopsy may be done, but the yield is low *(92)*. Blood cultures will occasionally be positive and in more severe infections should be obtained prior to initiation of treatment.

Therapy for cellulitis may be initiated with an antistaphylococcal penicillin or cefazolin; in the β-lactam allergic patient clindamycin may be used. Gram-negative organisms are an unusual cause of cellulitis even in diabetes, but when suspected, a fluoroquinolone may be added *(93)*. Recently, methicillin-resistant *S. aureus* (MRSA) have been identified as a cause of cellulitis and abscesses with increasing frequency. These organisms can be acquired not only within the health care system but also in the community. The potential for skin and soft-tissue infection to be caused by MRSA requires initiation of therapy with antibiotics such as vancomycin, deptomycin, or linezolid in severely ill patients.

NECROTIZING FASCIITIS

Necrotizing fasciitis is the most severe soft-tissue infection in patients with diabetes and is associated with mortality rates approaching 40% *(1,94,95)*. Patients with diabetes make up 20–30% of patients in case series of necrotizing fasciitis *(96)*. Necrotizing fasciitis typically starts in the subcutaneous space, spreads along fascial planes, and causes rapidly progressive necrosis of the superficial fascia and overlying skin. Systemic toxicity and high fever are common. The arms, legs, perineum and buttocks, and abdominal wall are common sites for this infection. Fournier's gangrene is a form of necrotizing fasciitis that involves the scrotum and may extend to the penis and adjacent soft tissue.

Necrotizing fasciitis has been classified by the causative organisms: in type 1 infection it is caused by a combination of anaerobic and one or more facultative aerobic organisms, whereas in type 2, group A streptococci, with or without staphylococci, are involved. Others suggest classifying necrotizing fasciitis as polymicrobial when caused by facultative Gram-negative bacilli such as *E. coli* and strict anaerobes such as *Bacteroides fragilis* or clostridium species (90% of cases) or monomicrobial when caused by streptococci (10% of cases) *(97–99)*.

Diagnosis and Treatment of Necrotizing Fasciitis: Pain, which is notably disproportionate to the severity of the clinical findings of infection, is a hallmark of necrotizing fasciitis and should bring the diagnosis to mind. Bullous lesions appear later in the course of the disease and are not painful; wounds or eschars are also noted often. Crepitus associated with polymicrobial infection can be detected in about half of cases. Laboratory tests usually show an elevated white blood cell (WBC) count with a left shift, and creatinine phosphokinase levels are often elevated. Plain X-rays are more sensitive than physical examination in detecting soft-tissue gas, but CT or magnetic resonance imaging (MRI) scanning is most useful to detect deep tissue and fascial plane involvement in cases in which clinical suspicion is not very strong. If clinical suspicion is high, urgent surgical exploration is indicated and has potentially a dual role, diagnostic and therapeutic *(97–99)*.

Aggressive surgical exploration and debridement of nonviable tissue is the mainstay of therapy. Broad-spectrum iv antibiotic therapy should be initiated empirically and can subsequently be refined based on Gram stain and culture results. Clindamycin is more effective than penicillin in the treatment of group A streptococcal infection in animal models. For this reason, as well as to inhibit bacterial exotoxin production, clindamycin is administered in combination with a broad-spectrum penicillin B lactamase inhibitor (e.g., piperacillin-tazobactam) or a carbapenem. In penicillin-allergic patients, a newer fluoroquinolone can be added to clindamycin.

Pyomyositis

Pyomyositis, a bacterial infection of the skeletal muscle, manifests clinically with fever and localized muscle pain and swelling *(26,100)*, and in a large series of pyomyositis cases in the United States, approx 15% of patients had diabetes mellitus *(101–103)*, and almost all cases (90%) were owing to *S. aureus*.

CT or MRI scanning is used to delineate the extent of muscle involvement. Although diabetic muscle infarction has a similar MRI appearance, muscle biopsy either open or percutaneous allows a definitive diagnosis *(95,104–106)*. Treatment includes iv antibiotics with good *S. aureus*, and possibly MRSA coverage (in areas or settings in which these strains are prevalent), and surgical drainage or debridement when there is abscess formation or significant tissue necrosis. The outcome is usually good with minimal long-term sequelae *(100)*.

Diabetic Foot Infections

Foot infections are frequent in patients with diabetes (Table 2), accounting for up to 20% of diabetes-related hospital admissions *(107–111)*. Infection frequently develops in existing neuropathic diabetic foot ulcers and is a major cause of morbidity *(111–113)*, and approx 15% of diabetic patients with foot ulcers may subsequently develop underlying osteomyelitis *(114)*. Infection, especially when it coexists with significant peripheral vascular disease (PVD), is a major risk factor for lower-extremity amputation *(109,115–118)*.

Table 2
Diabetic Foot Infections

Infected foot ulcer
Superficial structure infections
    Skin infection, e.g., local or extended cellulitis
    Nail changes, e.g., fungal paronychia
Deeper-structure infection
    Fasciitis, necrotizing fasciitis, gas gangrene
    Myositis
    Abscess
    Septic arthritis
    Tendinitis
    Osteomyelitis

PATHOGENESIS: ETIOLOGY

Diabetic foot infections most commonly develop when bacteria invade soft tissue adjacent to trauma-induced ulcerations. Neuropathy, PVD and local ischemia, and decreased resistance to infection, which is often referred to as immunopathy (119–122), are established risk factors for diabetes foot infections.

Sensory and motor neuropathy lead to foot deformities, abnormal weight bearing, and trauma, with resulting ulceration. Autonomic neuropathy results in impaired thermoregulation and anhidrosis leading to dry skin with fissuring, which, in turn, can serve as portals for bacterial invasion. Ischemia, which commonly results from intrapopliteal arterial stenosis or occlusion, contributes to tissue necrosis, a process accelerated by local soft-tissue infection. Finally, in the setting of hyperglycemia and acidosis, immunopathy, particularly defects in leukocyte function, has been implicated in the diabetic patient's susceptibility to infection (6,120), and several studies have reported an inadequate leukocytic response to severe foot infection in patients with diabetes (123). Improving glycemic control improves immune function, including the efficiency of intracellular killing of microorganisms (124).

Administration of granulocyte colony-stimulating factor may improve granulocyte counts, but any effects of stimulating WBC production on clinical outcomes has not yet been fully established (125,126). Polymicrobial involvement is the rule in severe diabetic foot infections associated with ulcers that penetrate deep into subcutaneous tissue, whereas infections involving skin and more superficial sc tissue are often monomicrobial, mainly owing to S. aureus or streptococci (usually group B). Thus, Gram-positive cocci predominate in most infections, but Gram-negative rods and anaerobic organisms are also frequently isolated from deeper or limb-threatening infections (127–130). The most common organisms cultured are aerobic Gram-positive cocci, mainly S. aureus, but also coagulase-negative staphylococci and group B streptococci. MRSA has become increasingly prevalent in diabetic foot wounds (131,132), having been isolated from up to 30% of all ulcers cultured (132). Enterococcus spp. are often encountered (Enterococcus faecalis was found in 29% of all wounds) (133) but may or may not be significant pathogens. Corynebacterium species, commonly known as diphtheroids, are also frequently recovered but are not likely pathogens in this setting (134). The facultative Gram-negative bacilli most frequently cultured include Proteus species, E. coli, and other Enterobacteriaceae (135). P. aeruginosa is recovered in approx 10–20% of cultures taken and is usually encountered in chronic ulcers that have failed to heal during prior antimicrobial treatment *(133,136,137)*. Anaerobic organisms, although rarely occurring in pure culture, can be found in as many as 80% of patients with severe polymicrobial infections *(137,138)*. Peptostreptococci (anaerobic Gram-positive cocci) and *Bacteroides* species are the major anaerobic pathogens.

CLINICAL DIAGNOSIS: CLASSIFICATION

The clinical diagnosis of foot infection is based on the presence of the classic signs of inflammation around the ulcer together with purulent discharge from the ulcer. Pain and tenderness may be absent, owing to neuropathy. Erythema may also be absent in the diabetic foot because of the inability to increase blood supply in response to infection *(107)*. Moreover, systemic signs of fever and leukocytosis may be absent in up to 50% of patients with deep foot infections *(107,115,123,139,140)*. Poor glycemic control might be the only systemic finding indicating an underlying infection *(119)*. In fact, leukocytosis, fever, malaise, and extreme hyperglycemia are associated with severe infection often complicated by bacteremia.

Several schemas have been proposed for the clinical classification of diabetic foot infections based on severity, extent or depth of involvement, clinical characteristics, anatomic location, and etiology *(107,111,120,141–143)*. A simple approach is to categorize infections as mild, moderate, or severe *(111)*. Infections can also be classified as non limb threatening or limb threatening *(1)*. Mild infections are usually associated with superficial ulcers without bone or deep-tissue involvement and can be managed on an outpatient basis. Moderate infections might have varying degrees of deep-tissue involvement with little necrosis and no systemic toxicity and may or may not require hospitalization. Severe infections can have extensive or rapidly progressive cellulitis, deep-tissue necrosis, bone infection, gangrene, ischemia, and systemic toxicity. These are limb threatening and require hospitalization *(107,111,119,127,141)*. Non-limb-threatening infections are typically superficial with a small area (<2 cm) of surrounding cellulites; no ulceration or, at most, a superficial ulceration; and no signs of systemic toxicity. Outpatient management is generally appropriate. Conversely, limb-threatening infections show signs of extensive involvement including ulcerations that will probe deeply to bone, joint, or deep fascial compartments; a larger area of surrounding cellulitis (≥2 cm) with edema; erythema; and often concomitant lymphangitis. Fever, malaise, leukocytosis, and hyperglycemia are variable. Ulceration that probes to bone or joint prior to debridement is indirect evidence of osteomyelitis *(144)*. Limb-threatening infection or any infection associated with significant ischemia could be life-threatening and requires prompt hospitalization *(1)*.

DIAGNOSTIC EVALUATION

Evaluation of lower-extremity infection must be systematic and thorough *(145)*. Wounds should be probed to ascertain the presence of underlying sinus tracts or abscesses, as well as deep extension along fascial planes. Probing also helps to determine whether bones or joints are involved in deep infection. When bone is palpable by gently advancing a sterile steel surgical probe into the wound, treatment for osteomyelitis is recommended, because the positive predictive value for osteomyelitis is 89% *(144)*. If bone cannot be detected by probing and plain radiograph does not suggest osteomyelitis, the recommended treatment is a course of antibiotics directed at soft-tissue infection. However, because occult osteomyelitis may be present *(146)*, radiography should be repeated in 2 wk, in search of corrosive changes indicating bone infection.

Clinically uninfected ulcers should not be cultured and superficial swabs from an infected ulcer are not ideal for culturing, because both colonizing and infecting organisms are recovered. Infecting organisms are more reliably detected in specimens obtained by curettage of the base of the ulcer after debridement *(111,141,147–149)*, and needle aspiration is a reliable method of detection, although its sensitivity is low *(135,150)*. Culturing of bone specimens, obtained by percutaneous biopsy or surgical excision (through approaches that do not traverse the ulcer), is the best method for determining the cause of underlying osteomyelitis.

X-rays should be obtained and evaluated for evidence of osteomyelitis or soft-tissue gas. If gas is identified in the ankle or hind foot, radiographs of the lower leg should be obtained to assess the extent of the gas formation. Whereas X-rays are very insensitive indicators of acute osteomyelitis, they are fairly specific when classic erosive or lytic changes are present in concert with a positive probe test *(151,152)*. When plain-film images are negative and there is clinical suspicion for underlying osteomyelitis, radionuclide scanning with technetium-99m methylene diphosphonate ("bone scanning") can be used to detect bone infection *(153,154)*. Although the sensitivity of three- or four-phase bone scans approaches 90–100%, their usefulness is tempered by the high frequency of false-positive results that reduce the specificity to ≤50% *(146,155)*. The presence of Charcot arthropathy is especially problematic in diagnosing concurrent osteomyelitis because bone scans will uniformly be positive. Labeled leukocyte scintigraphy is somewhat more accurate in diagnosing pedal osteomyelitis but specificity remains suboptimal *(156)*. By contrast, MRI is both a very sensitive and specific indicator of bone infection. Sensitivity for osteomyelitis in diabetic foot infections ranges from 90 to 100%, and specificity ranges from 80 to 100% *(157)*.

Given that the absence of palpable pulses does not unequivocally indicate that ischemia is present, peripheral arterial circulation should be assessed through noninvasive testing in the absence of pedal pulses. Arterial segmental Doppler pressures with waveforms, including ankle and toe pressures and calculation of the ankle/brachial indices (ABIs), are very useful in the evaluation of peripheral foot ischemia *(119)*. Transcutaneous oxygen tension measurements can also be a fairly reliable indicator, wherein levels <20–25 mmHg would portend a poorer prognosis for healing *(158)*. Finally, in all patients with nonhealing ulcers, vascular surgical consultation and angiography should be obtained to determine the need for limb-salvaging arterial revascularization. Infection in a foot wherein arterial insufficiency compromises wound healing is always limb threatening.

MANAGEMENT OF DIABETIC FOOT INFECTIONS

Antimicrobial therapy alone is rarely sufficient in the management of diabetic foot infections, especially when ulcers are present. Adjunctive management should always include avoidance of weight bearing (off-loading), debridement, control of hyperglycemia, and management of ischemia *(111,159–161)*. Careful follow-up is necessary in non-limb-threatening infections that are managed on an outpatient basis, because lack of a favorable response or nonadherence to prescribed treatments could lead to hospitalization.

Management of Nonlimb-Threatening Infections. Non-limb-threatening infections can usually be managed without hospitalization. These infections are primarily monomicrobial and are caused by *S. aureus* and *Streptococcus* spp. especially group B streptococci *(1,160,161)*. Thus, after culturing, empiric oral antibiotic therapy can be initiated using penicillinase-resistant antistaphylococcal penicillins (cloxacillin, dicloxacillin), cephalexin, clindamycin, fluoroquinolones, and TMP/SMZ. A patient's response should be assessed 48–72 h later and antibiotic therapy adjusted, if necessary, based on culture results and the clinical response to treatment. Appropriate wound care, including debridement, sterile dressings, and off-loading is essential. Topical agents have been used adjunctively on infected wounds (e.g., silver dressings, silver sulfadiazine cream, mafenide acetate, povidone-iodine solution, ciprofloxacin solution), but their benefit over systemic antibiotics and sterile dressings has not been proven *(133,148,162)*. If improvement is not noted, hospitalization aiming at more aggressive care should be considered *(111,159–161,163–165)*.

Management of Limb-Threatening Infections. Patients with limb-threatning infections require immediate hospitalization for debridement, metabolic control, and parenteral antibiotic therapy *(111,119,166,167)*. Delays in appropriate treatment can result in more proximal levels of amputation *(1)*. Surgical management of limb-threatening infections is vital and includes debridement of necrotic tissue, drainage of abscess cavities, and securing of deep specimens for aerobic and anaerobic cultures *(159)*. In patients with severe neuropathy, this can often be performed at the bedside. After debridement, patients are kept on bed rest to allow further dependent drainage and reduction of edema. In many cases, limb salvage depends on restoring perfusion to an ischemic foot, but sepsis should be controlled before revascularization. In severe, difficult-to-control infections, an open amputation (one or more toes) or in cases of life-threatening sepsis, guillotine amputation of the foot may prove to be necessary, although preservation of foot structure, which is necessary for weight bearing once the episode is finally resolved, is the primary goal *(119,168)*. Multiple debridements may be required on occasion, and special measures for wound closure such as plastic flaps, grafts, or negative-pressure dressings may be necessary *(169)*. Hyperbaric oxygen therapy is frequently considered an adjunctive measure to enhance oxygenation of peripheral tissues, but there is a paucity of controlled trials to prove its efficacy *(170)*.

It is not unusual to recover three to five organisms from deep-tissue cultures of limb-threatening foot wounds, especially when these are complicated by ischemia and gangrene *(1)*. Empirical antibiotic therapy should include broad-spectrum coverage for common Gram-positive and Gram-negative isolates as well as anaerobes *(111,148,159)*. Previous culture results, when available, may also assist in choosing initial antimicrobial regimens. Antimicrobial agents useful in this setting include β-lactam and β-lactamase inhibitor combinations, carbapenems, fluoroquinolones, or third-generation cephalosporins or cefepime in combination with agents to enhance antistaphylococcal or antianaerobic therapy *(111,128,129,151,161,171)*. Since single-agent treatment often fails to cover all responsible organisms, frequently several antibiotics need to be administered for more severe infections until culture results allow specific target therapy. Because limb-threatening infections often occur in patients who have been either treated previously or hospitalized frequently, attention must be given to infections caused by resistant organisms, especially MRSA, *P. aeruginosa,* and resistant Gram-negative rods.

Management of Osteomyelitis. Osteomyelitis frequently accompanies severe diabetic foot infections *(115,151,152)* and in addition to antimicrobial therapy usually requires resection of infected bone with or without local amputation *(172)*. When the infected bone has been completely resected (or amputated), the antibiotic therapy may be directed at residual soft-tissue infection; prolonged antibiotic therapy recommended for osteomyelitis is thus avoided. However, if residual infected bone remains, prolonged (at least 6 wk) antibiotic therapy based on the culture results is advised. Moderate success rates (63–77%) in managing osteomyelitis have been reported with prolonged antibiotic therapy alone *(173,174)*. Parenteral or oral agents may be used, often in combination, depending on the microbial isolates, and antimicrobial treatment with *(154,173,174)* antibiotic-impregnated polymethylmethacrylate beads or absorbable calcium sulfate pellets has been advocated as adjunctive treatment of osteomyelitis *(175)*. These devices produce high concentrations of an antibiotic locally with no concerns about systemic toxicity. Typically, gentamicin, tobramycin, or vancomycin is used. Nonabsorbable beads are removed in 2–4 wk. Absorbable beads, although not requiring removal, have the disadvantage of leaking calcium sulfate for several weeks. Further research is necessary to define the utility of these adjunctive measures *(175,176)*.

Candida Skin Infections

Superficial yeast such as candidal balanitis and vulvovaginitis are frequently seen in patients with diabetes and not infrequently are the presenting manifestation of diabetes *(177)*. Vulvovaginal candidal infection is a common cause of pruritus vulvae. Other presenting signs include vulvar erythema that may be accompanied by fissuring with or without satellite pustules. Vaginitis is usually accompanied by a white discharge. Traditional treatment involves normalizing blood sugar and treating both the vagina and vulva with topical antifungals. Vaginal candidiasis can also be treated with one 150-mg oral dose of fluconazole.

Angular stomatitis owing to *Candida* spp. is common in children and is seen occasionally in adults with diabetes *(177)*. It presents as white, curdlike material that adheres to erythematous, fissured areas at the angle of the mouth or as white patches on the buccal mucosa and palate. Diagnosis is readily confirmed by examination of a KOH preparation. Successful treatment may depend on normalization of blood sugar and the use of topical antifungals or oral fluconazole.

Paronychia caused by *Candida* spp. usually involves the hands but may also occur in the feet. It usually manifests as erythema, swelling, and separation of the fold from the lateral margin of the nail. The proximal nail fold can be involved, and then separation of the cuticle from the nail can ensue. Repeated episodes of inflammation are common. Bacterial paronychia indicated by purulent discharge can complicate the clinical picture. A positive KOH preparation on extruded serous material from the affected area confirms the diagnosis *(178)*. Candida infection of the web spaces appears as a white patch of skin, often with central peeling, and although it may be difficult to differentiate from its dermatophyte infection, its diagnosis can be confirmed on KOH preparation. Finally, candidal nail plate infections present with distal yellowing or whitening and thickening of the toenail resembling dermatophyte infections *(178)*.

Dermatophytosis (Tinea Pedis)

Candida spp. and more frequently tinea pedis may lead to inflammation and fissuring in the toe web spaces that serve as a portal of entry for bacteria and subsequent development of diabetic foot infections. Thus, tinea pedis should be aggressively managed in patients with diabetes especially when neuropathy and ischemic changes are present *(179–182)*. The nail dystrophy resulting from tinea infections may make proper nail care more difficult for the patient. Itraconazole (200 mg/d for 1 wk a month for 4 mo) and terbinafine (250 mg/d for 3 mo) can be used for treatment *(179–182)*.

OTHER SERIOUS INFECTIONS SEEN IN PATIENTS WITH DIABETES

Zygomycosis-Mucormycosis

Rhizopus spp., which is the most common organism causing zygomycosis in humans, as well as *Rhizomucor* spp., *Mucor* spp., and *Absidia* spp., are commonly found on fruits, on bread, and in the soil and are common components of decaying organic debris *(183)*. They are generally saprophytic and do not cause disease in immunocompetent hosts, although they are the third most frequent cause of invasive fungal infection in immuno-compromised patients. The pathogenesis involves invasion of major blood vessels, with subsequent ischemia, necrosis, and infarction of adjacent tissues, resulting in the production of a black eschar. Particularly at risk are granulocytopenic and acidotic patients, including those with renal insufficiency, diarrhea, and aspirin intake. Approximately 50% of cases of mucormycosis are seen in patients with type 1 diabetes mellitus *(1)* usually in the setting of ketoacidosis *(184)*. In addition, patients on glucocorticoid or desferoxamine therapy and those who have had previous splenectomy are at risk *(185,186)*.

In rhinocerebral mucormycosis, infection typically begins in the paranasal sinuses and extends by contiguous spread through bone and along vascular structures into the orbit and brain. Patients typically present with a history of fever, unilateral facial pain or headaches, nasal congestion, epistaxis, visual disturbances, and lethargy. Physical examination may reveal facial or periorbital cellulitis, proptosis, chemosis, and loss of extraocular movement. Palsies of cranial nerves II, III, IV, and VI are frequently noted, owing to cavernous sinus invasion. Occasionally, paralysis of the seventh nerve may also occur. Black necrotic lesions are generally observed on the hard palate or nasal mucosa *(187,188)*. Cavernous sinus thrombosis (patients typically present with severe headache, ophthalmoplegia, visual loss, and corneal anesthesia) or internal carotid artery thrombosis with hemiparesis occur in about one-third of cases *(189)*, and patients who present with these central nervous system (CNS) complications are at a very high risk of death *(186)*. Finally, zygomycetes may also cause pulmonary infection in patients with diabetes *(188)*.

A major pitfall in treating zygomycosis is differentiating it from more common bacterial infections, which may delay diagnosis, surgical resection, and appropriate antifungal therapy *(190–193)*. Diagnosis requires a high index of suspicion and is established with evidence of tissue invasion by fungal organisms. Scrapings from necrotic nasal tissue examined with KOH may reveal the characteristic appearance of broad, irregularly shaped nonseptate hyphae with right-angle branching. Fungal stains revealing these organisms in biopsy material obtained from necrotic tissue remain the mainstay for a definitive diagnosis. Fungal culture of biopsy tissue may be helpful, but results are only positive in 15–25% of cases despite positive histopathology. No serological tests are available, and blood cultures are not useful. Findings on radiographs of sinuses and orbits are nonspecific, but contrast-enhanced CT or MRI scans may demonstrate erosion or destruction of bone or sinuses and delineate the extent of disease, including CNS involvement *(187)*.

Successful treatment requires correction of the underlying risk factors, antifungal therapy with high doses of liposomal amphotericin B, or one of the newer azole agents (posaconazole but not voriconazole) together with aggressive surgery to debride all affected tissue *(194,195)*. Surgeons must remove all devitalized tissue and consider wide surgical debridement, if feasible. Endoscopic sinus surgery has been recently used successfully in the management of rhinocerebral mucormycosis *(196)*. Liposomal amphotericin B derivatives administered for prolonged periods are utilized more frequently nowadays in an effort to lessen renal toxicity. Aggressive measures to control hyperglycemia and ketoacidosis are crucial.

Mortality rates are very high because the infection has frequently spread and caused extensive tissue destruction by the time of diagnosis. The mortality rate is approx 85% for patients with the rhinocerebral form, whereas the overall mortality rate is approx 50% *(197,198)*.

Malignant (Necrotizing) External Otitis

Malignant external otitis is an invasive infection of the external auditory canal and skull base that usually develops in elderly patients with diabetes. Malignant otitis externa can on rare occasions be seen in patients who are immunocompromised owing to malignancy, acquired immunodeficiency syndrome, and malnutrition *(199–201)*.

Malignant external otitis is caused by *P. aeruginosa* in nearly all cases *(199,202)*. Other isolates often represent normal auditory canal flora. However, *S. aureus (203)*, *Proteus mirabilis*, *Klebsiella oxytoca*, *(204)* and *Pseudomonas cepacia (205)* have been reported to cause malignant external otitis. In rare cases, fungi, most often *Aspergillus fumigatus,* cause this infection *(206–209)*.

CLINICAL PRESENTATION

Severe otalgia unresponsive to routine analgesics and worse at night accompanied by otorrhea unresponsive to local agents is the presenting manifestation. Tenderness and swelling in the periauricular area often extending to the temporomandibular joint is common, and pain is aggravated by chewing. Inflammation and edema are present in the auditory canal, and granulation tissue is characteristically present at the bony-cartilaginous junction (at the site of the fissures of Santorini). Frequently, the ear canal is occluded, with resultant mild conductive hearing loss *(202,210,211)*. The tympanic membrane is almost always intact. Disease progression is associated with osteomyelitis of the skull base and temporomandibular joint *(202,210,211)*.

Cranial nerve palsies generally indicate advancing infection, with facial nerve palsy the most common presentation. CNS complications, including meningitis, brain abscess, and dural sinus thrombophlebitis, are rare but can be fatal *(202,210,211)*.

DIAGNOSIS

There is no single pathognomonic criterion that defines malignant external otitis. The diagnosis is generally made on the basis of a range of clinical, laboratory, and radiographic findings. Typical signs of infection such as fever and blood count abnormalities are notably absent. Although nonspecific, erythrosyte sedimentation rate is usually markedly increased and can be used to monitor disease activity *(199,211)*. Certain imaging modalities can be useful in the diagnosis and follow-up of malignant external otitis. Contrast-enhanced CT or MRI scans are ideal for the initial assessment of soft-tissue involvement, bone erosion, and dural inflammation. A quantitative bone scan can distinguish malignant external otitis from more benign infections and can correlate with disease activity *(212)*, but newer scans with single-photon emission computed tomography may be more helpful *(213)*. The differential diagnosis includes squamous cell carcinoma that can occasionally present as a painful, draining ear. Therefore, a biopsy to distinguish invasive infection from cancer is advised.

TREATMENT

Systemic antipseudomonal antibiotics are the primary therapy for malignant external otitis caused by *P. aeruginosa*. Ceftazidime or imipenem may be used, but ciprofloxacin (750 mg orally twice per day), if the isolate is susceptible, seems to be the antibiotic of choice, based on clinical experience; however, comparative trials of several antibiotics have not been performed to date *(214–216)*. Despite the relief of symptoms (pain and otorrhea), prolonged treatment for 6–8 wk is still recommended. Surgical debridement of the auditory canal and topical antipseudomonal therapy provide adjunctive treatment. Extensive surgical debridement is rarely undertaken given the efficacy of modern antimicrobial therapy. If organisms other than *P. aeruginosa* are causative, antimicrobial therapy based on in vitro susceptibility and treatment of osteomyelitis at other sites should be administered for several months.

In the past few years, ciprofloxacin-resistant *P. aeruginosa* strains have been isolated from patients with malignant external otitis *(217)*. Most cases have been effectively treated with a prolonged (>12 wk) course of an antipseudomonal β-lactam agent (ceftazidime, piperacillin, imipenem) with or without an aminoglycoside.

Emphysematous Cholecystitis

Emphysematous cholecystitis is a rare variant of acute cholecystitis. This infection is characterized by the presence of gas in the gallbladder lumen, gallbladder wall, or pericholecystic tissues. Compared with those with typical acute cholecystitis, patients with emphysematous cholecystitis are at greater risk of gallbladder necrosis, perforation, and peritonitis, for which diabetes is frequently a risk factor, its frequency ranging between 38 and 55% of patients with emphysematous cholecystitis *(218)*. The most common organisms isolated from patients were Clostridial species (46%), especially *Clostridia welchii*, and *E. coli* (33%) *(219)*. Symptoms are typical of acute cholecystitis, unless there is gallbladder perforation. Diagnosis is made by radiological imaging, because an abdominal radiograph may detect gas in the gallbladder, as can ultrasonography *(220)*. CT scan is probably the most sensitive radiological test for emphysematous cholecystitis, however. Prompt cholecystectomy is required in conjunction with broad-spectrum antibiotic therapy, including coverage for anaerobes and Gram-negative bacilli. Combinations of β-lactams and β-lactamase inhibitors, carbapenems, or multidrug combinations are usually effective. The mortality rate is much higher for patients with emphysematous cholecystitis than for acute nonemphysematous cholecystitis. In patients under age 60, mortality of emphysematous cholecystitis is 15%, compared with 1.4% in patients with acute nonemphysematous cholecystitis.

Periodontitis

Periodontitis is a chronic inflammatory bacterial disease of the tissues that surround and support the teeth. The disease results in loss of attachment of ligament fibers and supporting alveolar bone, which if left untreated can increase the mobility of a tooth and necessitate extraction. Diabetes may complicate the pathogenesis of periodontitis by causing abnormalities in the vasculature of the gingival tissues, deregulating the normal production of cytokines and growth factors, decreasing the synthesis and crosslinking of collagen, increasing collagenase levels, and depressing immune responses *(221)*. The risk of oral infections, particularly periodontitis, among patients with uncontrolled or poorly controlled diabetes is two to four times higher than that noted among healthy persons or patients with well-controlled diabetes *(221)*. Aggressive, more rapidly progressive, and difficult-to-treat forms of periodontitis develop in approx 30–45% of adult patients with diabetes mellitus and are concentrated primarily among those with poor glucose control. The prevalence of periodontal disease among patients with well-controlled diabetes is no higher than that in healthy nondiabetic subjects. This relationship suggests that poor control of blood glucose facilitates the development of periodontitis. Conversely, recent reports suggest that periodontitis may result in destabilization of metabolic balance in patients with diabetes. These findings suggest that prevention of and therapy for periodontitis and possibly other oral infections must be part of the overall care of patients with diabetes *(222,223)*.

CONCLUSIONS

We have provided a short synopsis of infections frequently seen in patients with diabetes. Infections in patients with diabetes may result in increased morbidity and mortality because of immune defects associated with hyperglycemia or because of other comorbidities frequently accompanying or complicating diabetes. Consequently, physicians should have a low threshold for aggressively pursuing the diagnosis and treatment of infection in patients with diabetes.

REFERENCES

1. Joshi N, Caputo GM, Weitekamp MR, Karchmer AW. Infections in patients with diabetes mellitus. N Engl J Med 1999;341:1906–1912.
2. Wheat LJ. Infection and diabetes mellitus. Diabetes Care 1980;3:187–197.
3. Shah B, Hux J. Quantifying the risk of infectious diseases for people with diabetes. Diabetes Care 2003;26:510–513.
4. File TM Jr, and Tan JS. Infectious complications in diabetic patients. Curr Ther Endocrinol Metab 1997;6:491–495.
5. McMahon MM, Bistrian BR. Host defenses and susceptibility to infection in patients with diabetes mellitus. Infect Dis Clin North Am 1995;9:1–9.
6. Delamaire M, Maugendre D, Moreno M, Le Goff M, Allannic H, and Genetet B. Impaired leucocyte functions in diabetic patients. Diabet Med 1997;14:29–34.
7. Geerlings SE, Hoepelman AI. Immune dysfunction in patients with diabetes mellitus (DM). FEMS Immunol Med Microbiol 1999;26:259–265.
8. Muchova J, Liptakova , A., Orszaghova Z, et al. Antioxidant systems in polymorphonuclear leucocytes of type 2 diabetes mellitus. Diabet Med 1999;16:74–78.
9. Pozzilli P, Leslie RD. Infections and diabetes: mechanisms and prospects for prevention. Diabet Med 1994;11:935–941.
10. Breen JD, Karchmer AW. Staphylococcus aureus infections in diabetic patients. Infect Dis Clin North Am 1995;9:11–24.
11. Cooper G, Platt R. Staphylococcus aureus bacteremia in diabetic patients: endocarditis and mortality. Am J Med 1982;73:658–662.
12. Farley MM, Harvey RC, Stull T. A population-based assessment of invasive disease due to group B streptococcus in nonpregnant adults. N Engl J Med 1993;328:1807–1811.
13. Leibovici L, Samra Z, Konisberger H, Kalter-Leibovici O, Pitlik S, Drucker M. Bacteremia in adult diabetic patients. Diabetes Care 1991;14:89–94.
14. Chee S, Ang C. Endogenous Klebsiella endophthalmitis—a case series. Ann Acad Med Singapore 1995;24:473–478.
15. Telzak E, Greenberg M, Budnick L, Singh T, Blum S. Diabetes mellitus—a newly described risk factor for infection from Salmonella enteritidis. J Infect Dis 1991;164:538–541.
16. Koziel H, Koziel MJ. Pulmonary complications of diabetes mellitus: pneumonia. Infect Dis Clin North Am 1995;9:65–96.

17. Valdez R, Narayan K, Geiss L, Engelgau M. Impact of diabetes mellitus on mortality associated with pneumonia and influenza among non-Hispanic black and white US adults. Am J Public Health 1999;89:1715–1721.

18. Fine MJ, Smith MA, Carson CA, Mutha SS, Sankey SS, Weissfeld LA, Kapoor WN. Prognosis and outcomes of patients with community-acquired pneumonia. A meta-analysis. JAMA 1996; 275:134–141.

19. Lipsky B, Boyko E, Inui T, Koepsell T. Risk factors for acquiring pneumonococcal infections. Arch Intern Med 1986;146:2179–2185.

20. Ewig S, Torres A. Severe community-acquired pneumonia. Clin Chest Med 1999;20:575–587.

21. Hansen LA, Prakash UB, Colby TV. Pulmonary complications in diabetes mellitus. Mayo Clin Proc 1989;64:791–799.

22. Leibovici L, Yehezkelli Y, Porter A, Regev A, Krauze I, Harell D. Influence of diabetes mellitus and glycaemic control on the characteristics and outcome of common infections. Diabet Med 1996;13:457–463.

23. Thomsen RW, Hundborg HH, Lervang HH, Johnsen SP, Sorensen HT, Schonheyder HC. Diabetes and outcome of community-acquired pneumococcal bacteremia: a 10-year population-based cohort study. Diabetes Care 2004;27:70–76.

24. Gleckman RA, al-Wawi M. A review of selective infections in the adult diabetic. Compr Ther 1999;25:109–113.

25. Silwer H, Oscarsson P. Incidence and coincidence of diabetes mellitus and pulmonary tuberculosis in Swedish county. Acta Med Scand Suppl 1958;335:1–48.

26. Fine M, Auble T, Yealy D, et al. A prediction rule to identify low-risk patients with community-acquired pneumonia. N Engl J Med 1997;336:243–250.

27. Bridges CB, Fukuda K, Cox NJ, Singleton JA. Prevention and control of influenza: recommendations of the Advisory Committee on Immunization Practices (ACIP). MMWR Recomm Rep 2001;50:1–44.

28. Patterson JE, Andriole VT. Bacterial urinary tract infections in diabetes. Infect Dis Clin North Am 1997;11:735–750.

29. Patterson JE, Andriole VT. Bacterial urinary tract infections in diabetes. Infect Dis Clin North Am 1995;9:25–51.

30. Hoepelman I. Urinary tract infection in patients with diabetes mellitus. Int J Antimicrob Agents 1994;4:113–116.

31. Andriole V. Asymptomatic bacteriuria in patients with diabetes—enemy or innocent visitor? N Engl J Med 2002;347:1617–1618.

32. Nicolle, L. Asymptomatic bacteriuria in diabetic women. Diabetes Care 2000;23:722–723.

33. Hoepelman AI, Meiland R, Geerlings SE. Pathogenesis and management of bacterial urinary tract infections in adult patients with diabetes mellitus. Int J Antimicrob Agents 2003;22(Suppl 2): 35–43.

34. Geerlings SE, Meiland R, Hoepelman AI. Pathogenesis of bacteriuria in women with diabetes mellitus. Int J Antimicrob Agents 2002;19:539–545.

35. Menendez V, Cofan F, Talbot-Wright R, Ricart MJ, Gutierrez R, Carretero P. Urodynamic evaluation in simultaneous insulin-dependent diabetes mellitus and end stage renal disease. J Urol 1996;155: 2001–2004.

36. Ronald A, Ludwig. Urinary tract infections in adults with diabetes. Int J Antimicrob Agents 2001;17:287–292.

37. Balasoiu D, van Kessel KC, van Kats-Renaud HJ, Collet TJ, Hoepelman AI. Granulocyte function in women with diabetes and asymptomatic bacteriuria. Diabetes Care 1997;20:392–395.

38. Zozulinska D, Majchrzak A, Sobieska M, Wiktorowicz K, Wierusz-Wysocka B. Serum interleukin-8 level is increased in diabetic patients [letter]. Diabetologia 1999;42:117–118.

39. Geerlings SE, Brouwer EC, Van Kessel KC, Gaastra W, Stolk RP, Hoepelman AI. Cytokine secretion is impaired in women with diabetes mellitus. Eur J Clin Invest 2000;30:995–1001.

40. Brauner A, Flodin U, Hylander B, Ostenson CG. Bacteriuria, bacterial virulence and host factors in diabetic patients. Diabet Med 1993;10:550–554.

41. Hansen DS, Gottschau A, Kolmos HJ. Epidemiology of Klebsiella bacteraemia: a case control study using Escherichia coli bacteraemia as control. J Hosp Infect 1998;38:119–132.

42. Lye WC, Chan RK, Lee EJ, Kumarasinghe G. Urinary tract infections in patients with diabetes mellitus. J Infect 1992;24:169–174.

43. Ling TK, Ng JM, Cheng AF, Norrby SR. A retrospective study of clinical characteristics of Acinetobacter bacteremia. Scand J Infect Dis 1996;101:26–32.

44. Munoz P, Llancaqueo A, Rodriguez-Creixems M, Pelaez T, Martin L, Bouza E. Group B streptococcus bacteremia in nonpregnant adults. Arch Intern Med 1997;157:213–216 .

45. Zhanel GG, Nicolle LE, Harding GK. Prevalence of asymptomatic bacteriuria and associated host factors in women with diabetes mellitus.The Manitoba Diabetic Urinary Infection Study Group. Clin Infect Dis 1995;21:316–322.

46. Geerlings S.E, Stolk RP, Camps , M.J, et al. Consequences of asymptomatic bacteriuria in women with diabetes mellitus. Arch Intern Med 2001;161:1421–1427.

47. Hooton TM, DS, AE., S.et al. A prospective study of asymptomatic bacteriuria in sexually active young women. N Engl J Med 2000;343:992–997.

48. Ooi ST, Frazee LA, Gardner WG. Management of asymptomatic bacteriuria in patients with diabetes mellitus. Ann Pharmacother 2004;38:490–493.

49. Raz R. Asymptomatic bacteriuria. Clinical significance and management. Int J Antimicrob Agents 2003;22(Suppl 2):45–47.

50. Harding GK, Zhanel GG, Nicolle LE, Cheang M. Antimicrobial treatment in diabetic women with asymptomatic bacteriuria. N Engl J Med 2002;347:1576–1583.

51. Zhanel GG, Harding GK, Guay DR. Asymptomatic bacteriuria. which patients should be treated? Arch Intern Med 1990;150:1389–1396.

52. Semethkowska-Jurkiewicz E, Horoszek-Maziarz S, Galinski J, Manitius A, Krupa-Wojciechowska B. The clinical course of untreated asymptomatic bacteriuria in diabetic patients—14 year follow-up. Mater Med Pol 1995;27:91–95.

53. Bonadio M, Meini M, Gigli C, Longo B, Vigna A. Urinary tract infection in diabetic patients. Urol Int 1999;63:215–219.

54. Nicolle L, Friesen , D., Harding G, Roos L. Hospitalization for acute pyelonephritis in Manitoba, Canada during the period from 1989–1992: impact of diabetes, pregnancy, and aboriginal origin. Clin Infect Dis 1995;22:1051–1056.

55. Forland M, Thomas V, Shelokov A. Urinary tract infections in patients with diabetes mellitus: studies on antibody coating of bacteria. JAMA 1977;238:1924–1926.

56. Carton J, Maradona J, Nuno F, Fernandez-Alvarez R, Perez-Gonzalez F, Arsensi V. Diabetes mellitus and bacteraemia: a comparative study between diabetic and non-diabetic patients. Eur J Med 1992;1:281–287.

57. Rahav G, Levinger S, and Frucht-Pery J. 1994. Escherichia coli endophthalmitis secondary to pyelonephritis: another complication of diabetes? Clin Infect Dis 18:117–118.

58. Walmsley RS, David DB, Allan RN, Kirkby GR. Bilateral endogenous Escherichia coli endophthalmitis: a devastating complication in an insulin-dependent diabetic. Postgrad Med J 1996;72:361–363.

59. Thomsen RW, Hundborg HH, Lervang HH, Johnsen SP, Schonheyder HC, Sorensen HT. Diabetes mellitus as a risk and prognostic factor for community-acquired bacteremia due to enterobacteria: a 10-year, population-based study among adults. Clin Infect Dis 2005;40:628–631.

60. Toyota T. Vertebral osteomyelitis in diabetes mellitus. Intern Med 1997;36:382, 383.

61. Griffin M, Bergstralhn E, Larson T. Renal papillary necrosis - a sixteen-year clinical experience. J Am Soc Nephrol 1995;6:248–256.

62. Smitherman KO, and Peacock JE, Jr. Infectious emergencies in patients with diabetes mellitus. Med Clin North Am 1995;79:53–77.

63. Edelstein H, McCabe R. Perinephric abscess: modern diagnosis and treatment in 47 cases. Medicine (Baltimore) 1988;67:118–131.

64. Goichot B, Andres E. Emphysematous pyelonephritis. N Engl J Med. 2000;342:60–61.

65. Huang J, Tseng C. Emphysematous pyelonephritis: clinico-radiological classification, management, prognosis, and pathogenesis. Arch Intern Med 2000;160:797–805.

66. Evanoff G, Thompson C, Foley R, et al. Spectrum of gas within the kidney: emphysematous pyelonephritis and emphysematous pyelitis. Am J Med 1987;83:149–154.

67. Cook D, Achong M, Dobranowski J. Emphysematous pyelonephritis: complicated urinary tract infection in diabetes. Diabetes Care 1989;12:229–232.

68. Pontin A, Barnes R, Joffe J, Kahn D. Emphysematous pyelonephritis in diabetic patients. Br J Urol 1995;75:71–74.

69. Tang H, Li C, Yen M, et al. Clinical characteristics of emphysematous pyelonephritis. J Microbiol Immunol Infect 2001;34:125–130.

70. Pappas S, Peppas T, Sotiropoulos A, Katsadoros D. Emphysematous pyelonephritis: a case report and review of the literature. Diabet Med. 1993;10:574–576.
71. Shokeir A, El-Azab M, Mohsen T, El-Diasty T. Emphysematous pyelonephritis: a 15-year experience with 20 cases. Urology 1997;49:343–346.
72. Zabbo A, Montie J, and Popowniak K, et al. Bilateral emphysematous pyelonephritis. Urology 1985;25:293–296.
73. Emphysematous pyelonephritis. Lancet. 1985;2:314–315.
74. Mydlo J, Maybee G, Ali-Khan M. Percutaneous drainage and/or nephrectomy in the treatment of emphysematous pyelonephritis. Urol Int. 2003;70:147–150.
75. Ahlering T, Boyd S, Hamilton C, et al. Emphysematous pyelonephritis: a 5-year experience with 13 patients. J Urol 1985;134:1086–1088.
76. Joris L, van Daele G, Timmermans U, Rutsaert RJ. Emphysematous pyelonephritis. Intensive Care Med 1989;15:206–208.
77. Tahir H, Thomas G, Sheerin N, et al. Successful medical treatment of acute bilateral emphysematous pyelonephritis. Am J Kidney Dis 2000;36:1267–1270.
78. Punnose J, Yahya T, Premchandran J, et al. Emphysematous pyelonephritis responding to medical therapy. Int J Clin Pract 1997;51:468–470.
79. Jain S, Agarwal N, Chaturvedi S. Emphysematous pyelonephritis: a rare presentation. J Postgrad Med 2000;46:31–32.
80. Best C, Terris M, Tacker J, et al. Clinical and radiological findings in patients with gas forming renal abscess treated conservatively. J Urol 1999;162:1273–1276.
81. Singh C, Lytle WJ. Cystitis emphysematosa caused by Candida albicans. J Urol 1983;130:1171–1173.
82. High KP, Quagliarello VJ. Yeast perinephric abscess: report of a case and review. Clin Infect Dis 1992;15:128–133.
83. Fisher J, Newman C, Sobel J. Yeast in the urine: solutions for a budding problem. Clin Infect Dis 1995;20:183–189.
84. Wong-Beringer A, Jacobs R, Guglielmo J. Treatment of funguria. JAMA 1992;20:2780–2785.
85. Jacobs LG. Fungal urinary tract infections in the elderly: treatment guidelines. Drugs Aging 1996;8:89–96.
86. Kauffman CA, Vazquez JA, Sobel JD, et al. Prospective multicenter surveillance study of funguria in hospitalized patients. The National Institute for Allergy and Infectious Diseases (NIAID) Mycoses Study Group. Clin Infect Dis 2000;30:14–18.
87. Leu H, Huang C. Clearance of funguria with short-course antifungal regimens: a prospective, randomized, controlled study. Clin Infect Dis 1995;20:1152–1157.
88. Sobel JD, Kauffman CA, McKinsey D, Zervos M, Vazquez JA, Karchmer AW, Lee J, Thomas C, Panzer H, Dismukes WE. Candiduria: a randomized, double-blind study of treatment with fluconazole and placebo. The National Institute of Allergy and Infectious Diseases (NIAID) Mycoses Study Group. Clin Infect Dis 2000;30:19–24.
89. Kemmerly SA. Dermatologic manifestations of infections in diabetics. Infect Dis Clin North Am 1994;8:523–532.
90. Bisno A, Stevens D. Streptococcal infections of skin and soft tissues. N Engl J Med 1996;334:240–245.
91. Brogan T, Nizet V, Waldhausen, J. Streptococcal skin infections. N Engl J Med 1996;334:1478.
92. Brook I, Frazier E. Clinical features and aerobic and anaerobic microbiological characteristics of cellulitis. Arch Surg 1995;130:786–792.
93. File T, Tan J. Treatment of skin and soft-tissue infections. Am J Surg 1995;169:27S-33S.
94. Balbierz JM, Ellis K. Streptococcal infection and necrotizing fasciitis—implications for rehabilitation: a report of 5 cases and review of the literature. Arch Phys Med Rehabil 2004;85:1205–1209.
95. Sentochnik DE. Deep soft-tissue infections in diabetic patients. Infect Dis Clin North Am 1995;9:53–64.
96. Gozal D, Ziser A, Shupak A, Ariel A, Melamed Y. Necrotizing fasciitis. Arch Surg 1986;121:233–235.
97. McArdle P, Gallen I. Necrotising fasciitis in diabetics. Lancet 1996;348:552.
98. Rajbhandari S, Wilson R. Unusual infections in diabetes. Diabetes Res Clin Pract 1998;39:123–128.
99. Prakash PK, Biswas M, ElBouri K, Braithwaite PA, Hanna FW. Pneumococcal necrotizing fasciitis in a patient with Type 2 diabetes. Diabet Med 2003;20:899–903.
100. Collazos J, Fernandez A, Martinez E, Mayo J, de la Viuda J. Pneumococcal pyomyositis: case report, review of the literature and comparison with classic pyomyositis caused by other bacteria. Arch Intern Med 1996;156:1470–1474.

101. Walling DM, Kaelin WG, Jr. Pyomyositis in patients with diabetes mellitus. Rev Infect Dis 1991;13:797–802.
102. Bonafede P, Butler J, Kimbrough R, Loveless M. Temperate zone pyomyositis. West J Med 1992;156:419–432.
103. Brown, R. Pyomyositis in patients with diabetes. Postgrad Med J 1989;86:79–89.
104. Claudepierre P, Saint-Marcoux B, Larget-Piet B, Allain J, Montazel J, Chevalier X. Clinical images: value of magnetic resonance imaging in extensive pyomyositis. Arthritis Rheum 1996;39:1760–1763.
105. Fam A, Rubenstein J, Saibil F. Pyomyositis: early detection and treatment. J Rheumatol 1993;20:521–524.
106. Sagar M, Bowerfind W, Wigley F. A man with diabetes and a swollen leg. Lancet 1999;353:116–118.
107. Gibbons G, Eliopoulos G. Infection of the diabetic foot. In: Habershaw G, ed. Management of Diabetic Foot Problems. WB Saunders, Philadelphia1995;121–129.
108. Frykberg RG. Diabetic foot ulcerations: management and adjunctive therapy. Clin Podiatr Med Surg 2003;20:709–728.
109. Ulbrecht J, Cavanagh P, Caputo G. Foot problems in diabetes: an overview. Clin Infect Dis. 2004;39:S73–82.
110. Foster A, Edmonds M. An overview of foot disease in patients with diabetes. Nurs Stand 2001;16:45–52; quiz 54–45.
111. Lipsky BA, Berendt AR, Deery HG, et al. Diagnosis and treatment of diabetic foot infections. Clin Infect Dis 2004;39:885–910.
112. Frykberg RG. Diabetic foot ulcers: pathogenesis and management. Am Fam Physician 2002;66: 1655–1662.
113. Senior C. Assessment of infection in diabetic foot ulcers. J Wound Care 2000;9:313–317.
114. Ramsey SD, Newton K, Blough D, et al. Incidence, outcomes, and cost of foot ulcers in patients with diabetes. Diabetes Care 1999;22:382–387.
115. Eneroth M, Apelqvist J, Stenstrom A. Clinical characteristics and outcome in 223 diabetic patients with deep foot infections. Foot Ankle Int 1997;18:716–722.
116. Adler AI, Boyko EJ, Ahroni J, Smith DG. Lower-extremity amputation in diabetes: the independent effects of peripheral vascular disease, sensory neuropathy, and foot ulcers. Diabetes Care 1999;22:1029–1035.
117. Eneroth M, Larsson J, Apelqvist J. Deep foot infections in patients with diabetes and foot ulcer: an entity with different characteristics, treatments, and prognosis. J Diabetes Complications 1999;13: 254–263.
118. Jeffcoate W, Harding K. Diabetic foot ulcers. Lancet 2003;361:1545–1551.
119. Caputo GM, Cavanagh PR, Ulbrecht JS, Gibbons GW, Karchmer AW. Assessment and management of foot disease in patients with diabetes. N Engl J Med 1994;331:854–860.
120. Laing P. The development and complications of diabetic foot ulcers. Am J Surg 1998;176:11S-19S.
121. Saltzman CL, Pedowitz WJ. Diabetic foot infections. Instr Course Lect 1999;48:317–320.
122. Caballero E, Frykberg RG. Diabetic foot infections. J Foot Ankle Surg 1998;37:248–255.
123. Armstrong DG, Perales TA, Murff RT, Edelson GW, Welchon JG. Value of white blood cell count with differential in the acute diabetic foot infection. J Am Podiatr Med Assoc 1996;86:224–227.
124. Gallacher S, Thomson G, Fraser W, Fisher B, Gemmell C, Mac- Cuish A. Neutrophil bactericidal function in diabetes mellitus: evidence for association with blood glucose control. Diabet Med 1995;12:916–920.
125. Gough A, Clapperton M, Rolando N, Foster AVM, Howard JP, Ediabetes mellitusonds ME. Randomised placebo-controlled trial of granulocyte-colony-stimulating factor in diabetic foot infection. Lancet 1997;35:855–859.
126. Kastenbauer TB, Hornlein G, Sokol, Irsigle K. Evaluation of granulocyte-colony stimulating factor (Filgrastim) in infected diabetic foot ulcers. Diabetologia 2003;46:27–30.
127. Karchmer AW, Gibbons GW. Foot infections in diabetes: evaluation and management. Curr Clin Top Infect Dis 1994;14:1–22.
128. Grayson ML, Gibbons GW, Habershaw GM, et al. Use of ampicillin/sulbactam versus imepenem/cilistatin in the treatment of limb-threatening foot infections in diabetic patients. Clin Infect Dis 1994;18:683–693.
129. Lipsky B, Itani K, Norden C. Linezolid versus ampicillin-sulbactam/amoxicillin-clavulanate for treatment of diabetic foot infections. Clin Infect Dis 2004;38:17–24.
130. Brunner UV, Hafner J. Diabetic foot infection. Curr Probl Dermatol 1999;27:252–258.

131. Tentolouris N, Jude EB, Smirnof I, Knowles EA, Boulton AJM. Methicillin-resistant Staphylococcus aureus: an increasing problem in a diabetic foot clinic. Diabet Med 1999;16:767–771.

132. Dang CN, Prasad YDM, Boulton A.J.M, Jude EB. Methicillin-resistant Staphylococcus aureus in the diabetic foot clinic: a worsening problem. Diabet Med 2003;20:159–161.

133. Ge Y, MacDonald D, Hait H, Lipsky B, Zasloff M, Holroyd K. Microbiological profile of infected diabetic foot ulcers. Diabet Med 2002;19:1032–1035.

134. Bessman AN, Geiger PJ, Canawati H. Prevalence of corynebacteria in diabetic foot infections. Diabetes Care 1992;15:1531–1533.

135. Wheat LJ, Allen SD, Henry M, et al. Diabetic foot infections: bacteriologic analysis. Arch Intern Med 1986;146:1935–1940.

136. Goldstein EJ, Citron DM, Nesbit CA. Diabetic foot infections: bacteriology and activity of 10 oral antimicrobial agents against bacteria isolated from consecutive cases. Diabetes Care 1996;19:638–641.

137. Grayson ML. Diabetic foot infections: antimicrobial therapy. Infect Dis Clin North Am 1995;9:143–161.

138. Gerding DN. Foot infections in diabetic patients: the role of anaerobes. Clin Infect Dis 1995;20(Suppl 2):S283–288.

139. Sumpio BE. Foot ulcers. N Engl J Med 2000;343:787–793.

140. Frykberg RG, Veves A. Diabetic foot infections. Diabetes Metab Rev 1996;12:255–270.

141. American Diabetes Association. Consensus Development Conference on diabetic foot wound care. Diabetes Care 1999;22:1354–1360.

142. Armstrong DG, Lavery LA, Harkless LB. Validation of a diabetic wound classification system: the contribution of depth, infection, and ischemia to risk of amputation. Diabetes Care 1998;21:855–859.

143. Oyibo SO, Jude EB, Tarawneh I, Nguyen HC, Harkless LB, Boulton AJM. A comparison of two diabetic foot ulcer classification systems; the Wagner and the University of Texas wound classification systems. Diabetes Care 2001;24:84–88.

144. Grayson ML, Gibbons GW, Balogh K, Levin E, Karchmer AW. Probing to bone in infected pedal ulcers: a clinical sign of underlying osteomyelitis in diabetic patients. JAMA 1995;273:721–723.

145. Edelson GW, Armstrong DG, Lavery LA, Caicco G. The acutely infected diabetic foot is not adequately evaluated in an inpatient setting. Arch Intern Med 1996;156:2373–2378.

146. Newman LG, Waller J, Palestro CJ, et al. Unsuspected osteomyelitis in diabetic foot ulcers: diagnosis and monitoring by leukocyte scanning with indium 111 oxyquinolone. JAMA 1991;266:1246–1251.

147. McGuckin M, Goldiabetes mellitusan R, Bolton L, Salcido R. The clinical relevance of microbiology in acute and chronic wounds. Adv Skin Wound Care 2003;16:12–25.

148. Lipsky BA. Antibiotic therapy of diabetic foot infections. Wounds Suppl B 2000;12:55B–63B.

149. Pellizzer G, Strazzabosco M, Presi S, et al. Deep tissue biopsy vs. superficial swab culture monitoring in the microbiological assessment of limb-threatening diabetic foot infection. Diabet Med 2001;18:822–827.

150. Sapico FL, Witte JL, Canawati HN, et al. The infected foot of the diabetic patient: quantitative microbiology and analysis of clinical features. Rev Infect Dis suppl 1984;1 6:S171–S176.

151. Lipsky BA. Osteomyelitis of the foot in diabetic patients. Clin Infect Dis 1997;25:1318–1326.

152. Calhoun JS, Dowling JPF, Mader JT. Osteomyelitis of the diabetic foot. Wounds Suppl B 2000;12:48B–54B.

153. Jacobson AF, Williams JE. Bone scintigraphic findings in patients with foot ulcers and normal plain film radiographs. J Am Podiatr Med Assoc 2003;93:91–96.

154. Snyder RJ, Cohen MM, Sun C, Livingston J. Osteomyelitis in the diabetic patient: diagnosis and treatment. Part 2001;1: Overview, diagnosis, and microbiology. Ostomy Wound Manage 2001: 47:18–22, 25–30; quiz 31–32.

155. Keenan AM, Tindel NL, Alavi A. Diagnosis of pedal osteomyelitis in diabetic patients using current scintigraphic techniques. Arch Intern Med 1989;149:2262–2266.

156. Palestro CJ, Caprioli R, Love C, et al. Rapid diagnosis of pedal osteomyelitis in diabetics with a technetium-99m-labeled monoclonal antigranulocyte antibody. J Foot Ankle Surg 2003;42:2–8.

157. Morrison WB, Ledermann HP. Work-up of the diabetic foot. Radiol Clin North Am 2002;40:1171–1192.

158. Kalani M, Brismar K, Fagrell B, Ostergren J, Jorneskog G. Transcutaneous oxygen tension and toe blood pressure as predictors for outcome of diabetic foot ulcers. Diabetes Care 1999;22:147–151.

159. Tan JS, File TM, Jr. Diagnosis and treatment of diabetic foot infections. Baillieres Best Pract Res Clin Rheumatol 1999;13:149–161.

160. Caputo GM, Joshi N, Weitekamp MR. Foot infections in patients with diabetes. Am Fam Physician 1997;56:195–202.

161. Ge Y, MacDonald D, Henry MM, Hait HI, Nelson KA, Lipsky BA, Zasloff MA, Holroyd KJ. In vitro susceptibility to pexiganan of bacteria isolated from infected diabetic foot ulcers. Diagn Microbiol Infect Dis 1999;35:45–53.

162. Wakefield MC, Kan VL, Arora S, Weiswasser J, Sidawy AN. Nonoperative management of diabetic foot infections. Semin Vasc Surg 2003;16:79–85.

163. Shea KW. Antimicrobial therapy for diabetic foot infections. A practical approach. Postgrad Med 1999;106:85–86, 89–94.

164. Frykberg RG. Diabetic foot infections: evaluation and management. Adv Wound Care 1998;11:329–331.

165. van der Meer JW, Koopmans PP, Lutterman JA. Antibiotic therapy in diabetic foot infection. Diabet Med 1996;13(Suppl 1):S48–S51.

166. Tan JS, Friediabetes mellitusan NM, Hazelton-Miller C, Flanagan JP, File TP. Can aggressive treatment of diabetic foot infections reduce the need for above-ankle amputation?. Clin Infect Dis 1996;23:286–291.

167. Lipsky BA, Berendt AR. Principles and practice of antibiotic therapy of diabetic foot infections. Diabetes Metab Res Rev 2000;16 Suppl 1:S42–46.

168. Bridges RM, Jr, Deitch EA. Diabetic foot infections. pathophysiology and treatment. Surg Clin North Am 1994;74:537–555.

169. Clare MP, Fitzgibbons TC, McMullen ST, Stice RC, Hayes DF, Henkel A.L. Experience with vacuum assisted closure negative pressure technique in the treatment of non-healing diabetic and dysvascular wounds. Foot Ankle Int 2002;23:896–901.

170. Wang C, Schwaitzberg S, Berliner E, Zarin DA, Lau J. Hyperbaric oxygen for treating wounds: a systematic review of the literature. Arch Surg 2003;138:272–279; discussion 280.

171. Edmonds M, Foster A. The use of antibiotics in the diabetic foot. Am J Surg 2004;187:25S-28S.

172. Ha Van G, Martini J, Danan JP, Tauber JP, Grimaldi A. [Role of conservative orthopedic surgery in the treatment of the diabetic foot]. Diabetes Metab 1996;22:80–86.

173. Venkatesan P, Lawn S, Macfarlane RM, Fletcher EM, Finch RG, Jeffcoate WJ. Conservative management of osteomyelitis in the feet of diabetic patients. Diabetic Med 1997;14:487–490.

174. Pittet D, Wyssa B, Herter-Clavel C, Kursteiner K, Vaucher J, Lew PD. Outcome of diabetic foot infections treated conservatively: a retrospective cohort study with long-term follow-up. Arch Intern Med 1999;159:851–856.

175. Roeder B, Van Gils CC, Maling S. Antibiotic beads in the treatment of diabetic pedal osteomyelitis. J Foot Ankle Surg 2000;39:124–130.

176. Armstrong DG, Findlow AH, Oyibo SO, Boulton AJM. The use of absorbable antibiotic impregnated calcium sulphate pellets in the management of diabetic foot infections. Diabet Med 2001;18:942–943.

177. Vazquez JA, Sobel JD. Fungal infections in diabetes. Infect Dis Clin North Am 1995;9:97–116.

178. Tan JS, Joseph WS. Common fungal infections of the feet in patients with diabetes mellitus. Drugs Aging 2004;21:101–112.

179. Robbins J. Treatment of onychomycosis in the diabetic patient population. J Diabetes Complications 2003;17:98–104.

180. Rich P. Onychomycosis and tinea pedis in patients with diabetes. J Am Acad Dermatol 2000;43:S130–S134.

181. Gupta AK, Humke S. The prevalence and management of onychomycosis in diabetic patients. Eur J Dermatol 2000;10:379–384.

182. Albreski DA, Gupta AK, Gross EG. 1999. Onychomycosis in diabetes. Management considerations. Postgrad Med Spec No:26–30.

183. Ribes JA, Vanover-Sams CL, Baker DJ. Zygomycetes in human disease. Clin Microbiol Rev 2000;13:236–301.

184. Khanna S, Sourmekh B, Bradley J, Billman G, Kearns D, Spear R, Peterson BA case of fatal rhinocerebral mucormycosis with new onset diabetic ketoacidosis. J Diabetes Complications 1998;12:224–227.

185. Sugar A. Mucormycosis. Clin Infect Dis. 1992;14:S126–129.

186. Butugan O, Sanchez T, Goncelez F, Venosa A, Miniti A. Rhinocerebral mucormycosis: predisposing factors, diagnosis, therapy, complications and survival. Rev Laryngol Otol Rhinol (Bord) 1996;117:53–55.

187. Harril WC, Stewart MG, Lee AG, Cernoch P. Chronic rhinocerebral mucormycosis. Laryngoscope 1996;106:1292–1297.

188. Lee F, Mossad S, Adal K. Pulmonary mucormycosis: the last 30 years. Arch Intern Med 1999;159:1301–1309`.

189. Rinaldi M. Zygomycosis. Inf Dis Clin North Am 1989;3:19–41.

190. Mondy K, Haughey B, Custer P, Wippold FN, Ritchie D, Mundy L. Rhinocerebral mucormycosis in the era of lipid-based amphotericin B: case report and literature review. Pharmacotherapy 2002;22:519–526.

191. Raj P, Vella E, Bickerton R. Successful treatment of rhinocerebral mucormycosis by a combination of aggressive surgical debridement and the use of systemic liposomal amphotericin B and local therapy with nebulized amphotericin: a case report. J Laryngol Otol 1998;112:367–370.

192. Saltoglu N, Tasova Y, Zorludemir S, Dundar I. Rhinocerebral zygomycosis treated with liposomal amphotericin B and surgery. Mycoses 1998;41:45–49.

193. Strasser M, Kennedy R, Adam R. Rhinocerebral mucormycosis: therapy with amphotericin B lipid complex. Arch Intern Med. 1996;156:337–339.

194. Greenberg R, Anstead G, Herbrecht R, et al. Posaconazole (POS) Experience in the treatment of zygomycosis. In: Proceedings of the 43rd Interscience Conference on Antimicrobial Agents and Chemotherapy, 2003;abstract M-1757.

195. Langford J, McCartney D, Wang R. Frozen section-guided surgical debridement for management of rhino-orbital mucormycosis. Am J Ophthalmol 1997;124:265–267.

196. Avet P, Kline L, Sillers M. Endoscopic sinus surgery in the management of mucormycosis. J Neuroophthalmol 1999;19:56–61.

197. Parfrey, N. Improved diagnosis and prognosis of mucormycosis. A clinicopathologic study of 33 cases. Medicine (Baltimore) 1986;65:113–123.

198. Tedder M, Spratt JA, Anstadt MP, Hegde SS, Tedder SD, Lowe JE. Pulmonary mucormycosis: results of medical and surgical therapy. Ann Thorac Surg 1994;57:1044–1050.

199. Rubin J, Yu VL. Malignant external otitis: insights into pathogenesis, clinical manifestations, diagnosis, and therapy. Am J Med 1988;85:391–398.

200. Ress B, Luntz M, Telischi F, Balkany T, Whiteman, M. Necrotizing external otitis in patients with AIDS. Laryngoscope 1997;107:456–460.

201. Weinroth S, Schessel D, Tuazon C. Malignant otitis externa in AIDS patients: case report and review of the literature. Ear Nose Throat J 1994;73:772–774, 777, 778.

202. Rubin Grandis J, Branstetter BFT, Yu VL. The changing face of malignant (necrotising) external otitis: clinical, radiological, and anatomic correlations. Lancet Infect Dis 2004;4:34–39.

203. Bayardelle P, Jolivet-Granger M, Larochelle, D. Staphylococcal malignant external otitis. Can Med Assoc J 1982;126:155–156.

204. Garcia Rodriguez J, Montes Martinez I, Gomez Gonzalez J, Ramos Macias A, Lopez Alburquerque, T. A case of malignant external otitis involving Klebsiella oxytoca. Eur J Clin Microbiol Infect Dis 1992;11:75–77.

205. Dettelbach M, Hirsch B, Weissman J. Pseudomonas cepacia of the temporal bone: malignant external otitis in a patient with cystic fibrosis. Otolaryngol Head Neck Surg 1994;111:528–532.

206. Harley W, Dummer J, Anderson T, Goodiabetes mellitusan, S. Malignant external otitis due to Aspergillus flavus with fulminant dissemination to the lungs. Clin Infect Dis 1995;20:1052–1054.

207. Chai FC, Auret K, Christiansen K, Yuen PW, Gardam D. Malignant otitis externa caused by Malassezia sympodialis. Head Neck 2000;22:87–89.

208. Yao M, Messner, A. Fungal malignant otitis externa due to Scedosporium apiospermum. Ann Otol Rhinol Laryngol 2001;110:377–380.

209. Bellini C, Antonini P, Ermanni S, Dolina M, Passega E, Bernasconi E. Malignant otitis externa due to Aspergillus niger. Scand J Infect Dis 2003;35:284–288.

210. Dousary S, Attallh M, al Rabah, A. Otitis externa malignant.A case report and review of literature. Otolaryngol Pol. 1998;52:19–22.

211. Bhandary S, Karki P, Sinha B. Malignant otitis externa: a review. Pac Health Dialog. 2002;9:64–67.

212. Stokkel M, Takes R, van Eck-Smit B, Baatenburg de Jong, R. The value of quantitative gallium-67 single-photon emission tomography in the clinical management of malignant external otitis. Eur J Nucl Med 1997;24:1429–1432.

213. Amorosa L, Modugno G, Pirodda, A. Malignant external otitis: review and personal experience. Acta Otolaryngol Suppl 1996;521:3–16.

214. Wiseman L, Balfour J. Ciprofloxacin. A review of its pharmacological profile and therapeutic use in the elderly. Drugs Aging 1994;4:145–173.

215. Gehanno P. Ciprofloxacin in the treatment of malignant external otitis. Chemotherapy. 1994;40 (Suppl 1):35–40.

216. Hickey S, Ford G, O'Connor A, Eykyn S, Sonksen P. Treating malignant otitis with oral ciprofloxacin. BMJ 1989;299:550–551.
217. Berenholz L, Katzenell U, Harell M. Evolving resistant pseudomonas to ciprofloxacin in malignant otitis externa. Laryngoscope 2002;112:1619–1622.
218. Tellez L, Rodriguez-Montes J, deLis S, Martin L. Acute emphysematous cholecystitis: report of twenty cases. Hepatogastroenterology 1999;46:2144–2148.
219. Jolly B, Love J. Emphysematous cholecystitis in an elderly woman: case report and review of the literature. J Emerg Med. 1993;11:593–597.
220. Gill K, Chapman A, Weston M. The changing face of emphysematous cholecystitis. Br J Radiol 1997;70:986–990.
221. Collin H, Uusitupa M, Niskanen L, et al. Periodontal findings in elderly patients with non-insulin dependent diabetes mellitus. J Periodontol 1998;69:962–966.
222. Grossi SG, Genco RJ. Periodontal disease and diabetes mellitus: a two-way relationship. Ann Periodontol 1998;3:51–61.
223. Pucher J, Stewart J. Periodontal disease and diabetes mellitus. Curr Diab Rep 2004;4:46–50.

23 The HAART-Induced Metabolic Syndrome

Sotirios Tsiodras, MD, Theodoros Kelesidis, MD, and Christos S. Mantzoros, MD, DSc

INTRODUCTION

The presence of abnormalities of glucose metabolism *(1)*, hyperlipidemia *(2–5)*, and body fat redistribution *(6–9)* were first recognized in patients with human immunodeficiency virus (HIV) taking antiretrovirals approx 7 yr ago. Thus, acquired lipodystrophy and the associated metabolic syndrome, an extremely rare entity in the past, is now commonly seen in patients with HIV *(10)*.

Although the term *lipodystrophy*, mostly but not exclusively applying to body fat redistribution, was initially used to describe this syndrome, the term HIV/highly active antiretroviral therapy (HAART)–associated metabolic syndrome is currently being increasingly used. This syndrome increases morbidity and probably mortality, impairs quality of life, and affects patients' adherence to antiretrovirals. Thus, this syndrome is of considerable clinical interest. Both clinical and research efforts are confounded, however, by the lack of a widely accepted definition and diagnostic criteria for HIV/HAART-associated metabolic syndrome *(11–14)*. In this review, we describe the components of the syndrome and discuss the risk factors, pathogenesis (Fig. 1), clinical manifestations and implications, as well as the therapeutic approaches to this syndrome.

From: *Contemporary Diabetes: Obesity and Diabetes*
Edited by: C. S. Mantzoros © Humana Press Inc., Totowa, NJ

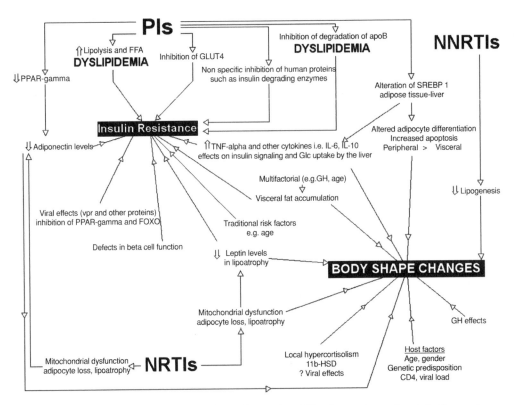

Fig. 1. Mechanisms operating in HIV/HAART-associated lipodystrophy and metabolic syndrome. PPARγ, peroxisome proliferator activated receptor type gamma. GLUT4, glucose transporter 4; Glc, glucose; vpr, HIV-1 accessory protein; IL, interleukin; 11β-HSD, 11β-hydroxysteroid dehydrogenase; apoB, apolipoprotein B; FOXO, family of Forkhead box class O (FOXO) transcription factors; SREBP, sterol regulatory element binding protein; PIs, protein inhibitors; NRTIs, nucleoside reverse transcriptase inhibitors; NNRTIs, non-nucleoside reverse transcriptase inhibitors; TNF, tumor necrotizing factor; GH, growth hormone; FFA, free fatty acids.

LIPODYSTROPHY

Clinical Presentation of Lipodystrophy

Lipodystrophy is characterized clinically by lipoatrophy/fat loss, lipohypertrophy/fat accumulation, or both and is associated with various other components of the HIV/HAART-associated metabolic syndrome *(15)*. Lipoatrophy typically includes decreased subcutaneous (SC) fat in the upper or lower extremities, with prominent veins, loss of SC fat in the buttocks, and facial atrophy *(15)*. Although facial and peripheral lipoatrophy are reminiscent of fat loss in extremely old individuals as well as patients experiencing HIV wasting, fat wasting should be differentiated from other wasting conditions associated with HIV infection, including the acquired immunodeficiency syndrome–wasting syndrome, malnutrition, cachexia, adrenal insufficiency, and severe chronic infections.

Fat accumulation can be seen in the area of the neck, dorsocervical region, abdomen, and trunk *(16,17)*, or it can manifest as SC fat deposits (i.e., lipomas), particularly in the dorsocervical area *(18)*. These findings can be either symmetric or asymmetric. Breast enlargement has also been observed *(19)*.

These clinical manifestations of fat redistribution make patients presenting with this syndrome feel that they could be recognized as HIV positive on the basis of their physical appearance, and this may result in stigmatizing effects.

Epidemiology of Lipodystrophy

The prevalence of HIV-associated "lipodystrophy" syndrome has been reported to be as high as 60–80% in patients receiving HAART (20), but the prevalence of lipodystrophy differs among different studies. This may be explained by the lack of a standard definition of the syndrome, differences in study design (e.g., cohort vs prospective studies), inherent differences among the populations studied, and, most importantly, the duration of observation in each study. A representative study has reported that the prevalence of any change in body habitus was 62% in protease inhibitor-experienced patients, 33% in protease inhibitor-naive patients and 21% in antiretroviral-naive patients (21). The prevalence of fat redistribution seems to be lower in HIV-infected children, however (22).

Risk Factors and Pathogenesis of HAART-Induced Lipoatrophy

The development of lipoatrophy is strongly associated with the use of combination antiretroviral regimens, the type of antiretrovirals used, and the duration of therapy (23). Exposure to nucleoside reverse transcriptase inhibitors (NRTIs) seems to be the most important risk factor for the development of lipoatrophy (23,24). Dual NRTI therapy is more likely to cause fat wasting than is therapy with a single NRTI, and lipoatrophy tends to get worse with increasing duration of therapy (25–28). Stavudine likely has a greater effect on lipoatrophy compared with other NRTIs (29,30) whereas newer NRTIs, such as abacavir (30,31), emtricitabine, and tenofovir (32,33), appear much better in this regard. Other important risk factors for lipoatrophy include increasing age (24,27), as well as racial (34) and probably other host factors, since lipoatrophy does not develop in the majority of NRTI-treated patients (26,34). Higher baseline HIV RNA (23) and CD4 T-lymphocyte counts <100 cells/mm^3 (26,34) have also been associated with HAART-associated lipoatrophy. NRTIs likely induce fat loss via interference with adipocyte differentiation whereas efavirenz, a nonnucleoside reverse transcriptase inhibitor (NNRTI), may contribute to fat atrophy through decreased lipogenesis (35). The effect of NRTIs is explained in part by effects on DNA polymerase γ that lead to mitochondrial toxicity and dysfunction (28,36) and a subsequent decrease in mitochondrial DNA (mtDNA) levels in various tissues, including adipose tissue (36,37). Depletion of mtDNA has recently been associated with fat tissue loss (38), which could lead to peripheral lipoatrophy. This process of mtDNA depletion may be difficult to reverse even with discontinuation of NRTIs (39).

Combination regimens of NRTIs with protease inhibitors may exacerbate fat wasting (27) but contribution of the protease inhibitors seems to be less significant than that of NRTIs. Protease inhibitors probably act via effects on transcription factors involved in the activation of genes responsible for long-chain fatty acid synthesis and adipocyte differentiation such as sterol-regulatory element-binding protein-1c (SREBP-1c) (40,41). SREBP-1c is a natural stimulatory ligand of peroxisome proliferator-activated receptor γ (PPARγ) and, thus, the adipocyte expression of PPARγ, a nuclear factor playing essential roles in adipogenesis, adiponectin production and glucose and lipid metabolism (42,43), is inhibited by protease inhibitors (44,45). The fact that PPARγ gene mutations result in lipodystrophy associated with metabolic abnormalities in patients without HIV too emphasizes the important role of this nuclear factor in the pathogenesis of metabolic syndrome (10). Since PPARγ is preferentially expressed in peripheral adipose tissue *(46)*, inhibition of PPARγ expression by protease inhibitors would result in apoptosis and impaired differentiation of peripheral adipocytes, with relative sparing of intra-abdominal visceral adipocytes. This contributes to body fat redistribution, abnormal secretion and circulating levels of adipokines, and subsequently to biochemical changes associated with the HAART-induced metabolic syndrome.

Risk Factors and Pathogenesis of HAART-Induced Fat Accumulation and Metabolic Syndrome

There is significant overlap between manifestations of increased fat accumulation in patients with HIV treated with HAART and the general population. In general, abdominal circumference increases with age *(47)* and, thus, HIV-infected patients may develop abdominal obesity as a result of not only their HAART therapy but also increasing age *(47,48)*. Protease inhibitors were the first class of agents to be associated with this syndrome, and efavirenz also appears to be strongly associated with gynecomastia and regional fat accumulation in HIV-infected patients receiving HAART *(49)*. Fat accumulation has been reported to be more common in female than male patients *(50,51)* and is also associated with low viral load levels *(52)* and smoking *(53)*.

In addition to the increased fat accumulation in the abdomen, which is mainly owing to an increase in visceral fat, hepatic steatosis and increased intramyocellular lipids may also contribute to the metabolic changes in HIV-infected patients receiving HAART *(54–57)*. This could also be associated with increased circulating fatty acids and subsequently increased storage of fatty acids and/or impaired fatty acid oxidation *(54,57,58)*.

Fat accumulation in the dorsocervical region of this population is morphologically very similar to that seen in Cushing disease, but the hypothalamic–pituitary–adrenal axis is not activated in this syndrome *(6,59)*. Changes in the expression of important enzymes in glucocorticoid production locally in the adipose tissue, such as 11β-hydroxysteroid dehydrogenase type 1, may induce local hypercortisolemia, however, and could thus lead to fat accumulation and regional adiposity *(60)*.

Diagnostic Assessment of Fat Redistribution

All patients who begin HAART should undergo regular assessment of their body morphology. Simple anthropometric measures including waist circumference are easily performed clinical measures of central fat accumulation that may provide valuable information about future cardiovascular risk *(61)*. More sophisticated and accurate estimates of body fat distribution include the use of skin-fold calipers, bioelectrical impedance, regional dual energy X-ray absorptiometry, ultrasonography, and whole-body/single-slice computed tomography (CT) or magnetic resonance imaging (MRI) *(62–65)*. Single-slice CT or MRI at the L4–5 level correlates well with whole-body fat *(66)*, but, in contrast to MRI, CT is associated with radiation exposure. At present, these techniques are only used in research settings.

LIPID ABNORMALITIES: DYSLIPIDEMIA

Epidemiology of Lipid Abnormalities

A cohort study that we performed showed a cumulative incidence of hypercholesterolemia and hypertriglyceridemia of 24 and 19%, respectively, over a 5-yr period after the initiation of protease inhibitor therapy *(5)*. Cholesterol elevations were noted in 27% of patients receiving a protease inhibitor, 23% of those receiving an NNRTI, and 10% of those receiving an NRTI in a large study, whereas these abnormalities were seen in only 8% of antiretroviral naive HIV patients *(67)*. The respective percentages were 40, 32, 23, and 15% for hypertriglyceridemia and 27, 19, 25, and 26% for low high-density lipoprotein (HDL) cholesterol, respectively *(67)*. The development of dyslipidemia may precede the development of body fat redistribution by 3–6 mo *(68,69)*. Since decreases in total HDL and low-density lipoprotein (LDL) cholesterol might exist at the time of infection before any treatment is given to patients with HIV, increasing total cholesterol and LDL cholesterol levels after initiation of HAART may actually reflect a return to "baseline preinfection" serum levels *(70)*, and, thus, the HAART-induced dyslipidemia may be only relative in nature.

Risk Factors and Pathogenesis of Lipid Abnormalities

The development of dyslipidemia is strongly associated with the use of antiretrovirals, but changes in lipid and lipoprotein were also observed prior to the introduction of HAART *(71,72)* and were probably associated with both immune modulation, disease progression *(72)*, and genetic predisposition *(73,74)*. Traditional risk factors such as age and changes in baseline lipid are also important predictors of HIV/HAART-related dyslipidemia *(5)*. Finally, viral progression may be an important risk factor for dyslipidemia, and low HDL has been associated with higher HIV RNA values *(29)*.

By contrast, younger age, female sex, black race, and NNRTI-containing antiretroviral therapy regimens appear to be protective against low HDL cholesterol in HIV-positive patients receiving antiretrovirals *(29)*. Therapy with NRTIs or NNRTIs has also been associated with dyslipidemia. Nevirapine may have a more favorable lipid profile than the other commonly used NNRTI, such as efavirenz *(75)*, and more favorable lipid effects for triglyceride and HDL cholesterol levels have also been reported with the nonstavudine-containing regimens *(29)*.

Hypercholesterolemia, hypertriglyceridemia, and increased apoB lipoprotein levels appear to have a greater association with the use of protease inhibitor-based regimens *(5,76)*. Specific protease inhibitors differ in their effects on lipid levels, with ritonavir characteristically associated with hypertriglyceridemia *(76)*. The pathogenesis includes protease inhibitor effects of SREBPs in the liver and adipocytes (as discussed earlier) *(77)*. In addition, protease inhibitors inhibit the proteasome-mediated breakdown of apolipoprotein B in hepatocytes and adipocytes *(77,78)*. This leads to the overproduction of triglyceride-rich lipoproteins that circulate freely in the serum, inducing metabolic effects *(77)*. Additional mechanisms include the enhanced formation of very low-density lipoproteins (VLDLs) *(76)* by ritonavir, a reduction in lipoprotein lipase activity that has been observed with saquinavir *(79)*, and an increased mobilization of the lipid stores *(29,80)*.

Implications of Lipid Abnormalities

Hepatomegaly owing to fatty liver is associated with increased lipid biosynthesis in the liver and chronic hypertriglyceridemia *(81)*; extremely high levels of serum triglycerides may contribute to the development of acute pancreatitis *(82)*. Dyslipidemia can also predispose patients to accelerated atherosclerosis and premature coronary artery disease (CAD) *(83,84)*, as well as increased risk of cardiovascular *(67,85)* and cerebrovascular *(86)* events. Other traditional risk factors may interact with hyperlipidemia to increase the risk of atherosclerosis, including elevated diastolic blood pressure (DBP), decreased tissue plasminogen activator (tPA) levels, and increased plasminogen activator inhibitor-1 (PAI-1) levels *(87,88)*.

Diagnostic Evaluation for Lipid Abnormalities

A fasting panel that includes total cholesterol LDL, and HDL cholesterol as well as triglyceride levels should be obtained in all patients annually before the institution of antiretrovirals. The measurements can then be repeated at regular intervals such as 1 to 2 mo after initiation of any regimen, and subsequently in longer intervals unless lipid abnormalities are detected and/or lipid-lowering therapy is initiated.

INSULIN RESISTANCE AND ABNORMAL GLUCOSE HOMEOSTASIS

Epidemiology

The development of insulin resistance and the subsequent development of impaired glucose metabolism are major components of HIV-associated metabolic syndrome (1) and are closely associated with changes in fat redistribution. Longitudinal studies have reported a 5% cumulative incidence of hyperglycemia 5 yr after the initiation of protease inhibitor therapy (5), and/or that diabetes mellitus or impaired glucose tolerance (IGT) is approximately threefold as likely to develop in HIV-infected men receiving combination antiretroviral therapy as it is in control subjects (89).

Risk Factors and Pathogenesis

Traditional risk factors such as family history of diabetes, increased age, and smoking may play an important role in the pathogenesis of insulin resistance (29), as does previous use of pentamidine (5) or coinfection with hepatitis C (90). The presence of fat redistribution abnormalities and/or other metabolic changes (i.e., dyslipidemia, as well as decreased levels of the adipokines leptin and adiponectin [see below]) are among the independent risk factors associated with the development of insulin resistance (15). Visceral fat accumulation is linked to insulin resistance in patients with HIV/HAART-associated metabolic syndrome (91), as is SC fat loss in patients with lipoatrophy (61).

In addition, antiretroviral therapy seems to be one of the main risk factors mediating insulin resistance in HIV patients treated with HAART (15). The use of protease inhibitors mediates insulin resistance by affecting glucose uptake, adipogenesis, and lipolysis (92). Protease inhibitors directly inhibit the translocation and intrinsic activity of glucose transporter 4 (GLUT4) (93,94), an effect that may be accompanied by impaired glucose phosphorylation (58). The newer protease inhibitor atazanavir does not appear to have an effect on GLUT4 in vivo, however; and thus, it may have little effect on insulin resistance (95). In addition, protease inhibitor-induced increased lipolysis and elevated free fatty acid (FFA) levels lead to impaired insulin sensitivity (96,97). A detrimental short-term effect on insulin sensitivity has been described for indinavir (98) and lopinavir (99) even in the absence of HIV infection. Finally, treatment with protease inhibitors may also have an inhibitory effect on insulin secretion (100).

Virally mediated mechanisms may also be implicated in the development of insulin resistance in HIV lipodystrophy. The HIV-1 accessory protein Vpr not only plays an important role in mediating viral replication and host cell functions, but also appears to increase tissue sensitivity to glucocorticoids (101). Vpr may also inhibit PPARγ activity, (102) and the Foxo proteins that function as negative transcription factors for insulin (103), thus contributing to insulin resistance and adipocyte apoptosis. Other mechanisms include defects in β-cell function (91) as well as impaired negative feedback of insulin on β-cells (104) and sustained CD36 deficiency induced by antiretroviral therapy (105).

Adipokines (Adiponectin, Leptin, and Tumor Necrosis Factor-α) and Other Proinflammatory Cytokines in HIV/HAART-Associated Insulin Resistance and Abnormal Glucose Homeostasis

Transgenic mouse models of lipoatrophy provide important insights into the development of metabolic syndrome. These include (1) transgenic mice overexpressing nuclear SREBP-1c, resulting in disordered adipocyte differentiation and a significant decrease in white adipose tissue (WAT) *(106)*; (2) transgenic mice expressing protein AZIP/F-1, leading to inhibition of transcription factors critical for fat development and absence of WAT *(107)*; and (3) transgenic PPARγ–/– mice, which also lack adipose tissue treated with an inhibitor of PPARγ/retinoid X receptor *(108)*. All these mouse models have lipoatrophy associated with marked insulin resistance; hyperlipidemia; and decreased expression and/or activation of several molecules, including leptin, adiponectin, and PPARγ *(106–109)*. In accordance with the hypothesis that dysfunction of adipose tissue is the cause of the constellation of metabolic findings, transplantation of near-physiological amounts of fat tissue to AZIP/F-1 mice results in reversal of insulin resistance and improvement of dyslipidemia *(110)*.

In humans, rare syndromes of congenital lipoatrophic diabetes exist, which show metabolic changes similar to the mouse models just described *(111–113)*. Similarly, HIV-positive patients treated with HAART may develop generalized fat depletion or lipoatrophy, associated with low adiponectin and leptin levels and features of metabolic syndrome *(114,115)*.

Leptin, a 16-kDa adipocyte-secreted polypeptide, circulates at levels directly proportional to body fat mass and acute changes in nutritional status. Leptin acts primarily on hypothalamic receptors to regulate energy homeostasis, body weight, and neuroendocrine and immune function *(116)*. Moreover, leptin regulates insulin action and lipid profile in animals and humans, acting through several mechanisms, including a decrease in food intake, a decrease in intrahepatic or intramyocellular lipids, and/or by direct and indirect neural stimulation of skeletal muscle adenosine monophosphate-activated protein kinase *(117,118)*. Ob/ob mice, which completely lack leptin, and rodents and humans with congenital lipoatrophy have low leptin levels, which are associated with profound insulin resistance and hyperlipidemia *(116,118,119)*. In humans with congenital lipodystrophy and metabolic syndrome, administration of leptin at physiological doses decreased fasting glucose by 45%, HbA1c by 16%, fasting triglycerides by 61%, and FFAs by 61% in a 4-mo open-label pilot trial *(119)*. These changes were maintained after 8–10 mo of leptin treatment in another smaller study *(120)*. Fasting leptin levels have been shown to correlate well with total body fat concentrations in HIV-infected patients *(121,122)*; thus, patients with HAART-induced lipoatrophy and metabolic syndrome also have decreased leptin levels that are associated with insulin resistance *(114)*, suggesting that leptin deficiency may play a role in the pathogenesis of this syndrome.

Adiponectin (AdipoQ, ACRP30, apM1), a 30-kDa adipocyte-secreted hormone that circulates in high concentrations in the bloodstream, has also been proposed to be a link between central obesity and insulin resistance *(116)*. Adiponectin expression and serum levels correlate negatively with total and visceral fat mass and insulin resistance and return to normal after long-term weight loss *(123)*. Other adipokines (tumor necrosis factor-α [TNF-α], IL-6), β-adrenergic agonists, glucocorticoids, and testosterone, which induce insulin resistance, have also been shown to inhibit adiponectin expression

(124,125). At the molecular level, adiponectin expression is stimulated through the SREBP-1/PPARγ pathway *(126,127)*; humans with inactivating PPARγ mutations have very low adiponectin levels and severe diabetes, and administration of PPARγ agonists, such as thiazolidinediones (TZDs), increases adiponectin levels by binding to specific adiponectin receptors *(128)* and in this way improves insulin resistance *(125)*. Adiponectin acts by enhancing insulin-induced suppression of glucose production in the liver, while increasing insulin-dependent glucose transport and FFA oxidation in muscle *(129)*. The insulin-sensitizing effects in muscle, like those of leptin, involve activation of AMP-activated protein kinase *(129)*. In addition to its beneficial effects on insulin sensitivity, adiponectin improves the lipid profile and has anti-inflammatory and antiatherogenic effects *(116,125)*.

Adiponectin knockout mice develop insulin resistance *(130,131)*, whereas transgenic mice overexpressing adiponectin have improved insulin sensitivity, independent of body adiposity *(132)*. Obese and lipoatrophic mice have low circulating adiponectin levels, insulin resistance, and hyperlipidemia, and administration of adiponectin improves their metabolic profile *(108,131)*. In humans, low circulating adiponectin levels have been consistently linked to obesity and several components of the metabolic syndrome, including intra-abdominal fat, insulin resistance/type 2 diabetes, elevated triglycerides, low HDL levels, and the presence of coronary artery disease *(123,133)*. More important, low adiponectin levels precede and correlate well with the decline in insulin sensitivity in previously healthy individuals *(134,135)*. This suggests that hypoadiponectinemia may contribute to the pathogenesis of insulin resistance. We and others have shown that low adiponectin levels and mRNA expression are also seen in conditions associated with fat redistribution and insulin resistance, such as congenital lipodystrophy and HIV/HAART-induced metabolic syndrome *(113,115,136)*. A previous study showed that administration of protease inhibitors to mice results in decreased adiponectin expression and circulating levels as well as dyslipidemia, and administration of adiponectin ameliorates the lipid abnormalities *(137)*.

Leptin and adiponectin may have additive effects in normalizing insulin sensitivity and metabolic abnormalities in animals, because administration of each hormone alone is only partially effective, whereas a combination of physiological doses of adiponectin and leptin completely reverses the insulin resistance of lipoatrophic mice, which have low adiponectin and leptin levels *(108)*. These observations suggest that the adipocyte-secreted hormones leptin and adiponectin may be critical mediators of the insulin resistance and metabolic syndrome associated with lipoatrophy and that the combined effects of these two hormones might be necessary to maintain a normal metabolic state. Initial studies involving administration of leptin or adiponectin to subjects with HIV/HAART metabolic syndrome are presently under way.

Clinical Findings Related to Insulin Resistance and Abnormal Glucose Homeostasis

Insulin resistance commonly manifests as hyperinsulinemia in normoglycemic subjects preceding the development of glucose intolerance and diabetes *(61)*. The latter may manifest with the classic signs of polydipsia and increased hunger, polyuria, fatigue, poor concentration, blurred vision, changes in weight, and slow wound healing *(51,115)*. When insulin resistance is severe, acanthosis nigricans, possibly hypertrichosis, and hirsutism can be observed. Hyperinsulinemia is also associated with dyslipidemia, increased diastolic blood pressure, and markedly increased levels of PAI-1 *(61,138)*, as well as with increased waist circumference and loss of peripheral SC fat.

Diagnostic Evaluation of Insulin Resistance and Abnormal Glucose Homeostasis

Patients receiving HAART should be closely monitored for the development of diabetes. The order of events is progression from the normal state to normoglycemic hyperinsulinemia, to impaired fasting glucose and IGT, and later to frank diabetes. The detection of hyperglycemia is based on determinations of fasting glucose levels and when appropriate an oral glucose tolerance test and a glycosylated hemoglobin measurement.

Recent recommendations, based on empirical evidence, suggest that fasting glucose should be measured before initiating HAART, 3–6 mo after starting or switching drugs, and at least annually during protease inhibitor therapy *(139)*. The formal evaluation of insulin resistance is more complex and currently not recommended outside research settings. Such evaluation may range from simple fasting insulin levels to more complex tests such as the hyperinsulinemic euglycemic clamp, which serves as the "gold standard" technique in the research setting.

Hyperinsulinemia and insulin resistance have been associated with increased cardiovascular risk in the general population *(140,141)* and may act synergistically with other risk factors such as lipid changes, metabolic changes, and associated endothelial dysfunction to produce accelerated atherosclerosis *(142)*.

THERAPEUTIC STRATEGIES FOR HIV/HAART METABOLIC SYNDROME

Treatment of Lipoatrophy

Therapeutic attempts have focused on antiretroviral switch strategies *(143,144)*, plastic or dermatology surgery for replacement of facial fat loss *(145,146)*, and the use of insulin sensitizers *(147–150)*. Avoiding NRTIs that have been associated with lipoatrophy and fat loss *(143)* and switching from an NRTI to an NRTI-sparing regimen, such as indinavir and efavirenz, may lead to significant increases in visceral and SC fat, although this could also possibly lead to significant decreases in lean body mass *(151)*. When necessary, the substitution of stavudine with abacavir or zidovudine may be another effective strategy *(143,144)*. Caution should be exercised, however, in switching antiretroviral regimens to treat fat redistribution changes in HIV patients who have achieved good immunological status and viral suppression *(152,153)*.

In HIV-negative patients with diabetes, both the TZDs pioglitazone and rosiglitazone have been reported to increase total body and SC fat with a concomitant decrease in visceral fat *(154–156)*. Although initial results from studies on the insulin sensitizer rosiglitazone replicated these findings in patients with HIV/HAART metabolic syndrome *(147,148)*, subsequent studies revealed conflicting and rather disappointing results *(149,150,157)*. By contrast, a study evaluating pioglitazone found a trend toward an increase in total body and abdominal fat over 12 mo of pioglitazone use *(158)*.

Recently, administration of leptin to patients with congenital and acquired (non-HIV) lipodystrophy *(119)* resulted in significant metabolic improvements *(119)*. We have shown in a pilot proof-of-concept study that leptin replacement therapy for 2 mo improved the insulin resistance of HIV-positive lipoatrophic and leptin-deficient subjects without having any adverse effects on lipoatrophy *(159)*. Thus, administration of leptin alone or in combination with TZDs or switch strategies could reverse many of the metabolic abnormalities observed in HIV/HAART metabolic syndrome.

Anabolic steroids cannot be currently recommended for the therapy of lipoatrophy because there is evidence that their use may be associated with a decrease in peripheral fat *(160,161)*. Finally, costly procedures such as surgical implants, ranging from polymeric substances *(162)*, liquid injectable silicone *(163)*, Dermafat grafts *(164)* to lipoinjection of autologous fat *(165)*, have also been tried and injections of polylactic acid, a bioabsorbable material that stimulates collagen formation in the buccal area, have also been used to improve facial appearance *(166)*. These methods need to be further studied before they can be recommended as established safe and effective treatment options.

Treatment of Lipohypertrophy

Approaches that have been used for cases of HIV-related fat accumulation, include diet and exercise, antiretroviral switching, anabolic steroids, recombinant human growth hormone (rhGH), growth hormone-releasing hormone (GHRH), metformin, and insulin-sensitizing agents *(15,167)*. Antiretroviral discontinuation and plastic surgery have also been suggested. The role of diet in the pathogenesis of HIV/HAART-associated metabolic syndrome has not yet been fully elucidated *(168)*; however, individualized nutrition care plans are becoming an increasingly common feature of the medical management of HIV-infected patients with body fat redistribution *(169,170)*. Although modification of diet may theoretically have a beneficial effect in some, if not most, subjects with the syndrome, two cross-sectional studies of HIV-infected patients failed to show a clear association between total or saturated fat intake and lipodystrophic changes even though total energy intake was higher in the fat redistribution compared with the nonfat redistribution group *(171,172)*. A combination of a diet high in fiber and an aerobic exercise program may be effective in partially reversing abdominal obesity *(173)*, but these results have not yet been replicated. Thus, in anticipation of future, more detailed studies, one could possibly recommend a decrease in the intake of saturated fat and excess calories to subjects with lipohypertrophy.

Intensive aerobic exercise in subjects without HIV can decrease intra-abdominal adipose tissue *(174)*, and several small studies have shown a beneficial effect of physical activity on metabolic parameters associated with HIV/HAART syndrome *(175–179)*. An improvement in lipohypertrophy and dyslipidemia by individualized light aerobic training was noted in a study of HIV-infected patients with lipodystrophy and/or dyslipidemia *(180)*; thus, physical activity may also be a significant protective factor for the development of fat redistribution syndromes *(181)*.

Metformin, a medication with insulin-sensitizing properties, has been associated with decreased body weight and visceral adipose tissue in HIV-infected subjects with central obesity *(182,183)*. Because its use can be complicated by lactic acidosis extreme caution should be used in administrating it especially in patients receiving NRTIs and/or having liver or renal dysfunction. TZDs are discussed in more detail in the "Lipoatrophy" and the "Insulin Resistance" sections, because their role in lipohypertrophy *per se* has not yet been clearly elucidated in HIV/HAART syndrome. A recent review of available data concluded that rosiglitazone has no major effect on lipohypertrophy *(184)*, and the only available randomized study on pioglitazone did not have the power to analyze data according to lipodystrophy category *(185)*.

Since its first approval for use in HIV-associated wasting *(186)*, rhGH has been successfully used in HIV-negative adults to reduce abdominal adiposity *(187,188)*. Administration of GHRH results in a reduction in total body and visceral fat mass in HIV-negative patients *(189–193)*, and improvements in total and regional body composition, increased lean mass, and reduced truncal and visceral fat in patients with HIV and lipodystrophy *(194)*. One should be extremely cautious in presenting rhGH for patients with HIV, however, because high doses of rhGH may lead to worsening of glucose tolerance as well as significant increases in circulating insulin-like growth factor-1, which may potentially lead to long-term adverse effects *(15)*.

The use of anabolic steroids in patients with HIV/HAART-associated metabolic syndrome may result in reduction of truncal fat in a manner similar to that in non-HIV-infected patients *(195)*. However, because the use of steroids is also associated with peripheral fat loss *(see* Treatment of Lipoatrophy) and may induce insulin resistance, especially in women, these agents should probably be reserved only for selected subgroups of patients.

Surgical procedures have been used in an attempt to improve lipohypertrophy and treat excess dorsocervical fat with successful results especially in cases with prominent "buffalo humps" *(196,197)*. Because only small case series describe these invasive and expensive approaches, one should carefully review available follow-up data, surgeons' experience, and cost before recommending them.

Treatment of Hyperlipidemia

The Infectious Diseases Society of America and the Adult AIDS Clinical Trials Group have recently published guidelines on the evaluation and management of dyslipidemia in HIV-infected adults receiving antiretrovirals *(198)*. Dietary approaches, exercise, antihyperlipidemic medications, and antiretroviral switch strategies are among the therapeutic modalities suggested. Risk stratification is important in selecting lipid-lowering targets in these subjects *(198)*. Patients with coronary heart disease (CHD), risk equivalents of CHD, or risk factors for CHD should have lower target LDL cholesterol values. For example, for a patient with CHD, the target LDL cholesterol level is <100 mg/dL, whereas for individuals with zero to one risk factor, the target LDL cholesterol level is <160 mg/dL *(198)*. For patients with triglyceride levels >200 mg/dL, the LDL cholesterol target should be achieved first; then the focus becomes the non-HDL cholesterol values *(198)*. The initial step in treating HIV-related dyslipidemia is dietary intervention, and dietary management should be individualized *(170)*.

Patients with severe hypertriglyceridemia should consume low-fat diets with the caution that diets high in carbohydrates may actually exacerbate hyperinsulinemia. Fish oil preparations contain high doses of omega-3 polyunsaturated fatty acids, which may lower plasma triglyceride concentrations *(199,200)*. Total and aerobic exercise was significantly and inversely associated with fasting plasma triglyceride levels in an observational study performed at our institution *(172)*, but well-designed interventional studies are not available. Thus, a combination of diet and exercise is recommended in anticipation of further more detailed interventional studies.

For patients for whom diet and exercise are not sufficient and in whom the LDL cholesterol level is the primary target, a statin is the first choice of therapy, but potential significant interactions with the cytochrome-P450 liver enzyme system and antiretrovirals used should always be considered. Pravastatin, atorvastatin, and fluvastatin seem to be better choices in this regard *(198,201)*. Regular follow-up of liver enzymes as well as for any evidence of muscle toxicity is necessary when coadministering protease inhibitors with statins. For patients with hypertriglyceridemia, a fibrate (e.g., gemfibrozil or fenofibrate) is preferred, the alternative being niacin or fish oil capsules *(198,202)*. Fibrates have not been extensively evaluated in HIV-infected patients

(83,158,203). Fenofibrate had no statistically significant effect in a randomized clinical trial, whereas gemfibrozil may have a less detrimental effect on fat loss *(204).* Niacin may also be used, but its use in HIV-infected patients could possibly be limited by its effect of inducing moderate increases in insulin resistance *(205).*

Insulin sensitizers may also affect lipid levels favorably in patients with HIV. For example, the use of metformin may lead to mild reductions in triglyceride levels through decreased hepatic VLDL production *(61,96).* TZDs, and especially pioglitazone, which has a more favorable effect on the lipid profile compared with rosiglitazone *(206,207),* also affect favorably the lipid profile by increasing HDL levels *(158,184),* as they do in patients without HIV *(208).*

Antiretroviral switch strategies have also been used in the treatment of hyperlipidemia, whereas interruption of HAART improves dyslipidemia. The latter carries extreme risks in immunologically and virologically compromised patients *(209).* Thus, switch strategies have been used only in patients with favorable treatment histories *(198).* Because ritonavir regimens are most commonly associated with hyperlipidemia, substituting ritonavir for other protease inhibitors, namely, nelfinavir, indinavir *(210),* or the newer atazanavir *(211),* may prove to have positive effects on hyperlipidemia. Improvement in serum triglycerides has been noted with switches from a protease inhibitor to an NNRTI but these effects are not consistently seen across all studies *(212,213),* although NNRTIs, such as nevirapine or efavirenz, have beneficial effects on HDL cholesterol levels over time *(26,214,215).* Although an increase in HDL cholesterol observed after switching from a protease inhibitor to nevirapine may be owing to a decreased catabolism of the HDL lipoprotein *(216),* replacement of a protease inhibitor or NNRTI with the NRTI abacavir may result in modest improvements in both cholesterol and triglycerides *(144).*

Treatment of IGT and Diabetes

Nonpharmacological approaches such as diet and exercise, as well as antihyperglycemic agents such as insulin-sensitizing agents, and insulin are the mainstays of therapy. Substitution of an NNRTI, such as nevirapine, for a protease inhibitor may improve insulin resistance in patients with HIV *(217,218)* whereas moderate effects on glucose metabolism are noted for a switch from abacavir to a protease inhibitor *(219).* Switch strategies are not generally used for patients with insulin resistance or glucose intolerance.

Diet and exercise are the initial steps in the management of IGT and diabetes. Nutritional counseling is important in these patients and should be individualized *(170).* Aerobic exercise in a manner similar to that observed in obese HIV-negative patients *(220,221)* could increase peripheral glucose disposal and improve insulin sensitivity in HIV patients with insulin resistance thus delaying and probably preventing the onset of diabetes mellitus *(173),* possibly by reducing muscle lipid content *(222).*

Metformin has been shown to increase insulin sensitivity by decreasing plasma insulin, triglycerides, and FFA levels in both HIV-negative and -positive patients with insulin resistance *(182,223).* Metformin therapy in HIV patients with lipodystrophy and insulin resistance has been associated with reductions in insulin, weight, waist circumference, diastolic blood pressure, and concentrations of tPA and PAI-1 *(183,224,225).* Although no significant adverse events have been reported to date, one should be cautious about potential side effects.

TZDs are PPARγ agonists that initiate a cascade of events leading to increased transcription or inhibition of genes involved in the regulation of adipocyte differentiation, lipid metabolism, and insulin action *(226–228)*. One of the major effects seen with TZDs is their insulin-sensitizing action in peripheral tissues, liver, and adipose tissue *(226)*. TZDs increase adiponectin levels and facilitate fatty acid uptake and storage by adipocytes *(226)*, leading to a decrease in the levels of circulating FFAs and further enhancement of insulin sensitivity. In the adipose tissue, TZDs regulate several enzymes mediating insulin sensitivity such as adiponectin, tumor necrosis factor-α, resistin, and 11β-HSD1 *(226–228)*. In vitro experiments demonstrate that PPARγ agonists increase adiponectin expression in adipose tissue *(227)*, and treatment with TZDs in vivo markedly increases circulating adiponectin levels *(229,230)*. Rosiglitazone has been shown to improve insulin resistance in patients with HIV-associated metabolic syndrome but at the expense of increased triglyceride and cholesterol concentrations *(147–150,231)*. We have shown, in a small interventional study, that administration of pioglitazone has favorable effects on insulin sensitivity, lipid abnormalities, blood pressure levels, and body fat distribution, possibly by increasing adiponectin levels of HIV-infected patients with metabolic syndrome *(185)*. Thus, the presence of frank diabetes requires lifestyle modifications and therapy with insulin-sensitizing agents and/or antihyperglycemic agents with or without insulin *(232,233)*. Finally, targeting dyslipidemia may ameliorate insulin resistance by decreasing circulating plasma FFAs that are negatively associated with glucose uptake *(234)*.

Future research efforts will need to pursue aggressively new potent therapies that could target insulin resistance in HIV patients with HIV/HAART-associated metabolic syndrome. Novel medications that could enhance insulin-stimulated glucose transport need to be tested *(235)*, and the role of leptin therapy needs to be further evaluated by larger studies on insulin resistance in lipoatrophic subjects. Finally, because patients with HIV lipodystrophy have both leptin and adiponectin deficiencies *(74,115)*, administration of medications that increase adiponectin, either alone or in combination with leptin, could be tested as another treatment option for this syndrome.

CONCLUSIONS

Direct medication toxicity and complex interactions between HIV infection and combination antiretroviral therapy and/or possibly other factors (e.g., genetic, environmental) influence an individual's risk of developing HIV/HAART-induced metabolic syndrome. HIV/HAART-associated metabolic syndrome currently affects the majority of patients treated with potent combinations of antiretrovirals. Significant metabolic disturbances including insulin resistance and hyperlipidemia have been identified in association with lipodystrophic changes and fat redistribution in these patients. It is extremely important for the clinician to diagnose, monitor, and treat the manifestations of HIV/HAART metabolic syndrome, because this syndrome may be associated with an increased risk of cardiovascular disease and other complications. Individualized diet and exercise programs as well as treatment with appropriate medications could ameliorate some of these abnormalities and, it is hoped, prevent the development of complications. Finally, research exploring the pathogenesis of the syndrome is continuously evolving, and it is expected that in the not too distant future it will be translated into tangible benefits for HIV-positive patients with HAART-induced metabolic syndrome.

REFERENCES

1. Behrens G, Dejam A, Schmidt H, et al. Impaired glucose tolerance, beta cell function and lipid metabolism in HIV patients under treatment with protease inhibitors. AIDS 1999;13:F63–F70.

2. Carr A, Samaras K, Burton S, et al. A syndrome of peripheral lipodystrophy, hyperlipidaemia and insulin resistance in patients receiving HIV protease inhibitors. AIDS 1998;12:F51–F58.

3. Vigouroux C, Gharakhanian S, Salhi Y, et al. Adverse metabolic disorders during highly active anti-retroviral treatments (HAART) of HIV disease. Diabetes Metab 1999;25:383–392.

4. Struble K, Piscitelli SC. Syndromes of abnormal fat redistribution and metabolic complications in HIV-infected patients. Am J Health Syst Pharm 1999;56:2343–2348.

5. Tsiodras S, Mantzoros C, Hammer S, Samore M. Effects of protease inhibitors on hyperglycemia, hyperlipidemia, and lipodystrophy: a 5-year cohort study. Arch Intern Med 2000;160:2050–2056.

6. Miller KK, Daly PA, Sentochnik D, et al. Pseudo-Cushing's syndrome in human immunodeficiency virus–infected patients. Clin Infect Dis 1998;27:68–72.

7. Stocker DN, Meier PJ, Stoller R, Fattinger KE. "Buffalo hump" in HIV-1 infection. Lancet 1998;352:320, 321.

8. Carr A, Samaras K, Thorisdottir A, Kaufmann GR, Chisholm DJ, Cooper DA. Diagnosis, prediction, and natural course of HIV-1 protease-inhibitor-associated lipodystrophy, hyperlipidaemia, and diabetes mellitus: a cohort study. Lancet 1999;353:2093–2099.

9. Engelson ES, Kotler DP, Tan Y, et al. Fat distribution in HIV-infected patients reporting truncal enlargement quantified by whole-body magnetic resonance imaging. Am J Clin Nutr 1999;69:1162–1169.

10. Garg A. Acquired and inherited lipodystrophies. N Engl J Med 2004;350:1220–1234.

11. Carter VM, Hoy JF, Bailey M, Colman PG, Nyulasi I, Mijch AM. The prevalence of lipodystrophy in an ambulant HIV-infected population: it all depends on the definition. HIV Med 2001;2:174–180.

12. Ioannidis JP, Trikalinos TA, Law M, Carr A. HIV lipodystrophy case definition using artificial neural network modelling. Antiviral Ther 2003;8:435–441.

13. Moyle G. Lipodystrophy: lack of agreement on definition and etiology presents a challenge to research and therapy. AIDS Read 2002;12:438, 440–432.

14. Carr A, Emery S, Law M, Puls R, Lundgren JD, Powderly WG. An objective case definition of lipodystrophy in HIV-infected adults: a case-control study. Lancet 2003;361:726–735.

15. Leow MK, Addy CL, Mantzoros CS. Clinical review 159: human immunodeficiency virus/highly active antiretroviral therapy–associated metabolic syndrome: clinical presentation, pathophysiology, and therapeutic strategies. J Clin Endocrinol Metab 2003;88:1961–1976.

16. Hengel RL, Watts NB, Lennox JL. Benign symmetric lipomatosis associated with protease inhibitors. Lancet 1997;350:1596.

17. Carr A, Cooper DA. Lipodystrophy associated with an HIV-protease inhibitor. N Engl J Med 1998;339:1296.

18. Lo JC, Mulligan K, Tai VW, et al. "Buffalo hump" in men with HIV-1 infection. Lancet 1998;351:871–875.

19. Mann M, Piazza-Hepp T, Koller E, Struble K, Murray J. Unusual distributions of body fat in AIDS patients: a review of adverse events reported to the Food and Drug Administration. AIDS Patient Care STDS 1999;13:287–295.

20. Behrens GM, Stoll M, Schmidt RE. Lipodystrophy syndrome in HIV infection: what is it, what causes it and how can it be managed? Drug Safety 2000;23:57–76.

21. Miller J, Carr A, Emery S, et al. HIV lipodystrophy: prevalence, severity and correlates of risk in Australia. HIV Med 2003;4:293–301.

22. European Paediatric Lipodystrophy Group. Antiretroviral therapy, fat redistribution and hyperlipidaemia in HIV-infected children in Europe. AIDS 2004;18:1443–1451.

23. Mallon PW, Miller J, Cooper DA, Carr A. Prospective evaluation of the effects of antiretroviral therapy on body composition in HIV-1-infected men starting therapy. AIDS 2003;17:971–979.

24. Murphy R, Katlama C, Weverling G-J, et al. Fat redistribution and metabolic study (FRAMS) in patients receiving a nucleoside reverse transcriptase inhibitor, or protease inhibitor–based regimen over 4 years: FRAMS II substudy of the Atlantic Study. In: Program and abstracts of the 11th Conference on Retroviruses and Opportunistic Infections (abstract 718).

25. Lichtenstein KA, Ward DJ, Moorman AC, et al. Clinical assessment of HIV-associated lipodystrophy in an ambulatory population. AIDS 2001;15:1389–1398.

26. McComsey G, Bhumbra N, Ma JF, Rathore M, Alvarez A. Impact of protease inhibitor substitution with efavirenz in HIV-infected children: results of the First Pediatric Switch Study. Pediatrics 2003;111:e275–e281.

27. Mallal S, John M, Moore C, James I, McKinnon E. Contribution of nucleoside analogue reverse transcriptase inhibitors to subcutaneous fat wasting in patients with HIV infection. AIDS 2000;14:1309–1316.

28. Reiss P, Casula M, de Ronde A, Weverling G, Goudsmit J, Lange J. Greater and more rapid depletion of mitochondrial DNA in blood of patients treated with dual (zidovudine+didanosine or zidovudine+zalcitabine) vs. single (zidovudine) nucleoside reverse transcriptase inhibitors. HIV Med 2004;5:11–14.

29. Currier JS, Havlir DV. Complications of HIV disease and antiretroviral therapy. Highlights of the 11th Conference on Retroviruses and Opportunistic Infections, February 8–11, 2004, San Francisco, California, USA. Top HIV Med 2004;12:31–45.

30. McComsey GA, Ward DJ, Hessenthaler SM, et al. Improvement in lipoatrophy associated with highly active antiretroviral therapy in human immunodeficiency virus-infected patients switched from stavudine to abacavir or zidovudine: the results of the TARHEEL study. Clin Infect Dis 2004;38:263–270.

31. Martin A, Smith DE, Carr A, et al. Reversibility of lipoatrophy in HIV-infected patients 2 years after switching from a thymidine analogue to abacavir: the MITOX Extension Study. AIDS 2004;18: 1029–1036.

32. Gallant JE, Staszewski S, Pozniak AL, et al. Efficacy and safety of tenofovir DF vs stavudine in combination therapy in antiretroviral-naive patients: a 3-year randomized trial. JAMA 2004;292:191–201.

33. Saag MS, Cahn P, Raffi F, et al. Efficacy and safety of emtricitabine vs stavudine in combination therapy in antiretroviral-naive patients: a randomized trial. JAMA 2004;292:180–189.

34. Lichtenstein KA, Delaney KM, Armon C, et al. Incidence of and risk factors for lipoatrophy (abnormal fat loss) in ambulatory HIV-1-infected patients. J Acquir Immune Defic Syndr 2003;32:48–56.

35. Hadri K, Glorian M, Monsempes C, et al. In vitro suppression of the lipogenic pathway by the non-nucleoside reverse transcriptase inhibitor efavirenz in 3T3 and human preadipocytes or adipocytes. J Biol Chem 2004;279:15,130–15,141.

36. Shikuma CM, Hu N, Milne C, et al. Mitochondrial DNA decrease in subcutaneous adipose tissue of HIV-infected individuals with peripheral lipoatrophy. AIDS 2001;15:1801–1809.

37. Cherry C, Gahan M, McArthur J, Lewin S, Hoy J, Wesselingh S. Exposure to dideoxynucleosides is reflected in lowered mitochondrial DNA in subcutaneous fat. J Acquir Immune Defic Syndr 2002;30:271–277.

38. Nolan D, Hammond E, James I, McKinnon E, Mallal S. Contribution of nucleoside-analogue reverse transcriptase inhibitor therapy to lipoatrophy from the population to the cellular level. Antiviral Ther 2003;8:617–626.

39. Hoy JF, Gahan ME, Carr A, et al. Changes in mitochondrial DNA in peripheral blood mononuclear cells from HIV-infected patients with lipoatrophy randomized to receive abacavir. J Infect Dis 2004;190:688–692.

40. Yokoyama C, Wang X, Briggs MR, et al. SREBP-1, a basic-helix-loop-helix-leucine zipper protein that controls transcription of the low density lipoprotein receptor gene. Cell 1993;75:187–197.

41. Tontonoz P, Kim JB, Graves RA, Spiegelman BM. ADD1: a novel helix-loop-helix transcription factor associated with adipocyte determination and differentiation. Mol Cell Biol 1993;13:4753–4759.

42. Lee CH, Olson P, Evans RM. Minireview: lipid metabolism, metabolic diseases, and peroxisome proliferator-activated receptors. Endocrinology 2003;144:2201–2207.

43. He W, Barak Y, Hevener A, et al. Adipose-specific peroxisome proliferator-activated receptor gamma knockout causes insulin resistance in fat and liver but not in muscle. Proc Natl Acad Sci USA 2003, 100:15,712–15,717.

44. Bastard JP, Caron M, Vidal H, et al. Association between altered expression of adipogenic factor SREBP1 in lipoatrophic adipose tissue from HIV-1-infected patients and abnormal adipocyte differentiation and insulin resistance. Lancet 2002;359:1026–1031.

45. Caron M, Auclair M, Vigouroux C, Glorian M, Forest C, Capeau J. The HIV protease inhibitor indinavir impairs sterol regulatory element-binding protein-1 intranuclear localization, inhibits preadipocyte differentiation, and induces insulin resistance. Diabetes 2001;50:1378–1388.

46. Adams M, Montague CT, Prins JB, et al. Activators of peroxisome proliferator-activated receptor gamma have depot-specific effects on human preadipocyte differentiation. J Clin Invest 1997;100:3149–3153.

47. Amorosa V, Synnestvedt M, Gross R, et al. A tale of 2 epidemics: the intersection between obesity and HIV infection in the urban United States. In: Program and abstracts of the 11th Conference on Retroviruses and Opportunistic Infections (abstract 879).

48. Kotler DP, Rosenbaum K, Wang J, Pierson RN. Studies of body composition and fat distribution in HIV-infected and control subjects. J Acquir Immune Defic Syndr Hum Retrovirol 1999;20:228–237.

49. Rahim S, Ortiz O, Maslow M, Holzman R. A case-control study of gynecomastia in HIV-1-infected patients receiving HAART. AIDS Read 2004;14:23–24, 29–32, 35–40.

50. Thiebaut R, Daucourt V, Mercie P, et al. Lipodystrophy, metabolic disorders, and human immunodeficiency virus infection: Aquitaine Cohort, France, 1999. Groupe d'Epidemiologie Clinique du Syndrome d'Immunodeficience Acquise en Aquitaine. Clin Infect Dis 2000;31:1482–1487.

51. Hadigan C, Miller K, Corcoran C, Anderson E, Basgoz N, Grinspoon S. Fasting hyperinsulinemia and changes in regional body composition in human immunodeficiency virus-infected women. J Clin Endocrinol Metab 1999;84:1932–1937.

52. Galli M, Cozzi-Lepri A, Ridolfo AL, et al. Incidence of adipose tissue alterations in first-line antiretroviral therapy: the LipoICoNa Study. Arch Intern Med 2002;162:2621–2628.

53. Forrester JE, Gorbach SL. Fat distribution in relation to drug use, human immunodeficiency virus (HIV) status, and the use of antiretroviral therapies in Hispanic patients with HIV infection. Clin Infect Dis 2003;37(Suppl 2):S62–S68.

54. Gan SK, Samaras K, Thompson CH, et al. Altered myocellular and abdominal fat partitioning predict disturbance in insulin action in HIV protease inhibitor–related lipodystrophy. Diabetes 2002;51:3163–3169.

55. Luzi L, Perseghin G, Tambussi G, et al. Intramyocellular lipid accumulation and reduced whole body lipid oxidation in HIV lipodystrophy. Am J Physiol Endocrinol Metab 2003;284:E274–E280.

56. Torriani M, Hadigan C, Jensen ME, Grinspoon S. Psoas muscle attenuation measurement with computed tomography indicates intramuscular fat accumulation in patients with the HIV-lipodystrophy syndrome. J Appl Physiol 2003;95:1005–1010.

57. Sutinen J, Hakkinen AM, Westerbacka J, et al. Increased fat accumulation in the liver in HIV-infected patients with antiretroviral therapy-associated lipodystrophy. AIDS 2002;16:2183–2193.

58. Behrens GM, Boerner AR, Weber K, et al. Impaired glucose phosphorylation and transport in skeletal muscle cause insulin resistance in HIV-1-infected patients with lipodystrophy. J Clin Invest 2002;110:1319–1327.

59. Yanovski JA, Miller KD, Kino T, et al. Endocrine and metabolic evaluation of human immunodeficiency virus–infected patients with evidence of protease inhibitor-associated lipodystrophy. J Clin Endocrinol Metab 1999;84:1925–1931.

60. Sutinen J, Kannisto K, Korsheninnikova E, et al. In the lipodystrophy associated with highly active antiretroviral therapy, pseudo-Cushing's syndrome is associated with increased regeneration of cortisol by 11beta-hydroxysteroid dehydrogenase type 1 in adipose tissue. Diabetologia 2004;47:1668–1671.

61. Hadigan C, Meigs JB, Corcoran C, et al. Metabolic abnormalities and cardiovascular disease risk factors in adults with human immunodeficiency virus infection and lipodystrophy. Clin Infect Dis 2001;32:130–139.

62. Mazess RB, Barden HS, Bisek JP, Hanson J. Dual-energy x-ray absorptiometry for total-body and regional bone-mineral and soft-tissue composition. Am J Clin Nutr 1990;51:1106–1112.

63. Lambrinoudaki I, Georgiou E, Douskas G, Tsekes G, Kyriakidis M, Proukakis C. Body composition assessment by dual-energy x-ray absorptiometry: comparison of prone and supine measurements. Metabolism 1998;47:1379–1382.

64. Weits T, van der Beek EJ, Wedel M, ter haar Romeny BM. Computer tomography measurement of abdominal fat deposition in relation to anthropometry. Int J Obes 1988;12:217–225.

65. van der Kooy K, Seidell JC. Techniques for the measurement of visceral fat: a practical guide. Int J Obes 1993;17:187–196.

66. Schoen RE, Thaete FL, Sankey SS, Weissfeld JL, Kuller LH. Saggital diameter in comparison with single slice CT as a predictor of total visceral adipose tissue volume. Int J Obes Relat Metab Disord 1998;22:338–342.

67. Friis-Moller N, Weber R, Reiss P, et al. Cardiovascular disease risk factors in HIV patients—association with antiretroviral therapy: results from the DAD study. AIDS 2003;17:1179–1193.

68. Keruly J, Mehta S, Chaisson R, Moore R. Incidence of and factors associated with the development of hypercholesterolemia and hyperglycemia in HIV-infected patients using a protease inhibitor. In: Proceedings of the 38th Interscience Conference on Antimicrobial Agents and Chemotherapy, 1998 (abstract I–95).

69. Mann M, Piazza-Hepp T, Koller E, Gibert C. Abnormal fat distribution in AIDS patients following protease inhibitor therapy: FDA summary. In: Proceedings of the Fifth Conference on Retroviruses and Opportunistic Infections, 1998 (abstract 412).

70. Riddler SA, Smit E, Cole SR, et al. Impact of HIV infection and HAART on serum lipids in men. JAMA 2003;289:2978–2982.

71. Grunfeld C, Kotler DP, Hamadeh R, Tierney A, Wang J, Pierson RN. Hypertriglyceridemia in the acquired immunodeficiency syndrome. Am J Med 1989;86:27–31.

72. Grunfeld C, Kotler DP, Shigenaga JK, et al. Circulating interferon-alpha levels and hypertriglyceridemia in the acquired immunodeficiency syndrome. Am J Med 1991;90:154–162.

73. Fauvel J, Bonnet E, Ruidavets JB, et al. An interaction between apo C-III variants and protease inhibitors contributes to high triglyceride/low HDL levels in treated HIV patients. AIDS 2001;15:2397–2406.

74. Nagy G, Karchmer A, Tsiodras S, Mantzoros C, Welty FK. The effects of apolipoprotein E genotype and protease inhibitors on plasma lipoproteins in HIV-infected men and women on HAART. In: Proceedings of the 41st Annual Meeting of the Infectious Diseases Society of America, 2003 (abstract 111).

75. van Leth F, Phanuphak P, Gazzard B, et al. Lipid changes in a randomized comparative trial of first-line antiretroviral therapy with regimens containing either nevirapine alone, efavirenz alone or both drugs combined, together with stavudine and lamivudine (2NN Study). In: Proceedings of the 10th Conference on Retroviruses and Opportunistic Infections, 2003 (abstract 752).

76. Purnell JQ, Zambon A, Knopp RH, et al. Effect of ritonavir on lipids and post-heparin lipase activities in normal subjects. AIDS 2000;14:51–57.

77. Hui DY. Effects of HIV protease inhibitor therapy on lipid metabolism. Prog Lipid Res 2003;42:81–92.

78. Liang JS, Distler O, Cooper DA, Jamil H, Deckelbaum RJ, Ginsberg HN, Sturley SL. HIV protease inhibitors protect apolipoprotein B from degradation by the proteasome: a potential mechanism for protease inhibitor-induced hyperlipidemia. Nat Med 2001;7:1327–1331.

79. Ranganathan S, Kern PA. The HIV protease inhibitor saquinavir impairs lipid metabolism and glucose transport in cultured adipocytes. J Endocrinol 2002;172:155–162.

80. Reeds DN, Mittendorfer B, Patterson BW, Powderly WG, Yarasheski KE, Klein, S. Alterations in lipid kinetics in men with HIV-dyslipidemia. Am J Physiol Endocrinol Metab 2003:285:E490–E497.

81. Riddle TM, Kuhel DG, Woollett LA, Fichtenbaum CJ, Hui DY. HIV protease inhibitor induces fatty acid and sterol biosynthesis in liver and adipose tissues due to the accumulation of activated sterol regulatory element-binding proteins in the nucleus. J Biol Chem 2001;276:37,514–37,519.

82. Routy JP, Smith GH, Blank DW, Gilfix BM. Plasmapheresis in the treatment of an acute pancreatitis due to protease inhibitor–induced hypertriglyceridemia. J Clin Apheresis 2001;16:157–159.

83. Henry K, Melroe H, Huebsch J, et al. Severe premature coronary artery disease with protease inhibitors. Lancet 1998;351:1328.

84. Flynn T, Bricker L. Myocardial infarction in HIV-infected men receiving protease inhibitors. Ann Intern Med 1999;131:548.

85. Friis-Moller N, Sabin CA, Weber R, et al. Combination antiretroviral therapy and the risk of myocardial infarction. N Engl J Med 2003;349:1993–2003.

86. Currie J, Havlir D. Conference highlights—complications of HIV disease and antiretroviral therapy. Top HIV Med 2004;12:31–39.

87. Mary-Krause M, Cotte L, Partisani M, Simon A, Costagliola D. Impact of treatment with protease inhibitor (PI) on myocardial infarction (MI) occurrence in HIV-infected men. In: Proceedings of the Eighth Conference on Retroviruses and Opportunistic Infections, 2001 (abstract 657).

88. Klein D, Hurley L, Sorel M, Sidney S. Do protease inhibitors increase the risk for coronary heart disease among HIV positive patients—follow-up. In: Proceedings of the Eighth Conference on Retroviruses and Opportunistic Infections, 2001 (abstract 655).

89. Brown T, Cole SR, Li X, et al. Prevalence and incidence of prediabetes and diabetes in the Multicenter AIDS Cohort Study. In: Proceedings of the 11th Conference on Retroviruses and Opportunistic Infections, 2004:73 (Abstract).

90. Duong M, Petit JM, Piroth L, et al. Association between insulin resistance and hepatitis C virus chronic infection in HIV-hepatitis C virus–coinfected patients undergoing antiretroviral therapy. J Acquir Immune Defic Syndr 2001;27:245–250.

91. Andersen O, Haugaard SB, Andersen UB, et al. Lipodystrophy in human immunodeficiency virus patients impairs insulin action and induces defects in beta-cell function. Metabolism 2003;52: 1343–1353.

92. Janneh O, Hoggard PG, Tjia JF, et al. Intracellular disposition and metabolic effects of zidovudine, stavudine and four protease inhibitors in cultured adipocytes. Antiviral Ther 2003;8:417–426.

93. Murata H, Hruz PW, Mueckler, M. The mechanism of insulin resistance caused by HIV protease inhibitor therapy. J Biol Chem 2000;275:20,251–20,254.

94. Nolte L, Yarasheski K, Kawanaka K, Fisher J, Le N, Holloszy J. The HIV protease inhibitor indinavir decreases insulin- and contraction-stimulated glucose transport in skeletal muscle. Diabetes 2001;50:1397–1401.

95. Noor M, Grasela D, Parker R, et al. The effect of atazanavir vs lopinavir/ritonavir on insulin-stimulated glucose disposal rate in healthy subjects. In: Proceedings of the 11th Conference on Retroviruses and Opportunistic Infections, 2004 (abstract 702).

96. Hadigan C, Borgonha S, Rabe J, Young V, Grinspoon, S. Increased rates of lipolysis among human immunodeficiency virus–infected men receiving highly active antiretroviral therapy. Metabolism 2002;51:1143–1147.

97. Meininger G, Hadigan C, Laposata M, et al. Elevated concentrations of free fatty acids are associated with increased insulin response to standard glucose challenge in human immunodeficiency virus-infected subjects with fat redistribution. Metabolism 2002;51:260–266.

98. Noor MA, Seneviratne T, Aweeka FT, et al. Indinavir acutely inhibits insulin-stimulated glucose disposal in humans: a randomized, placebo-controlled study. AIDS 2002;16:F1–F8.

99. Lee GA, Seneviratne T, Noor MA, et al. The metabolic effects of lopinavir/ritonavir in HIV-negative men. AIDS 2004;18:641–649.

100. Beatty G, Khalili M, Abbasi F, et al. Quantification of insulin-mediated glucose disposal in HIV-infected individuals: comparison of patients treated and untreated with protease inhibitors. J Acquir Immune Defic Syndr 2003;33:34–40.

101. Kino T, Gragerov A, Slobodskaya O, Tsopanomichalou M, Chrousos G, Pavlakis G. Human immunodeficiency virus type 1 (HIV-1) accessory protein Vpr induces transcription of the HIV-1 and glucocorticoid-responsive promoters by binding directly to p300/CBP coactivators. J Virol 2002;76: 9724–9734.

102. Shrivastav S, Kino T, Chrousos GP, Kopp JB. HIV-1 Vpr binds and inhibits PPAR-gamma: implications for HIV-associated insulin resistance and lipodystrophy. In: Proceedings of the International Meeting of the Institute of Human Virology, 2000.

103. Kino T, Chrousos GP. Human immunodeficiency virus type-1 accessory protein Vpr: a causative agent of the AIDS-related insulin resistance/lipodystrophy syndrome? Ann N Y Acad Sci 2004;1024:153–167.

104. Haugaard SB, Andersen O, Storgaard H, et al. Insulin secretion in lipodystrophic HIV-infected patients is associated with high levels of nonglucose secretagogues and insulin resistance of beta-cells. Am J Physiol Endocrinol Metab 2004;287:E677–E685.

105. Serghides L, Nathoo S, Walmsley S, Kain KC. CD36 deficiency induced by antiretroviral therapy. AIDS 2002;16:353–358.

106. Shimomura I, Hammer RE, Richardson JA, et al. Insulin resistance and diabetes mellitus in transgenic mice expressing nuclear SREBP-1c in adipose tissue: model for congenital generalized lipodystrophy. Genes Dev 1998;12:3182–3194.

107. Moitra J, Mason MM, Olive M, et al. Life without white fat: a transgenic mouse. Genes Dev 1998;12:3168–3181.

108. Yamauchi T, Kamon J, Waki H, et al. The fat-derived hormone adiponectin reverses insulin resistance associated with both lipoatrophy and obesity. Nat Med 2001;7:941–946.

109. Colombo C, Cutson JJ, Yamauchi T, et al. Transplantation of adipose tissue lacking leptin is unable to reverse the metabolic abnormalities associated with lipoatrophy. Diabetes 2002;51:2727–2733.

110. Gavrilova O, Marcus-Samuels B, Graham D, et al. Surgical implantation of adipose tissue reverses diabetes in lipoatrophic mice. J Clin Invest 2000;105:271–278.

111. Pardini VC, Victoria IM, Rocha SM, et al. Leptin levels, beta-cell function, and insulin sensitivity in families with congenital and acquired generalized lipoatropic diabetes. J Clin Endocrinol Metab 1998;83:503–508.

112. Hegele RA. Familial partial lipodystrophy: a monogenic form of the insulin resistance syndrome. Mol Genet Metab 2000;71:539–544.

113. Haque WA, Shimomura I, Matsuzawa Y, Garg A. Serum adiponectin and leptin levels in patients with lipodystrophies. J Clin Endocrinol Metab 2002;87:2395.

114. Nagy GS, Tsiodras S, Martin LD, et al. Human immunodeficiency virus type 1-related lipoatrophy and lipohypertrophy are associated with serum concentrations of leptin. Clin Infect Dis 2003;36:795–802.

115. Addy CL, Gavrila A, Tsiodras S, Brodovicz K, Karchmer AW, Mantzoros CS. Hypoadiponectinemia is associated with insulin resistance, hypertriglyceridemia, and fat redistribution in human immunodeficiency virus–infected patients treated with highly active antiretroviral therapy. J Clin Endocrinol Metab 2003;88:627–636.

116. Kershaw EE, Flier JS. Adipose tissue as an endocrine organ. J Clin Endocrinol Metab 2004;89: 2548–2556.

117. Minokoshi Y, Kim YB, Peroni OD, et al. Leptin stimulates fatty-acid oxidation by activating AMP-activated protein kinase. Nature 2002;415:339–343.
118. Muzzin P, Eisensmith RC, Copeland KC, Woo SL. Correction of obesity and diabetes in genetically obese mice by leptin gene therapy. Proc Natl Acad Sci USA 1996;93:14804–14808.
119. Oral EA, Simha V, Ruiz E, et al. Leptin-replacement therapy for lipodystrophy. N Engl J Med 2002;346:570–578.
120. Simha V, Szczepaniak LS, Wagner AJ, DePaoli AM, Garg A. Effect of leptin replacement on intrahepatic and intramyocellular lipid content in patients with generalized lipodystrophy. Diabetes Care 2003;26:30–35.
121. Mynarcik DC, Combs T, McNurlan MA, Scherer PE, Komaroff E, Gelato MC. Adiponectin and leptin levels in HIV-infected subjects with insulin resistance and body fat redistribution. J Acquir Immune Defic Syndr 2002;31:514–520.
122. Kosmiski LA, Kuritzkes DR, Lichtenstein KA, et al. Fat distribution and metabolic changes are strongly correlated and energy expenditure is increased in the HIV lipodystrophy syndrome. AIDS 2001;15:1993–2000.
123. Weyer C, Funahashi T, Tanaka S, et al. Hypoadiponectinemia in obesity and type 2 diabetes: close association with insulin resistance and hyperinsulinemia. J Clin Endocrinol Metab 2001;86:1930–1935.
124. Nishizawa H, Shimomura I, Kishida K, et al. Androgens decrease plasma adiponectin, an insulin-sensitizing adipocyte-derived protein. Diabetes 2002;51:2734–2741.
125. Havel PJ. Update on adipocyte hormones: regulation of energy balance and carbohydrate/lipid metabolism. Diabetes 2004;53(Suppl 1):S143–S151.
126. Iwaki M, Matsuda M, Maeda N, Funahashi T, Matsuzawa Y, Makishima M, Shimomura, I. Induction of adiponectin, a fat-derived antidiabetic and antiatherogenic factor, by nuclear receptors. Diabetes 2003;52:1655–1663.
127. Seo JB, Moon HM, Noh MJ, et al. Adipocyte determination- and differentiation-dependent factor 1/sterol regulatory element-binding protein 1c regulates mouse adiponectin expression. J Biol Chem 2004;279:22,108–22,117.
128. Yamauchi T, Kamon J, Ito Y, et al. Cloning of adiponectin receptors that mediate antidiabetic metabolic effects. Nature 2003;423:762–769.
129. Rajala MW, Scherer PE. Minireview: the adipocyte—at the crossroads of energy homeostasis, inflammation, and atherosclerosis. Endocrinology 2003;144:3765–3773.
130. Maeda N, Shimomura I, Kishida K, et al. Diet-induced insulin resistance in mice lacking adiponectin/ACRP30. Nat Med 2002;8:731–737.
131. Kubota N, Terauchi Y, Yamauchi T, et al. Disruption of adiponectin causes insulin resistance and neointimal formation. J Biol Chem 2002;277:25,863–25,866.
132. Combs TP, Pajvani UB, Berg AH, et al. A transgenic mouse with a deletion in the collagenous domain of adiponectin displays elevated circulating adiponectin and improved insulin sensitivity. Endocrinology 2004;145:367–383.
133. Hotta K, Funahashi T, Arita Y, et al. Plasma concentrations of a novel, adipose-specific protein, adiponectin, in type 2 diabetic patients. Arterioscler Thromb Vasc Biol 2000;20:1595–1599.
134. Stefan N, Vozarova B, Funahashi T, et al. Plasma adiponectin concentration is associated with skeletal muscle insulin receptor tyrosine phosphorylation, and low plasma concentration precedes a decrease in whole-body insulin sensitivity in humans. Diabetes 2002;51:1884–1888.
135. Lindsay RS, Funahashi T, Hanson RL, et al. Adiponectin and development of type 2 diabetes in the Pima Indian population. Lancet 2002;360:57–58.
136. Lihn AS, Richelsen B, Pedersen SB, et al. Increased expression of TNF-alpha IL-6, and IL-8 in HALS: implications for reduced adiponectin expression and plasma levels. Am J Physiol Endocrinol Metab 2003;285:E1072–E1080.
137. Xu A, Yin S, Wong L, Chan KW, Lam KS. Adiponectin ameliorates dyslipidemia induced by the human immunodeficiency virus protease inhibitor ritonavir in mice. Endocrinology 2004;145:487–494.
138. Sattler FR, Qian D, Louie S, et al. Elevated blood pressure in subjects with lipodystrophy. AIDS 2001;15:2001–2010.
139. Schambelan M, Benson CA, Carr A, et al. Management of metabolic complications associated with antiretroviral therapy for HIV-1 infection: recommendations of an International AIDS Society–USA panel. J Acquir Immune Defic Syndr 2002;31:257–275.
140. Despres JP, Lamarche B, Mauriege P, et al. Hyperinsulinemia as an independent risk factor for ischemic heart disease. N Engl J Med 1996;334:952–957.

141. Pyorala M, Miettinen H, Laakso M, Pyorala K. Hyperinsulinemia predicts coronary heart disease risk in healthy middle-aged men: the 22-year follow-up results of the Helsinki Policemen Study. Circulation 1998;98:398–404.

142. de Larranaga GF, Bocassi AR, Puga LM, Alonso BS, Benetucci JA. Endothelial markers and HIV infection in the era of highly active antiretroviral treatment. Thromb Res 2003;110:93–98.

143. Carr A, Workman C, Smith DE, et al. Abacavir substitution for nucleoside analogs in patients with HIV lipoatrophy: a randomized trial. JAMA 2002;288:207–215.

144. Moyle GJ, Baldwin C, Langroudi B, Mandalia S, Gazzard BG. A 48-week, randomized, open-label comparison of three abacavir-based substitution approaches in the management of dyslipidemia and peripheral lipoatrophy. J Acquir Immune Defic Syndr 2003;33:22–28.

145. Jones DH, Carruthers A, Orentreich D, et al. Highly purified 1000-cSt silicone oil for treatment of human immunodeficiency virus-associated facial lipoatrophy: an open pilot trial. Dermatol Surg 2004;30:1279–1286.

146. Moyle GJ. Bridging a gap: surgical management of HIV-associated lipoatrophy. AIDS Read 2004;14:472–475.

147. Hadigan C, Yawetz S, Thomas A, Havers F, Sax PE, Grinspoon S. Metabolic effects of rosiglitazone in HIV lipodystrophy: a randomized, controlled trial. Ann Intern Med 2004;140:786–794.

148. Gelato MC, Mynarcik DC, Quick JL, et al. Improved insulin sensitivity and body fat distribution in HIV-infected patients treated with rosiglitazone: a pilot study. J Acquir Immune Defic Syndr 2002;31:163–170.

149. Sutinen J, Hakkinen AM, Westerbacka J, et al. Rosiglitazone in the treatment of HAART-associated lipodystrophy—a randomized double-blind placebo-controlled study. Antiviral Ther 2003;8:199–207.

150. Carr A, Workman C, Carey D, et al. No effect of rosiglitazone for treatment of HIV-1 lipoatrophy: randomised, double-blind, placebo-controlled trial. Lancet 2004;363:429–438.

151. Boyd M, Bien D, van Warmerdam P, et al. Lipodystrophy in patients switched to indinavir/ritonavir 800/100 mg BID and efavirenz 600 mg QD after failing nucleoside combination therapy: a prospective, 48-week observational sub-study of HIV-NAT 009. In: Proceedings of the 10th Conference on Retroviruses and Opportunistic Infections, 2003 (abstract 738).

152. Martinez E, Arnaiz JA, Podzamczer D, et al. Substitution of nevirapine, efavirenz, or abacavir for protease inhibitors in patients with human immunodeficiency virus infection. N Engl J Med 2003;349:1036–1046.

153. Diabetes, Prevention, Program, Research, and Group. Reduction in the incidence of type 2 diabetes with lifestyle intervention or metformin. N Engl J Med 2002;346:393–403.

154. Miyazaki Y, Mahankali A, Matsuda M, et al. Effect of pioglitazone on abdominal fat distribution and insulin sensitivity in type 2 diabetic patients. J Clin Endocrinol Metab 2002;87:2784–2791.

155. Virtanen KA, Hallsten K, Parkkola R, et al. Differential effects of rosiglitazone and metformin on adipose tissue distribution and glucose uptake in type 2 diabetic subjects. Diabetes 2003;52:283–290.

156. Carey DG, Cowin GJ, Galloway GJ, et al. Effect of rosiglitazone on insulin sensitivity and body composition in type 2 diabetic patients [corrected]. Obes Res 2002;10:1008–1015.

157. Kannisto K, Sutinen J, Korsheninnikova E, et al. Expression of adipogenic transcription factors, peroxisome proliferator-activated receptor gamma co-activator 1, IL-6 and CD45 in subcutaneous adipose tissue in lipodystrophy associated with highly active antiretroviral therapy. AIDS 2003;17:1753–1762.

158. Gavrila A, Hsu W, Tsiodras S, Doweiko J, Martin L, Moses A, Karchmer A, Mantzoros CS. Effect of Pioglitazone and/or Fenofibrate on the HIV-associated metabolic syndrome: A 2x2 factorial, randomized, double-blinded, placebo-controlled trial. In: Proceedings of the Endocrine Society 86th Annual Meeting, 2004 (abstract).

159. Lee JH, Chan JL, Murphy R, DePaoli AM, Mantzoros CS. Leptin Replacement Therapy Improves Insulin Resistance in Highly Active Antiretroviral Therapy (HAART). Paper presented at the Endocrine Fellows Foundation Forum Advances in the Diagnosis and Treatment of Diabetes June 3, 2004, Rosen Centre Hotel, Orlando FL. Available at www.endocrinefellows.org/poster.html.

160. Katznelson L, Finkelstein J, Schoenfeld D, Rosenthal D, Anderson E, Klibanski A. Increase in bone density and lean body mass during testosterone administration in men with acquired hypogonadism. J Clin Endocrinol Metab 1996;81:4358–4365.

161. Jaque S, Schroeder E, Azen S, et al. Regional body composition changes during anabolic therapy. Clin Exerc Physiol 2002;4:50–59.

162. Protopapa C, Sito G, Caporale D, Cammarota N. Bio-Alcamid in drug-induced lipodystrophy. J Cosmet Laser Ther 2003;5:226–230.

163. Orentreich D, Leone AS. A case of HIV-associated facial lipoatrophy treated with 1000-cs liquid injectable silicone. Dermatol Surg 2004;30:548–551.

164. Strauch B, Baum T, Robbins N. Treatment of human immunodeficiency virus-associated lipodystrophy with dermafat graft transfer to the malar area. Plast Reconstr Surg 2004;113:363–370; discussion 371–362.

165. Serra-Renom JM, Fontdevila J. Treatment of facial fat atrophy related to treatment with protease inhibitors by autologous fat injection in patients with human immunodeficiency virus infection. Plast Reconstr Surg 2004;114:551–555; discussion 556, 557.

166. Moyle G, Lysakova L, Brown S, et al. A randomized open-label study of immediate versus delayed polylactic acid injections for the cosmetic management of facial lipoatrophy in persons with HIV infection. HIV Med 2004;5:82–87.

167. Koutkia P, Grinspoon S. HIV-associated lipodystrophy: pathogenesis, prognosis, treatment, and controversies. Annu Rev Med 2004;55:303–317.

168. Ross R, Dagnone D, Jones P, et al. Reduction in obesity and related comorbid conditions after diet-induced weight loss or exercise-induced weight loss in men. A randomized, controlled trial. Ann Intern Med 2000;133:92–103.

169. Roubenoff R, Weiss L, McDermott A, et al. A pilot study of exercise training to reduce trunk fat in adults with HIV-associated fat redistribution. AIDS 1999;13:1373–1375.

170. Fields-Gardner C, Fergusson P. Position of the American Dietetic Association and Dietitians of Canada: nutrition intervention in the care of persons with human immunodeficiency virus infection. J Am Diet Assoc 2004;104:1425–1441.

171. Batterham MJ, Garsia R, Greenop PA. Dietary intake, serum lipids, insulin resistance and body composition in the era of highly active antiretroviral therapy 'Diet FRS Study'. AIDS 2000;14:1839–1843.

172. Gavrila A, Tsiodras S, Doweiko J, et al. Exercise and vitamin E intake are independently associated with metabolic abnormalities in human immunodeficiency virus-positive subjects: a cross-sectional study. Clin Infect Dis 2003;36:1593–1601.

173. Roubenoff R, Schmitz H, Bairos L, et al. Reduction of abdominal obesity in lipodystrophy associated with human immunodeficiency virus infection by means of diet and exercise: case report and proof of principle. Clin Infect Dis 2002;34:390–393.

174. Schwartz R, Shuman W, Larson V, et al. The effect of intensive endurance exercise training on body fat distribution in young and older men. Metabolism 1991;40:545–551.

175. Yarasheski KE, Tebas P, Stanerson B, et al. Resistance exercise training reduces hypertriglyceridemia in HIV-infected men treated with antiviral therapy. J Appl Physiol 2001;90:133–138.

176. Jones SP, Doran DA, Leatt PB, Maher B, Pirmohamed M. Short-term exercise training improves body composition and hyperlipidaemia in HIV-positive individuals with lipodystrophy. AIDS 2001;15:2049–2051.

177. Roubenoff R, McDermott A, Weiss L, et al. Short-term progressive resistance training increases strength and lean body mass in adults infected with human immunodeficiency virus. AIDS 1999;13:231–239.

178. Smith BA, Neidig JL, Nickel JT, Mitchell GL, Para MF, Fass RJ. Aerobic exercise: effects on parameters related to fatigue, dyspnea, weight and body composition in HIV-infected adults. AIDS 2001;15:693–701.

179. Hadigan C, Jeste S, Anderson EJ, Tsay R, Cyr H, Grinspoon S. Modifiable dietary habits and their relation to metabolic abnormalities in men and women with human immunodeficiency virus infection and fat redistribution. Clin Infect Dis 2001;33:710–717.

180. Thoni GJ, Fedou C, Brun JF, et al. Reduction of fat accumulation and lipid disorders by individualized light aerobic training in human immunodeficiency virus infected patients with lipodystrophy and/or dyslipidemia. Diabetes Metab 2002;28:397–404.

181. Domingo P, Sambeat MA, Perez A, Ordonez J, Rodriguez J, Vazquez G. Fat distribution and metabolic abnormalities in HIV-infected patients on first combination antiretroviral therapy including stavudine or zidovudine: role of physical activity as a protective factor. Antiviral Ther 2003;8:223–231.

182. Saint-Marc T, Touraine J. Effects of metformin on insulin resistance and central adiposity in patients receiving effective protease inhibitor therapy. AIDS 1999;13:1000–1002.

183. Hadigan C, Corcoran C, Basgoz N, Davis B, Sax P, Grinspoon S. Metformin in the treatment of HIV lipodystrophy syndrome: a randomized controlled trial. JAMA 2000;284:472–477.

184. Grinspoon S, Carr A. Cardiovascular risk and body-fat abnormalities in HIV-infected adults. N Engl J Med 2005;352:48–62.

185. Gavrila A, Hsu W, Tsiodras S, et al. Improvement in highly active antiretroviral therapy-induced metabolic syndrome by treatment with pioglitazone but not with fenofibrate: A 2 x 2 factorial, randomized, double-blinded, placebo-controlled trial. Clin Infect Dis 2005;40:745–749.

186. Schambelan M, Mulligan K, Grunfeld C, et al. Recombinant human growth hormone in patients with HIV-associated wasting: a randomized, placebo-controlled trial. Serostim Study Group. Ann Intern Med 1996;125:873–882.

187. Cuneo R, Judd S, Wallace J, et al. The Australian Multicenter Trial of Growth Hormone (GH) Treatment in GHDeficient Adults. J Clin Endocrinol Metab 1998;83:107–116.

188. Johannsson G, Marin P, Lonn L, et al. Growth hormone treatment of abdominally obese men reduces abdominal fat mass, improves glucose and lipoprotein metabolism, and reduces diastolic blood pressure. J Clin Endocrinol Metab 1997;83:727–734.

189. Torres R, Unger K. The effect of recombinant human growth hormone on protease-inhibitor-associated fat maldistribution syndrome. In: Proceedings of the Sixth Conference on Retroviruses and Opportunistic Infections, 1999 (abstract 675).

190. Wanke C, Gerrior J, Kantaros J, Coakley E, Albrecht M. Recombinant human growth hormone improves the fat redistribution syndrome (lipodystrophy) in patients with HIV. AIDS 1999;13: 2099–2103.

191. Nguyen Q-V, Malinverni R, Furrer H. Treatment of HAART associated fat accumulation disease with recombinant human growth hormone: results of a randomised double blind placebo controlled crossover trial. In: Proceedings of the XIII International AIDS Conference, 2000 (abstract LbPp114).

192. Lo JC, Mulligan K, Noor MA, et al. The effects of recombinant human growth hormone on body composition and glucose metabolism in HIV-infected patients with fat accumulation. J Clin Endocrinol Metab 2001;86:3480–3487.

193. Engelson ES, Glesby MJ, Mendez D, et al. Effect of recombinant human growth hormone in the treatment of visceral fat accumulation in HIV infection. J Acquir Immune Defic Syndr 2002;30:379–391.

194. Koutkia P, Canavan B, Breu J, Torriani M, Kissko J, Grinspoon S. Growth hormone-releasing hormone in HIV-infected men with lipodystrophy: a randomized controlled trial. JAMA 2004;292:210–218.

195. Marin P, Oden B, Bjorntorp P. Assimilation and mobilization of triglycerides in subcutaneous abdominal and femoral adipose tissue in vivo in men: effects of androgens. J Clin Endocrinol Metab 1995;80:239–243.

196. Piliero PJ, Hubbard M, King J, Faragon JJ. Use of ultrasonography-assisted liposuction for the treatment of human immunodeficiency virus-associated enlargement of the dorsocervical fat pad. Clin Infect Dis 2003;37:1374–1377.

197. Gervasoni C, Ridolfo AL, Vaccarezza M, et al. Long-term efficacy of the surgical treatment of buffalo hump in patients continuing antiretroviral therapy. AIDS 2004;18:574–576.

198. Dube MP, Stein JH, Aberg JA, et al. Guidelines for the evaluation and management of dyslipidemia in human immunodeficiency virus (HIV)–infected adults receiving antiretroviral therapy: recommendations of the HIV Medical Association of the Infectious Disease Society of America and the Adult AIDS Clinical Trials Group. Clin Infect Dis 2003;37:613–627.

199. Griffin B, Zampelas A. Influence of dietary fatty acids on the atherogenic lipoprotein phenotype. Nutr Res Rev 1997;8:1–26.

200. Berry E. Dietary fatty acids in the management of diabetes mellitus. Am J Clin Nutr 1997;66:S991–S997.

201. Fichtenbaum C, Gerber J, Rosenkranz S, et al. Pharmacokinetic interactions between protease inhibitors and selected HMG-CoA reductase inhibitors. In: Proceedings of the Seventh Conference on Retroviruses and Opportunistic Infections, 2000 (abstract LB6).

202. Rao A, D'Amico S, Balasubramanyam A, Maldonado M. Fenofibrate is effective in treating hypertriglyceridemia associated with HIV lipodystrophy. Am J Med Sci 2004;327:315–318.

203. Hewitt R, Shelton M, Esch L. Gemfibrozil effectively lowers protease inhibitor-associated hypertriglyceridemia in HIV-1-positive patients. AIDS 1999;13:868, 869.

204. Martinez E, Domingo P, Ribera E, et al. Effects of metformin or gemfibrozil on the lipodystrophy of HIV-infected patients receiving protease inhibitors. Antiviral Ther 2003;8:403–410.

205. Gerber M, Yarasheski K, Dreschsler H, et al. Niacin in HIV-infected individuals with hyperlipidemia receiving potent antiretroviral therapy. In: Proceedings of the 10th Conference on Retroviruses and Opportunistic Infections, 2003 (abstract 726).

206. Khan MA, St Peter JV, Xue JL. A prospective, randomized comparison of the metabolic effects of pioglitazone or rosiglitazone in patients with type 2 diabetes who were previously treated with troglitazone. Diabetes Care 2002;25:708–711.

207. van Wijk JP, de Koning EJ, Martens EP, Rabelink TJ. Thiazolidinediones and blood lipids in type 2 diabetes. Arterioscler Thromb Vasc Biol 2003;23:1744–1749.

208. Winkler K, Konrad T, Fullert S, et al. Pioglitazone reduces atherogenic dense LDL particles in nondiabetic patients with arterial hypertension: a double-blind, placebo-controlled study. Diabetes Care 2003;26:2588–2594.

209. Hatano H, Miller KD, Yoder CP, et al. Metabolic and anthropometric consequences of interruption of highly active antiretroviral therapy. AIDS 2000;14:1935–1942.

210. Periard D, Telenti A, Sudre P, et al. Atherogenic dyslipidemia in HIV-infected individuals treated with protease inhibitors. Circulation 1999;100:700–705.

211. Gazzard BG, Moyle G. Does atazanavir cause lipodystrophy? J HIV Ther 2004;9:41–44.

212. Viciana P, Alarcon A, Martin D, et al. Partial improvement of lipodystrophy after switching from HIV-1 protease inhibitors (PI) to efavirenz. In: Proceedings of the 7th Conference on Retroviruses and Opportunistic Infections, 2000 (abstract 84).

213. Barreiro P, Soriano V, Blanco F, Casimiro C, de la Cruz JJ, Gonzalez-Lahoz J. Risks and benefits of replacing protease inhibitors by nevirapine in HIV-infected subjects under long-term successful triple combination therapy. AIDS 2000;14:807–812.

214. Tebas PKY, Powderly WG, Kane E, Marin D, Simpson J, Claxton S, Klebert M, Henry KA prospective open label pilot trial of a maintenance nevirapine-containing regimen in patients with undetectable viral loads on protease inhibitor regimens for at least 6 months. In: Proceedings of the Seventh Conference on Retroviruses and Opportunistic Infections, 2000 (abstract 45).

215. Martinez E, Blanco J, Garcia M, et al. Impact of switching from HIV-1 protease inhibitors to efavirenz in patients with lipodystrophy. In: Proceedings of the Seventh Conference on Retroviruses and Opportunistic Infections, 2000 (abstract 50).

216. Petit JM, Duong M, Masson D, et al. Serum adiponectin and metabolic parameters in HIV-1-infected patients after substitution of nevirapine for protease inhibitors. Eur J Clin Invest 2004;34:569–575.

217. Martinez E, Conget I, Lozano L, Casamitjana R, Gatell JM. Reversion of metabolic abnormalities after switching from HIV-1 protease inhibitors to nevirapine. AIDS 1999;13:805–810.

218. Domingo P, Matias-Guiu X, Pujol RM, et al. Switching to nevirapine decreases insulin levels but does not improve subcutaneous adipocyte apoptosis in patients with highly active antiretroviral therapy-associated lipodystrophy. J Infect Dis 2001;184:1197–1201.

219. van der Valk M, Allick G, Weverling GJ, et al. Markedly diminished lipolysis and partial restoration of glucose metabolism, without changes in fat distribution after extended discontinuation of protease inhibitors in severe lipodystrophic human immunodeficient virus-1–infected patients. J Clin Endocrinol Metab 2004;89:3554–3560.

220. Krotkiewski M, Bjorntorp P. Muscle tissue in obesity with different distribution of adipose tissue: effects of physical training. Int J Obes 1986;10:331–341.

221. Lamarche B, Despres J, Pouliot M, et al. Is body fat loss a determinant factor in the improvement of carbohydrate and lipid metabolism following aerobic exercise training in obese women? Metabolism 1992;41:1249–1256.

222. Driscoll SD, Meininger GE, Ljungquist K, et al. Differential effects of metformin and exercise on muscle adiposity and metabolic indices in human immunodeficiency virus–infected patients. J Clin Endocrinol Metab 2004;89:2171–2178.

223. Stumvoll M, Nurjhan N, Perriello G, Dailey G, Gerich J. Metabolic effects of metformin in non-insulin-dependent diabetes mellitus. N Engl J Med 1995;333:550–554.

224. Hadigan C, Meigs JB, Rabe J, et al. Increased PAI-1 and tPA antigen levels are reduced with metformin therapy in HIV-infected patients with fat redistribution and insulin resistance. J Clin Endocrinol Metab 2001;86:939–943.

225. Hadigan C, Rabe J, Grinspoon S. Sustained benefits of metformin therapy on markers of cardiovascular risk in human immunodeficiency virus–infected patients with fat redistribution and insulin resistance. J Clin Endocrinol Metab 2002;87:4611–4615.

226. Yki-Jarvinen, H. Thiazolidinediones. N Engl J Med 2004;351:1106–1118.

227. Maeda N, Takahashi M, Funahashi T, et al. PPARgamma ligands increase expression and plasma concentrations of adiponectin, an adipose-derived protein. Diabetes 2001;50:2094–2099.

228. Yang WS, Jeng CY, Wu TJ, et al. Synthetic peroxisome proliferator-activated receptor-gamma agonist, rosiglitazone, increases plasma levels of adiponectin in type 2 diabetic patients. Diabetes Care 2002;25:376–380.

229. Phillips SA, Ciaraldi TP, Kong AP, et al. Modulation of circulating and adipose tissue adiponectin levels by antidiabetic therapy. Diabetes 2003;52:667–674.

230. Yu JG, Javorschi S, Hevener AL, et al. The effect of thiazolidinediones on plasma adiponectin levels in normal, obese, and type 2 diabetic subjects. Diabetes 2002;51:2968–2974.

231. Yki-Jarvinen H, Sutinen J, Silveira A, et al. Regulation of plasma PAI-1 concentrations in HAART-associated lipodystrophy during rosiglitazone therapy. Arterioscler Thromb Vasc Biol 2003;23:688–694.

232. Keruly J, Chaisson R, Moore R. Diabetes and hyperglycemia in patients receiving protease inhibitors. Prog of the Fifth Conference on Retroviruses and Opportunistic Infections, Chicago, IL, 1998 (abstract 415).

233. Rothstein A, Caldwell R, Allmon C, Zolopa A, Montoya J. Investigation of protease inhibitor-associated hypercholesterolemia in a university based HIV clinic. In: Proceedings of the 38th Interscience Conference on Antimicrobial Agents and Chemotherapy. American Society for Microbiology, 2004, p. 390.

234. Nystrom T, Bratt G, Sjoholm A. Bezafibrate-induced improvement in glucose uptake and endothelial function in protease inhibitor–associated insulin resistance. J Intern Med 2002;252:570–574.

235. Cheng M, Chen S, Schow SR, et al. In vitro and in vivo prevention of HIV protease inhibitor–induced insulin resistance by a novel small molecule insulin receptor activator. J Cell Biochem 2004;92:1234–1245.

IV TREATMENT

24

Diet and Lifestyle in Prevention and Management of Type 2 Diabetes

Frank B. Hu, MD, PhD

CONTENTS

INTRODUCTION

The prevalence of type 2 diabetes is increasing rapidly in the United States *(1)* and worldwide *(2)*. It is estimated that the prevalence of diabetes in adults will reach 5.4% and the number of adults with diabetes worldwide will reach 300 million in the year 2025 *(2)*. The diabetes epidemic closely parallels the worldwide epidemic of obesity *(3)*. Whereas genotypes resulting in a thrifty metabolism may have been an advantage in times of nutrient scarcity, in most parts of the world these same genes when combined with an increasingly inactive and hypercaloric lifestyle may now contribute to obesity and diabetes *(4)*.

Diabetes is associated with serious health consequences. It is a major risk factor for coronary heart disease (CHD) and stroke. In fact, the vast majority of patients with diabetes die of cardiovascular complications. Diabetes is also the leading cause of blindness, kidney failure, and nontraumatic amputations, resulting from microvascular complications. The economic toll of diabetes is enormous, exceeding $132 billion in 2002 *(5)*.

Diet and lifestyle modifications are considered the cornerstone in the prevention and management of type 2 diabetes *(6)*. In this chapter, we describe recent developments in the prevention and treatment of diabetes through diet and lifestyle modifications from observational studies and clinical trials.

From: *Contemporary Diabetes: Obesity and Diabetes*
Edited by: C. S. Mantzoros © Humana Press Inc., Totowa, NJ

PREVENTABILITY OF TYPE 2 DIABETES

Both epidemiological studies and clinical trials have demonstrated that type 2 diabetes is largely preventable through diet and lifestyle. Using data from the Nurses' Health Study, we defined a low-risk group according to five variables:

1. A body mass index ([BMI]; the weight in kilograms divided by the square of the height in meters) of <25.
2. A diet high in cereal fiber and polyunsaturated fat and low in *trans* fat and glycemic load (which reflects the effect of diet on blood glucose level).
3. Engagement in moderate to vigorous physical activity for at least half an hour per day.
4. No current smoking.
5. The consumption of an average of at least a half serving of an alcoholic beverage per day.

Compared with the rest of the cohort, women in the low-risk group (3.4% of the women) had a relative risk (RR) of diabetes of 0.09 (95% confidence interval [CI]: 0.05–0.17). A total of 91% of the cases of diabetes in this cohort (95% CI: 83–95%) could be attributed to the five factors listed. Thus, these data provide strong epidemiological evidence that the majority of cases of type 2 diabetes could be prevented by the adoption of a healthier lifestyle.

The preventability of diabetes has also been demonstrated by several randomized trials. In a Chinese trial, 577 subjects who had impaired glucose tolerance (IGT) were randomly assigned to either the control group or to one of three different intervention groups (diet, exercise, or diet plus exercise) *(7)*. Participants in the diet intervention group were prescribed a diet with a specific fat content and with individual goals for cereal, vegetables, meat, milk, and oil intake. Compared with the control group, the diet-alone, exercise-alone, and diet-plus-exercise interventions were associated with 31, 46, and 42% reductions in risk of developing diabetes, respectively. In the Finnish Diabetes Prevention Study *(8)*, 522 persons with IGT were randomly assigned to either the control group or an intervention group in which each individual received counseling aimed at reducing weight, total intake of fat, and intake of saturated fat and increasing both intake of fiber and physical activity. The intervention resulted in an overall risk reduction of 58%. In the US-based Diabetes Prevention Program *(9)*, 3234 nondiabetic persons with IGT were randomly assigned to placebo, metformin (a biguanide that lowers blood glucose levels primarily by decreasing hepatic glucose production) (850 mg twice daily), or a lifestyle modification program with the goals of at least a 7% weight loss and at least 150 min of physical activity per week. In this study, 50% of the participants in the lifestyle intervention group had achieved the goal of weight loss of 7% or more by the end of the curriculum (at 24 wk), and 38% had a weight loss of at least 7% at the time of the most recent visit; the proportion of participants who met the goal of at least 150 min of physical activity per week was 74% at 24 wk and 58% at the most recent visit. During 2.8 yr of follow-up, the lifestyle intervention group reduced the incidence of diabetes by 58% (95% CI: 48–66%) compared with the placebo group. Lifestyle intervention was equally effective in men and women and in different ethnic groups.

BODY WEIGHT AND CARDIOVASCULAR RISK PROFILE

Excessive body weight, even at "normal range," increases the risk of diabetes. In the Nurses' Health Study *(10)*, the single most important risk factor for type 2 diabetes was overweight and obesity; the RRs were 38.8 for women with BMIs of ≥ 35 kg/m^2 and

20.1 for those with BMIs of 30.0–34.9 kg/m^2, compared with women with BMIs <23 kg/m^2. Even a BMI within a normal range (23–24.9 kg/m^2) substantially elevated the risk (RR = 2.67). In this cohort of women, 61% (95% CI: 58–64%) of cases of type 2 diabetes could be attributed to overweight and obesity (using 25 kg/m^2 as a cut point).

Obesity not only increases the risk of developing type 2 diabetes but also augments the risk of CHD among patients with diabetes (11). Weight gain during adulthood is a powerful predictor of type 2 diabetes, hypertension, and CHD. By contrast, weight loss improves glucose tolerance and lipid profile and decreases blood pressure (BP). In a review of 33 studies of obese patients with type 2 diabetes, hypertension, or hypercholesterolemia, moderate weight loss (<10% of initial body weight) improved the cardiovascular risk factor profile, including glycemic control, in both nondiabetic and diabetic individuals (12).

BODY WEIGHT AND ENERGY BALANCE

Because body weight is determined primarily by the critical balance between energy intake and energy expenditure, weight loss can be achieved by effectively decreasing total energy intake and/or increasing physical activity. A moderate energy restriction (250–500 calories less than the average daily intake) has been associated with increased insulin sensitivity and improved glycemic control (13). In addition, a rapid weight loss results in excessive breakdown of muscle instead of fat. Thus, it has been suggested that weight loss should not exceed 2 kg/wk.

Recently, a multicenter randomized clinical trial (dubbed "Look AHEAD" [Action for Health in Diabetes]) has been launched to examine the effects of achieving and maintaining weight loss over the long-term through decreased caloric intake and exercise among 5000 obese patients with type 2 diabetes in 16 clinical centers in the United States. The results from this trial will not be available for several years. Nonetheless, the available evidence suggests that aiming for modest or moderate weight loss among both nondiabetic and diabetic patients with obesity seems warranted when larger reductions in body weight are difficult to achieve and/or maintain (12).

PHYSICAL ACTIVITY

Convincing epidemiological data support the role of physical activity in preventing diabetes, and physical activity is clearly a cornerstone of weight maintenance. Aerobic exercise by overweight and obese adults results in modest weight loss independent of the effect of caloric reduction through diet (14). However, only part of the beneficial effect of physical activity on diabetes is mediated through changes in body weight. Physical activity improves insulin sensitivity (15–17), and a reduced risk of developing diabetes with increased activity has been demonstrated in several prospective studies (10,17–25). In most studies, a significant inverse association between physical activity and diabetes remained even after adjustment for BMI. Besides the benefits of vigorous activity, daily walking for >30 min has been found to be associated with a 20–45% risk reduction (17,21,23,24,26), and a faster walking pace predicted lower risk independent of the time spent walking (17,21,23). In addition, regular physical activity, including brisk walking, has been associated with significantly lower risk of cardiovascular events among women with type 2 diabetes (27).

Sedentary behaviors such as prolonged television watching have also been found to be strongly associated with obesity, weight gain, and risk of diabetes, with the increased

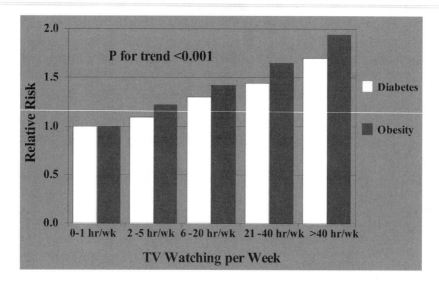

Fig. 1. Multivariate relative risks (RRs) of obesity and type 2 diabetes according to hours spent watching television per week (Nurses' Health Study 1986–1998). RRs for obesity were adjusted for age, smoking, alcohol consumption, and dietary covariates. RRs for diabetes were adjusted for age, smoking, alcohol consumption, family history of diabetes, and dietary covariates. (Data are based on those from ref. *26*.)

risk not entirely explained by the decreased physical activity and unhealthy eating patterns associated with watching television *(26)*. In the Health Professionals' Follow-up Study *(23)*, men who watched television more than 40 h/wk had a nearly threefold increase in the risk of type 2 diabetes compared with those who spent <1 h/wk watching television. In the Nurses' Health Study *(26)*, time spent watching television was directly associated with risk of obesity and type 2 diabetes (Fig. 1). In particular, each 2-h/d increment in television watching was associated with a 23% (95% CI: 17–30%) increase in obesity and a 14% (95% CI: 5–23%) increase in risk of diabetes. By contrast, each hour per day of brisk walking was associated with a 24% (95% CI: 19–29%) reduction in obesity and a 34% (95% CI: 27–41%) reduction in diabetes. It was estimated that 30% (95% CI: 24–36%) of new cases of obesity and 43% (95% CI: 32–52%) of new cases of diabetes could be prevented by adopting a relatively active lifestyle (<10 h/wk of television watching and ≥30 min/d of brisk walking). Thus, public health campaigns to reduce the risk of obesity and type 2 diabetes should promote not only increasing exercise levels but also decreasing sedentary behaviors, especially prolonged television watching.

SMOKING

Several prospective studies demonstrated that smoking is associated with a modestly increased risk of developing diabetes *(28–33)*. Prospective studies clearly demonstrated that the beneficial effects of smoking cessation on risk of diabetes outweigh the adverse effects of weight gain *(32,33)*. Cigarette smoking markedly augmented the risk of CHD in patients with diabetes. In the Nurses' Health Study *(34)*, compared with individuals who had never smoked, the RRs for CHD across categories of smoking were 1.21 (95% CI: 0.97–1.51) for past smokers, 1.66 (95% CI: 1.10–2.52) for current smokers of 1–14 cigarettes/d, and 2.68 (95% CI: 2.07–3.48) for current smokers of 15 or more cigarettes/d in multivariate analyses adjusting for age, history of high BP and cholesterol, and other cardiovascular risk factors ($p < 0.0001$ for trend). The multivariate RR of CHD among women with diabetes who had stopped smoking for more than 10 yr was similar to that among women with diabetes who had never smoked (RR = 1.01 [95% CI: 0.73–1.38]).

ALCOHOL

Moderate alcohol consumption (one to three drinks per day) has been consistently associated with lower incidence of diabetes compared with abstinence or occasional alcohol consumption *(10,28,30,35–53)*. Most studies have observed a U-shaped association, with heavy alcohol consumption being associated with increased risk compared with moderate consumption *(38,41,43,45–47,51,52)*. Five experimental studies investigated the effect of chronic alcohol consumption on insulin sensitivity. One study with 51 postmenopausal women showed a significant increase in insulin sensitivity after 8 wk of moderate alcohol consumption *(54)*. In another study among 23 healthy middle-aged men, insulin sensitivity seemed to increase over a 17-d period in an insulin-resistant subgroup but not among men with normal insulin sensitivity *(55)*. However, the other three intervention trials found no effect of alcohol consumption on insulin sensitivity *(56–58)*.

Several prospective studies examined the association between moderate alcohol intake and risk of CHD in patients with diabetes and all found an inverse association *(59,60)*. The associations observed among patients with diabetes appear to be stronger than those observed in the general population, suggesting that moderate alcohol consumption may have a particular cardiovascular benefit in this high-risk group.

A major concern with alcohol consumption among individuals with diabetes is the potential danger of hypoglycemia, especially among those who use sulfonylureas. However, in several clinical studies, no alteration in glucose homeostasis occurred in patients with diabetes when moderate alcohol was consumed with meals *(61)*. Christiansen et al. *(62)* also showed that a dose of 0.66 g of ethanol/kg followed by a continuous iv infusion of 0.1 g of ethanol/kg did not induce aberrations in carbohydrate metabolism in diet-treated patients with type 2 diabetes. They concluded that even when alcohol is not part of a meal, the effect of alcohol on glucose homeostasis may be less than previously expected. In addition, whereas heavy drinking is associated with diabetic neuropathy *(63)* and retinopathy *(64)*, moderate alcohol intake poses little if any additional risk for these complications *(65)*. Thus, for patients with diabetes who choose to drink, light to moderate drinking (e.g., one to two drinks per day) with a meal should not be discouraged.

MAJOR DIETARY FACTORS

Amount and Types of Fat

Higher total fat intake has been hypothesized to contribute to diabetes. However, results from metabolic studies on the relationship between total fat intake and insulin sensitivity in humans with no change in the fatty acid profile are inconsistent and generally do not support the hypothesis that high-fat diets have detrimental effects on insulin sensitivity *(66)*. Similarly, whereas some earlier prospective observational studies suggested a positive association between total fat intake and risk of diabetes *(67,68)*, most large cohort studies with validated food frequency questionnaires found no significant association *(69–75)*.

More important than the total fat intake may be the specific types of fat consumed *(76)*. Substituting unsaturated fat for saturated fat was shown to increase insulin sensitivity in intervention studies in diabetic *(77)*, overweight *(78)*, and healthy subjects *(79)*. Higher intake of vegetable fat or polyunsaturated fat was found to be inversely associated with risk of diabetes in the Nurses' Health Study and the Iowa Women's Study, two large cohort studies among women *(72,73)*. A higher ratio of polyunsaturated to saturated fat was significantly associated with risk of diabetes in the EPIC-Norfolk Study, although the association was attenuated after adjustment for BMI *(75)*. In the Health Professionals Follow-up Study *(74)*, a significant inverse association between polyunsaturated fat and diabetes was observed only among lean men.

The data on the relationship between dietary fat intake and risk of CHD among patients with diabetes are lacking. However, it is widely agreed that intake of saturated fat should be restricted. The point of controversy lies in whether saturated fats should be replaced with unsaturated fats or with carbohydrates. Current guidelines from the American Diabetes Association (ADA) *(80)* and the European Association for the Study of Diabetes *(13)* do not specify the percentage of calories from carbohydrate and fat and recommend that the diet composition for patients with diabetes be based on individualized nutritional assessment and treatment goals. However, because most patients with diabetes are overweight or obese, reduction in total fat is still the most commonly recommended approach for patients with diabetes. Because low-fat, high-carbohydrate diets can exacerbate diabetic dyslipidemia by reducing high-density lipoprotein (HDL) levels and raising triglycerides *(81)*, the overall value of high-carbohydrate diets for diabetic nutrition therapy is questionable. In a recent study of diabetic women in the Nurses' Health Study *(82)*, a diet characterized by higher cholesterol and saturated fat and lower polyunsaturated:saturated fat ratio was associated with increased risk of cardiovascular disease (CVD), whereas total fat intake was not related to risk of CVD. We estimated that the replacement of saturated fat with monounsaturated fat was associated with a greater reduction in risk than replacement with carbohydrates.

Fish and n-3 Fatty Acids

Although higher intakes of fish and marine n-3 fatty acids have been associated with reduced risk of fatal CHD *(83)* and sudden cardiac death *(84)* in the general population, debate persists about the effects of long-chain n-3 fatty acids (EPA and DHA, primary components of fish oil) among patients with diabetes. The low rates of diabetes among populations with a high fish intake, such as Eskimos, raised the possibility that fish oils may be protective against this condition *(85)*. In support of this notion, limited data have suggested that fish n-3 fatty acids may improve insulin sensitivity *(86)* and glucose tolerance *(87)*. However, other investigators found no appreciable relationship between fish consumption and risk of type 2 diabetes *(88)*. Several studies have reported no improvement *(89)* or even worsening *(90)* of glycemic control among subjects with type 2 diabetes treated with fish oil, which was attributed to an increase in hepatic glucose output. On the other hand, studies have consistently shown that fish oil significantly lowers triglyceride levels in both nondiabetic and diabetic subjects *(91)*. A recent meta-analysis of 26 trials *(92)* found that among patients with diabetes, fish oil lowers triglyceride levels significantly, by about 30%, without adverse effects on glycosylated hemoglobin A_{1c} (HbA$_{1c}$,) but also leads to a 5% increase in low-density lipoprotein (LDL) cholesterol.

Few data are available on the relationship between intake of n-3 fatty acids and risk of CHD among patients with diabetes. In the Nurses' Health Study, compared with the risk among women who seldom consumed fish (less than one serving per month), the RRs (95% CI) of CHD adjusted for age, smoking, and other established coronary risk factors were 0.70 (0.48–1.03) for fish consumption one to three times per month, 0.60 (0.42–0.85) for consumption once per week, 0.64 (0.42–0.99) for consumption two to four times per week, and 0.36 (0.20–0.66) for consumption five or more times per week (p for trend = 0.002). These results support the role of regular fish consumption in preventing CHD among diabetic patients. The effects of fish oil supplementation on cardiovascular end points among patients with diabetes need to be studied in future trials.

Trans-*Fatty Acids*

Trans-fatty acids are formed when vegetable oils are hardened by partial hydrogenation. The major sources of *trans*-fatty acids are stick margarine, commercially baked products, and deep-fried fast food. Consumption of these foods should be limited among patients with diabetes.

Metabolic studies have shown that *trans*-fatty acids, compared with *cis*-unsaturated fatty acids, raise levels of LDL cholesterol and triglyceride and decrease levels of HDL cholesterol (93). In several prospective cohort studies, a higher intake of *trans*-fatty acids was associated with a significantly elevated risk of CHD. Recent studies have also suggested potential adverse effects of *trans*-fat on glucose metabolism. In a 6-wk intervention study, a diet very high in *trans*-monounsaturated fat (20% of energy) was associated with a higher postprandial insulin response than was a *cis*-monounsaturated fat diet in 16 obese persons with type 2 diabetes (94). In the Nurses' Health Study, a high intake of *trans*-fatty acids was associated with a higher risk of type 2 diabetes during 14 yr of follow-up (95). Among diabetic patients, *trans*-fat, as well as saturated fat, should be replaced with monounsaturated and polyunsaturated fats.

Quality and Quantity of Carbohydrates

Low-fat, high-carbohydrate diets generally produce higher postprandial glucose and insulin responses. However, similar to total fat, the total percentage of energy derived from carbohydrates in the diet has generally not been found to predict risk of diabetes (88). Metabolic consequences of carbohydrate intake depend not only on their quantity but also on their quality. The glycemic response of a given carbohydrate load depends on the food sources, which has led to the development of the glycemic index (GI), which ranks foods by their ability to raise postprandial blood glucose levels (96). The GI quantifies the glycemic response by a standard amount of carbohydrates from a food relative to the response by the same amount of carbohydrates from white bread or glucose. The overall GI of a diet has been found to be associated with an increased risk of diabetes in some prospective observational studies (70,71,97), although findings have been inconsistent (98,99). However, the relevance of the concept of GI is indirectly supported by the reduction in the incidence of diabetes observed with acarbose, an α-glucosidase inhibitor that slows down the digestion of carbohydrates (100).

The effects of carbohydrate-rich foods on insulin resistance and risk of diabetes may also depend on fiber content and type. Several epidemiological studies found that diets rich in whole grains (98,101–103) or cereal fiber (10,70,71,97–99,103) may protect against type 2 diabetes. Controlled feeding studies have found benefits of whole grains, compared with refined grains, on insulin sensitivity and glucose metabolism (104–107). This effect may be partially mediated by positive effects on body weight—studies generally support an inverse association between intake of whole grains and body weight *(108)*. In addition, fiber tends to slow down gastrointestinal absorption, resulting in a lower GI of whole-grain products compared with their refined-grain counterparts, but other mechanisms by which whole grains influence glucose metabolism are likely to play a role as well, such as short-chain fatty acid production *(109)* and micronutrient content *(110)*.

Several metabolic studies have evaluated the relatively long-term effects of low-GI diets. In a crossover study of six healthy adults over 4 wk, Jenkins et al. *(111)* found that a low-GI diet significantly reduced 24-h urinary C-peptide levels (a 32% reduction) compared with a high-GI diet. Meanwhile, serum fructosamine levels decreased by 7%. In a 4-wk study of 30 patients with CHD, Frost et al. *(112)* found that a low-GI diet improved glucose tolerance and insulin sensitivity. Insulin-stimulated glucose uptake in isolated fat cells was significantly greater following the low-GI diet. The same group subsequently reported an improvement in insulin sensitivity, as determined by the short insulin tolerance test, with a low-GI diet among 28 premenopausal women in a 3-wk randomized study *(113)*. Studies conducted among patients with diabetes have also found improved glycemic control with a low-GI diet *(114,115)*.

The GI and glycemic load concept has not been incorporated into dietary recommendations in the United States. One reason the ADA did not recommend the use of the GI in its dietary recommendations was the perception that this concept is too complex for the health professional, let alone patients with diabetes. Available evidence, however, suggests that reducing dietary GI and glycemic load is not as difficult as perceived. In a recent randomized trial lasting 12 mo, Gilbertson et al. *(116)* compared the effect of low-GI dietary advice vs the carbohydrate-exchange diet among 104 children with type 2 diabetes. The study found that flexible dietary instruction with an emphasis on low-GI foods improved HbA_{1c} levels without increasing the risk of hypoglycemia. In contrast to conventional belief, twice as many parents of children in the low-GI group reported that their children had no difficulties selecting their own meals at the 12-mo time point (51 vs 24%; $p = 0.01$), and most parents and children chose to continue the low-GI diet after completion of the study.

In dietary practice, the GI values are probably most useful for selecting foods that contain a high amount of carbohydrates, especially starchy foods, but they have limited utility for ranking fruits and vegetables and other foods containing small amounts of carbohydrates. In evaluating the health effects of individual foods, GI values should never be used in isolation; nutrient composition of the foods and overall dietary patterns are clearly important.

Individual Foods

The relationship between consumption of specific foods or beverages and risk of diabetes has been examined in the past decade. An inverse association between coffee consumption and risk of type 2 diabetes has been observed in several *(117–120)*, but not all *(121)*, prospective cohort studies. The beneficial effect of coffee consumption on the development of diabetes has been attributed mainly to caffeine, but other constituents of coffee, such as potassium, niacin, magnesium, and antioxidant substances, may have beneficial effects on glucose metabolism and insulin resistance as well.

Frequent consumption of meat, in particular processed meat, has been consistently shown to increase the risk of diabetes in prospective studies *(74,122,123)*. Although processed meats are a major component of the so-called Western diet pattern in these study populations, these associations were found to be independent of the "Western"

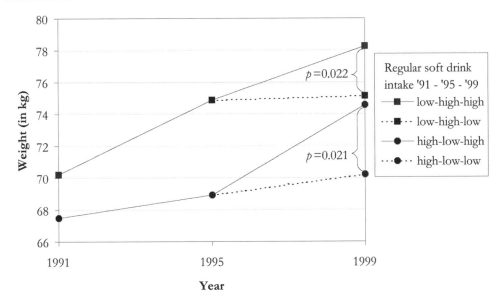

Fig. 2. Mean weight in 1991, 1995, and 1999 according to trends in sugar-sweetened soft drink consumption in 1969 women who changed consumption between 1991 and 1995 and either changed or maintained level of consumption until 1999. Low and high intakes were defined as ≤ 1/wk and ≥ 1/d. The number of subjects was as follows: low-high-high = 323, low-high-low = 461, high-low-high = 110, and high-low-low = 746. Groups with similar intake in 1991 and 1995 were combined for estimates for these time points. Means were adjusted for age, alcohol intake, physical activity, smoking, postmenopausal hormone use, oral contraceptive use, cereal fiber intake, and total fat intake at each time point. (Modified from ref. *131*.)

pattern *(122,123)*. Furthermore, while the associations between red meat consumption and risk of diabetes were largely attenuated by controlling for fat intake, processed meats remained significantly associated with risk *(122)*, indicating that constituents of processed meats other than fatty acids, such as nitrite or advanced glycation end products, may be relevant in the development of diabetes.

Recent findings from prospective studies also indicate that consumption of nuts *(124)* and dairy products *(125)* may have beneficial effects in the development of diabetes. Consumption of fruits and vegetables has been found to be inversely associated with risk of diabetes in the National Health and Nutrition Examination Survey *(126)* but not among older women in the Iowa Women's Health Study *(98)*.

Several epidemiological studies found that diets rich in whole grains may protect against type 2 diabetes *(98,101–103)*. Controlled feeding studies found benefits of whole grains, compared with refined grains, on insulin sensitivity and glucose *(105)*.

Sugar-sweetened beverages are receiving growing attention as potential contributors to the obesity and diabetes epidemic *(127)*. Energy contained in beverages seems less well detected by the body, and subsequent food intake is poorly adjusted to account for the energy intake from beverages. Sugar-sweetened beverages have been associated with weight gain in clinical studies *(128,129)* and observational studies among children *(130)* and adults *(131)*. The high sugar loads from sugar-sweetened beverages may also have detrimental effects on glucose metabolism leading to diabetes, which is beyond their potential contribution to obesity *(131)*. In the Nurses' Health Study II, a higher consumption of sugar-sweetened beverages was associated with a greater magnitude of weight gain and an increased risk of developing of type 2 diabetes in women (Fig. 2).

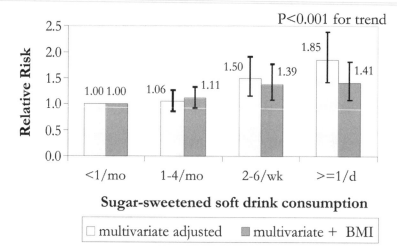

Fig. 3. Multivariate relative risks (RRs) of type 2 diabetes according to sugar-sweetened soft drink consumption in Nurses' Health Study II 1991–1999. Multivariate RRs were adjusted for age; alcohol consumption (0, 0.1–4.9, 5.0–9.9, 10+ g/d); physical activity (quintiles); family history of diabetes; smoking (never, past, current); postmenopausal hormone use (never, ever); oral contraceptive use (never, past, current); intake (quintiles) of cereal fiber; magnesium; *trans*=fat; polyunsaturated:saturated fat; and consumption of sugar-sweetened soft drinks, diet soft drinks, fruit juice, and fruit punch (other than the main exposure, depending on model). (Data based on those in ref. *131*.)

After adjustment for potential confounders, women consuming one or more sugar-sweetened soft drinks per day had an RR of type 2 diabetes of 1.83 (95% CI: 1.42–2.36; $p < 0.001$ for trend) compared with those who consumed less than one of these beverages per month. The RR for extreme categories further controlling for BMI was 1.39 (95% CI: 1.07–1.76; $p = 0.012$ for trend) (Fig. 3). This finding suggests that BMI accounted for about half of the excess risk.

CONCLUSIONS

Compelling evidence from metabolic studies, large prospective observational studies, and clinical trials indicate that unhealthy diets, obesity, and sedentary lifestyles are major contributors to the diabetes epidemic. Obesity is the strongest risk factor for diabetes, and maintenance of a healthy weight by avoiding energy overconsumption and by engaging in regular physical activity is clearly the key to diabetes prevention. Substitution of unsaturated fat for saturated and *trans*-fats and of whole-grain foods for refined-grain foods is an effective and important strategy to prevent diabetes. A diet rich in fruits, vegetables, legumes, whole grains, and healthy sources of protein (poultry and fish) and with unsaturated vegetable fats as the main source of fat but low in red and processed meats, refined grains, and sugar-sweetened beverages can offer significant protection against type 2 diabetes and CVD. Similarly, dietary recommendations for the management of diabetes should focus more on the quality of fat and carbohydrate in the diet than quantity (percentage of energy) alone, in addition to balancing total energy intake with energy expenditure. There is convincing evidence that alcohol in moderation with a meal can be a healthy choice, unless contraindicated. Finally, stopping smoking is one of the most effective ways to reduce the risk of CHD among patients with diabetes.

REFERENCES

1. Mokdad AH, Ford ES, Bowman BA, et al. Diabetes trends in the U.S.: 1990–1998 [in process citation]. Diabetes Care 2000;23:1278–1283.
2. King H, Aubert RE, Herman WH. Global burden of diabetes, 1995–2025: prevalence, numerical estimates, and projections [see comments]. Diabetes Care 1998;21:1414–1431.
3. No authors listed. Diet, nutrition and the prevention of chronic diseases: report of a joint WHO/FAO expert consultation. WHO Technical Report Series No. 916. World Health Organization, Geneva, Switzerland, 2002.
4. Neel JV. Diabetes mellitus: a "thrifty" genotype rendered detrimental by "progress"? Am J Hum Genet 1962;14:353–362.
5. No authors listed. Economic costs of diabetes in the U.S. in 2002. Diabetes Care 2003;26:917–932.
6. Schulze MB, Hu FB. Primary prevention of diabetes: what can be done and how much can be prevented? Ann Rev Public Health 2005;26:445–467.
7. Pan XR, Li GW, Hu YH, et al. Effects of diet and exercise in preventing NIDDM in people with impaired glucose tolerance: the Da Qing IGT and Diabetes Study. Diabetes Care 1997;20: 537–544.
8. Tuomilehto J, Lindstrom J, Eriksson JG, et al. Prevention of type 2 diabetes mellitus by changes in lifestyle among subjects with impaired glucose tolerance. N Engl J Med 2001;344:1343–1350.
9. Knowler WC, Barrett-Connor E, Fowler SE, et al. Reduction in the incidence of type 2 diabetes with lifestyle intervention or metformin. N Engl J Med 2002;346:393–403.
10. Hu FB, Manson JE, Stampfer MJ, et al. Diet, lifestyle, and the risk of type 2 diabetes mellitus in women. N Engl J Med 2001;345:790–797.
11. Manson JE, Colditz GA, Stampfer MJ, et al. A prospective study of maturity-onset diabetes mellitus and risk of coronary heart disease and stroke in women. Arch Intern Med 1991;151:1141–1147.
12. Goldstein DJ. Beneficial effects of modest weight loss. Int J Obes 1992;16:397–415.
13. Ha TK, Lean ME. Recommendations for the nutritional management of patients with diabetes mellitus. Eur J Clin Nutr 1998;52:467–481.
14. No authors listed. Clinical guidelines on the identification, evaluation, and treatment of overweight and obesity in adults—the evidence report. National Institutes of Health. Obes Res 1998; 6(Suppl 2):51S–209S.
15. Mayer-Davis EJ, D'Agostino R Jr, Karter AJ, et al. Intensity and amount of physical activity in relation to insulin sensitivity: the Insulin Resistance Atherosclerosis Study. JAMA 1998; 279:669–674.
16. Duncan GE, Perri MG, Theriaque DW, Hutson AD, Eckel RH, Stacpoole PW. Exercise training, without weight loss, increases insulin sensitivity and postheparin plasma lipase activity in previously sedentary adults. Diabetes Care 2003;26:557–562.
17. Wannamethee SG, Shaper AG, Alberti KG. Physical activity, metabolic factors, and the incidence of coronary heart disease and type 2 diabetes. Arch Intern Med 2000;160:2108–2116.
18. Manson JE, Rimm EB, Stampfer MJ, et al. Physical activity and incidence of non-insulin-dependent diabetes mellitus in women. Lancet 1991;338:774–778.
19. Helmrich SP, Ragland DR, Leung RW, Paffenbarger RS Jr. Physical activity and reduced occurrence of non-insulin-dependent diabetes mellitus. N Engl J Med 1991;325:147–152.
20. Haapanen N, Miilunpalo S, Vuori I, Oja P, Pasanen M. Association of leisure time physical activity with the risk of coronary heart disease, hypertension and diabetes in middle-aged men and women. Int J Epidemiol 1997;26:739–747.
21. Hu FB, Sigal RJ, Rich-Edwards JW, et al. Walking compared with vigorous physical activity and risk of type 2 diabetes in women: a prospective study. JAMA 1999;282:1433–1439.
22. Okada K, Hayashi T, Tsumura K, Suematsu C, Endo G, Fujii S. Leisure-time physical activity at weekends and the risk of Type 2 diabetes mellitus in Japanese men: the Osaka Health Survey. Diabet Med 2000;17:53–58.
23. Hu FB, Leitzmann MF, Stampfer MJ, Colditz GA, Willett WC, Rimm EB. Physical activity and television watching in relation to risk for type 2 diabetes mellitus in men. Arch Intern Med 2001;161:1542–1548.
24. Hu G, Qiao Q, Silventoinen K, et al. Occupational, commuting, and leisure-time physical activity in relation to risk for Type 2 diabetes in middle-aged Finnish men and women. Diabetologia 2003;46:322–329.
25. Kriska AM, Saremi A, Hanson RL, et al. Physical activity, obesity, and the incidence of type 2 diabetes in a high-risk population. Am J Epidemiol 2003;158:669–675.

26. Hu FB, Li TY, Colditz GA, Willett WC, Manson JE. Television watching and other sedentary behaviors in relation to risk of obesity and type 2 diabetes mellitus in women. JAMA 2003;289:1785–1791.

27. Hu FB, Stampfer MJ, Solomon C, et al. Physical activity and risk for cardiovascular events in diabetic women. Ann Intern Med 2001;134:96–105.

28. Feskens EJ, Kromhout D. Cardiovascular risk factors and the 25-year incidence of diabetes mellitus in middle-aged men: the Zutphen Study. Am J Epidemiol 1989;130:1101–1108.

29. Rimm EB, Manson JE, Stampfer MJ, et al. Cigarette smoking and the risk of diabetes in women. Am J Public Health 1993;83:211–214.

30. Rimm EB, Chan J, Stampfer MJ, Colditz GA, Willett WC. Prospective study of cigarette smoking, alcohol use, and the risk of diabetes in men. BMJ 1995;310:555–559.

31. Kawakami N, Takatsuka N, Shimizu H, Ishibashi H. Effects of smoking on the incidence of non-insulin-dependent diabetes mellitus: replication and extension in a Japanese cohort of male employees. Am J Epidemiol 1997;145:103–109.

32. Wannamethee SG, Shaper AG, Perry IJ. Smoking as a modifiable risk factor for type 2 diabetes in middle-aged men. Diabetes Care 2001;24:1590–1595.

33. Will JC, Galuska DA, Ford ES, Mokdad A, Calle EE. Cigarette smoking and diabetes mellitus: evidence of a positive association from a large prospective cohort study. Int J Epidemiol 2001;30:540–546.

34. Al-Delaimy WK, Manson JE, Solomon CG, et al. Smoking and risk of coronary heart disease among women with type 2 diabetes. Arch Intern Med 2002;162:273–279.

35. Stampfer MJ, Colditz GA, Willett WC, et al. A prospective study of moderate alcohol drinking and risk of diabetes in women. Am J Epidemiol 1988;128:549–558.

36. Holbrook TL, Barrett-Connor E, Wingard DL. A prospective population-based study of alcohol use and non-insulin-dependent diabetes mellitus. Am J Epidemiol 1990;132:902–909.

37. Hodge AM, Dowse GK, Collins VR, Zimmet PZ. Abnormal glucose tolerance and alcohol consumption in three populations at high risk of non-insulin-dependent diabetes mellitus. Am J Epidemiol 1993;137:178–189.

38. Gurwitz JH, Field TS, Glynn RJ, et al. Risk factors for non-insulin-dependent diabetes mellitus requiring treatment in the elderly. J Am Geriatr Soc 1994;42:1235–1240.

39. Monterrosa AE, Haffner SM, Stern MP, Hazuda HP. Sex difference in lifestyle factors predictive of diabetes in Mexican-Americans. Diabetes Care 1995;18:448–456.

40. Sugimori H, Miyakawa M, Yoshida K, et al. Health risk assessment for diabetes mellitus based on longitudinal analysis of MHTS database. J Med Syst 1998;22:27–32.

41. Tsumura K, Hayashi T, Suematsu C, Endo G, Fujii S, Okada K. Daily alcohol consumption and the risk of type 2 diabetes in Japanese men: the Osaka Health Survey. Diabetes Care 1999;22:1432–1437.

42. Ajani UA, Hennekens CH, Spelsberg A, Manson JE. Alcohol consumption and risk of type 2 diabetes mellitus among US male physicians. Arch Intern Med 2000;160:1025–1030.

43. Wei M, Gibbons LW, Mitchell TL, Kampert JB, Blair SN. Alcohol intake and incidence of type 2 diabetes in men. Diabetes Care 2000;23:18–22.

44. Conigrave KM, Hu BF, Camargo CA Jr, Stampfer MJ, Willett WC, Rimm EB. A prospective study of drinking patterns in relation to risk of type 2 diabetes among men. Diabetes 2001;50:2390–2395.

45. Kao WH, Puddey IB, Boland LL, Watson RL, Brancati FL. Alcohol consumption and the risk of type 2 diabetes mellitus: atherosclerosis risk in communities study. Am J Epidemiol 2001;154:748–757.

46. de Vegt F, Dekker JM, Groeneveld WJ, et al. Moderate alcohol consumption is associated with lower risk for incident diabetes and mortality: the Hoorn Study. Diabetes Res Clin Pract 2002;57:53–60.

47. Wannamethee SG, Shaper AG, Perry IJ, Alberti KG. Alcohol consumption and the incidence of type II diabetes. J Epidemiol Community Health 2002;56:542–548.

48. Watanabe M, Barzi F, Neal B, et al. Alcohol consumption and the risk of diabetes by body mass index levels in a cohort of 5,636 Japanese. Diabetes Res Clin Pract 2002;57:191–197.

49. Carlsson S, Hammar N, Grill V, Kaprio J. Alcohol consumption and the incidence of type 2 diabetes: a 20-year follow-up of the Finnish twin cohort study. Diabetes Care 2003;26:2785–2790.

50. Lu W, Jablonski KA, Resnick HE, et al. Alcohol intake and glycemia in American Indians: the strong heart study. Metabolism 2003;52:129–135.

51. Nakanishi N, Suzuki K, Tatara K. Alcohol consumption and risk for development of impaired fasting glucose or type 2 diabetes in middle-aged Japanese men. Diabetes Care 2003;26:48–54.

52. Wannamethee SG, Camargo CA Jr, Manson JE, Willett WC, Rimm EB. Alcohol drinking patterns and risk of type 2 diabetes mellitus among younger women. Arch Intern Med 2003;163:1329–1336.

53. Howard AA, Arnsten JH, Gourevitch MN. Effect of alcohol consumption on diabetes mellitus: a systematic review. Ann Intern Med 2004;140:211–219.

54. Davies MJ, Baer DJ, Judd JT, Brown ED, Campbell WS, Taylor PR. Effects of moderate alcohol intake on fasting insulin and glucose concentrations and insulin sensitivity in postmenopausal women: a randomized controlled trial. JAMA 2002;287:2559–2562.

55. Sierksma A, Patel H, Ouchi N, et al. Effect of moderate alcohol consumption on adiponectin, tumor necrosis factor-alpha, and insulin sensitivity. Diabetes Care 2004;27:184–189.

56. Cordain L, Melby CL, Hamamoto AE, et al. Influence of moderate chronic wine consumption on insulin sensitivity and other correlates of syndrome X in moderately obese women. Metabolism 2000;49:1473–1478.

57. Flanagan DE, Pratt E, Murphy J, et al. Alcohol consumption alters insulin secretion and cardiac autonomic activity. Eur J Clin Invest 2002;32:187–192.

58. Zilkens RR, Burke V, Watts G, Beilin LJ, Puddey IB. The effect of alcohol intake on insulin sensitivity in men: a randomized controlled trial. Diabetes Care 2003;26:608–612.

59. Solomon CG, Hu FB, Stampfer MJ, et al. Moderate alcohol consumption and risk of coronary heart disease among women with type 2 diabetes mellitus [see comments]. Circulation 2000; 102:494–499.

60. Tanasescu M, Hu FB. Alcohol consumption and risk of coronary heart disease among individuals with type 2 diabetes. Curr Diabetes Rep 2001;1:187–191.

61. Burge MR, Zeise TM, Sobhy TA, Rassam AG, Schade DS. Low-dose ethanol predisposes elderly fasted patients with type 2 diabetes to sulfonylurea-induced low blood glucose. Diabetes Care 1999;22:2037–2043.

62. Christiansen C, Thomsen C, Rasmussen O, et al. Effect of alcohol on glucose, insulin, free fatty acid and triacylglycerol responses to a light meal in non-insulin-dependent diabetic subjects. Br J Nutr 1994;71:449–454.

63. Bell DS. Alcohol and the NIDDM patient. Diabetes Care 1996;19:509–513.

64. Christiansen C, Thomsen C, Rasmussen O, Hansen C, Hermansen K. The acute impact of ethanol on glucose, insulin, triacylglycerol,and free fatty acid responses and insulin sensitivity in type 2 diabetes. Br J Nutr 1996;76:669–675.

65. Moss SE, Klein R, Klein BE. The association of alcohol consumption with the incidence and progression of diabetic retinopathy. Ophthalmology 1994;101:1962–1968.

66. Lichtenstein AH, Schwab US. Relationship of dietary fat to glucose metabolism. Atherosclerosis 2000;150:227–243.

67. Marshall JA, Hoag S, Shetterly S, Hamman RF. Dietary fat predicts conversion from impaired glucose tolerance to NIDDM:the San Luis Valley Diabetes Study. Diabetes Care 1994;17:50–56.

68. Feskens EJ, Virtanen SM, Rasanen L, et al. Dietary factors determining diabetes and impaired glucose tolerance: a 20-year follow-up of the Finnish and Dutch cohorts of the Seven Countries Study. Diabetes Care 1995;18:1104–1112.

69. Colditz GA, Manson JE, Stampfer MJ, Rosner B, Willett WC, Speizer FE. Diet and risk of clinical diabetes in women. Am J Clin Nutr 1992;55:1018–1023.

70. Salmeron J, Ascherio A, Rimm EB, et al. Dietary fiber, glycemic load, and risk of NIDDM in men. Diabetes Care 1997;20:545–550.

71. Salmeron J, Manson JE, Stampfer MJ, Colditz GA, Wing AL, Willett WC. Dietary fiber, glycemic load, and risk of non-insulin-dependent diabetes mellitus in women. JAMA 1997;277:472–477.

72. Salmeron J, Hu FB, Manson JE, et al. Dietary fat intake and risk of type 2 diabetes in women. Am J Clin Nutr 2001;73:1019–1026.

73. Meyer KA, Kushi LH, Jacobs DR Jr, Folsom AR. Dietary fat and incidence of type 2 diabetes in older Iowa women. Diabetes Care 2001;24:1528–1535.

74. van Dam RM, Willett WC, Rimm EB, Stampfer MJ, Hu FB. Dietary fat and meat intake in relation to risk of type 2 diabetes in men. Diabetes Care 2002;25:417–424.

75. Harding AH, Day NE, Khaw KT, et al. Dietary fat and the risk of clinical type 2 diabetes: the European prospective investigation of Cancer-Norfolk study. Am J Epidemiol 2004;159:73–82.

76. Hu FB, van Dam RM, Liu S. Diet and risk of Type II diabetes: the role of types of fat and carbohydrate. Diabetologia 2001;44:805–817.

77. Summers LK, Fielding BA, Bradshaw HA, et al. Substituting dietary saturated fat with polyunsaturated fat changes abdominal fat distribution and improves insulin sensitivity. Diabetologia 2002;45:369–377.

78. Lovejoy JC, Smith SR, Champagne CM, et al. Effects of diets enriched in saturated (palmitic), monounsaturated (oleic), or trans (elaidic) fatty acids on insulin sensitivity and substrate oxidation in healthy adults. Diabetes Care 2002;25:1283–1288.

79. Vessby B, Unsitupa M, Hermansen K, et al. Substituting dietary saturated for monounsaturated fat impairs insulin sensitivity in healthy men and women: the KANWU Study. Diabetologia 2001; 44:312–319.

80. American Diabetes Association. Nutrition recommendations and principles for people with diabetes mellitus. Diabetes Care 2001;24(Suppl 1):S44–S47.

81. Parks EJ, Hellerstein MK. Carbohydrate-induced hypertriacylglycerolemia: historical perspective and review of biological mechanisms. Am J Clin Nutr 2000;71:412–433.

82. Tanasescu M, Cho E, Manson JE, Hu FB. Dietary fat and cholesterol and the risk of cardiovascular disease among women with type 2 diabetes. Am J Clin Nutr 2004;79:999–1005.

83. Kromhout D, Bosscheiter EB, de Lezenne Coulander C. The inverse relation between fish consumption and 20-year mortality from coronary heart disease. N Engl J Med 1985;312:1205–1209.

84. Albert CM, Hennekens CH, O'Donnell CJ, et al. Fish consumption and risk of sudden cardiac death. JAMA 1998;279:23–28.

85. Kromann N, Green A. Epidemiologic studies in the Upernavik District, Greenland. Acta Med Scand 1980;208:401–406.

86. Popp-Snijders C, Shouten JA, Heine RJ, van der Meer J, van der Veen EA. Dietary supplementation of omega-3 polyunsaturated fatty acids improve insulin sensitivity in non-insulin-dependent diabetes mellitus. Diabetes Care 1987;4:141–147.

87. Feskens EJM, Virtanen SM, Rasanen L, et al. Dietary factors determining diabetes and impaired glucose tolerance. Diabetes Care 1995;18:1104–1112.

88. Hu FB, van Dam RM, Liu S. Diet and risk of Type II diabetes: the role of types of fat and carbohydrate. Diabetologia 2001;44:805–817.

89. Axelrod L, Camuso J, Williams E, Kleinman K, Briones E, Schoenfeld D. Effects of a small quantity of omega-3 fatty acids on cardiovascular risk factors in NIDDM: a randomized, prospective, double-blind, controlled study. Diabetes Care 1994;17:37–44.

90. Glauber H, Wallace P, Griver K, Brechtel G. Adverse metabolic effects of omega-3 fatty acids in non-insulin-dependent diabetes mellitus. Ann Intern Med 1988;108:663–668.

91. Connor WE. Diabetes, fish oil, and vascular disease. Ann Intern Med 1995;123:950–952.

92. Friedberg CE, Janssen MJFM, Heine RJ, Grobbee DE. Fish oil and glycemic control in diabetes: a meta-analysis. Diabetes Care 1998;21:494–500.

93. Ascherio A, Katan MB, Zock PL, Stampfer MJ, Willett WC. Trans fatty acids and coronary heart disease. N Engl J Med 1999;340:1994–1998.

94. Christiansen E, Schnider S, Palmvig B, Tauber-Lassen E, Pedersen O. Intake of a diet high in trans monounsaturated fatty acids or saturated fatty acids: effects on postprandial insulinemia and glycemia in obese patients with NIDDM. Diabetes Care 1997;20:881–887.

95. Salmeron J, Hu FB, Manson JE, et al. Dietary fat intake and risk of type 2 diabetes in women. Am J Clin Nutr 2001;73:1019–1026.

96. Jenkins DJ, Wolever TM, Taylor RH, et al. Glycemic index of foods: a physiological basis for carbohydrate exchange. Am J Clin Nutr 1981;34:362–366.

97. Schulze MB, Liu S, Rimm EB, Manson JE, Willett WC, Hu FB. Glycemic index, glycemic load, and dietary fiber intake and incidence of type 2 diabetes in younger and middle-aged women. Am J Clin Nutr 2004;80:348–356.

98. Meyer KA, Kushi LH, Jacobs DR Jr, Slavin J, Sellers TA, Folsom AR. Carbohydrates, dietary fiber, and incident type 2 diabetes in older women. Am J Clin Nutr 2000;71:921–930.

99. Stevens J, Ahn K, Juhaeri, Houston D, Steffan L, Couper D. Dietary fiber intake and glycemic index and incidence of diabetes in African-American and white adults: the ARIC study. Diabetes Care 2002;25:1715–1721.

100. Chiasson JL, Josse RG, Gomis R, Hanefeld M, Karasik A, Laakso M. Acarbose for prevention of type 2 diabetes mellitus: the STOP-NIDDM randomised trial. Lancet 2002;359:2072–2077.

101. Liu S, Manson JE, Stampfer MJ, et al. A prospective study of whole-grain intake and risk of type 2 diabetes mellitus in US women. Am J Public Health 2000;90:1409–1415.

102. Fung TT, Hu FB, Pereira MA, et al. Whole-grain intake and the risk of type 2 diabetes: a prospective study in men. Am J Clin Nutr 2002;76:535–540.

103. Montonen J, Knekt P, Jarvinen R, Aromaa A, Reunanen A. Whole-grain and fiber intake and the incidence of type 2 diabetes. Am J Clin Nutr 2003;77:622–629.

104. Fukagawa NK, Anderson JW, Hageman G, Young VR, Minaker KL. High-carbohydrate, high-fiber diets increase peripheral insulin sensitivity in healthy young and old adults. Am J Clin Nutr 1990;52:524–528.

105. Pereira MA, Jacobs DR Jr, Pins JJ, et al. Effect of whole grains on insulin sensitivity in overweight hyperinsulinemic adults. Am J Clin Nutr 2002;75:848–855.

106. Keenan JM, Pins JJ, Frazel C, Moran A, Turnquist L. Oat ingestion reduces systolic and diastolic blood pressure in patients with mild or borderline hypertension: a pilot trial. J Fam Pract 2002;51:369.

107. Chandalia M, Garg A, Lutjohann D, von Bergmann K, Grundy SM, Brinkley LJ. Beneficial effects of high dietary fiber intake in patients with type 2 diabetes mellitus. N Engl J Med 2000;342: 1392–1398.

108. Pereira MA, Ludwig DS. Dietary fiber and body-weight regulation: observations and mechanisms. Pediatr Clin North Am 2001;48:969–980.

109. Thorburn A, Muir J, Proietto J. Carbohydrate fermentation decreases hepatic glucose output in healthy subjects. Metabolism 1993;42:780–785.

110. Liu S. Intake of refined carbohydrates and whole grain foods in relation to risk of type 2 diabetes mellitus and coronary heart disease. J Am Coll Nutr 2002;21:298–306.

111. Jenkins DJ, Wolever TM, Collier GR, et al. Metabolic effects of a low-glycemic-index diet. Am J Clin Nutr 1987;46:968–975.

112. Frost G, Keogh B, Smith D, Akinsanya K, Leeds A. The effect of low-glycemic carbohydrate on insulin and glucose response in vivo and in vitro in patients with coronary heart disease. Metabolism 1996;45:669–672.

113. Frost G, Leeds A, Trew G, Margara R, Dornhorst A. Insulin sensitivity in women at risk of coronary heart disease and the effect of a low glycemic diet. Metabolism 1998;47:1245–1251.

114. Jenkins DJ, Wolever TM, Buckley G, et al. Low-glycemic-index starchy foods in the diabetic diet. Am J Clin Nutr 1988;48:248–254.

115. Wolever TM, Jenkins DJ, Vuksan V, et al. Beneficial effect of a low glycaemic index diet in type 2 diabetes. Diabet Med 1992;9:451–458.

116. Gilbertson HR, Brand-Miller JC, Thorburn AW, Evans S, Chondros P, Werther GA. The effect of flexible low glycemic index dietary advice versus measured carbohydrate exchange diets on glycemic control in children with type 1 diabetes. Diabetes Care 2001;24:1137–1143.

117. van Dam RM, Feskens EJ. Coffee consumption and risk of type 2 diabetes mellitus. Lancet 2002;360:1477–1478.

118. Salazar-Martinez E, Willett WC, Ascherio A, et al. Coffee consumption and risk for type 2 diabetes mellitus. Ann Intern Med 2004;140:1–8.

119. Rosengren A, Dotevall A, Wilhelmsen L, Thelle D, Johansson S. Coffee and incidence of diabetes in Swedish women: a prospective 18-year follow-up study. J Intern Med 2004;255:89–95.

120. Tuomilehto J, Hu G, Bidel S, Lindstrom J, Jousilahti P. Coffee consumption and risk of type 2 diabetes mellitus among middle-aged Finnish men and women. JAMA 2004;291:1213–1219.

121. Saremi A, Tulloch-Reid M, Knowler WC. Coffee consumption and the incidence of type 2 diabetes. Diabetes Care 2003;26:2211, 2212.

122. Schulze MB, Manson JE, Willett WC, Hu FB. Processed meat intake and incidence of Type 2 diabetes in younger and middle-aged women. Diabetologia 2003;46:1465–1473.

123. Fung TT, Schulze MB, Manson JE, Willett WC, Hu FB. Dietary patterns, meat intake and the risk of type 2 diabetes in women. Arch Intern Med 2004;164:2235–2240.

124. Jiang R, Manson JE, Stampfer MJ, Liu S, Willett WC, Hu FB. Nut and peanut butter consumption and risk of type 2 diabetes in women. JAMA 2002;288:2554–2560.

125. Pereira MA, Jacobs DR Jr, Van Horn L, Slattery ML, Kartashov AI, Ludwig DS. Dairy consumption, obesity, and the insulin resistance syndrome in young adults: the CARDIA Study. JAMA 2002;287:2081–2089.

126. Ford ES, Mokdad AH. Fruit and vegetable consumption and diabetes mellitus incidence among U.S. adults. Prev Med 2001;32:33–39.

127. Bray GA, Nielsen SJ, Popkin BM. Consumption of high-fructose corn syrup in beverages may play a role in the epidemic of obesity. Am J Clin Nutr 2004;79:537–543.

128. Tordoff MG, Alleva AM. Effect of drinking soda sweetened with aspartame or high-fructose corn syrup on food intake and body weight. Am J Clin Nutr 1990;51:963–969.

129. Raben A, Vasilaras TH, Moller AC, Astrup A. Sucrose compared with artificial sweeteners: different effects on ad libitum food intake and body weight after 10 wk of supplementation in overweight subjects. Am J Clin Nutr 2002;76:721–729.

130. Ludwig DS, Peterson KE, Gortmaker SL. Relation between consumption of sugar-sweetened drinks and childhood obesity: a prospective, observational analysis. Lancet 2001;357:505–508.

131. Schulze MB, Manson JE, Ludwig DS, et al. Sugar-sweetened beverages, weight gain, and incidence of type 2 diabetes in young and middle-aged women. JAMA 2004;292(8):927–934.

25 Diet, Exercise, and Behavioral Treatment of Obesity

George L. Blackburn, MD, PhD

Contents

INTRODUCTION

Approximately 18.2 million Americans had diabetes in 2002 *(1)*. An estimated 70% of type 2 diabetes risk in the United States is attributable to overweight and obesity, with each kilogram of weight gain over 10 yr increasing risk by 4.5% *(2)*. Modest weight loss, often achievable by a combination of reduced caloric intake and increased physical activity, lowers the risk of diabetes and insulin resistance and improves measures of glycemia and dyslipidemia in those with diabetes *(3–8)*.

Lifestyle interventions that change eating behavior, increase physical activity, and result in modest weight loss are known to prevent or delay diabetes in persons at high risk for the disease *(3,5)*. Even modest weight loss (5–10% of body weight) *(9)* and physical activity (30 min daily) *(10)* have been found to have a positive impact on diabetes risk and management *(4)*. The proven benefits of reduced caloric intake, consumption of a prudent diet, and physical activity strongly suggest that lifestyle modification (Table 1) should be the first choice to prevent or delay diabetes *(3,5)*, and more effectively manage disease in individuals with diabetes.

DIET

Overview

Insulin sensitivity is known to improve rapidly after the start of an energy-deficit diet, even before much weight loss occurs, and continues to improve with ongoing weight reduction *(11)*. The magnitude of improvement appears to be primarily related

From: *Contemporary Diabetes: Obesity and Diabetes*
Edited by: C. S. Mantzoros © Humana Press Inc., Totowa, NJ

Table 1
Diet, Exercise, and Behavioral Treatment of Obesity[a]

- Get regular exercise—at least 30 min/d of brisk walking, sports, or active games.
- Eat a healthful diet rich in vegetables, fruits, and whole grains and low in refined carbohydrates, such as sweets and white bread.
- Limit the amount of high-sugar beverages you drink, such as soft drinks and fruit punches.
- Avoid high-fat foods, such as ice cream, butter, and high-fat meats.
- Limit alcohol to no more than one drink per day for women, two per day for men, and none if you have any difficulty controlling alcohol intake.
- Eat several small meals throughout the day instead of three large meals.
- Always eat a balanced breakfast.
- If you are overweight, aim to lose no more than 2 lb/wk—losing more than that can be unhealthy and often leads to rebound weight gain.
- Get your family and friends involved by encouraging them to eat healthful foods and exercise together.
- Realize that your diet and exercise regimen are lifestyle changes that must be maintained in the long term to keep weight off.

[a]Sources: National Institute of Diabetes and Digestive and Kidney Diseases, American Diabetes Association, Centers for Disease Control and Prevention (13,36).

to the amount of weight lost (12). In patients with obesity and type 2 diabetes, a 5% weight loss at the end of 1 yr of dietary therapy is known to decrease fasting blood glucose, insulin, hemoglobin A1c concentrations, and the dose of oral hypoglycemic therapy (12). Although many different diets are used to treat obesity, energy content is the primary determinant of weight loss (13,14), with a low-fat approach considered the treatment standard (15).

High-Protein/Low-Carbohydrate Diets

Data indicate that weight loss from low-carbohydrate diets is associated with duration of diet and reduction in energy intake, but not with the restriction of carbohydrates (16). Studies that compared a low-carbohydrate diet with a low-fat calorie-reduced diet in obese patients (17,18) found greater short-term weight loss on the low-carbohydrate diet, but no significant difference in weight loss between the two groups after 1 yr (17,18).

Structured Meal Plans/Meal Replacements

Evidence suggests a direct relation between portion size served and amount of food consumed (19). Portion-controlled diets provide servings of food with fixed-calorie and macronutrient content. Data show several kilograms more weight loss in obese persons who consume prepackaged prepared meals or liquid-formula meal replacements compared with subjects on a standard diet (20–22).

Dairy Diet

An antiobesity effect of dietary calcium and dairy foods has been identified in animal studies, observational and population studies, and clinical trials (23). Evidence suggests an inverse relation between intake of dietary calcium and dairy products and body fat (24–26). These data are consistent with those from other studies (27–32).

Weight Maintenance

The key to successful weight management is to provide patients with a dietary regimen that results in long-term compliance *(13)*. Observational studies show that physical activity is also critical for preventing weight regain *(33,34)*. Evidence suggests that it is unlikely that one approach is appropriate for all patients *(13,35)*.

Healthy Diet

Achieving energy balance and maintaining a healthy body weight are critical for the prevention and treatment of type 2 diabetes, and limiting saturated fat intake can help prevent the vascular complications of diabetes *(36)*. Higher consumption of whole grains and dietary fiber is associated with reduced risk of diabetes in some studies *(37)*. The evidence that micronutrients influence the risk of diabetes is limited, although some studies suggest that certain micronutrients may affect glucose and insulin metabolism *(38)*.

The *Dietary Guidelines for Americans 2005 (39)* features Institute of Medicine reference intakes for macronutrients *(40)* and recommends a diet rich in fruits, vegetables, whole grains, and lean meats *(41)*. Dietary patterns *(42)* that emphasize these foods and limit red meat, full-fat dairy products, and foods and beverages high in added sugars are associated with decreased risk of a variety of chronic diseases *(14,43,44)*. Physicians can employ practical tools to teach their patients the key elements of the Dietary Guidelines *(96)*.

EXERCISE

Benefits

Data show that weight loss programs that combine diet and exercise produce greater improvements in cardiovascular risk factors than those that rely on diet alone *(45,46)*, including significant reductions in the incidence of diabetes *(47,48)*. Physical activity has been found to contribute to the maintenance of long-term weight loss *(49)*, improve cardiorespiratory and muscular fitness, and reduce risk factors for cardiovascular and metabolic diseases *(10,50)*. Accumulating evidence indicates that physical activity reduces the risk of chronic disease both directly, through its impact on hormones, and indirectly, through its impact on weight control *(36,51)*.

Physical Activity and Weight Change

Six large studies, including four randomized controlled trials, have tested whether progression from prediabetes to diabetes could be delayed or prevented by intensive lifestyle modification (nutrition and exercise interventions) or by use of commercially available glucose-lowering drugs *(2,4,47,48,52,53)*. All of the interventions were effective to varying degrees. In the lifestyle-modification studies, results were obtained by a modest reduction in body weight and moderate exercise (e.g., walking) *(36)*.

Recommended Treatment

TYPE OF EXERCISE

Data from the Diabetes Prevention Program *(3)* showed that a 5–7% weight loss achieved through diet and exercise reduced the incidence of diabetes by 58% in participants randomized to lifestyle intervention; those in this group lowered their intake of fat and calories, and exercised at moderate intensity, usually by walking an average of 30 min/d, 5 d/wk. This level of exercise is consistent with a consensus public health recommendation for physical activity developed in the mid-1990s *(50,54,55)*. It is also known to reduce the risk of diabetes *(56–59)*. Current recommendations for physical activity call for 30–60 min/d of moderate-intensity activity (e.g., brisk walking) *(10)*.

DURATION: LONG OR SHORT BOUTS

Studies show that total exercise time is greater when daily physical activity is divided into many short bouts (e.g., 10-min bouts, three to four times a day) compared with one long bout (e.g., 30–40 min once per day) *(60)*. Although many short rounds of activity produce greater adherence to an exercise program, most data suggest that the total volume of physical activity is the only factor of importance to weight management *(13)*.

INTENSITY

The beneficial effect of exercise is dose related, increasing with the duration and amount of energy expended. Available evidence suggests that a high volume of physical activity—80–90 min of moderate-intensity activity, such as walking, or 35 min of vigorous exercise, such as jogging—is needed to maintain weight loss *(33)*. Data show that physical activity is critical for preventing weight regain *(33,34,51)*.

MOTIVATION

Several strategies have been used to enhance long-term maintenance of physical activity *(13)*. These include patient participation in a traditionally structured gymnasium-based program or a behaviorally-based intervention *(61)*, increased contact by mail or telephone *(62)*, development of a home-based walking program (i.e., the use of a treadmill), *(63)* and incorporation of exercise into activities of daily living (e.g., taking the stairs instead of an elevator). These initiatives notwithstanding, all studies report a decline in exercise adherence over time *(61–64)*.

BEHAVIOR MODIFICATION

Behavior Therapy

Behavior modification is a goal-oriented therapy that helps patients identify and change behaviors that prevent them from achieving their objectives for weight loss and increased physical activity. The approach is based on teaching patients how to set and achieve realistic and measurable goals. Behavior modifications involves making small rather than large changes so that incremental steps are taken toward more important and more distant goals *(65–67)*. Table 2 identifies and describes various strategies that patients can use to help them achieve positive long-term behavior change.

Self-Monitoring

Self-monitoring, the systematic observation and recording of target behaviors, is the cornerstone of behavioral treatment *(66)*. Self-monitoring tools include food diaries to record intake, types, amounts, calorie content, as well as times, places, and feelings; physical activity logs to track frequency, duration, and intensity of exercise; and body weight scales to record changes in body weight. Self-monitoring increases patients' awareness of behaviors, creates records that can be reviewed by health-care professionals, and identifies targets for intervention *(13)*.

Cognitive-Behavior Therapy

Cognitive restructuring takes place within the framework of behavior modification. It involves changing perceptions, thoughts, or beliefs that undermine efforts to manage

Table 2
Behavioral Strategies to Improve Weight Management[a]

Strategy	Description
Self-monitoring	Record "what, where, and when" of eating and physical activity to increase patients' awareness of their own behavior.
Goal setting	Set specific short-term targets in eating and exercise habits to achieve incremental improvements.
Stimulus control	Identify triggers associated with poor eating and physical activity behaviors, and design strategies to break the link.
Cognitive restructuring	Change perceptions, thoughts, or beliefs undermining weight control efforts, and help patients develop realistic expectations about weight loss.
Problem solving	Analyze situations preventing maintenance of a healthier lifestyle and identify possible solutions to problems; maintain a philosophy that planning, not willpower, is key to weight management.
Relapse prevention	Develop skills based on the premise that lapses in weight control behavior can be anticipated in certain situations (e.g., travel, celebrations, bad mood); identify triggers that lead to overeating.
Stress management	Decrease psychological stress to prevent dysfunctional eating.
Contingency management	Use rewards (tangible or verbal) to increase performance of specific behaviors or when specified goals are reached.
Social support	Use assistance from family members and friends in modifying lifestyle behaviors.
Ongoing contact	Maintain visits, telephone calls, or Internet communication with physicians and office staff or other health care professionals to promote adherence with recommended lifestyle changes.

[a]Adapted from ref. *13*.

weight, and helping patients develop realistic expectations about weight loss. Formal behavior therapy can take place in group or one-on-one sessions with a health-care professional who is skilled in the delivery of behavioral techniques used to modify lifestyle habits *(65,68)*.

Motivational Interviewing

STAGES OF CHANGE

According to the transtheoretical or stages of change model, the process of change is seen as a series of steps (Table 3), each with certain tasks and characteristics. These have been successfully incorporated into smoking cessation program and are now being used to help people lose weight *(69)* and increase physical activity *(70)*. The stages are precontemplation, contemplation, preparation, action, maintenance, and relapse/recycling. Clinicians can help patients move from one level to the next by providing stage-appropriate information support, or tools.

PATIENT READINESS TO CHANGE

Motivational interviewing is a client-centered, directive method for enhancing intrinsic motivation to change by exploring and resolving ambivalence. Compared with nondirective counseling, it is more focused and goal directed. The examination and resolution of ambivalence is its central purpose, and the counselor is intentionally directive in pursuit of this goal *(71)*. By identifying and defusing resistances, physicians can create opportunities for change, as well as agendas for achieving it.

Table 3
Stages of Change Model[a]

- Precontemplation—not ready for change
- Contemplation—thinking about change
- Preparation—getting ready to make a change, planning, and commitment
- Action—making the change, implementing the plan, and taking the action
- Maintenance—sustaining and integrating behavior change
- Relapse/recycling—slipping back to previous behavior and reentering the cycle of change

[a]Adapted from ref. 95.

PATIENT-CENTERED COUNSELING

Patient-centered counseling is an approach that encourages patients to set goals and express their own ideas for therapy, with input from their health care provider. Treatment plans include realistic goals that take into account the patient's readiness for therapy and ability to comply with the proposed plan. Frequently scheduled follow-up visits are necessary to monitor progress, modify the treatment plan as called for, and provide encouragement (13,67).

TEAMWORK

Effective therapy requires a long-term structured approach with continued support from the physician and other caregivers, particularly during periods of patient recidivism and weight regain (13). Regular (65) and ongoing contact with patients (72,73) is known to promote long-term adherence and help prevent weight regain (67).

PROMOTING CHANGE

Data indicate that patients usually seek out and respect advice from their primary care physicians, and that such advice can motivate them to change unhealthy behavior (74–76). Studies show that the process of change is gradual, especially in adults (77). Most people are unable to convert new behavior into habitual practice without guided application of a significant length of time (78).

In the Look AHEAD (Action for Health in Diabetes) Trial, for example, obese patients are randomly assigned to Lifestyle or Diabetes Support and Education interventions for 4 yr, with 7.5 yr of follow-up (79). Similarly, the Women's Intervention Nutrition Study protocol includes randomization to intensive dietary intervention with long-term counseling followed by monthly group sessions (80).

Although there are no formulas for changing minds or behaviors, certain similarities apply to most individuals. Data indicate that people learn and change through successive approximation (81), and that they need to hear a message several times and in a variety of ways before it can become an impetus to action. Other ways to move patients toward new eating and activity behaviors include implementing interpersonal sensitivity, setting up patient-important (82) encounters, confronting resistances, participating in give-and-take, and fostering bonds by engaging individuals or group members in a common enterprise (35,67,77).

CONCLUSIONS

From 1990 to 2001, the prevalence of diabetes increased by 61%, with approx 1.3 million Americans developing diabetes each year (83). The increase in type 2 diabetes, which accounts for 90–95% of all diagnosed cases, is a result of the epidemic increase in excess body weight that occurred in the US population during that period *(84)*. Weight loss can improve many obesity-related comorbidities, including insulin resistance and type 2 diabetes. It can also prevent the development of new diabetes in high-risk persons who are overweight or obese *(84–87)*.

Weight loss resulting from negative energy balance can be achieved by decreasing energy intake, increasing energy expenditure, or both *(13)*. Data have shown that lifestyle dietary and activity modifications leading to approx 5% weight loss decreased the 4- to 6-yr cumulative incidence of diabetes by more than 50% in men and women who are overweight or obese and have impaired glucose tolerance *(3,5)*. The Swedish Obese Subjects Study demonstrated similar outcomes *(88)*.

Twenty-eight percent of American adults lead sedentary lifestyles *(89)*. Current recommendations for physical activity call for 30–60 min/d of moderate activity *(90)*. Efforts to achieve the goals of *Healthy People 2010 (91)* require new strategies for delivering primary and secondary prevention via intensive lifestyle modifications, i.e., nutritional and exercise interventions. At present, the preventive health care model receives only sporadic attention in the context of office visits for acute and chronic medical problems *(92)*.

To successfully attack the interrelated diseases of obesity and diabetes, health-care providers and medical organizations need to transform that model into a system that provides preventive care and early detection as an integral part of standard medical practice *(93)*. A treatment strategy based on the National Heart, Lung, and Blood Institute's clinical guidelines on obesity and the Surgeon General's reports on physical activity *(55)* and obesity *(94)* offers clinicians an easily adapted, evidence-based blueprint for incorporating information about weight and exercise into discussions with patients *(95)*. One helpful approach that summarizes these key recommendations into an easily remembered acronym is "CQE:" Cut Calories, Choose Quality Foods, and Exercise daily for good health and weight loss *(97)*.

ACKNOWLEDGMENT

The author would like to acknowledge the support of the S. Daniel Abraham Teaching Fund and the Harvard Center for Healthy Living at Harvard Medical School, the National Institute of Diabetes and Digestive and Kidney Diseases Grant P30-DK-40561, Look AHEAD: Action for Health in Diabetes P30-DK-57154, and the Boston Obesity Nutrition Research Center (BONRC) P30-DK-46200.

There is no conflict of interest. The author thanks Rita Buckley for assistance with medical writing.

REFERENCES

1. Centers for Disease Control and Prevention. National Diabetes Fact Sheet: General Information and National Estimates on Diabetes in the United States, 2003. U.S. Department of Health and Human Services, Centers for Disease Control and Prevention, Atlanta, 2004.
2. National Institute of Diabetes and Digestive Kidney Diseases. Diabetes Mellitus Interagency Coordinating Committee. Diabetes Prevention Program Meeting Summary. National Institutes of Health, Bethesda, MD, 2001.
3. Knowler WC, Brrett-Connor E. Diabetes Prevention Program Research Group, Fowler SE, Hamman RF, Lachin JM, Walker EA, Nathan DM. Reduction in the incidence of type 2 diabetes with lifestyle intervention or metformin. N Engl J Med 2002;346:393–403.
4. Sherwin RS, Anderson RM, Buse JB, et al. The prevention or delay of type 2 diabetes. American Diabetes Association. National Institute of Diabetes and Digestive and Kidney Diseases. Diabetes Care 2004;27(Suppl 1):S47–S54.

5. Tuomilehto J, Lindstrom J, Eriksson JG, et al. Prevention of type 2 diabetes mellitus by changes in lifestyle among subjects with impaired glucose tolerance. N Engl J Med 2001;344:1343–1350.

6. UKPDS Group. UK Prospective Diabetes Study 7: response of fasting plasma glucose to diet therapy in newly presenting type II diabetic patients, Metabolism 1990;39:905–912.

7. Dattilo AM, Kris-Etherton PM. Effects of weight reduction on blood lipids and lipoproteins: a meta-analysis. Am J Clin Nutr 1992;56:320–328.

8. Williams KV, Kelley DE. Metabolic consequences of weight loss on glucose metabolism and insulin action in type 2 diabetes. Diabetes Obes Metab 2000;2:121–129.

9. Blackburn G. Effect of degree of weight loss on health benefits. Obes Res 1995;3:211s–216s.

10. NHLBI. The Practical Guide to the Identification, Evaluation, and Treatment of Overweight and Obesity in Adults, National Heart, Lung, and Blood Institute, Bethesda, MD, 2000.

11. Kelley DE, Wing R, Buonocore C, Sturis J, Polonsky K, Fitzsimmons M. Relative effects of calorie restriction and weight loss in noninsulin-dependent diabetes mellitus. J Clin Endocrinol Metab 1993;77:1287–1293.

12. Wing RR, Koeske R, Epstein LH, Nowalk MP, Gooding W, Becker D. Long-term effects of modest weight loss in type II diabetic patients. Arch Intern Med 1987;147:1749–1753.

13. Klein S, Burke LE, Bray GA, et al. American Heart Association Council on Nutrition, Physical Activity, and Metabolism; American College of Cardiology Foundation. Clinical implications of obesity with specific focus on cardiovascular disease: a statement for professionals from the American Heart Association Council on Nutrition, Physical Activity, and Metabolism: endorsed by the American College of Cardiology Foundation. Circulation 2004;110:2952–2967.

14. Ello-Martin JA, Ledikwe JH, Roe LS, Rolls BJ. The influence of food portion size and energy density on energy intake: implications for weight management. Am J Clin Nutr 2005;82:236S–241S.

15. Clinical Guidelines on the Identification, Evaluation, and Treatment of Overweight and Obesity in Adults—The Evidence Report. National Institutes of Health. Obes Res 1998;6(Suppl 2):51S–209S.

16. Astrup A, Meinert Larsen T, Harper A. Atkins and other low-carbohydrate diets: hoax or an effective tool for weight loss? Lancet 2004;364:897–899.

17. Foster GD, Wyatt HR, Hill JO, et al. A randomized trial of a low-carbohydrate diet for obesity. N Engl J Med 2003;348:2082–2090.

18. Stern L, Iqbal N, Seshadri P, et al. The effects of low-carbohydrate versus conventional weight loss diets in severely obese adults: one-year follow-up of a randomized trial. Ann Intern Med 2004;140:778–785.

19. Rolls BJ, Morris EL, Roe LS. Portion size of food affects energy intake in normal-weight and overweight men and women. Am J Clin Nutr 2002;76:1207–1213.

20. Jeffery RW, Wing RR, Thorson C, Burton LR, Raether C, Harvey J, Mullen M. Strengthening behavioral interventions for weight loss: a randomized trial of food provision and monetary incentives. J Consult Clin Psychol 1993;61:1038–1045.

21. Ditschuneit HH, Flechtner-Mors M, Adler G. Metabolic and weight loss effects of long-term dietary intervention in obese subjects. Am J Clin Nutr 1999;69:198–204.

22. Flechtner-Mors M, Ditschuneit HH, Johnson TD, Suchard MA, Adler G. Metabolic and weight-loss effects of a long-term dietary intervention in obese patients: a four-year follow-up. Obes Res 2000;8:399–402.

23. Zemel MB. Role of calcium and dairy products in energy partitioning and weight management. Am J Clin Nutr 2004;79:709S–912S.

24. Lin YC, Lyle RM, McCabe LD, McCabe GP, Weaver CM, Teegarden D. Dairy calcium is related to changes in body composition during a two-year exercise intervention in young women. J Am Coll Nutr 2000;19:754–760.

25. Lovejoy JC, Champagne CM, Smith SR, de Jonge L, Xie H. Ethnic differences in dietary intakes, physical activity, and energy expenditure in middle-aged, premenopausal women: the Healthy Transitions Study. Am J Clin Nutr 2001;74:90–95.

26. Buchowski MS, Semenya J, Johnson AO. Dietary calcium intake in lactose maldigesting intolerant and tolerant African-American women. J Am Coll Nutr 2002;21:47–54.

27. Heaney RP, Davies KM, Barger-Lux MJ. Calcium and weight: clinical studies. J Am Coll Nutr 2002;21:152S–155S.

28. Heaney RP. Normalizing calcium intake: projected population effects for body weight. J Nutr 2003;133:268S–270S.

29. Pereira MA, Jacobs DR Jr, Van Horn L, Slattery ML, Kartashov AI, Ludwig DS. Dairy consumption, obesity, and the insulin resistance syndrome in young adults: the CARDIA Study. JAMA 2002;287:2081–2089.

30. Zemel MB, Thompson W, Milstead A, Morris K, Campbell P. Calcium and dairy acceleration of weight and fat loss during energy restriction in obese adults. Obes Res 2004;12:582–590.

31. Zemel MB, Nocton AM, Richards JD. Dairy (yogurt) augments fat loss and reduces central adiposity during energy restriction in obese subjects. FASEB J 2003;A1088:(abstract).

32. Zemel MB, Nocton AM, Richards JD. Increasing dairy calcium intake reduces adiposity in obese African-American adults. Circulation 2002;106 (Suppl):II-610 (abstract).

33. Saris WH, Blair SN, van Baak MA, et al. How much physical activity is enough to prevent unhealthy weight gain? Outcome of the IASO 1st Stock Conference and consensus statement. Obes Rev 2003;4:101–114.

34. Jakicic JM, Clark K. American College of Sports Medicine, Coleman E, Donnelly JE, Foreyt J, Melanson E, Volek J, Volpe SL. American College of Sports Medicine position stand: appropriate intervention strategies for weight loss and prevention of weight regain for adults. Med Sci Sports Exerc 2001;33:2145–2156.

35. Wing RR, Phelan S. Long-term weight loss maintenance. Am J Clin Nutr 2005;82:222S–225S.

36. Eyre H, Kahn R. American Cancer Society. American Diabetes Association. American Heart Association Collaborative Writing Committee, Robertson RM, Clark NG, Doyle C, et al. Preventing cancer, cardiovascular disease, and diabetes: a common agenda for the American Cancer Society, the American Diabetes Association, and the American Heart Association. Stroke 2004;35: 1999–2010.

37. Hu FB, Manson JE, Stampfer MJ, Colditz G, Liu S, Solomon CG, Willett WC. Diet, lifestyle, and the risk of type 2 diabetes mellitus in women. N Engl J Med 2001;345:790–797.

38. Franz MJ, Bantle JP, Beebe CA, et al. Evidence-based nutrition principles and recommendations for the treatment and prevention of diabetes and related complications. Diabetes Care 2002;25:148–198.

39. Dietary Guidelines Advisory Committee. 2005 Dietary Guidelines Advisory Committee Report. The U.S. Departments of Health and Human Services (HHS) and Agriculture (USDA), Washington DC, 2005.

40. Institute of Medicine. Food and Nutrition Board. Dietary Reference Intakes for Energy, Carbohydrate, Fiber, Fat, Fatty Acids, Cholesterol, Protein, and Amino Acids (Macronutrients). The National Academies of Sciences, Washington DC, 2004.

41. Fung TT, Rimm EB, Spiegelman D, Rifai N, Tofler GH, Willett WC, Hu FB. Association between dietary patterns and plasma biomarkers of obesity and cardiovascular disease risk. Am J Clin Nutr 2001;73:61–67.

42. Dietary patterns for weight management and health. Proceedings of a symposium. Dallas, Texas, USA. April 27–29, 2001. Obes Res 2001;9(Suppl 4):217S–358S.

43. Krauss RM, Eckel RH, Howard B, et al. AHA Dietary Guidelines: revision 2000: A statement for healthcare professionals from the Nutrition Committee of the American Heart Association. Circulation 2000;102:2284–2299.

44. Byers T, Nestle M, McTiernan A, et al. American Cancer Society 2001 Nutrition and Physical Activity Guidelines Advisory Committee. American Cancer Society guidelines on nutrition and physical activity for cancer prevention: Reducing the risk of cancer with healthy food choices and physical activity. CA Cancer J Clin 2002;52:92–119.

45. Stefanik ML. Physical activity for preventing and treating obesity-related dyslipoproteinemias. Med Sci Sports 1999;31:609–618.

46. Wing RR. Physical activity in the treatment of adult overweight and obesity. Med Sci Sports 1999;31:547–552.

47. Pan XR, Li GW, Hu YH, et al. Effects of diet and exercise in preventing NIDDM in people with impaired glucose tolerance: the Da Qing IGT and Diabetes Study. Diabetes Care 1997;20:537–544.

48. Eriksson J, Lindgarde F. Prevention of type 2 diabetes mellitus by diet and physical exercise. Diabetologia 1991;34:891–898.

49. Wing RR, Jeffery RW. Benefits of recruiting participants with friends and increasing social support for weight loss and maintenance. J Consult Clin Psychol 1999;67:132–138.

50. Pate RR, Pratt M, Blair SN, et al. Physical activity and public health: a recommendation from the Centers for Disease Control and Prevention and the American College of Sports Medicine. JAMA 1995;273:402–407.

51. Jakicic JM, Otto AD. Physical activity considerations for the treatment and prevention of obesity. Am J Clin Nutr 2005;82:226S–229S.

52. Buchanan TA, Xiang AH, Peters RK, et al. Preservation of pancreatic beta-cell function and prevention of type 2 diabetes by pharmacological treatment of insulin resistance in high-risk hispanic women. Diabetes 2002;51:2796–2803.

53. Chiasson JL, Josse RG, Gomis R, Hanefeld M, Karasik A, Laakso M. STOP-NIDDM Trial Research Group. Acarbose for prevention of type 2 diabetes mellitus: the STOP-NIDDM randomised trial. Lancet 2002;359:2072–2077.

54. NIH Consensus Development Panel on Physical Activity and Cardiovascular Health. Physical activity and cardiovascular health. JAMA 1996;276:241–246.

55. Physical Activity and Health: A Report of the Surgeon General. US Department of Health and Human Services, Centers for Disease Control and Prevention, Washington, DC, 1996.

56. National Cholesterol Education Program (NCEP) Expert Panel on Detection, Evaluation and Treatment of High Blood Cholesterol in Adults (Adult Treatment Panel III). Third Report of the National Cholesterol Education Program (NCEP) Expert Panel on Detection, Evaluation, and Treatment of High Blood Cholesterol in Adults (Adult Treatment Panel III) final report. Circulation 2002;106:3143–3421.

57. Yang D, Fontaine KR, Wang C, Allison DB. Weight loss causes increased mortality: cons. Obes Rev 2003;4:9–16.

58. Fontaine KR, Redden DT, Wang C, Westfall AO, Allison DB. Years of life lost due to obesity. JAMA 2003;289:187–193.

59. Miller WC, Koceja DM, Hamilton EJ. A meta-analysis of the past 25 years of weight loss research using diet, exercise or diet plus exercise intervention. Int J Obes Relat Metab Disord 1997;21: 941–947.

60. Jakicic JM, Wing RR, Butler BA, Robertson RJ. Prescribing exercise in multiple short bouts versus one continuous bout: effects on adherence, cardiorespiratory fitness, and weight loss in overweight women. Int J Obes Relat Metab Disord 1995;19:893–901.

61. Dunn AL, Marcus BH, Kampert JB, Garcia ME, Kohl HW 3rd, Blair SN. Comparison of lifestyle and structured interventions to increase physical activity and cardiorespiratory fitness: a randomized trial. JAMA 1999;281:327–334.

62. Castro CM, King AC, Brassington GS. Telephone versus mail interventions for maintenance of physical activity in older adults. Health Psychol 2001;20:438–444.

63. Jakicic JM, Winters C, Lang W, Wing RR. Effects of intermittent exercise and use of home exercise equipment on adherence, weight loss, and fitness in overweight women: a randomized trial. JAMA 1999;282:1554–1560.

64. King AC, Taylor CB, Haskell WL, Debusk RF. Strategies for increasing early adherence to and long-term maintenance of home-based exercise training in healthy middle-aged men and women. Am J Cardiol 1988;61:628–632.

65. Foreyt JP, Poston WS 2nd. The role of the behavioral counselor in obesity treatment. J Am Diet Assoc 1998;98(10)(Suppl 2):S27–S30.

66. Wing RR. Behavioral approaches to the treatment of obesity. In: Bray GA, Bouchard C, James WPT eds. Handbook of Obesity. New York, Marcel Dekker, 1998;855–873.

67. Foster GD, Makris AP, Bailer BA. Behavioral treatment of obesity. Am J Clin Nutr 2005;82:2305–2355.

68. Wadden TA, Sarwer DB, Berkowitz RI. Behavioural treatment of the overweight patient. Baillieres Best Pract Res Clin Endocrinol Metab 1999;13:93–107.

69. Greene GW, Rossi SR, Rossi JS, Velicer WF, Fava JL, Prochaska JO. Dietary applications of the stages of change model. J Am Diet Assoc 1999;99:673–678.

70. Sarkin JA, Johnson SS, Prochaska JO, Prochaska JM. Applying the transtheoretical model to regular moderate exercise in an overweight population: validation of a stages of change measure. Prev Med 2001;33:462–469.

71. Rollnick S, Miller WR. What is motivational interviewing? Behav Cognitive Psychother 1995; 23:325–334.

72. Perri MG, Nezu AM, Patti ET, McCann KL. Effect of length of treatment on weight loss. J Consult Clin Psychol 1989;57:450–452.

73. Perri MG, Shapiro RM, Ludwig WW, Twentyman CT, McAdoo WG. Maintenance strategies for the treatment of obesity: an evaluation of relapse prevention training and posttreatment contact by mail and telephone. J Consult Clin Psychol 1984;52:404–413.

74. Stead LF. 2001. Physician advice for smoking cessation (Cochrane Review). Cochrane Database Syst Rev:CD000165.

75. Kreuter MW, Chheda SG, Bull FC. How does physician advice influence patient behavior? Evidence for a priming effect. Arch Fam Med 2000;9:426–433.

76. Bull FC, Jamrozik K. Advice on exercise from a family physician can help sedentary patients to become active. Am J Prev Med 1998;15:85–94.

77. Gardner H. Changing Minds: The Art and Science of Changing Our Own and Other People's Minds. Harvard Business School Press, Boston, 2004.

78. Blackburn GL. Teaching, learning, doing—best practices in education. Am J Clin Nutr 2005;82: 218S–221S.

79. Ryan DH, Espeland MA, Foster GD, et al. Look AHEAD Research. Look AHEAD (Action for Health in Diabetes): design and methods for a clinical trial of weight loss for the prevention of cardiovascular disease in type 2 diabetes. Control Clin Trials 2003;24:610–628.

80. The Women's Health Initiative Study Group. Design of the Women's Health Initiative clinical trial and observational study. Control Clin Trials 1998;19:61–109.

81. DiClemente CC. Motivational enhancement therapy. In: Programs and abstracts of the American Society of Addiction Medicine 2003, Session 1. In The State of the Art in Addiction Medicine. Washington, DC.

82. Guyatt G, Montori V, Devereaux PJ, Schunemann H, Bhandari M. Patients at the center: in our practice, and in our use of language. ACP J Club 2004;140:A11.

83. US Department of Health and Human Services, Centers for Disease Control and Prevention. National Diabetes Fact Sheet: United States, 2003. Centers for Disease Control, Silver Spring, MD, 2003.

84. Mokdad AH, Ford ES, Bowman BA, Nelson DE, Engelgau MM, Vinicor F, Marks JS. Diabetes trends in the U.S.: 1990–1998. Diabetes Care 2000;23:1278–1283.

85. Jemal A, Tiwari RC, Murray T, Ghafoor A, Samuels A, Ward E, Feuer EJ, Thun MJ, with the American Cancer Society. Cancer statistics, 2004. CA Cancer J Clin 2004;54:8–29.

86. Mokdad AH, Marks JS, Stroup DF, Gerberding JL. Actual causes of death in the United States, 2000. JAMA 2004;291:1238–1245.

87. Centers for Disease Control and Prevention (CDC). Annual smoking-attributable mortality, years of potential life lost, and economic costs: United States, 1995–1999. MMWR Morb Mortal Wkly Rep 2002;51:300–303.

88. Sjostrom CD, Peltonen M, Wedel H, Sjostrom L. Differentiated long-term effects of intentional weight loss on diabetes and hypertension. Hypertension 2000;36:20–25.

89. USDA Center for Nutrition Policy and Promotion. Interactive Healthy Eating Index, Washington DC, 2004.

90. National Task Force on the Prevention and Treatment of Obesity. Overweight, obesity, and health risk. Arch Intern Med 2000;160:898–904.

91. Office of Disease Prevention and Health Promotion US. Department of Health and Human Services. Healthy People 2010. (Conference Edition in Two Volumes). Washington DC. January 2000.

92. Smith RA, Wender RC. Cancer screening and the periodic health examination. Cancer 2004;100: 1553–1557.

93. Blackburn GL, Walker WA. Introduction. Symposium: science-based solutions to obesity. What are the roles of academia, government, industry, and healthcare? Am J Clin Nutr 2005;82:207S–210S.

94. US Department of Health and Human Services. The Surgeon General's Call to Action to Prevent and Decrease Overweight and Obesity. US Department of Health and Human Services, Public Health Service, Office of the Surgeon General, Rockville, MD, 2001.

95. Manson JE, Skerrett PJ, Greenland P, VanItallie TB. The escalating pandemics of obesity and sedentary lifestyle: a call to action for clinicians. arch Intern Med 2004;164:249–258.

96. Blackburn GL, Waltman BA. Physician's guide to the new dietary guidelines 2005; now best to counsel patients. Cleve Clin J Med 2005;72:609–618.

97. Blackburn GL, Waltman BA. Expanding the limits of treatment-new strategies initiatives. J Am Diet Assoc 2005;105:S131–S135.

26 Medical Approaches to Treatment of the Obese Patient

George A. Bray, MD and Donna H. Ryan, MD

INTRODUCTION

Obesity has become a major focus of modern medicine, driven by the pandemic of overweight and obesity. The prevalence of obesity is rising to epidemic proportions around the world at an alarming rate. Current prevalence data from individual European national studies suggest rates of body mass index (BMI) ≥ 30 kg/m^2 for men are 10–20% and for women, 10–25% (1). In 2002, the National Health and Nutrition Examination Survey identified 64.5% of the US population with a BMI ≥ 25 kg/m^2 and 30.5% with obesity (BMI ≥ 30 kg/m^2) (2). More important, in this survey, 4.7% of the population had a BMI >40 kg/m^2 (2), and met the BMI criteria for bariatric surgery (3).

What is of concern about the obesity epidemic, of course, is the morbidities that accompany obesity. While there is alarm over the links among the obesity, diabetes, and cardiovascular risks, there is an appreciation by public health officials that even modest weight reduction can produce substantial health benefits. The US Diabetes Prevention Program (DPP) (4) and the Finnish Diabetes Prevention Study (5) both demonstrated significant reduction in risk of diabetes in persons with impaired glucose tolerance (IGT) who lost as little as 5–7% of baseline weight. Thus, physicians must develop effective office-based approaches to the management of obesity. Medicating for obesity is a tool unique to

From: *Contemporary Diabetes: Obesity and Diabetes*
Edited by: C. S. Mantzoros © Humana Press Inc., Totowa, NJ

physicians, and if they are to stem the tide of obesity-related morbidities, physicians must be knowledgeable about the use of medications in at-risk patients. This chapter is an updated guide to current practices in medicating for the management of obesity.

REALITIES OF TREATMENT

Obesity is a chronic, relapsing disease that has many causes. Environmental, biological, and psychological factors all play a role in the current prevalence of obesity. In most patients presenting with obesity, a clear etiological diagnosis is usually not possible. Because of its chronic nature and relative unknown cause, curing obesity is rare, but palliation is a realistic clinical goal. Weight loss occurs with most treatments, and except for surgery or very low-calorie diets it is usually slow, meaning 0.5–1.0 kg/wk. Recidivism, or regain of body weight, is common after a weight loss program is terminated. In contrast to the relatively slow rate of weight loss, weight regain may be rapid. A regain in weight after termination of drug or other treatment is often ascribed to a failure of the drugs or other treatment. A more appropriate interpretation is that medications do not work if not taken. This is true of medications for the treatment of obesity, just as it is for medications used to treat hypertension, diabetes, heart disease, or asthma. Lifestyle approaches to weight management also must be consistently implemented if they are to be of benefit. As clinicians, we do not expect to cure such diseases as hypertension or hypercholesterolemia with medications. Rather, we expect to palliate them. When the medications for any of these diseases are discontinued, we expect the disease to recur. This means that medications only work when used. The same arguments go for medications used to treat overweight. It is a chronic, incurable disease for which drugs only work when used.

Many physicians and laypeople are leery of treatments for obesity. This concern stems from problems associated with the use of drugs and some diets. First, almost every drug and some diets that have been used to treat obesity have been associated with undesirable outcomes that have resulted in injury or death (6). One of the most serious was the appearance of cardiac valvulopathy following treatment with fenfluramine and dexfenfluramine (7–11). Fenfluramine and dexfenfluramine were subsequently withdrawn from the market. Second, some medications, particularly amphetamines and methamphetamines, are addictive, and this has tarnished the use of drugs with similar chemical structures, whether or not they have been demonstrated to be addictive (12). For example, abuse of either phentermine or diethylpropion is rare (6). Fenfluramine, a drug with a chemical structure similar to that of amphetamine, has not been reported to be addictive. Even though sibutramine has no abuse potential (13), the drug was given a class IV designation by the Food and Drug Administration (FDA). Finally, weight-loss medications are infrequently reimbursed by health insurers and frequently marketed at prices nearing $100/mo. Because patients often must pay out of pocket for these medications, high cost is a barrier to continued use. In weighing the options for treatment of obesity, physicians must be cognizant of these barriers to success.

EVALUATION OF THE OBESE PATIENT: CLASSIFICATION AND RISK ASSESSMENT OF OBESITY

The first step in assessing the obese patient is to consider potential causes of the condition. Table 1 outlines an etiological classification of obesity. Whereas secondary causes of obesity are rare, endocrine and hypothalamic syndromes, such as leptin

Table 1
Etiological Classification of Obesity

- Genetic
- Hypothalamic
- Endocrine
- Dietary
- Sedentary lifestyle
- Drug-induced
- Idiopathic

Table 2
Drugs Associated With Weight Gain

Psychiatric/neurological
    Antipsychotics: olazapine, clozapine, risperidone
    Antidepressants: selective serotonin reuptake inhibitors,
      tricyclic antidepressants
    Lithium
    Antiepileptics: valproate, gabapentin, carbamazepine
Diabetes treatment
    Insulin
    Sulfonylureas
    Thiazolidinediones
Others
    Hormonal contraceptives
    Corticosteroids
    Progestational agents
    Antihistamines
    β-Blockers, α-blockers

deficiency, hypothyroidism, Cushing syndrome, growth hormone deficiency, Prader-Willi syndrome, and hypothalamic injury, must be considered.

Although diet and a sedentary lifestyle are always contributory, physicians must remember that the amount of energy imbalance required to result in significant weight gain does not usually manifest as sloth or gluttony. With an excess energy intake of only 100 kcal/d, >5 kg will be gained in 1 yr, and 50 kg in 10 yr. Whereas there are strong genetic influences on weight and body habitus, the cause of the obesity epidemic of the last 30 yr is an environmental, rather than a genetic, shift.

Table 2 lists drugs that may be associated with weight gain. Many common medications promote weight gain, and physicians must be cognizant of the additional health risks imposed by such weight gain and seek alternative therapy for susceptible individuals. A recent review of this subject is helpful (*see* ref. *14*). Another problem is the excessive gain and weight retention that can follow pregnancy or that is associated with menopause. Not all women are susceptible, but at least a subset report the onset of obesity with these life events.

Operationally, BMI is a useful way of communicating the degree of overweight. Table 3 shows BMI values for various heights and weights. Whereas BMI may be elevated in bodybuilders without a concomitant increase in body fat, it generally reflects an increased percentage of total body fat. BMI may overestimate health risks from obesity

Table 3

A Table of Body Mass Index Using Either Pounds and Inches or Kilograms and Centimeters[a]

Height in inches		19	20	21	22	23	24	25	26	27	28	29	30	31	32	33	34	35	36	37	38	39	40	Centimeters
											Body mass index (kg/m^2)													
58	(lb)	91	95	100	105	110	115	119	124	129	134	138	143	148	153	158	162	167	172	177	181	186	191	
	(kg)	41	43	45	48	50	52	54	56	58	61	63	65	67	69	71	73	76	78	80	82	84	86	147
59	(lb)	94	99	104	109	114	119	124	128	133	138	143	148	153	158	163	168	173	178	183	188	193	198	
	(kg)	43	45	47	50	52	54	56	59	61	63	65	68	70	72	74	77	79	81	83	86	88	90	150
60	(lb)	97	102	107	112	118	123	128	133	138	143	148	153	158	164	169	174	179	184	189	194	199	204	
	(kg)	44	46	49	51	53	55	58	60	62	65	67	69	72	74	76	79	81	83	85	88	90	92	152
61	(lb)	100	106	111	116	121	127	132	137	143	148	153	158	164	169	174	180	185	190	195	201	206	211	
	(kg)	46	48	50	53	55	58	60	62	65	67	70	72	74	77	79	82	84	86	89	91	94	96	155
62	(lb)	104	109	115	120	125	131	136	142	147	153	158	164	169	175	180	186	191	196	202	207	213	218	
	(kg)	47	50	52	55	57	60	62	65	67	70	72	75	77	80	82	85	87	90	92	95	97	100	158
63	(lb)	107	113	118	124	130	135	141	146	152	158	163	169	175	180	186	192	197	203	208	214	220	225	
	(kg)	49	51	54	56	59	61	64	67	69	72	74	77	79	82	84	87	90	92	95	97	100	102	160
64	(lb)	110	116	122	128	134	140	145	151	157	163	169	174	180	186	192	198	203	209	215	221	227	233	
	(kg)	50	52	55	58	60	63	66	68	71	73	76	79	81	84	87	89	92	94	97	100	102	105	162
65	(lb)	114	120	126	132	138	144	150	156	162	168	174	180	186	192	198	204	210	216	222	228	234	240	
	(kg)	52	54	57	60	63	65	68	71	74	76	79	82	84	87	90	93	95	98	101	103	106	109	165
66	(lb)	117	124	130	136	142	148	155	161	167	173	179	185	192	198	204	210	216	223	229	235	241	247	
	(kg)	54	56	59	62	65	68	71	73	76	79	82	85	87	90	93	96	99	102	104	107	110	113	168
67	(lb)	121	127	134	140	147	153	159	166	172	178	185	191	198	204	210	217	223	229	236	242	248	255	
	(kg)	55	58	61	64	66	69	72	75	78	81	84	87	90	92	95	98	101	104	107	110	113	116	170

460

(in)		19	20	21	22	23	24	25	26	27	28	29	30	31	32	33	34	35	36	37	38	39	40	(cm)
68	(lb)	125	131	138	144	151	158	164	171	177	184	190	197	203	210	217	223	230	236	243	249	256	263	
	(kg)	57	60	63	66	69	72	75	78	81	84	87	90	93	96	99	102	105	108	111	114	117	120	173
69	(lb)	128	135	142	149	155	162	169	176	182	189	196	203	209	216	223	230	237	243	250	257	264	270	
	(kg)	58	61	64	67	70	74	77	80	83	86	89	92	95	98	101	104	107	110	113	116	119	123	175
70	(lb)	132	139	146	153	160	167	174	181	188	195	202	209	216	223	230	236	243	250	257	264	271	278	
	(kg)	60	63	67	70	73	76	79	82	86	89	92	95	98	101	105	108	111	114	117	120	124	127	178
71	(lb)	136	143	150	157	165	172	179	186	193	200	207	215	222	229	236	243	250	258	265	272	279	286	
	(kg)	62	65	68	71	75	78	81	84	87	91	94	97	100	104	107	110	113	117	120	123	126	130	180
72	(lb)	140	147	155	162	169	177	184	191	199	206	213	221	228	235	243	250	258	265	272	280	287	294	
	(kg)	64	67	70	74	77	80	84	87	90	94	97	100	104	107	111	114	117	121	124	127	131	134	183
73	(lb)	144	151	159	166	174	182	189	197	204	212	219	227	234	242	250	257	265	272	280	287	295	303	
	(kg)	65	68	72	75	79	82	86	89	92	96	99	103	106	110	113	116	120	123	127	130	133	137	185
74	(lb)	148	155	163	171	179	187	194	202	210	218	225	233	241	249	256	264	272	280	288	295	303	311	
	(kg)	67	71	74	78	81	85	88	92	95	99	102	106	110	113	117	120	124	127	131	134	138	141	188
75	(lb)	152	160	168	176	184	192	200	208	216	224	232	240	247	255	263	271	279	287	295	303	311	319	
	(kg)	69	72	76	79	83	87	90	94	97	101	105	108	112	116	119	123	126	130	134	137	141	144	190
76	(lb)	156	164	172	180	189	197	205	213	221	230	238	246	254	262	271	279	287	295	303	312	320	328	
	(kg)	71	74	78	82	86	89	93	97	101	104	108	112	115	119	123	127	130	134	138	142	145	149	193
BMI		19	20	21	22	23	24	25	26	27	28	29	30	31	32	33	34	35	36	37	38	39	40	BMI

[a]BMI is shown as bold underlined numbers at the top and bottom. To determine your BMI, select your height in either inches or centimeters and move across the row until you find your weight in pounds or kilograms. Your BMI can be read at the top or bottom. Italics denote pounds and inches; bold denotes kilograms and centimeters. (Copyright 1999 George A. Bray.)

Table 4
Metabolic Syndrome Criteria/NCEP *(16)* Criteria[a]

Risk factor	Defining level
Abdominal obesity	
Men	WC > 40 in. (102 cm)
Women	WC > 35 in. (88 cm)
Fasting glucose	≥110 mg/dL
Triglycerides	≥150 mg/dL
HDL cholesterol	
Men	<40 mg/dL
Women	<50 mg/dL
BP	≥130/85 mmHg

[a]The presence of three or more risk factors indicates metabolic syndrome.

in African American women and underestimate them in all Asians and Indians. On a practical level, clinical judgment usually suffices in interpreting BMI in relation to health risk. In particular, consideration of waist circumference (WC), in addition to BMI, can aid in risk assessment.

Intra-abdominal fat increases with age and carries the highest risk of developing cardiovascular and other disease consequences. Visceral fat distribution can be estimated by several techniques. The ratio of the circumference of the waist to the circumference of the hips has been widely used in epidemiological studies, but this is no better than the waist circumference alone. A WC >102 cm (40 in.) in men and >88 cm (35 in.) in women puts them in the high-risk category.

From epidemiological data, it is clear that increased abdominal fat, particularly visceral fat, carries increased risks. The top tertile in abdominal fat distribution nearly doubles the risk of mortality and morbidity from heart disease, diabetes, and hypertension. This extra risk is observed in men and women and rises sharply for the top 10th percentile of abdominal fat distribution *(15)*. When the difference in fat distribution is corrected, the excess mortality observed between men and women is largely, if not completely, eliminated. The risk associated with excess central accumulation of fat probably reflects the increase in visceral fat. Abnormal glucose tolerance, hypertension, and hyperlipidemia are more closely associated with the amount of visceral fat than with total body fat. The sagittal diameter has been proposed as a way to estimate visceral fat, but currently the only reliable way to determine visceral fat is with a computed tomography or magnetic resonance imaging scan. When newer, less-expensive methods become available, this will be an important clinical advance.

METABOLIC SYNDROME

In the United States, the definition of metabolic syndrome that is most commonly used is that derived from the 2001 National Cholesterol Education Program (NCEP) *(16)*. In Europe, the World Health Organization (WHO) has a different set of criteria *(17)*. Tables 4 and 5 provide the criteria proposed by each group for defining metabolic syndrome. The aim of using either of these sets of criteria is to identify persons with insulin resistance and the accompanying dyslipidemia (small, dense low-density lipoprotein [LDL] particles; low levels of high-density lipoprotein [HDL] cholesterol;

Table 5
WHO Definition *(17)* of Metabolic Syndrome, 1998[a]

1. Antihypertensive treatment and/or elevated BP (>160 mmHg systolic or >90 mmHg diastolic)
2. Elevated plasma triglyceride (>1.7 mmol/L) and/or low HDL cholesterol (<0.9 mmol/L in men, <1.0 mmol/L in women)
3. Elevated BMI (>30 kg/m^2 and/or WHR >0.90 in men and >0.85 in women)
4. Microalbuminuria urinary albumin excretion rate >20 mg/mL

[a]Insulin resistance (IR) plus any two of the listed conditions indicates metabolic syndrome. IR is defined as having type 2 diabetes, impaired fasting glucose, IGT (for those with normal fasting glucose values, <110 mg/dL), and being in the highest quartile of the homeostasis model of IR (HOMA-IR) index.

and elevated triglycerides), vascular dysfunction (elevations in blood pressure [BP]), and increased risk of developing of type 2 diabetes. Metabolic syndrome is best managed by weight reduction, as evidenced by the results of the DPP *(4)* and Finnish Diabetes Prevention trials *(5)*. We believe that the presence of metabolic syndrome is an indication for medical interventions to aid weight loss, because the health risks of the disorder justify that approach.

EVALUATION OF RISK TO GUIDE TREATMENT

Because all treatments for obesity entail some risk, it is important to decide whether drug treatment is appropriate for the risks involved. To do this requires an assessment of the risk associated with total fat and fat distribution, as well as an assessment of metabolic fitness and complicating factors. In general, clinical judgment can be used to "adjust" BMI to assess risk. We propose here a scheme that relies on fat distribution assessed by waist circumference and evaluation of other risk factors. Our scheme helps physicians codify the judgment decisions.

Body weights associated with a BMI of 19–25 kg/m^2 are good weights for most people. Body weights associated with a BMI >30 kg/m^2 are almost invariably associated with increasing risk. Risk assessment for a BMI of 25–30 kg/m^2 should include an accounting for visceral fat and other comorbid factors that are affected by body weight, such as diabetes, hypertension, and dyslipidemia. Table 6 shows how a BMI <30 kg/m^2 can be adjusted to reflect the risk imposed by visceral fat deposition as reflected in the WC. It also illustrates the adjustment that one may make to reflect the increased risk imparted by the presence of comorbid conditions, such as hyperlipidemia, hypertension, sleep apnea, and physical inactivity, and for degrees of weight gain since age 18.

Once relative risk is evaluated, the appropriateness of various treatments can be determined from Table 7, which uses BMI as an indicator of risk to suggest appropriate treatments. Lifestyle, diet, and exercise are appropriate for all levels of BMI. As BMI increases, consideration of adding medications to lifestyle measures is appropriate. At higher BMI levels, surgery becomes a viable consideration for the concerned patient who has failed in other attempts to lose weight.

INITIATION OF PHARMACOLOGICAL THERAPY

Practice guidelines, such as the National Institutes of Health, National Heart, Lung, and Blood Institute "Clinical Guidelines on the Identification, Evaluation, and

Table 6
Risk-Adjusted BMI Using Metabolic and Anthropometric Variables[a]

	Your BMI			
	Adjustment scores added to BMI (kg/m^2)			*BMI*
Points to be added	0	+1	+3	—
Weight gain since age 18 (kg)	<5	5–15	>15	—
Triglycerides (mg/dL)	<150	150–300	>300	—
HDL cholesterol (mg/dL)				
Male	>50	35–50	<35	—
Female	>60	45–60	<45	—
WC (cm)				
Male	<80 cm (32 in.)	80–100 cm (32–42 in.)	>100 cm (42 in.)	—
Female	<70 cm (28 in.)	70–90 cm (28–35 in.)	>90 cm (35 in.)	—
BP (mmHg)	<130/<80	130–160/80–95	>160/>95	—
Sleep apnea	Absent	—	Present	—
Physical activity	Regular	Sedentary	—	—
	Total right-hand column = your adjusted BMI			

[a]In the top right-hand blank, enter your current BMI. Then, for each row, select the appropriate amount for each risk factor if you know it, and write the points to be added in the blank in the right-hand column. After filling in all of the blanks to the right, add the adjusted values to your BMI for your adjusted BMI.

Table 7
Use of BMI to Select Appropriate Treatments

	BMI category (kg/m^2)				
Treatment	25–29.9	27–29.9	30–34.9	35–39.9	≥40
Diet, exercise, lifestyle	+	+	+	+	+
Pharmacotherapy		With comorbidities	+	+	+
Surgery				With comorbidities	+

Treatment of Overweight and Obesity in Adults—The Evidence Report" *(3)*, recommend a trial of behavioral approaches before medications are initiated. We endorse this approach. In practice, however, most obese patients who are candidates for medications have had prior weight loss attempts without lasting success, and physicians need only document this history.

First, before initiating drug therapy, counseling sessions with patients are important. Because the amount of weight reduction is correlated with the degree of behavioral change, assessing readiness to change is an important first step. The medications will, through biological measures, reinforce the intention to restrict food intake and modify eating behavior. However, patients can override their biological signals. If patients are to maximize the amount of weight lost during the active weight loss phase, they must be ready to change entrenched behavior patterns. Second, patients must have a realistic weight loss goal. It is unrealistic for very obese patients to expect to achieve the ideal BMI of 25 kg/m^2. However, loss of 5–10% initial body weight can translate into significant health benefits. A focus on a realistic weight loss goal of 10% and on health, rather than cosmetic benefits, is essential for the very obese. Once reached, the patient can then establish a new weight loss goal. One theory to the success of lifestyle change is setting small, achievable goals to prevent failure.

A frank discussion of side effects must be preliminary to a patient's consent to undergo treatment. Sibutramine can cause blood pressure elevation and patients must be prepared to return to their doctor for monitoring. Orlistat causes fat malabsorption and anal leakage by blocking up to 30% of fat digestion, and occasional diarrheal steatorrhea must be anticipated. Another facet of the counseling interview is to describe the weight gain that is certain to occur if medications are stopped and there has not been permanent lifestyle adaptation to maintain weight loss.

MEDICATION AS ADJUNCTIVE TREATMENT

Medications for the treatment of obesity are considered adjuncts to the overall treatment plan. The other components of a standard treatment protocol include the following:

- The use of meal replacements (i.e., shakes, bars, frozen entrees) as means of portion and calorie control. These are important adjuncts in the active weight loss and weight loss maintenance phases.
- Counseling on how to reduce fat and calorie intake.
- An exercise program that will increase activity such as walking.
- The use of techniques for behavior modification that can help the patient monitor food intake, increase physical activity, and develop constructive cognitive strategies for dealing with the everyday demands to eat.

STRATEGIES FOR PREVENTION OF RELAPSE
FOLLOWING WEIGHT LOSS

Physicians should develop a list of local resources for weight loss and lifestyle adaptation. Health clubs, hospital- or clinic-based programs, commercial programs (e.g., Weight Watchers, Jenny Craig, Weight Loss Resources, Nutri/System), and support organizations (e.g., Overeaters Anonymous, TOPS Club) can all play a role.

If a patient is an appropriate candidate, treatment options are discussed and medications are initiated with the behavioral program. Failure to lose >4 lb after 4–8 wk of treatment is considered "treatment failure." Nonresponsive patients should not continue on medication. Evidence from clinical trials demonstrates that weight loss plateaus after 6 mo or less. When patients discontinue the treatment, as they often do, they regain weight unless lifestyle changes have become a permanent part of daily life. Enrollees in our weight loss programs must commit to 1 yr of treatment and then are given the option of either continued medication or an intensive lifestyle program that incorporates exercise (burning >2000 kcal/wk) and behavior modification techniques. We encourage them to resume medication whenever weight regain exceeds 5% and provide "refresher courses" of more intensive therapy.

Table 8
FDA-Approved Drugs for Treatment of Obesity

Drug	Trade names	Dosage	US Drug Enforcement Agency schedule
Pancreatic lipase inhibitor approved for long-term use			
Orlistat	Xenical	120 mg three times daily before meals	—
Norepinephrine-serotonin reuptake inhibitor approved for long-term use			
Sibutramine	Meridia Reductil	5–15 mg/d	IV
Noradrenergic drugs approved for short-term use			
Diethylpropion	Tenuate Tenuate Dospan	25 mg three times daily 75 mg every morning	IV
Phentermine	Adipex Ionamin Slow Release	15–37.5 mg/d 15–30 mg/d	IV
Benzphetamine	Didrex	25–50 mg three times daily	III
Phendimetrazine	Bontril Prelu-2	17.5–70 mg three times daily 105 mg every day	III

The physician plays an important role in monitoring progress by providing positive reinforcement for success and devising constructive strategies for problem areas. Once weight has plateaued, the physician must shift emphasis to the lifelong goal of weight maintenance.

DRUGS APPROVED FOR CLINICAL USE IN TREATMENT OF OBESITY

Only two drugs are approved for long-term management of obesity by the Committee on Proprietary Medicinal Products (CPMP) and FDA: sibutramine (Meridia in the United States and Reductil in Europe) and orlistat (Xenical). Phentermine is still widely prescribed in the United States but has approval for short-term management of obesity—usually interpreted as use for a few weeks—and has been taken off the market in Europe. Phentermine is no longer patent protected in the United States and is thus relatively inexpensive. Other noradrenergic drugs are still available in the United States but are rarely used. Table 8 gives all drugs currently listed in the U.S. *Physicians' Desk Reference* with an obesity indication. We recommend two comprehensive reviews of obesity pharmacotherapy (*see* refs. *18* and *19*).

Sibutramine

Sibutramine entered the American market in 1997. It is a β-phenethylamine with a cyclobutyl group on the side chain. Sibutramine inhibits the reuptake of serotonin and norepinephrine and produces weight loss by a dual mechanism of action. It promotes satiety and increases energy expenditure, blocking the reduction in metabolic rate that accompanies weight loss. One key to successful use of sibutramine is to prescribe an appropriate dietary approach. Because sibutramine promotes satiety—it does not produce anorexia—it works best in a program that enforces regular portion-controlled meals. One regimen for the active weight loss period is to use two meal replacements (breakfast and lunch), two small fruit snacks (150 kcal each), and a sensible dinner (approx 600–700 kcal or two frozen entrees) in addition to sibutramine.

There are three key factors to sibutramine's efficacy. First, weight loss is dose related. The usual starting dose is 10 mg, but the drug may be increased to 15 mg. An advantage is sibutramine's once-a-day dosing. Second, the amount of initial weight loss is related to the intensity of the behavioral intervention. Highly structured, portion-controlled schemes produce the most weight loss. Third, sibutramine is very effective at weight loss maintenance. Placebo-controlled studies demonstrate successful weight loss maintenance with sibutramine for up to 2 yr.

In general, clinical trials inform us that about three-fourths of patients treated with 15 mg/d of sibutramine will achieve >5% weight loss and 80% of those will maintain that loss for 2 yr. About 5% of patients will not tolerate the drug because of adverse effects on BP and pulse. Some patients (approx 20%) are non responders.

Sibutramine, like other sympathomimetic agents, produces a small increase in mean heart rate and mean BP, which has been observed in clinical trials. The BP response is variable, however. A subset, about 5%, of patients appear to be sensitive to the BP effects and cannot tolerate sibutramine. Some patients may need to discontinue sibutramine because of BP elevations to a hypertensive range. Other side effects, including dry mouth, insomnia, and asthenia, are similar to those of other drugs. Sibutramine is not associated with valvular heart disease, primary pulmonary hypertension, or substance abuse.

Sibutramine should be used with caution in patients with cardiovascular disease and in those taking selective serotonin reuptake inhibitors. It should not be used within 2 wk of taking monoamine oxidase inhibitors nor should it be used with other noradrenergic agents. For more information on sibutramine's clinical use, readers are directed to ref. *20,* for a recent review.

Orlistat

Orlistat is marketed as Xenical. Fat digestion can be inhibited by blocking the enzymatic action of pancreatic lipase. In experimental studies, orlistat (tetrahydrolipstatin) has been shown to be a potent inhibitor of lipase activity that decreases intestinal triglyceride hydrolysis in a dose-dependent manner. In clinical trials, it also has a dose-dependent effect on fat absorption and weight loss. After a high-fat meal, steatorrheal diarrhea is expected, but gastrointestinal (GI) events in practice are mild to moderate, resolve spontaneously, and are usually limited to one or two episodes per patient. Deficiency of fat-soluble vitamins can occur, and vitamin supplementation should be used. In general, patients tolerate the drug very well, especially if there is advance patient education.

Orlistat works best when given with a diet that has approx 30% fat content, so patient counseling is important. If a high-fat meal or snack is consumed, GI distress can result. For a very-low-fat meal, orlistat will not produce a caloric deficit and patients on a low-fat diet will not lose weight while taking orlistat.

Orlistat is effective in producing and sustaining weight loss. It is given at a dose of 120 mg before meals three times daily. Data from clinical trials support that about 70%

of patients will achieve >5% weight loss and at 2 yr 70% of them will have maintained that loss. There are clinical trials documenting the use of orlistat for up to 4 yr.

One advantage of the use of orlistat is its beneficial effect on LDL cholesterol. Because orlistat blocks fat absorption, the reduction in LDL is about twice that seen with weight loss alone. A recent review provides more detail on the clinical use of orlistat (*see* ref. *21*).

OTHER DRUGS IN CLINICAL TRIALS

Bupropion, a drug approved by the FDA for treatment of depression, produces weight loss *(22)*. A 6-mo randomized, double-blind, placebo-controlled trial *(22)* compared two doses of bupropion against placebo. Both doses of medication produced significantly more weight loss than placebo. Topiramate is a neurotherapeutic agent approved for the treatment of epilepsy. A placebo-controlled, double-blind, randomized dose-ranging clinical trial of topiramate at doses of 64, 96, 192, and 184 mg/d produced dose-related weight loss but was also associated with dose-related increases in the number of neurological side effects. Zonisamide is another neurotherapeutic drug used in the treatment of epilepsy. In a 16-wk randomized, placebo-controlled clinical trial, it produced significantly greater weight loss than placebo. Rimonabant, an antagonist to the cannabinoid receptor-1 (CB-1), produced significant weight loss in a double-blind, randomized, placebo-controlled trial. This drug also reduces weight gain in individuals who stop smoking. Leptin is a peptide produced almost exclusively in adipose tissue. Absence of leptin produces massive obesity in mice (ob/ob) and in humans *(23),* and treatment with this peptide decreases food intake in the ob/ob mouse and the leptin-deficient human *(24)*. A dose-ranging clinical trial with leptin produced modest loss of weight with doses ranging from 0.01 to 0.3 mg/kg. Axokine, a modified form of ciliary neurotrophic factor, acts through the same janus kinase signal for transduction and translation system as leptin, but also through leptin-independent mechanisms, since Axokine reduces food intake in animals that lack leptin or leptin receptors *(25)*. In a randomized clinical trial, it produced modest weight loss that was much smaller in people who developed antibodies to it.

Neuropeptide Y (NPY) is one of the most potent stimulators of food intake and appears to act through NPY Y-5 and/or Y-1 receptors *(18)*. Several pharmaceutical companies are attempting to identify antagonists to these receptors *(26)*. Nasally administered PYY is one of these antagonists currently in clinical trials. Pancreatic glucagon produces a dose-related decrease in food intake *(18)*. A fragment of glucagon (amino acids 6–29) called glucagon-like peptide-1 (GLP-1) reduced food intake when given either peripherally *(27)* or into the brain, and, thus, exendin, an analog of GLP-1, has been used in humans *(28)*.

SPECIAL ISSUES IN DIABETES

Regarding patients with diabetes, diabetic control improves with weight reduction, and hypoglycemia becomes a possibility for those patients taking insulin or oral hypoglycemic medications. Some patients may develop increased hunger owing to hypoglycemia, and weight loss may slow or stop. Physicians must remember to monitor glucose carefully and to reduce or stop diabetic medications as weight loss occurs. In our clinics, we halve or discontinue insulin and sulfonylureas at the start of the weight-loss program.

REFERENCES

1. www.iotf.org. International Obesity Task Force. WHO Report.
2. Flegal KM, Carroll MD, Ogden CL, Johnson CL. Prevalence and trends in obesity among US adults, 1999–2000. JAMA 2002;288:1723–1727.
3. National Institutes of Health. Clinical guidelines on the identification, evaluation, and treatment of overweight and obesity in adults—the evidence report. Obes Res 1998;6(Suppl 2):51S–209S.
4. Knowler WC, Barrett-Connor E, Fowler SE, et al. Reduction in the incidence of type 2 diabetes with lifestyle intervention or metformin. N Engl J Med 2002;346:393–403.
5. Tuomilehto J, Lindstrom J, Eriksson JG, et al. Prevention of type 2 diabetes mellitus by changes in lifestyle among subjects with impaired glucose tolerance. N Engl J Med 2001;344:1343–1350.
6. Connolly HM, Crary JL, McGoon MD, et al. Valvular heart disease associated with fenfluramine-phentermine. N Engl J Med 1997;337:581–588.
7. Mast ST, Jollis JG, Ryan T, Anstrom KJ, Crary JL. The progression of fenfluramine-associated valvular heart disease assessed by echocardiography. Ann Intern Med 2001;134:261–266.
8. Weintraub M, Bray GA. Drug treatment of obesity. Med Clin North Am 1989;73:237–249.
9. Bray GA. Obesity: a time bomb to be defused. Lancet 1998;352:160–161.
10. McMahon FG, Fujioka K, Singh BN, et al. Efficacy and safety of sibutramine in obese white and African American patients with hypertension: a 1-year, double-blind, placebo-controlled, multicenter trial. Arch Intern Med 2000;160:2185–2191.
11. Finer N, James WP, Kopelman PG, Lean ME, Williams G. One-year treatment of obesity: a randomized, double-blind, placebo-controlled, multicentre study of orlistat, a gastrointestinal lipase inhibitor. Int J Obes Relat Metab Disord 2000;24:306–313.
12. Ryan DH, Bray GA, Helmcke F, et al. Serial echocardiographic and clinical evaluation of valvular regurgitation before, during, and after treatment with fenfluramine or dexfenfluramine and mazindol or phentermine. Obes Res 1999;7:313–322.
13. Cole JO, Levin A, Beake B, Kaiser PE, Scheinbaum ML. Sibutramine: a new weight loss agent without evidence of the abuse potential associated with amphetamines. J Clin Psychopharmacol 1998;18:231–236.
14. A Practical Guide to Drug Induced Weight Gain. McGraw-Hill, New York, 2002.
15. Bray GA. Don't throw the baby out with the bath water. Am J Clin Nutr 2004;79:347–349.
16. Executive summary of the third report of the National Cholesterol Education Program (NCEP) Expert Panel on Detection, Evaluation, and Treatment of High Blood Cholesterol in Adults (Adult Treatment Panel III). JAMA 2001;285:2486–2497.
17. Alberti KG, Zimmet PZ. Definition, diagnosis and classification of diabetes mellitus and its complications. Part 1: diagnosis and classification of diabetes mellitus provisional report of a WHO consultation. Diabet Med 1998;15:539–553.
18. Bray GA, Greenway FL. Current and potential drugs for treatment of obesity. Endocr Rev 1999;20:805–875.
19. Yanovski SZ, Yanovski JA. Obesity. N Engl J Med 2002;346:591–602.
20. Ryan DH. The role of sibutramine in the clinical management of obesity. In: Medeiros-Neto G, Halpern A, Bouchard C, eds. Progress in Obesity Research. John Libbey Eurotext, London, UK, 1999, pp. 1051–1057.
21. Halpern A. Orlistat in the treatment of obesity. In: Medeiros-Neto G, Halpern A, Bouchard C, eds. Progress in Obesity Research. John Libbey Eurotext, London, UK, 1999, pp. 1045–1050.
22. Anderson JW, Greenway FL, Fujioka K, Gadde KM, McKenney J, O'Neil PM. Bupropion SR enhances weight loss: a 48-week double-blind, placebo-controlled trial. Obes Res 2002;10:633–641.
23. Montague CT, Farooqi IS, Whitehead JP, et al. Congenital leptin deficiency is associated with severe early-onset obesity in humans. Nature 1997;387:903–908.
24. Farooqi IS, Jebb SA, Langmack G, et al. Effects of recombinant leptin therapy in a child with congenital leptin deficiency. N Engl J Med 1999;341:879–884.
25. Lambert PD, Anderson KD, Sleeman MW, et al. Ciliary neurotrophic factor activates leptin-like pathways and reduces body fat, without cachexia or rebound weight gain, even in leptin-resistant obesity. Proc Natl Acad Sci USA 2001;98:4652–4657.
26. Bray GA, Tartaglia LA. Medicinal strategies in the treatment of obesity. Nature 2000;404:672–677.
27. Flint A, Raben A, Astrup A, Holst JJ. Glucagon-like peptide 1 promotes satiety and suppresses energy intake in humans. J Clin Invest 1998;101:515–520.
28. Al-Barazanji KA, Arch JR, Buckingham RE, Tadayyon M. Central exendin-4 infusion reduces body weight without altering plasma leptin in (fa/fa) Zucker rats. Obes Res 2000;8:317–323.

27 Treatment of the Obese Patients With Type 2 Diabetes

Jean L. Chan, MD, Christos S. Mantzoros, MD, DSc, and Martin J. Abrahamson, MD

CONTENTS

INTRODUCTION

Type 2 diabetes mellitus is a chronic disease often associated with obesity that is increasing at an alarming rate, with a projected prevalence of 366 million cases worldwide by 2030 *(1)*. In the United States, the lifetime risk of developing diabetes for individuals born in 2000 is a staggering 32.8% for males and 38.5% for females *(2)*. The rapid increase in the prevalence of this condition is likely related to several factors, including the concomitant escalation in the prevalence of obesity *(3)*, a sedentary lifestyle and high-fat diets, and an aging population. Type 2 diabetes is also increasing at epidemic proportions in children and adolescents in association with the increasing prevalence of obesity in this population as well *(4)*. These statistics are especially disturbing in light of the fact that diabetes is one of the leading causes of blindness, end-stage renal disease, and lower-extremity amputation and contributes significantly to cardiovascular death *(5,6)*. In this chapter, we focus on the medical treatment of type 2 diabetes, with a specific emphasis on the approach to the obese patient with this disease.

From: *Contemporary Diabetes: Obesity and Diabetes*
Edited by: C. S. Mantzoros © Humana Press Inc., Totowa, NJ

PATHOPHYSIOLOGY AND NATURAL HISTORY OF TYPE 2 DIABETES

A major pathophysiological defect in type 2 diabetes is insulin resistance, which occurs primarily at the level of skeletal muscle and the liver and leads to unrestrained hepatic glucose production and diminished insulin-stimulated glucose uptake and utilization *(7,8)*. The mechanism by which this occurs may be related to defects in insulin receptor binding, decreased numbers of insulin receptors; or, most commonly, postreceptor attenuation of insulin action *(7)*. The resulting hyperglycemia further impairs insulin secretion and worsens insulin resistance, through downregulation of the glucose transport system in β-cells and insulin-sensitive tissues, causing a state of "glucose toxicity" *(8)*. In addition, the high circulating free fatty acid levels associated with diabetes further aggravate insulin resistance and may adversely affect β-cell secretion, a phenomenon known as lipotoxicity *(9)*.

Although type 2 diabetes is typically considered a state of insulin resistance, impairment of β-cell secretory function (both basal and glucose stimulated) is a prerequisite and early manifestation of the condition *(7)*. Longitudinal studies in Pima Indians, a population with a particularly high incidence of type 2 diabetes, provide evidence that dual defects in insulin secretion and insulin action occur early in the course of the disease *(10)*. Serum glucose levels increase progressively over time, and it has been suggested that β-cell secretory dysfunction may be present in some patients as long as 9–12 yr before diagnosis *(11)*. Loss of the acute insulin response to a carbohydrate load generally occurs when fasting plasma glucose levels reach 115 mg/dL *(7)* and leads to postprandial hyperglycemia. By the time fasting glucose levels reach 140 mg/dL, 75% of β-cell function has been lost *(12)*, underscoring the important role that β-cell dysfunction, in addition to insulin resistance, plays in the pathogenesis of the disease.

Type 2 diabetes is a progressive disorder that often requires more pharmacological therapy over time. This was demonstrated in the United Kingdom Prospective Diabetes Study (UKPDS), in which patients receiving either conventional or intensive treatment had initial improvement in hemoglobin A1c (HbA1c) but secondary treatment failure ensued at the same rate for each group regardless of the therapy used *(13)*. The difficulty in maintaining HbA1c at target levels over time may be related to patient factors (e.g., lack of adherence to diet, exercise, and medication regimens) but primarily reflects the natural history of the disease, which is associated with a progressive decline in β-cell function *(14)*.

GOALS OF THERAPY AND MONITORING IN TYPE 2 DIABETES

It is important to establish goals for patients with type 2 diabetes early in the treatment plan and to provide guidelines for recognition of ineffective therapy so that appropriate modification of treatment can occur in order to optimize glycemic control and reduce risk of complications. The American Diabetes Association (ADA) and the American College of Endocrinology (ACE) have proposed target goals for fasting and postprandial plasma glucose levels and HbA1c (Table 1) *(15,16)*. Plasma glucose levels are generally 10% higher than capillary whole blood glucose, and postprandial glucose levels are defined as peak levels 1 to 2 h *(15)* or 2 h *(16)* after the beginning of a meal.

The recommendations for target goals by the ADA and ACE differ slightly, but the overall goal of therapy should be to achieve the best glycemic control without excessive risk of hypoglycemia and with consideration for patient-specific factors such as medical comorbidities and expected longevity. Thus, the optimal frequency and timing of self-monitored blood glucose levels requires tailoring to the needs of the individual patient

Table 1
Diabetes Treatment Goals *(15,16)*

	Normal	ADA goal	ACE goal
Preprandial glucose (mg/dL)[a]	<100	90–130	<100
Postprandial glucose (mg/dL)[a]	<140[c]	<180	<140[c]
HbA1c (%)[b]	<6.0	<7.0	<6.5

[a]Plasma glucose values.
[b]HbAIC, glycosylated hemoglobin.
[c]Two-hour postprandial.

but should be sufficient to facilitate the achievement of glycemic goals. HbA1c levels should be measured at least twice per year in patients who are meeting treatment goals but more frequently (every 3 mo) in those who are not meeting goals or in whom changes in therapy are being made *(15)*. When modifying treatment to meet targets for fasting and postprandial blood glucose levels and HbA1c, it is important to remember that postprandial glucose levels contribute more than fasting glucose levels to HbA1c at levels of HbA1c <7.3% *(17)*.

MEDICAL NUTRITION THERAPY AND EXERCISE

Lifestyle modification, in the form of medical nutrition therapy and exercise, is an essential and integral component, along with pharmacotherapy when necessary, of an optimal management program for patients with type 2 diabetes. Diet and lifestyle approaches to the management of diabetes are discussed in greater detail in Chapter 24, and, thus, we only briefly discuss this topic herein.

The Diabetes Prevention Program study of more than 3000 nondiabetic subjects with an average body mass index of 34 kg/m^2 illustrates the importance of lifestyle intervention in the prevention of diabetes *(18)*. Lifestyle modification (with a goal of at least 7% weight loss and 150 min of physical activity per week) had a greater effect (58% compared to placebo) on reduction in the incidence of diabetes than metformin (31% reduction) *(18)*. When type 2 diabetes is associated with obesity, modest weight loss can significantly improve insulin resistance and β-cell function *(19)*. Thus, dietary counseling focusing on appropriate carbohydrate intake and caloric reduction for weight loss is critical. Exercise is an essential counterpart to dietary changes for achieving weight loss and provides a number of synergistic metabolic benefits, including improvement in insulin sensitivity and glycemic control, maintenance of weight loss, reduction of cardiovascular risk, and increased psychological well-being *(20)*. In a recent meta-analysis, pharmacotherapy (including orlistat and sibutramine) for weight loss (discussed in greater detail in Chapter 26) in patients with type 2 diabetes resulted in a modest but statistically significant weight loss of 2.6–4.5 kg that was associated with an improvement in HbA1c of 0.4–0.7% *(21)*.

Recently, much attention has been directed in the popular media toward low-carbohydrate diets for weight loss. Several studies have been conducted to address the benefits of low-carbohydrate compared with more traditional, low-fat diets for the treatment of obesity *(22–25)*. There is evidence for greater weight loss at 6 mo on low-carbohydrate diets, but the weight loss achieved with low-carbohydrate and low-fat diets was not significantly different at 1 yr *(22,23)*. Although these diets do not appear to have deleterious effects on lipid profiles or blood pressure, the long-term effects of low-carbohydrate diets are not well understood. Thus, it is important to individualize recommendations for patients with a goal to achieve at least modest weight loss (5–10% of baseline body weight) *(19)*. Low glycemic index diets may be associated with more successful weight loss and improved glycemic control *(26)*.

ORAL ANTIHYPERGLYCEMIC AGENTS

Because attempts at lifestyle modification alone often fail to induce or maintain adequate glycemic control in the majority of patients *(27)*, pharmacotherapy is usually necessary. Several classes of oral agents are now available for clinical use (Table 2). These agents have been discussed in greater detail recently *(see refs. 28–30)* and, thus, are reviewed only briefly herein, with a focus on the practical use of these medications in the obese patient with diabetes. Most oral agents as monotherapy will lower HbA1c levels by 0.5–2%, and the addition of a second agent usually provides an additional lowering of 0.5–2%, depending on the agent used (Table 2) *(31–52)*.

Insulin Sensitizers

BIGUANIDES: METFORMIN (GLUCOPHAGE®)

Metformin increases insulin sensitivity at the level of the liver by inhibiting hepatic gluconeogenesis and reducing hepatic glucose production *(31)*. Metformin may decrease glucose absorption from the gastrointestinal (GI) tract and also increases peripheral insulin sensitivity through mechanisms that are not well understood.

THIAZOLIDINEDIONES: ROSIGLITAZONE (AVANDIA®) AND PIOGLITAZONE (ACTOS®)

Thiazolidinediones (TZDs) are an important, relatively newer class of insulin sensitizers that activate peroxisome proliferators-activated receptor γ receptors found primarily in adipose tissue and alter transcription of proteins involved in insulin resistance and glucose uptake *(32)*. TZDs also improve insulin sensitivity at the liver (by reducing hepatic glucose production) and muscle (by increasing glucose uptake), likely through indirect mechanisms.

Insulin Secretagogues

SULFONYLUREAS: GLYBURIDE (DIABETA®, MICRONASE®, GLYNASE®), GLIPIZIDE (GLUCOTROL®, GLUCOTROL XL®), CHLORPROPAMIDE (DIABINESE®), AND GLIMEPIRIDE (AMARYL®)

Sulfonylureas stimulate insulin secretion by the β-cell through activation of an adenosine triphosphate–dependent potassium channel on the β-cell plasma membrane, which results in cell membrane depolarization, an increase in intracellular calcium, and subsequent release of insulin *(33)*.

SHORT-ACTING NONSULFONYLUREA INSULIN SECRETAGOGUES: REPAGLINIDE (PRANDIN®) AND NATEGLINIDE (STARLIX®)

The meglitinide analog, repaglinide and the D-phenylalanine derivative nateglinide, are newer nonsulfonylurea agents that stimulate acute insulin secretion in response to nutrients *(34)*. They are rapidly absorbed from the GI tract and have a short half-life (approx 1.5 h) and duration of action (approx 2–4 h).

α-Glucosidase Inhibitors: Acarbose (Precose®) and Miglitol (Glyset®)

This class of medications, α-glucosidase inhibitors, delays the absorption of carbohydrates and, thus, primarily reduces postprandial hyperglycemia (by up to 50 mg/dL)

Table 2
Oral Antihyperglycemic Agents (31–52)[a]

Class	Agents	Major mechanism of action	HbA1c reduction	Additional agent	Additional HbA1c reduction
Biguanide	Metformin	Decreases hepatic glucose production	1.5–2.0	+ Sulfonylurea + Nonsulfonylurea secretagogue + TZD + α-GI	1.5–2.0 0.6–1.0 1.0–1.2 0.7–1.0
TZD	Pioglitazone Rosiglitazone	Decreases peripheral insulin resistance	1.0–1.5	+ Sulfonylurea + Nonsulfonylurea secretagogue	0.6–1.3 0.8–2.0
Sulfonylurea	Chlorpropamide Glimepiride Glipizide Glyburide	Increases insulin secretion	1.5–2.0	+ α-GI	1.0–1.5
Nonsulfonylurea secretagogue	Nateglinide Repaglinide	Increases prandial insulin secretion	1.0–2.0		
α-GI	Acarbose Miglitol	Delays carbohydrate absorption from GI tract	0.5–1.0		

[a]HbA1c, glycosylated hemoglobin; TZD, thiazolidinedione; α-GI, α-glucosidase inhibitor.

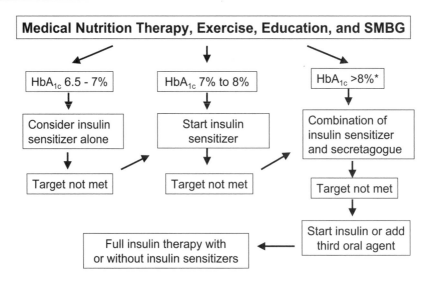

Fig. 1. New treatment paradigm for obese patient with type 2 diabetes. *Insulin therapy should be initiated if severe symptoms and ketonuria are present and in patients who are pregnant or planning to become pregnant in the near future. SMBG, self-monitoring of blood glucose; HbA1c, glycosylated hemoglobin. (© Martin J. Abrahamson, MD.)

without significant effects on fasting glucose levels yet can achieve a modest reduction in HbA1c (0.5–1%) *(35)*.

APPROACH TO USE OF ORAL ANTIHYPERGLYCEMIC AGENTS IN OBESE PATIENTS WITH TYPE 2 DIABETES

Type 2 diabetes has traditionally been treated in a stepwise manner, starting with lifestyle modification, proceeding to the use of one oral antihyperglycemic agent, followed by a combination of two or more oral agents before considering insulin *(53)*. However, data from the National Health and Nutrition Examination Survey of 1999–2000 demonstrated that <40% of patients with diabetes attained the ADA HbA1c goal of <7% *(54)*. Thus, a more aggressive approach is warranted to improve the percentage of patients reaching target goals for HbA1c.

In Fig. 1 and the section below, we present our general approach to the initiation of pharmacotherapy for the obese patient with type 2 diabetes. When medical nutrition therapy and exercise (as discussed earlier) fail to achieve glycemic goals, pharmacotherapy should be instituted and guided by the HbA1c and severity of symptoms. Consideration should be given to starting combination therapy simultaneously, rather than sequentially, in patients with suboptimal glycemic control whose HbA1c exceeds 8%. The selection of specific agents depends on the dominant underlying pathophysiology and should also be guided by efficacy of the drug, as well as its durability of effect, side effect profile, contraindications, and potential benefit for some of the other metabolic abnormalities associated with obesity and insulin resistance. For example, insulin sensitizers have a number of nonglycemic actions that ameliorate these metabolic abnormalities, including effects on body weight and fat distribution, lipid profiles, inflammatory markers, and thrombotic tendency (Table 3) *(55–77)*, in contrast to sulfonylureas, which have minimal effects on these parameters except for a tendency to increase body weight. TZDs lower triglycerides (pioglitazone more effectively than rosiglitazone) and increase high-density lipoprotein (HDL) and low-density

Table 3
Nonglycemic Effects of Insulin Sensitizers on Metabolic Abnormalities Associated
With Obesity and Insulin Resistance (55–69,71–77)[a]

	Metformin	TZDs
Body composition		
Body weight	↓/↔	↑
Body fat (total)	↓	↑[P]
Visceral fat	↓	↓/↔ [P,T]
Subcutaneous fat	↓	↑ [P,T]
Visceral/sc fat ratio	↔	↓
Lipid profile		
Total cholesterol	↓	↔[P] / ↑[R]
LDL-cholesterol	↓	↔[P] / ↑[R]
HDL-cholesterol	↔	↑ [P,R]
Triglycerides	↓/↔	↓[P]/↔[R]
Inflammatory markers		
C-reactive protein	↓/↔	↓[P,R,T]
Thrombotic factors		
PAI-1	↓	↓
Fibrinogen	↔	↓
Platelet aggregation	↓	↓

[a]↑ = increase; ↓ = decrease; ↔ = no significant effect; TZDs, thiazolidinediones
[P] = pioglitazone; [R] = rosiglitazone; [T] = troglitazone; PAI-1 = plasminogen activator inhibitor-1.

lipoprotein (LDL) cholesterol, although the increased LDL is due to a shift of small, dense LDL toward larger, less atherogenic particles (65,66). In some studies, the use of pioglitazone has been associated with more favorable improvements in lipid metabolism compared with rosiglitazone (63,64). However, the long-term relative efficacy and clinical outcomes of the nonglycemic, metabolic effects of these agents remain to be fully determined.

Patients with an HbA1c of <7% are at the ADA and ACE goals for therapy. However, one could consider the use of an insulin sensitizer in this situation, given the lack of hypoglycemia and the general favorable side effect profile associated with these medications, especially in patients with no other comorbid diseases. Data from the UKPDS study demonstrated a 21% risk reduction in any diabetes-related end point for each 1% reduction in HbA1c, with no threshold of risk observed for any end point. Thus, the lowest risk of any microvascular or macrovascular complication was observed in those patients with an HbA1c in the normal range of <6% (78).

In patients whose HbA1c is between 7 and 8%, an insulin sensitizer should be considered as the initial therapy of choice to address the insulin resistance typically present in the obese patient with diabetes. Metformin is often used in this situation because of its weight-neutral effect or tendency to induce a modest amount of weight loss. In addition, the use of metformin as monotherapy in overweight patients in the UKPDS was associated with a significant decrease in macrovascular events including mortality (79). TZDs have also been shown to be safe and effective agents as monotherapy in patients with type 2 diabetes inadequately controlled by lifestyle interventions (80). These medications may be particularly beneficial for the patient with signs of severe insulin resistance (e.g., acanthosis nigricans) or renal impairment (in whom metformin would be contraindicated).

In patients with suboptimally controlled diabetes whose HbA1c is >8%, initial combination therapy with two agents (an insulin sensitizer and a secretagogue) should be considered because greater glycemic control can be attained compared to monotherapy alone. The use of glyburide and metformin in a fixed-dose combination tablet (Glucovance™) as initial therapy in patients with inadequate control on diet and exercise alone has been shown to result in a greater reduction in HbA1c compared to monotherapy with metformin and glyburide alone *(81,82)*. Two other fixed-dose combinations recently approved by the Food and Drug Administration are glipizide and metformin (Metaglip™) and rosiglitazone and metformin (Avandamet™). These combination medications may facilitate adherence to therapeutic regimens.

The short-acting nonsulfonylurea secretagogues target mainly postprandial, rather than fasting, blood glucose levels and may be particularly attractive for patients with irregular meal schedules or frequently skipped meals. These medications are taken with meals but not taken when a meal is missed, thus reducing the risk of hypoglycemia, which may be more likely to occur when a meal is missed by someone taking a long-acting sulfonylurea. These medications can also be used safely in patients with renal impairment.

The use of α-glucosidase inhibitors can be considered as monotherapy *(83)* for patients with an HbA1c <7% or in combination with other classes of antihyperglycemic medications (metformin, sulfonylureas) to achieve an additional lowering of HbA1c of approx 0.5–1%. These medications also primarily decrease postprandial blood glucose levels and, thus, can be used in patients in whom postprandial hyperglycemia is the predominant problem.

AVAILABLE INSULIN FORMULATIONS: BASAL AND SHORT OR RAPID ACTING

Because of the progressive decline in β-cell function over time, many patients will eventually require insulin therapy. Use of insulin in patients with type 2 diabetes is often viewed by patients as a treatment of "last resort" after oral agents have failed and, thus, may carry negative connotations. Hence, it is important to recognize that insulin treatment is initiated as a consequence of the progressive nature of the disease, rather than secondary to noncompliance. Insulin remains an important part of the therapeutic regimen for these patients and should be utilized when appropriate to optimize glycemic control. In this section, we present a brief overview of the normal physiology of insulin secretion and currently available insulin formulations, which have been reviewed in greater detail elsewhere *(84,85)*. In the next major section, we present a practical approach for initiating and adjusting insulin regimens in obese patients with type 2 diabetes.

In individuals without diabetes, a basal amount of insulin is secreted at all times to regulate hepatic glucose production overnight and between meals *(8)*. At mealtime, ingestion of nutrients stimulates the acute, first-phase insulin response, followed by a second phase of insulin secretion that persists while blood glucose levels are elevated. Mealtime insulin secretion ensures inhibition of hepatic glucose production and promotion of glucose disposal. This maintains glucose levels within a normal range until they return to premeal levels, at which time insulin secretion also decreases to basal levels *(8)*.

Although the secretion of insulin in healthy individuals is complex and cannot be fully replicated in patients with diabetes, a combination of basal and short-acting, meal-related insulin provides the most physiological insulin replacement regimen. A basal insulin should ideally provide 24-h coverage without pronounced action peaks and with minimal risk of hypoglycemia. Similarly, a short-acting, meal-related insulin should ideally closely mimic the normal rapid rise in insulin after a meal with a subsequent rapid decline as glucose levels normalize in order to minimize postprandial hypoglycemia.

Basal Insulin Therapy: Neutral Protamine Hagedorn (NPH), Lente®, Ultralente®, and Insulin Analog Glargine (Lantus®)

NPH and Lente administered twice daily provide 24-h basal insulin coverage. Ultralente has a longer duration of action than NPH and Lente but does not provide 24-h coverage when administered once daily and is not commonly used owing to variability in absorption, inconsistent peak patterns, and erratic therapeutic outcomes (86).

Insulin glargine is an insulin analog with molecular modifications [Gly^{A21}, Arg^{B31}, Arg^{B32}] that shift the isoelectric point, resulting in reduced solubility at a physiological pH. After subcutaneous injection, glargine forms microprecipitates in the sc tissue, which delays its absorption into the systemic circulation (84). This results in a gradual and relatively constant-release pattern over approx 24 h with no pronounced peak in most patients (87,88).

Short- and Rapid-Acting Insulin Therapy: Regular Insulin, Lispro ([Lys^{B28}, Pro^{B29}], Humalog®), Aspart ([Asp^{B28}], NovoLog®), Glulisine ([Lys^{B3},Glu^{B29}], Apidra®)

Regular insulin has its peak action approx 2–4 h after administration and a duration of action of approx 4–6 h. In some patients, the relatively slow onset of action may result in early postprandial hyperglycemia, and the long duration of action may cause late postprandial hypoglycemia.

Rapid-acting insulin analogs (lispro, aspart, and glulisine) have been developed through modifications of the insulin molecule and are more rapidly absorbed with a shorter time to peak action and duration of action compared to regular insulin (84). Lispro, aspart, and glulisine are administered immediately before a meal in order to minimize mismatching of insulin action and carbohydrate absorption and thus reduce early postprandial hyperglycemia and late postprandial hypoglycemia. The pharmacokinetic profiles of these rapid-acting insulin analogs are similar, although aspart may have a slightly longer duration of action compared with lispro (89).

APPROACH TO USE OF INSULIN IN OBESE PATIENTS WITH TYPE 2 DIABETES

Insulin therapy should be considered initially in the following situations: (1) in patients presenting with severe symptoms and/or evidence of ketonuria or diabetic ketoacidosis; (2) in pregnant patients or patients undergoing preconception planning to become pregnant in the near future, because oral hyperglycemic agents cannot be used safely in pregnancy; and (3) in patients failing oral therapy with two agents. In the latter situation, a decision to add insulin or a third oral agent is often necessary. Addition of a TZD (troglitazone, which was withdrawn from the market because of hepatotoxicity, or rosiglitazone) to patients poorly controlled with a sulfonylurea and metformin resulted in a further reduction in HbA1c levels of 1% (rosiglitazone) (90) to 1.4% (troglitazone) (91). Thus, patients with an HbA1c of >8.5% may have a relatively slim chance of reaching target glycemic goals with the addition of a third oral agent, and institution of

Table 4
Starting Basal Insulin[a]

1. Add a single evening insulin dose (~10 U or 0.1 U/kg):
   • Use NPH or insulin glargine at bedtime or consider premixed insulin at dinner if post-dinner glucose is elevated.
2. Adjust the evening insulin dose based on FBG, increasing every 3–5 d as needed provided no nocturnal hypoglycemia occurs:
   • Increase by 2 U if FBG > 120 mg/dL.
   • Increase by 4 U if FBG > 140 mg/dL.
   • Increase by 6 U if FBG > 160 mg/dL.
3. Treat to target level (usually FBG < 120 mg/dL).

[a]FBG, fasting blood glucose.

insulin should be considered in this situation. A recent study evaluating the efficacy of adding a TZD (pioglitazone) vs bedtime NPH insulin to patients with suboptimal control on metformin and an insulin secretagogue found similar decreases in HbA1c with both treatments (1.9% with pioglitazone and 2.3% with insulin) but less hypoglycemia and increased HDL levels with pioglitazone compared to insulin (92).

If fasting blood glucose levels are elevated, basal insulin with NPH or insulin glargine should be started at bedtime. Addition of a basal bedtime insulin to oral monotherapy or combination therapy that is no longer effective has been shown to improve glycemic control (93–95). Table 4 outlines a simple approach to starting basal insulin. The majority of obese patients can be safely started on 10 U (≤0.1 U/kg) of NPH or glargine at bedtime although higher doses (e.g., 0.2 U/kg) can be considered initially in more obese, insulin-resistant individuals. Depending on whether fasting blood glucose levels remain consistently above 120, 140, or 160 mg/dL, dose adjustments of 2, 4, or 6 U, respectively, should be made every 3–5 d until a target fasting glucose of <120 mg/dL is reached provided that nocturnal hypoglycemia does not occur. The use of insulin glargine has been associated with less nocturnal hypoglycemia compared with NPH in some studies (94,95). Patients should continue their oral agents at the same dose after starting bedtime insulin, but the dose may eventually need to be reduced.

In addition to monitoring fasting blood glucose levels, postprandial glucose levels should be monitored in the patient receiving insulin therapy. Once fasting glucose levels are in the target range, a short-acting insulin or rapid-acting insulin analog should be considered if postprandial glucose levels remain consistently above goal and should be utilized before meals with the highest postprandial glucose excursions. The starting dose for the short- or rapid-acting insulin can be as low as 2 or 4 U, with titration up until target glucose levels have been reached. Although this approach may require more frequent administration of insulin, it also provides more flexibility for patients regarding timing of meals. Once patients require short-or rapid-acting insulin, oral secretagogues can be stopped but insulin sensitizers should be continued. A number of studies have demonstrated benefit (i.e., improved glycemic control on lower doses of insulin) with combination therapy of insulin and an insulin sensitizer. Both metformin (96–100) and TZDs (101–105) have been used with insulin although the combination of TZD with insulin was associated with more weight gain and edema (104,105) than metformin with insulin.

Multiple daily injection regimens with a rapid-acting insulin before meals and an intermediate- or long-acting insulin for basal supplementation have been associated with improved glycemic control in patients with type 2 diabetes *(106)*. Increasing the number of injections may help decrease the incidence of hypoglycemia by providing a more physiological insulin profile. For example, in patients using NPH and rapid-acting insulin twice daily, the risk of nocturnal hypoglycemia may be reduced by changing the time to take NPH from suppertime to bedtime *(107,108)*. This avoids waning of the insulin effect coinciding with the dawn phenomenon (an increase in insulin resistance during the early morning hours) *(108)*. The use of glargine insulin has been shown to provide a smoother metabolic effect and more physiological basal insulin coverage compared with NPH insulin, with no pronounced peak and lower intersubject variability *(87,88)*.

For patients who require both basal and prandial insulin but prefer to avoid multiple injections of insulin on a daily basis, combinations of rapid-acting analogs with intermediate-acting insulin using either premixed insulins or split-mix insulin regimens can be considered. Premixed fixed-dose insulin combinations administered twice daily before breakfast and dinner provide the simplest approach to using prandial and basal insulin but do not allow the dose of each component to be adjusted separately. Premixed insulin formulations containing rapid-acting insulin analogs have been associated with improved glycemic control compared with those containing regular insulin *(109)*. Alternatively, varying combinations of short- or rapid-acting and intermediate-acting insulins can be administered twice daily before breakfast and dinner. This requires that the insulins be mixed together in a syringe by the patient but also permits more flexibility in dose adjustment.

A LOOK TO THE FUTURE: UPCOMING THERAPIES

Significant advances have been made in the therapeutic armamentarium for the management of diabetes. However, the escalating prevalence of this chronic disease and the inexorable progressive nature of the condition compel the development of effective new agents for the treatment of diabetes. Thus, intensive efforts are being employed to develop novel agents, including agonists of glucagon-like peptide-1 (GLP-1), a hormone secreted from the GI tract after food ingestion that acts on β-cells to stimulate insulin secretion in a glucose-dependent fashion *(110)*. Similarly, compounds to inhibit dipeptidyl peptidase-IV, a proteolytic enzyme that degrades GLP-1, are being investigated *(110)*. These and other agents are discussed in more detail in Chapter 29.

CONCLUSIONS

Type 2 diabetes is a common chronic illness often associated with obesity and results from dual defects in β-cell secretion and peripheral insulin resistance. Improvement in glycemic control reduces the risk for the development and progression of microvascular and macrovascular complications. Hence, the goal of treatment should be to achieve and maintain near-normal glycemic control without increasing the risk of hypoglycemia. Medical nutrition therapy and exercise form the cornerstone of a comprehensive management program, but the vast majority of patients usually require pharmacological therapy to achieve and maintain an HbA1c of <7%. Oral antihyperglycemic agents and/or insulin should be initiated based on the HbA1c, severity of symptoms, and other patient-specific considerations. For the obese patient with diabetes, insulin sensitizers are effective medications, and combination therapy with insulin secretagogues and sensitizers should be considered in patients with suboptimal control. Insulin remains an important component of the therapeutic regimen for patients not achieving target glucose goals while taking oral agents or for those presenting with severe hyperglycemia and symptoms of diabetes. Newer insulin analogs with more physiological pharmacokinetic profiles are now available for clinical use. Adopting a more aggressive approach to the treatment of diabetes guided by ADA and ACE recommendations will increase the likelihood of achieving target glycemic goals and reduce the risk of developing diabetes-related complications.

REFERENCES

1. Wild S, Roglic G, Green A, Sicree R, King H. Global prevalence of diabetes: estimates for the year 2000 and projections for 2030. Diabetes Care 2004;27(5):1047–1053.
2. Narayan KM, Boyle JP, Thompson TJ, Sorensen SW, Williamson DF. Lifetime risk for diabetes mellitus in the United States. JAMA 2003;290(14):1884–1890.
3. Ford ES, Williamson DF, Liu S. Weight change and diabetes incidence: findings from a national cohort of US adults. Am J Epidemiol 1997;146(3):214–222.
4. Rosenbloom AL, Joe JR, Young RS, Winter WE. Emerging epidemic of type 2 diabetes in youth. Diabetes Care 1999;22(2):345–354.
5. Bjork S. The cost of diabetes and diabetes care. Diabetes Res Clin Pract 2001;54(Suppl 1):S13–S18.
6. Stern MP. The effect of glycemic control on the incidence of macrovascular complications of type 2 diabetes. Arch Fam Med 1998;7(2):155–162.
7. Kahn SE, Porte D Jr. The pathophysiology of type II (noninsulin-dependent) diabetes mellitus: implications for treatment. In: Porte D Jr, Sherwin RS, eds. Ellenberg & Rifkin's Diabetes Mellitus. Appleton & Lange, Stamford, CT, 1997, pp. 487–512.
8. DeFronzo RA, Bonadonna RC, Ferrannini E. Pathogenesis of NIDDM: a balanced overview. Diabetes Care 1992;15(3):318–368.
9. LeRoith D. Beta-cell dysfunction and insulin resistance in type 2 diabetes: role of metabolic and genetic abnormalities. Am J Med 2002;113(Suppl 6A):3S–11S.
10. Weyer C, Bogardus C, Mott DM, Pratley RE. The natural history of insulin secretory dysfunction and insulin resistance in the pathogenesis of type 2 diabetes mellitus. J Clin Invest 1999;104(6):787–794.
11. Harris MI, Klein R, Welborn TA, Knuiman MW. Onset of NIDDM occurs at least 4–7 yr before clinical diagnosis. Diabetes Care 1992;15(7):815–819.
12. Porte D Jr. Banting lecture 1990:beta-cells in type II diabetes mellitus. Diabetes 1991;40(2):166–180.
13. Turner RC, Cull CA, Frighi V, Holman RR. Glycemic control with diet, sulfonylurea, metformin, or insulin in patients with type 2 diabetes mellitus: progressive requirement for multiple therapies (UKPDS 49). UK Prospective Diabetes Study (UKPDS) Group. JAMA 1999;281(21):2005–2012.
14. U.K. Prospective Diabetes Study Group. U.K. prospective diabetes study 16. Overview of 6 years' therapy of type II diabetes: a progressive disease. Diabetes 1995;44(11):1249–1258.
15. American Diabetes Association. Standards of medical care in diabetes. Diabetes Care 2005;28(Suppl 1): S4–S36.
16. American College of Endocrinology consensus statement on guidelines for glycemic control. Endocr Pract 2002;8(Suppl 1):5–11.
17. Monnier L, Lapinski H, Colette C. Contributions of fasting and postprandial plasma glucose increments to the overall diurnal hyperglycemia of type 2 diabetic patients: variations with increasing levels of HbA(1c). Diabetes Care 2003;26(3):881–885.
18. Knowler WC, Barrett-Connor E, Fowler SE, et al. Reduction in the incidence of type 2 diabetes with lifestyle intervention or metformin. N Engl J Med 2002;346(6):393–403.
19. Klein S. Outcome success in obesity. Obes Res 2001;9(Suppl 4):354S–358S.
20. Hamdy O, Goodyear LJ, Horton ES. Diet and exercise in type 2 diabetes mellitus. Endocrinol Metab Clin North Am 2001;30(4):883–907.
21. Norris SL, Zhang X, Avenell A, et al. Efficacy of pharmacotherapy for weight loss in adults with type 2 diabetes mellitus: a meta-analysis. Arch Intern Med 2004;164(13):1395–1404.
22. Samaha FF, Iqbal N, Seshadri P, et al. A low-carbohydrate as compared with a low-fat diet in severe obesity. N Engl J Med 2003;348(21):2074–2081.
23. Foster GD, Wyatt HR, Hill JO, et al. A randomized trial of a low-carbohydrate diet for obesity. N Engl J Med 2003;348(21):2082–2090.
24. Stern L, Iqbal N, Seshadri P, et al. The effects of low-carbohydrate versus conventional weight loss diets in severely obese adults: one-year follow-up of a randomized trial. Ann Intern Med 2004; 140(10):778–785.

25. Yancy WS Jr, Olsen MK, Guyton JR, Bakst RP, Westman EC. A low-carbohydrate, ketogenic diet versus a low-fat diet to treat obesity and hyperlipidemia: a randomized, controlled trial. Ann Intern Med 2004;140(10):769–777.

26. Ludwig DS. Dietary glycemic index and the regulation of body weight. Lipids 2003;38(2):117–121.

27. UKPDS Group. UK Prospective Diabetes Study 7: response of fasting plasma glucose to diet therapy in newly presenting type II diabetic patients, Metabolism 1990;39(9):905–912.

28. DeFronzo RA. Pharmacologic therapy for type 2 diabetes mellitus. Ann Intern Med 1999;131(4): 281–303.

29. Ahmann AJ, Riddle MC. Current oral agents for type 2 diabetes: many options, but which to choose when? Postgrad Med 2002;111(5):32–40, 43.

30. Lebovitz HE. Oral antidiabetic agents: 2004. Med Clin North Am 2004;88(4):847–863.

31. Bell PM, Hadden DR. Metformin. Endocrinol Metab Clin North Am 1997;26(3):523–537.

32. Serdy S, Abrahamson MJ. Durability of glycemic control: a feature of the thiazolidinediones. Diabetes Technol Ther 2004;6(2):179–189.

33. Zimmerman BR. Sulfonylureas. Endocrinol Metab Clin North Am 1997;26(3):511–522.

34. Dornhorst A. Insulinotropic meglitinide analogues. Lancet 2001;358(9294):1709–1716.

35. Lebovitz HE. alpha-Glucosidase inhibitors. Endocrinol Metab Clin North Am 1997;26(3):539–551.

36. DeFronzo RA, Goodman AM. Efficacy of metformin in patients with non-insulin-dependent diabetes mellitus. The Multicenter Metformin Study Group. N Engl J Med 1995;333(9):541–549.

37. Einhorn D, Rendell M, Rosenzweig J, Egan JW, Mathisen AL, Schneider RL. Pioglitazone hydrochloride in combination with metformin in the treatment of type 2 diabetes mellitus: a randomized, placebo-controlled study. The Pioglitazone 027 Study Group. Clin Ther 2000;22(12):1395–1409.

38. Horton ES, Clinkingbeard C, Gatlin M, Foley J, Mallows S, Shen S. Nateglinide alone and in combination with metformin improves glycemic control by reducing mealtime glucose levels in type 2 diabetes. Diabetes Care 2000;23(11):1660–1665.

39. Moses R, Slobodniuk R, Boyages S, et al. Effect of repaglinide addition to metformin monotherapy on glycemic control in patients with type 2 diabetes. Diabetes Care 1999;22(1):119–124.

40. Jones TA, Sautter M, Van Gaal LF, Jones NP. Addition of rosiglitazone to metformin is most effective in obese, insulin-resistant patients with type 2 diabetes. Diabetes Obes Metab 2003;5(3):163–170.

41. Fonseca V, Rosenstock J, Patwardhan R, Salzman A. Effect of metformin and rosiglitazone combination therapy in patients with type 2 diabetes mellitus: a randomized controlled trial. JAMA 2000;283(13):1695–1702.

42. Rosenstock J, Brown A, Fischer J, et al. Efficacy and safety of acarbose in metformin-treated patients with type 2 diabetes. Diabetes Care 1998;21(12):2050–2055.

43. Halimi S, Le Berre MA, Grange V. Efficacy and safety of acarbose add-on therapy in the treatment of overweight patients with Type 2 diabetes inadequately controlled with metformin: a double-blind, placebo-controlled study. Diabetes Res Clin Pract 2000;50(1):49–56.

44. Phillips P, Karrasch J, Scott R, Wilson D, Moses R. Acarbose improves glycemic control in overweight type 2 diabetic patients insufficiently treated with metformin. Diabetes Care 2003;26(2):269–273.

45. Kipnes MS, Krosnick A, Rendell MS, Egan JW, Mathisen AL, Schneider RL. Pioglitazone hydrochloride in combination with sulfonylurea therapy improves glycemic control in patients with type 2 diabetes mellitus: a randomized, placebo-controlled study. Am J Med 2001;111(1):10–17.

46. Wolffenbuttel BH, Gomis R, Squatrito S, Jones NP, Patwardhan RN. Addition of low-dose rosiglitazone to sulphonylurea therapy improves glycaemic control in Type 2 diabetic patients. Diabet Med 2000;17(1):40–47.

47. Vongthavaravat V, Wajchenberg BL, Waitman JN, et al. An international study of the effects of rosiglitazone plus sulphonylurea in patients with type 2 diabetes. Curr Med Res Opin 2002;18(8):456–461.

48. Kerenyi Z, Samer H, James R, Yan Y, Stewart M. Combination therapy with rosiglitazone and glibenclamide compared with upward titration of glibenclamide alone in patients with type 2 diabetes mellitus. Diabetes Res Clin Pract 2004;63(3):213–223.

49. Hanefeld M, Brunetti P, Schernthaner GH, Matthews DR, Charbonnel BH. One-year glycemic control with a sulfonylurea plus pioglitazone versus a sulfonylurea plus metformin in patients with type 2 diabetes. Diabetes Care 2004;27(1):141–147.

50. Fonseca V, Grunberger G, Gupta S, Shen S, Foley JE. Addition of nateglinide to rosiglitazone monotherapy suppresses mealtime hyperglycemia and improves overall glycemic control. Diabetes Care 2003;26(6):1685–1690.

51. Raskin P, McGill J, Saad MF, et al. Combination therapy for type 2 diabetes: repaglinide plus rosiglitazone. Diabet Med 2004;21(4):329–335.

52. Jovanovic L, Hassman DR, Gooch B, et al. Treatment of type 2 diabetes with a combination regimen of repaglinide plus pioglitazone. Diabetes Res Clin Pract 2004;63(2):127–134.

53. Riddle MC. Tactics for type II diabetes. Endocrinol Metab Clin North Am 1997;26(3):659–677.

54. Saydah SH, Fradkin J, Cowie CC. Poor control of risk factors for vascular disease among adults with previously diagnosed diabetes. JAMA 2004;291(3):335–342.

55. Tiikkainen M, Hakkinen AM, Korsheninnikova E, Nyman T, Makimattila S, Yki-Jarvinen H. Effects of rosiglitazone and metformin on liver fat content, hepatic insulin resistance, insulin clearance, and gene expression in adipose tissue in patients with type 2 diabetes. Diabetes 2004;53(8):2169–2176.

56. Tankova T, Dakovska L, Kirilov G, Koev D. Metformin in the treatment of obesity in subjects with normal glucose tolerance. Rom J Intern Med 2003;41(3):269–275.

57. Shadid S, Jensen MD. Effects of pioglitazone versus diet and exercise on metabolic health and fat distribution in upper body obesity. Diabetes Care 2003;26(11):3148–3152.

58. Miyazaki Y, Mahankali A, Matsuda M, et al. Effect of pioglitazone on abdominal fat distribution and insulin sensitivity in type 2 diabetic patients. J Clin Endocrinol Metab 2002;87(6):2784–2791.

59. Pasquali R, Gambineri A, Biscotti D, et al. Effect of long-term treatment with metformin added to hypocaloric diet on body composition, fat distribution, and androgen and insulin levels in abdominally obese women with and without the polycystic ovary syndrome. J Clin Endocrinol Metab 2000;85(8):2767–2774.

60. Akazawa S, Sun F, Ito M, Kawasaki E, Eguchi K. Efficacy of troglitazone on body fat distribution in type 2 diabetes. Diabetes Care 2000;23(8):1067–1071.

61. Mori Y, Murakawa Y, Okada K, et al. Effect of troglitazone on body fat distribution in type 2 diabetic patients. Diabetes Care 1999;22(6):908–912.

62. Kelly IE, Han TS, Walsh K, Lean ME. Effects of a thiazolidinedione compound on body fat and fat distribution of patients with type 2 diabetes. Diabetes Care 1999;22(2):288–293.

63. Chiquette E, Ramirez G, Defronzo R. A meta-analysis comparing the effect of thiazolidinediones on cardiovascular risk factors. Arch Intern Med 2004;164(19):2097–2104.

64. Derosa G, Cicero AF, Gaddi A, et al. Metabolic effects of pioglitazone and rosiglitazone in patients with diabetes and metabolic syndrome treated with glimepiride: a twelve-month, multicenter, double-blind, randomized, controlled, parallel-group trial. Clin Ther 2004;26(5):744–754.

65. Lawrence JM, Reid J, Taylor GJ, Stirling C, Reckless JP. Favorable effects of pioglitazone and metformin compared with gliclazide on lipoprotein subfractions in overweight patients with early type 2 diabetes. Diabetes Care 2004;27(1):41–46.

66. Ovalle F, Bell DS. Lipoprotein effects of different thiazolidinediones in clinical practice. Endocr Pract 2002;8(6):406–410.

67. Despres JP. Potential contribution of metformin to the management of cardiovascular disease risk in patients with abdominal obesity, the metabolic syndrome and type 2 diabetes. Diabetes Metab 2003;29(4 Pt 2):6S53–6S61.

68. Grant PJ. Beneficial effects of metformin on haemostasis and vascular function in man. Diabetes Metab 2003;29(4 Pt 2):6S44–6S52.

69. Caballero AE, Delgado A, Aguilar-Salinas CA, et al. The differential effects of metformin on markers of endothelial activation and inflammation in subjects with impaired glucose tolerance: a placebo-controlled, randomized clinical trial. J Clin Endocrinol Metab 2004;89(8):3943–3948.

70. Satoh N, Ogawa Y, Usui T, et al. Antiatherogenic effect of pioglitazone in type 2 diabetic patients irrespective of the responsiveness to its antidiabetic effect. Diabetes Care 2003;26(9):2493–2499.

71. Mohanty P, Aljada A, Ghanim H, et al. Evidence for a potent antiinflammatory effect of rosiglitazone. J Clin Endocrinol Metab 2004;89(6):2728–2735.

72. Yatagai T, Nakamura T, Nagasaka S, et al. Decrease in serum C-reactive protein levels by troglitazone is associated with pretreatment insulin resistance, but independent of its effect on glycemia, in type 2 diabetic subjects. Diabetes Res Clin Pract 2004;63(1):19–26.

73. Haffner SM, Greenberg AS, Weston WM, Chen H, Williams K, Freed MI. Effect of rosiglitazone treatment on nontraditional markers of cardiovascular disease in patients with type 2 diabetes mellitus. Circulation 2002;106(6):679–684.

74. Sidhu JS, Cowan D, Kaski JC. The effects of rosiglitazone, a peroxisome proliferator-activated receptor-gamma agonist, on markers of endothelial cell activation, C-reactive protein, and fibrinogen levels in non-diabetic coronary artery disease patients. J Am Coll Cardiol 2003;42(10):1757–1763.

75. Akbar DH. Effect of metformin and sulfonylurea on C-reactive protein level in well-controlled type 2 diabetics with metabolic syndrome. Endocrine 2003;20(3):215–218.

76. Chu NV, Kong AP, Kim DD, et al. Differential effects of metformin and troglitazone on cardiovascular risk factors in patients with type 2 diabetes. Diabetes Care 2002;25(3):542–549.

77. Parulkar AA, Pendergrass ML, Granda-Ayala R, Lee TR, Fonseca VA. Nonhypoglycemic effects of thiazolidinediones. Ann Intern Med 2001;134(1):61–71.

78. Stratton IM, Adler AI, Neil HA, et al. Association of glycaemia with macrovascular and microvascular complications of type 2 diabetes (UKPDS 35): prospective observational study. BMJ 2000;321(7258):405–412.

79. UK Prospective Diabetes Study (UKPDS) Group. Effect of intensive blood-glucose control with metformin on complications in overweight patients with type 2 diabetes (UKPDS 34). Lancet 1998;352(9131):854–865.

80. Lebovitz HE, Dole JF, Patwardhan R, Rappaport EB, Freed MI. Rosiglitazone monotherapy is effective in patients with type 2 diabetes. J Clin Endocrinol Metab 2001;86(1):280–288.

81. Garber AJ, Larsen J, Schneider SH, Piper BA, Henry D. Simultaneous glyburide/metformin therapy is superior to component monotherapy as an initial pharmacological treatment for type 2 diabetes. Diabetes Obes Metab 2002;4(3):201–208.

82. Garber AJ, Donovan DS Jr, Dandona P, Bruce S, Park JS. Efficacy of glyburide/metformin tablets compared with initial monotherapy in type 2 diabetes. J Clin Endocrinol Metab 2003;88(8): 3598–3604.

83. Coniff RF, Shapiro JA, Robbins D, et al. Reduction of glycosylated hemoglobin and postprandial hyperglycemia by acarbose in patients with NIDDM: a placebo-controlled dose-comparison study. Diabetes Care 1995;18(6):817–824.

84. Bolli GB, Di Marchi RD, Park GD, Pramming S, Koivisto VA. Insulin analogues and their potential in the management of diabetes mellitus. Diabetologia 1999;42(10):1151–1167.

85. Vivian EM, Olarte SV, Gutierrez AM. Insulin strategies for type 2 diabetes mellitus. Ann Pharmacother 2004;38(11):1916–1923.

86. Lindstrom T, Olsson PO, Arnqvist HJ. The use of human ultralente is limited by great intraindividual variability in overnight plasma insulin profiles. Scand J Clin Lab Invest 2000;60(5):341–347.

87. Lepore M, Pampanelli S, Fanelli C, et al. Pharmacokinetics and pharmacodynamics of subcutaneous injection of long-acting human insulin analog glargine, NPH insulin, and ultralente human insulin and continuous subcutaneous infusion of insulin lispro. Diabetes 2000;49(12):2142–2148.

88. Heinemann L, Linkeschova R, Rave K, Hompesch B, Sedlak M, Heise T. Time-action profile of the long-acting insulin analog insulin glargine (HOE901) in comparison with those of NPH insulin and placebo. Diabetes Care 2000;23(5):644–649.

89. Hedman CA, Lindstrom T, Arnqvist HJ. Direct comparison of insulin lispro and aspart shows small differences in plasma insulin profiles after subcutaneous injection in type 1 diabetes. Diabetes Care 2001;24(6):1120, 1121.

90. Dailey GE III, Noor MA, Park JS, Bruce S, Fiedorek FT. Glycemic control with glyburide/metformin tablets in combination with rosiglitazone in patients with type 2 diabetes: a randomized, double-blind trial. Am J Med 2004;116(4):223–229.

91. Yale JF, Valiquett TR, Ghazzi MN, Owens-Grillo JK, Whitcomb RW, Foyt HL. The effect of a thiazolidinedione drug, troglitazone, on glycemia in patients with type 2 diabetes mellitus poorly controlled with sulfonylurea and metformin: a multicenter, randomized, double-blind, placebo-controlled trial. Ann Intern Med 2001;134(9 Pt 1):737–745.

92. Aljabri K, Kozak SE, Thompson DM. Addition of pioglitazone or bedtime insulin to maximal doses of sulfonylurea and metformin in type 2 diabetes patients with poor glucose control: a prospective, randomized trial. Am J Med 2004;116(4):230–235.

93. Groop LC, Widen E, Ekstrand A, et al. Morning or bedtime NPH insulin combined with sulfonylurea in treatment of NIDDM. Diabetes Care 1992;15(7):831–834.

94. Riddle MC, Rosenstock J, Gerich J. The treat-to-target trial: randomized addition of glargine or human NPH insulin to oral therapy of type 2 diabetic patients. Diabetes Care 2003;26(11):3080–3086.

95. Yki-Jarvinen H, Dressler A, Ziemen M. Less nocturnal hypoglycemia and better post-dinner glucose control with bedtime insulin glargine compared with bedtime NPH insulin during insulin combination therapy in type 2 diabetes. HOE 901/3002 Study Group. Diabetes Care 2000;23(8):1130–1136.

96. Yki-Jarvinen H, Ryysy L, Nikkila K, Tulokas T, Vanamo R, Heikkila M. Comparison of bedtime insulin regimens in patients with type 2 diabetes mellitus: a randomized, controlled trial. Ann Intern Med 1999;130(5):389–396.

97. Aviles-Santa L, Sinding J, Raskin P. Effects of metformin in patients with poorly controlled, insulin-treated type 2 diabetes mellitus: a randomized, double-blind, placebo-controlled trial. Ann Intern Med 1999;131(3):182–188.

98. Hermann LS, Kalen J, Katzman P, et al. Long-term glycaemic improvement after addition of metformin to insulin in insulin-treated obese type 2 diabetes patients. Diabetes Obes Metab 2001;3(6):428–434.

99. Fritsche A, Schmulling RM, Haring HU, Stumvoll M. Intensive insulin therapy combined with metformin in obese type 2 diabetic patients. Acta Diabetol 2000;37(1):13–18.
100. Jaber LA, Nowak SN, Slaughter RR. Insulin-metformin combination therapy in obese patients with type 2 diabetes. J Clin Pharmacol 2002;42(1):89–94.
101. Buse JB, Gumbiner B, Mathias NP, Nelson DM, Faja BW, Whitcomb RW. Troglitazone use in insulin-treated type 2 diabetic patients. The Troglitazone Insulin Study Group. Diabetes Care 1998;21(9): 1455–1461.
102. Schwartz S, Raskin P, Fonseca V, Graveline JF. Effect of troglitazone in insulin-treated patients with type II diabetes mellitus. Troglitazone and Exogenous Insulin Study Group. N Engl J Med 1998; 338(13):861–866.
103. Raskin P, Rendell M, Riddle MC, Dole JF, Freed MI, Rosenstock J. A randomized trial of rosiglitazone therapy in patients with inadequately controlled insulin-treated type 2 diabetes. Diabetes Care 2001;24(7):1226–1232.
104. Rosenstock J, Einhorn D, Hershon K, Glazer NB, Yu S. Efficacy and safety of pioglitazone in type 2 diabetes: a randomised, placebo-controlled study in patients receiving stable insulin therapy. Int J Clin Pract 2002;56(4):251–257.
105. Buch HN, Baskar V, Barton DM, Kamalakannan D, Akarca C, Singh BM. Combination of insulin and thiazolidinedione therapy in massively obese patients with Type 2 diabetes. Diabet Med 2002;19(7):572–574.
106. Ohkubo Y, Kishikawa H, Araki E, et al. Intensive insulin therapy prevents the progression of diabetic microvascular complications in Japanese patients with non-insulin-dependent diabetes mellitus: a randomized prospective 6-year study. Diabetes Res Clin Pract 1995;28(2):103–117.
107. Fanelli CG, Pampanelli S, Porcellati F, Rossetti P, Brunetti P, Bolli GB. Administration of neutral protamine Hagedorn insulin at bedtime versus with dinner in type 1 diabetes mellitus to avoid nocturnal hypoglycemia and improve control: a randomized, controlled trial. Ann Intern Med 2002; 136(7):504–514.
108. Bolli GB, Perriello G, Fanelli CG, De Feo P. Nocturnal blood glucose control in type I diabetes mellitus. Diabetes Care 1993;16(Suppl 3):71–89.
109. Roach P, Strack T, Arora V, Zhao Z. Improved glycaemic control with the use of self-prepared mixtures of insulin lispro and insulin lispro protamine suspension in patients with types 1 and 2 diabetes. Int J Clin Pract 2001;55(3):177–182.
110. Holst JJ, Deacon CF. Glucagon-like peptide 1 and inhibitors of dipeptidyl peptidase IV in the treatment of type 2 diabetes mellitus. Curr Opin Pharmacol 2004;4(6):589–596.

28 Surgical Treatment of Obesity and Diabetes

Benjamin E. Schneider, MD
and Edward C. Mun, MD

CONTENTS

INTRODUCTION

Obesity has increasingly been recognized as an epidemic in the United States. The incidence of obesity has risen such that the most recent National Health and Nutrition Examination Survey (NHANES 1999–2000) demonstrates that two-thirds of Americans are classified as overweight or obese *(1)*. A person's adiposity is typically described in terms of body mass index (BMI), defined as a person's weight (kg) divided by body surface area (m^2), at which obesity starts at a BMI of 30 kg/m^2. This rise in obesity is closely associated with increases in numerous related diseases such as type 2 diabetes mellitus, coronary artery disease, hypertension, dyslipidemia, asthma, obstructive sleep apnea, gastroesophageal reflux, stroke, certain types of cancer, degenerative joint disease, and depression *(2,3)*. Obese individuals may suffer from diminished life expectancy, depending on the age of onset of obesity (2–5 yr for those who are moderately obese and 5–20 yr for those with severe obesity) *(4)*. This increased mortality contributes to approx 280,000 deaths annually in the United States alone *(5)*. The economic cost of combating obesity and associated comorbidities is estimated to exceed $100 billion annually in the United States *(6)*.

SURGICAL THERAPY FOR MORBID OBESITY

Numerous lines of evidence confirm that weight loss reduces risk factors for obesity-induced comorbid diseases *(7)*. In response to the relatively poor weight loss attained by current nonoperative therapy (diet, exercise, behavior modification, pharmacotherapy),

From: *Contemporary Diabetes: Obesity and Diabetes*
Edited by: C. S. Mantzoros © Humana Press Inc., Totowa, NJ

Table 1
Criteria for Surgical Management of Morbid Obesity

Class II (BMI = 35–40 kg/m^2) obesity with significant comorbidities or Class III (BMI > 40 kg/m^2)
  obesity
Age 16–65 yr
Acceptable risk for surgery
Previous unsuccessful attempts at long-term weight loss by nonsurgical therapy
Realistic expectations of weight loss outcomes
A well-informed and motivated patient
Long-term commitment to lifestyle changes and follow-up
Supportive social environment
No active alcohol or substance abuse
Absence of psychosis and severe depression

surgical procedures have been developed to induce significant and durable weight loss. Despite the inherent perioperative risks, bariatric surgery has clearly demonstrated its superior weight loss capacity and resultant improvements in comorbidities. The goal of surgical therapy is to decrease the morbidity and mortality associated with severe obesity through sustained weight loss and improved metabolic and organ function. Various surgical techniques and management protocols by multiple centers led to the sometimes confusing practice of bariatric surgery. In 1991, the National Institutes of Health convened and established guidelines for the surgical management of severely obese individuals *(3)*. The resultant consensus statement established the criteria by which obese patients are selected and managed for surgical therapy (Table 1). To be eligible for surgical therapy, an obese patient must have a BMI >40 (or a BMI >35 with significant obesity-related comorbidities) along with acceptable surgical risk. Gradual acceptance of bariatric procedures by physicians and patients has led to dramatic growth in this field. In 2003, more than 100,000 bariatric procedures were performed *(8)*.

Surgical therapies for severe obesity are mechanistically either restrictive or malabsorptive in nature. The malabsorptive procedures are designed to bypass long segments of the small intestine, thereby reducing the intestinal absorptive surface area and resulting in less effective caloric uptake. Restrictive procedures are designed to reduce the capacity of the stomach by creating a small neostomach, thereby reducing the volume of food that a patient may be able to ingest. The combination of advances in technology and accumulated clinical experience has led to a better understanding of the surgical mechanisms as well as improved patient care and outcome. Whereas some techniques have evolved, others have become obsolete. An ideal bariatric operation would produce effective and durable weight loss with minimal morbidity and mortality to the patients.

MALABSORPTIVE PROCEDURES

Jejunoileal Bypass

Among malabsorptive procedures, jejunoileal bypass (JIB) was the first operation described (Fig. 1A). The JIB was created by dividing the proximal jejunum distal to the ligament of Treitz, then creating an anastomosis to the ileum 10 cm from the ileocecal valve *(9)*. Owing to the functional "short-gut syndrome" created by the procedure, only a fraction of the ingested nutrients was digested and absorbed in JIB, thus making it a purely malabsorptive procedure. Although effective in reducing

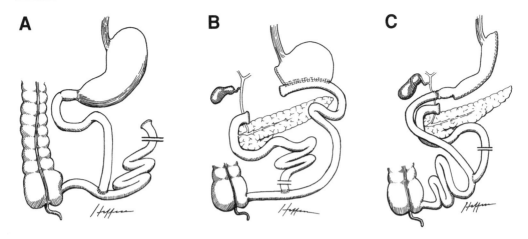

Fig. 1. Malabsorptive procedures: **(A)** JIB; **(B)** BPD; **(C)** BPD with DS.

absorptive capacity and thereby resulting in weight loss, late complications ultimately led to the need to reverse the procedure in 20–50% of patients and to abandon
this procedure completely *(10)*. Bacterial overgrowth in the stagnant blind intestinal
loop leading to translocation of the antigenic materials into the portal circulation is
thought to contribute to the major complications of this procedure. Patients often
developed nephrolithiasis, dental caries, renal failure, bypass enteritis, cirrhosis,
hepatic failure, arthritis, and severe metabolic deficiencies *(11–15)*. For survivors
of JIB, lifelong medical surveillance is necessary in order to monitor closely for
complications.

Biliopancreatic Diversion and Duodenal Switch

Biliopancreatic diversion (BPD) and duodenal switch (DS) operations were designed
to avoid the complications associated with the blind loop of the JIB while still maintaining the capacity to reduce absorption of nutrients. Thus, the blind intestinal segment was eliminated while the functional small bowel length was kept short in these
procedures, to maintain nutrient and caloric malabsorption. Both operations offer a
small degree of food volume restriction via either a distal gastrectomy (BPD) or sleeve
gastrectomy (DS) *(16)* (Fig. 1B,C) *(17)*. Passage of ingested food (via alimentary limb)
is diverted from contact with digestive enzymes and bile (via biliopancreatic limb) until
both reach the common intestinal channel for proper digestion and absorption. Both
BPD and DS rely on a short common channel to limit absorption of nutrients. As a
result, excess weight loss of 70–80% has been documented *(18,19)*. Conventionally, postoperative weight loss is described in terms of excess weight loss, defined as a person's
actual weight loss vs the amount of weight loss required to reach ideal body weight.
Although BPD and DS represent improvements over the JIB by eliminating the blind
intestinal loop, late nutritional complications may still occur. Diarrhea, hepatic failure,
and metabolic derangements such as metabolic bone disease, protein malnutrition, iron
deficiency anemia, and various vitamin deficiencies may occur *(20)*. In light of potential metabolic complications as well as a paucity of data comparing malabsorptive procedures to restrictive operations, the BPD and DS remain relatively uncommon bariatric
operations in the United States except in a few centers *(21)*.

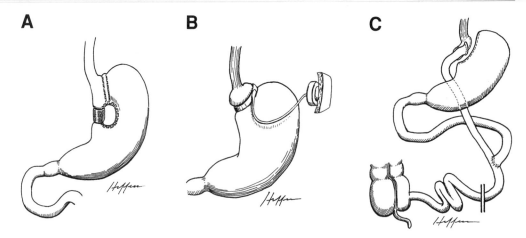

Fig. 2. Restrictive procedures: **(A)** VBG; **(B)** LAGB; **(C)** Roux-en-Y gastric bypass.

RESTRICTIVE PROCEDURES

Vertical Banded Gastroplasty

Vertical banded gastroplasty (VBG) evolved from earlier attempts to induce weight loss by gastric partitioning *(22,23)*. The procedure employs a vertical staple line to create a small gastric pouch and is often referred to as a "stomach-stapling" operation. The pouch outlet is then reinforced with a circumferential band of polypropylene mesh to ensure that the stoma does not dilate (Fig. 2A). It is purely restrictive in that it limits solid food intake by reducing the stomach's reservoir capacity, leaving the absorptive function of the small intestine unaltered. The small pouch gets filled quickly with solid food and limits the meal size. Weight loss occurs primarily owing to decreased solid food intake.

Early enthusiasm for VBG has gradually abated in light of a relatively high incidence of complications such as staple line dehiscence, stomal stenosis, weight regain, persistent vomiting, and need for revision *(24–27)*. Additionally, the weight loss following VBG has been shown to be inferior to that of gastric bypass in randomized prospective comparison. Sugerman et al. *(28)* reported excess weight loss at 1 yr following VBG to be 42%, vs 66% after gastric bypass. Furthermore, patients with a propensity to eat sweets (i.e., milkshakes, ice cream) tend to lose even less weight following VBG *(29)*. Because of the lack of sustained weight loss and high complication rates, VBG is no longer considered to be a first-line surgical option *(21)*.

Laparoscopic Adjustable Gastric Band

Laparoscopic adjustable gastric band (LAGB) represents another purely restrictive procedure. A band consisting of a silicon elastomer is placed circumferentially around the upper portion of the stomach in order to create a small gastric pouch (Fig. 2B). Because of the absence of the staple lines seen in VBG, many of the complications associated with the staple lines, such as staple line dehiscence, are avoided. An attached injection port is placed within a subcutaneous pocket, allowing adjustment of the inner diameter of the band by instilling or removing saline. This feature differentiates the LAGB from the VBG in that the aperture of the band may be adjusted, thus resulting in an increased degree of restriction and control. Furthermore, relative simplicity in placement, very low operative mortality (0–0.53%), and avoidance of gastric division or staple line make the LAGB an attractive surgical option *(30–32)*.

Despite Food and Drug Administration approval in 2001, the early experience with LAGB in the United States was disappointing in terms of complications and weight loss *(33)*. However, reports from international series as well as subsequent American experiences have demonstrated improved outcomes. One of the more common complications following LAGB is prolapse of the gastric wall through the band with resultant acute stomal obstruction and vomiting (2–14.2%) *(34–37)*. Other complications including device erosion through the gastric wall (0–2.8%) and device malfunction (0.4–11%); these complications generally require surgical revision (1–13.5%) *(30,35,38)*. Weight loss following LAGB tends to be slower than that following malabsorptive procedures or gastric bypass. Although more long-term follow-up data are necessary, the LAGB does appear to provide durable weight loss. Reports of excess weight loss at 12 mo (34.5–58%), 24 mo (36–87%), 36 mo (36.2–64%), 60 mo (46.7–54%), and 72 mo (30.4–62.6%) do support sustained weight loss following LAGB *(38–44)*. With the help of these encouraging data, LAGB continues to gain acceptance as a first-line procedure in the treatment of morbid obesity. It has largely replaced VBG as the main purely restrictive procedure.

GASTRIC BYPASS

Gastric bypass has undergone numerous technical changes since its first description as a weight loss procedure in 1969 *(45)*. Its development was based on the observation that patients who underwent partial gastrectomy for cancer and ulcer disease experienced significant long-term weight loss. Many of the subsequent modifications were aimed at improving postoperative weight loss and decreasing surgical complications. More recent advancement comes from application of laparoscopic techniques to gastric bypasss *(46)*. Currently, the operation entails construction of a small gastric pouch and a narrow stoma, and a Roux-en-Y rearrangement of the small intestine (Fig. 2C). Through division of the upper stomach, a very small gastric pouch (~30 cc) is created in order to restrict the volume of ingested food. This food-restriction mechanism is further enhanced by construction of a relatively tight outlet (gastrojejunostomy) to limit rapid emptying of the pouch's content into the rest of the gastrointestinal (GI) tract. The fundus of the stomach, which tends to dilate, is excluded to avoid excessive stretching of the pouch. Digestion and absorption of nutrients mostly occur in the common small bowel channel where alimentary Roux limb is joined by biliopancreatic limb (jejunojejunostomy). While gastric bypass is considered primarily a restrictive operation, additional mechanisms are also in play to induce weight loss. A direct passage of high-calorie food into the jejunum (Roux limb) is associated with dumping syndrome, characterized by nausea, light-headedness, palpitations, diaphoresis, and abdominal pain and/or diarrhea. Such unpleasant symptoms following ingestion of sweets provide negative conditioning against a diet high in sugar. More recently, the appetite-increasing hormone ghrelin was shown to be decreased and peptide YY increased (unpublished observations) in post–gastric bypass patients, offering additional clues to appetite reduction and excellent weight loss observed in these patients *(47)*.

Complications following gastric bypass such as GI leak, internal hernia, anastomotic stricture, and thromboembolic events are relatively infrequent *(48)*. Perioperative mortality may range from 0 to 2%, depending on the operative setting and surgeon's experience *(49–53)*. Weight loss following gastric bypass has been shown to be reliable and durable *(54)*. Early weight loss is typically rapid, and the maximum weight loss is usually reached in 1 to 2 yr. Excess weight loss 12 mo following gastric bypass has been described as ranging from 68 to 80% *(51,55–57)*. It is currently the most commonly performed bariatric procedure in the United States. The laparoscopic approach to gastric bypass is becoming more popular because of faster postoperative recovery, fewer wound infection and hernia complications, better cosmesis, and decreased incisional pain *(56)*.

OUTCOMES

For most patients, any of the current bariatric procedures may offer effective weight loss. While malabsorptive procedures may yield greater excess weight loss, restrictive procedures may result in fewer nutritional and metabolic complications and carry lower perioperative mortality. A recent meta-analysis of 136 studies on bariatric surgery found a progressive decrease in mortality from malabsorptive operations (1.1%) to gastric bypass (0.5%) to purely restrictive procedures (0.1%) *(58)*. By contrast, better weight loss is observed with purely restrictive operations, then decreases with gastric bypass to malabsorptive operations. In addition to weight loss benefit, patients enjoy improvement in or resolution of obesity-related comorbidies. Bariatric surgery has been clearly and repeatedly shown to reverse diabetes, hypertension, sleep apnea, and hyperlipidemia *(58)*. Following LAGB, the majority of patients with type 2 diabetes may expect remission of diabetes (64%) and improved glucose control (26%) *(36,59,60)*. In contrast to purely restrictive procedures, glycemic changes following gastric bypass may be even more profound, with many patients exhibiting resolution of diabetes well before maximum weight loss *(54)*. Although poorly understood at present, exclusion of the foregut (stomach and duodenum) from the food stream appears to influence the intestinal and hepatic hormonal milieu in a manner resulting in greater insulin sensitivity. Although almost all patients undergoing Roux-en-Y gastric bypass expect improvements in type 2 diabetes, complete resolution is more likely in those who achieve weight loss early in the course of their diabetes *(54,61–63)*.

Weight loss has long been the standard recommendation for morbidly obese patients, particularly those who experiernce associated comorbidity *(7)*. Given that current medical therapy is generally not effective in treating patients who reach morbid obesity, surgery offers a rational treatment option based on evidence from extensive studies. Bariatric procedures that are currently in use have been shown to achieve excellent weight loss unparalleled by any combinations of nonsurgical weight loss therapies. Surgically induced weight loss not only is durable but also results in improvements in and reversal of most of the medical conditions stemming from the underlying obesity, thereby improving quality of life. Various technological innovations and modifications of the techniques have made bariatric procedures more effective and safer. Although the current focus of the bariatric surgery field correctly targets reduction of surgical morbidity and improvement in patient safety, ongoing efforts must be made to better understand the pathophysiology of obesity and the physiological changes effected by bariatric surgery.

REFERENCES

1. Flegal KM, Ogden CM, Johnson CL. Prevalence and trends in obesity among US adults, 1999-2000. JAMA 2002;14:1723–1727.
2. Must A, Spadano J, Coakley EH, Field AE, Colditz G, Dietz WH. The disease burden associated with overweight and obesity. JAMA 1999;282:1523–1529.
3. Consensus Development Conference Panel. NIH conference: gastrointestinal surgery for severe obesity Ann Intern Med 1991;115:956–961.
4. Fontaine KR, et al. Years of life lost due to obesity. JAMA 2003;289:187–193.

5. Allison DB, Fontaine KR, Manson JE, Stevens J, VanItallie TB. Annual deaths attributable to obesity in the United States. JAMA 1999;282:1530–1538.

6. Wolf A, Colditz G. Current estimates of the economic cost of obesity in the United States. Obes Res 1998;6:97–106.

7. National Heart, Lung, and Blood Institute, Public Health Service, U.S. Department of Health and Human Services, eds. Expert Panel: Clinical Guidelines on the Identification, Evaluation, and Treatment of Overweight and Obesity in Adults: The Evidence Report. National Institutes of Health, Bethesda, MD:1998.

8. Steinbrook R. Surgery for severe obesity. N Engl J Med 2004;350:1075–1079.

9. Payne JH, DeWind LT. Surgical treatment of obesity. Am J Surg 1969;118:141–147.

10. Deitel M, Shahi B, Anand PK, Deitel FH, Cardinell DL. Long-term outcome in a series of jejunoileal bypass patients. Obes Surg 1993;3:247–252.

11. Requarth JA, Burchard KW, Colacchio TA, et al. Long-term morbidity following jejunoileal bypass: the continuing potential need for surgical reversal. Arch Surg 1995;130:318–325.

12. Kroyer JM, Talbert WM Jr. Morphologic liver changes in intestinal bypass patients. Am J Surg 1986;139:855–859.

13. Halverson JD, Wise L, Wazna MF, Ballinger WF. Jejunoileal bypass for morbid obesity: a critical appraisal. Am J Med 1978;64:461–475.

14. Greenway SE, G.F. Root surface caries: a complication of jejunoileal bypass. Obes Surg 2000;10:33–36.

15. Griffen WO Jr, Young VL, Stevenson CC. A prospective comparison of gastric and jejunoileal bypass procedures for morbid obesity. Ann Surg 1977;186:500–509.

16. Scopinaro N, Adami GF, Marinari GM, et al. Biliopancreatic diversion. World J Surg 1998;22: 936–946.

17. Mun EC, Blackburn GL, Matthews JB. Current status of medical and surgical therapy for obesity. Gastroenterology 2001;120:669–681.

18. Scopinaro N, Gianetta E, Adami GF, et al. Biliopancreatic diversion for obesity at eighteen years. Surgery 1996;119:261–268.

19. Hess DS, Hess DW. Biliopancreatic diversion with a duodenal switch. Obes Surg 1998;8:267–282.

20. Murr MM, Balsiger BM, Kennedy FP, Mai JL, Sarr MG. Malabsorptive procedures for severe obesity: comparison of pancreaticobiliary bypass and very very long limb Roux-en-Y gastric bypass. J Gastrointest Surg 1999;3:607–612.

21. Jones D, Provost D, De Maria EJ, Smith CD, Morgenstern L, Schirmer B. Optimal management of the morbidly obese patient SAGES appropirateness conference statement. Surg Endosc 2004;18: 1029–1037.

22. Mason EE. Vertical banded gastroplasty for obesity. Arch Surg 1982;117:701–706.

23. Pace WG, Martin EW Jr, Tetirick T, Fabri PJ, Carey LC. Gastric partitioning for morbid obesity. Ann Surg 1979;190:392–400.

24. MacLean LD, Rhode BM, Sampalis J, Forse RA. Results of the surgical treatment of obesity. Am J Surg 1993;165:155–160; discussion 160–152.

25. Nightengale ML, Sarr MG, Kelly KA, Jensen MD, Zinsmeister AR, Palumbo PJ. Prospective evaluation of vertical banded gastroplasty as the primary operation for morbid obesity [see comments]. Mayo Clin Proc 1991;66:773–782.

26. Balsiger BM, Poggio JL, Mai J, Kelly KA, Sarr MG. Ten and more years after vertical banded gastroplasty as primary operation for morbid obesity. J Gastrointest Surg 2000;4:598–605.

27. Balsiger BM, Murr MM, Mai J, Sarr MG. Gastroesophageal reflux after intact vertical banded gastroplasty: correction by conversion to Roux-en-Y gastric bypass. J Gastrointest Surg 2000;4:276–281.

28. Sugerman HJ, Starkey JV, Birkenhauer R. A randomized prospective trial of gastric bypass versus vertical banded gastroplasty for morbid obesity and their effects on sweets versus non-sweets eaters. Ann Surg 1987;205:613–624.

29. Sugerman HJ, Londrey GL, Kellum JM, et al. Weight loss with vertical banded gastroplasty and Roux-Y gastric bypass for morbid obesity with selective versus random assignment. Am J Surg 1989;157:93–102.

30. O'Brien PE, Dixon JB. Weight loss and early and late complications—the international experience. Am J Surg 2002;184:42S–45S.

31. Angrisani L, Furbetta F, Doldi B, et al. Lap-Band adjustable gastric banding system: the Italian experience with 1863 patients operated on 6 years. Surg Endosc 2003;17:409–412.

32. Schneider B, Sanchez V, Jones D. How to implant the laparoscopic adjustable gastric band for morbid obesity. Contemp Surg 2004;60:248–264.

33. FDA Trial Summary of Safety and Effectiveness Data: The Lap-Band Adjustable Gastric Banding System (P000008). www.fda.gov/cdrh/pdf/p000008.htm.

34. Ren CJ, Horgan S, Ponce J. US experience with the LAP-BAND System. Am J Surg 2002;184:46S–50S.

35. Rubenstein R. Laparoscopic adjustable gastric banding at a US center with up to 3-year follow-up. Obes Surg 2002;12:380–384.

36. Fielding GA, Rhodes M, Nathanson LK. Laparoscopic gastric banding for morbid obesity: surgical outcome in 335 cases. Surg Endosc 1999;13:550–554.

37. DeMaria EJ, Sugerman HJ, Kellum JM, Meador JG, Wolfe LG. Results of 281 consecutive total laparoscopic Roux-en-Y gastric bypasses to treat morbid obesity. Ann Surg 2002;235:640-645; discussion 645–647.

38. Angrisani L, Furbetta F, Doldi B, et al. Lap-Band adjustable gastric banding system: the Italian experience with 1863 patients operated on 6 years. Surg Endosc 2003;17:409–412.

39. DeMaria EJ. Laparoscopic adjustable silicone gastric banding. Surg Clin North Am 2001;81: 1129–1144, vii.

40. Weiner R, Wagner D, Bockhorn H. Laparoscopic gastric banding for morbid obesity. J Laparoendosc Adv Surg Tech A 1999;9:23–30.

41. Weiner R, Blanco-Engert R, Weiner S, et al. Outcome after laparoscopic adjustable gastric banding-8 years experience. Obes Surg 2003;13:427–434.

42. Dargent J. Laparoscopic adjustable gastric banding: lessons from the first 500 patients in a single institution. Obes Surg 1999;9:446–452.

43. O'Brien PE, Dixon JB. The extent of the problem of obesity. Am J Surg 2002;184:4S–8S.

44. Favretti F, Cadiere GB, Segato G, et al. Laparoscopic banding: selection and technique in 830 patients. Obes Surg 2002;12:385–390.

45. Mason EE, Ito C. Gastric bypass. Ann Surg 1969;170:329–339.

46. Wittgrove AC, Clark GW, Tremblay LJ. Laparoscopic gastric bypass, Roux-en-Y: preliminary report of five cases. Obes Surg 1994;4:353–357.

47. Cummings DE, Weigle DS, Frayo RS, et al. Plasma ghrelin levels after diet-induced weight loss or gastric bypass surgery. N Engl J Med 2002;346:1623–1630.

48. Schneider BE, Villegas L, Blackburn GL, Mun EC, Critchlow JF, Jones DB. Laparoscopic gastric bypass surgery: outcomes. J Laparoendosc Adv Surg Tech A 2003;13:247–255.

49. Flum DR, Dellinger EP. Impact of gastric bypass operation on survival: a population-based analysis. J Am Coll Surg 2004;199:543–551.

50. Higa KD, Boone KB, Ho T. Complications of the laparoscopic Roux-en-Y gastric bypass: 1,040 patients—what have we learned? Obes Surg 2000;10:509–513.

51. Schauer PR, Ikramuddin S, Gourash W, Ramanathan R, Luketich J. Outcomes after laparoscopic Roux-en-Y gastric bypass for morbid obesity. Ann Surg 2000;232:515–529.

52. Schauer P, Ikramuddin S., Hamad G, Gourash W. The learning curve for laparoscopic Roux-en-Y gastric bypass is 100 cases. Surg Endosc. 2003;17:212–215.

53. Wittgrove AC, Clark GW. Laparoscopic gastric bypass, Roux-en-Y-500 patients: technique and results, with 3–60 month follow-up. Obes Surg 2000;10:233–239.

54. Pories WJ, Swanson MS, MacDonald KG, et al. Who would have thought it? An operation proves to be the most effective therapy for adult-onset diabetes mellitus. Ann Surg 1995;222:339–350; discussion 350–352.

55. Matthews BD, Sing RF, DeLegge MH, Ponsky JL, Henniford BT. Initial results with a stapled gastrojejunostomy for the laparoscopic isolated Roux-en-Y gastric bypass. Am J Surg 2000;179:476–480.

56. Nguyen NT, Goldman C, Rosenquist CJ, et al. Laparoscopic versus open gastric bypass: a randomized study of outcomes, quality of life, and costs. Ann Surg 2001;234:279–289; discussion 289–291.

57. Higa KD, Boone KB, Ho T, Davies OG. Laparoscopic Roux-en-Y gastric bypass for morbid obesity: technique and preliminary results of our first 400 patients. Arch Surg 2000;135:1029–1033; discussion 1033–1034.

58. Buchwald H, Avidor Y, Braunwald E, et al. Bariatric surgery: a systematic review and meta-analysis. JAMA 2004;292:1724–1737.

59. Dixon JB, Dixon AF, O'Brien PE. Improvements in insulin sensitivity and beta-cell function (HOMA) with weight loss in the severely obese: homeostatic model assessment. Diabet Med 2003;20:127–134.

60. Dixon JB, O'Brien PE. Health outcomes of severely obese type 2 diabetic subjects 1 year after laparoscopic adjustable gastric banding. Diabetes Care 2002;25:358–363.

61. Schauer PR, Burguera B, Ikramuddin S, et al. Effect of laparoscopic Roux-en Y gastric bypass on type 2 diabetes mellitus. Ann Surg 2003;238:467–484.

62. Sjostrom CD, Lissner L, Wedel H, Sjostrom L. Reduction in incidence of diabetes, hypertension and lipid disturbances after intentional weight loss induced by bariatric surgery: the SOS Intervention Study. Obes Res 1999;7:477–484.

63. Sugerman HJ, Wolfe LG, Sica DA, Clore JN. Diabetes and hypertension in severe obesity and effects of gastric bypass-induced weight loss. Ann Surg 2003;237:751–756; discussion 757, 758.

29 Future Developments in the Area of Pharmacotherapy

Molecules in Early-Stage Preclinical Development and in Clinical Trials That May Affect Energy Homeostasis

Diana Barb, MD, *Greeshma K. Shetty,* MD, *and Christos S. Mantzoros,* MD, DSc

CONTENTS

INTRODUCTION
POTENTIAL TREATMENT OR TARGETS FOR PHARMACEUTICAL
    DEVELOPMENT
REFERENCES

INTRODUCTION

Obesity is a chronic and highly prevalent medical condition associated with increased risk of developing numerous comorbidities such as hypertension, type 2 diabetes, stroke, and heart disease. The etiology of obesity is multifactorial and the condition remains difficult to treat. In the United States, a nation of 60 million obese adults *(1)*, there are only a few antiobesity medications available or approved for the treatment of obesity. In addition, the short-term effect of these medications is modest and their long-term efficacy is doubtful, because rebound weight gain is common; therefore, the efforts of researchers and the pharmaceutical industry are currently focused on developing new potent antiobesity medications.

Pharmacotherapy should be considered for obese (body mass index [BMI] > 30 kg/m^2) or overweight individuals (BMI > 27 kg/m^2) with comorbidities. In addition to medications approved for short-term treatment (such as the noradrenergic agent phentermine), only two medications (the norepinephrine, dopamine, and serotonin reuptake inhibitor sibutramine and the lipase inhibitor orlistat) are currently approved for long-term treatment of obesity *(2)*. Moreover, an antidiabetic medication, metformin, results in approx 2 kg of weight loss over 2.8 yr *(3)* and can thus be considered an adjunctive antiobesity treatment. Since recent meta-analyses of published trials indicate that the effect of

From: *Contemporary Diabetes: Obesity and Diabetes*
Edited by: C. S. Mantzoros © Humana Press Inc., Totowa, NJ

available medications is only modest (on average 2.9 and 4.6% greater than placebo reduction in body weight after 1 yr of follow-up with orlistat and sibutramine, respectively) *(4)*, more effective medications are clearly needed. Thus, more than 100 molecules, mainly developed on the basis of recent discoveries in the physiology of energy homeostasis, are currently being tested in preclinical studies and clinical trials.

POTENTIAL TREATMENT OR TARGETS FOR PHARMACEUTICAL DEVELOPMENT

Current antiobesity agents and investigational antiobesity agents can be classified in the following main categories:

1. Agents acting on central nervous system (CNS) pathways including leptin and ciliary neurotrophic factor ([CNTF]; Axokine).
2. CNS agents that affect neurotransmitters or neural ion channels, including antidepressants, antiepileptic drugs, and cannabinoid-1 receptor antagonists.
3. Gastrointestinal (GI)-neural pathway agents, including those that increase cholecystokinin (CCK) or glucagon-like peptide-1 activity.
4. Agents that may increase resting metabolic rate.
5. Other diverse agents *(5)*.

Agents Acting on CNS Pathways

LEPTIN

Leptin, the product of the ob gene, a molecule produced almost exclusively by white adipose tissue, triggers anorexigenic circuits and is currently under investigation in phase III clinical trials in leptin-deficient humans. Treatment of children who are morbidly obese owing to congenital leptin deficiency (*n* = 13 to date; not all cases have been published) with daily sc injections of recombinant methionyl human leptin for up to 4 yr decreases appetite, fat mass, hyperinsulinemia, and hyperlipidemia; results in a rapid and sustained increase in thyroid hormone levels; and facilitates appropriately timed pubertal development *(6)*. Similarly, leptin treatment (0.03–0.04 mg/[kg·d]) of leptin-deficient patients with lipodystrophy for 4 mo improves glycemic control and decreases triglyceride levels, liver volume, and liver function tests *(7)*. However, in garden-variety obesity, which is a leptin-resistant state, phase II, randomized, double-blinded, placebo-controlled studies involving administration of recombinant leptin (0.1 and 0.3 mg/kg) have demonstrated a statistically significant, but modest in magnitude, weight loss (5.4–8.5 kg after 24 wk), mainly owing to fat loss *(8)*. Thus, elucidation of the mechanism responsible for the development of leptin resistance in these patients may lead to the development of "leptin sensitizers," including inhibitors of suppressor of cytokine signaling protein-3, a leptin-induced molecule, which impairs leptin signaling transduction through the Janus kinase/signal transducer and activator of transcription (JAK-STAT) pathway *(9)*. Moreover, whether administration of recombinant leptin to obese patients with relative leptin deficiency owing to heterogeneity of the leptin gene could be useful in the treatment of their obesity remains to be proven. Recent interventional studies in lean fasting humans have demonstrated that food deprivation–induced changes in several neuroendocrine axes can be reversed or blunted with the administration of leptin in replacement doses (0.025–0.1 mg/[kg·d]) *(10)*, raising the intriguing possibility that low-dose recombinant leptin replacement treatment may be useful as an adjunctive therapy for the maintenance of weight loss. Similarly, administration of leptin in replacement doses to women with exercise-induced hypothalamic amenorrhea normalizes their neuroendocrine axes, reproductive function, and bone metabolism, indicating that leptin may prove to be an effective treatment not only in this syndrome, but also possibly in anorexia nervosa *(11)*.

CILIARY NEUROTROPHIC FACTOR

CNTF is a 22-kDa protein and an endogenous neuroprotective factor present in the Schwann cells and astrocytes, but not in the peripheral circulation. CNTF is upregulated during injury to these cells *(12)*. The weight-reducing properties of this neuronal growth factor were originally discovered in the context of late-phase clinical trials for amyotrophic lateral sclerosis (ALS), in which CNTF did not affect the course of the disease, but, instead, induced marked weight loss in ALS patients who were not obese at the onset of the trial *(13)*. Although the exact molecular mechanism underlying CNTF's effects is not fully understood, similar to leptin, the anorectic effect is mediated by suppression of neuropeptide Y (NPY) production in the hypothalamus *(14)*. CNTF binds to the CNTF receptors and activates leptin-like intracellular signaling pathways of JAK–STAT and mitogen-activated protein kinase in hypothalamic nuclei, which regulate food intake and body weight. In animal models of obesity, CNTF has been proven to overcome the leptin resistance *(14–16)*.

Axokine, a second-generation recombinant human variant of CNTF that has improved activity and stability, was tested in a recent double-blind, randomized, parallel-group, multicenter study in which 173 obese patients received CNTF (0.3, 1.0, and 2.0 µg/kg) or placebo for 12 wk. Administration of CNTF resulted in significant weight loss (–1.5, –4.1, and –3.4 kg, respectively) with no major adverse effects except for injection site reaction and nausea at the highest doses *(17)*. Although the magnitude of the weight loss observed is not greater than that produced by currently available medications, 30% of participants who did not develop neutralizing antibodies lost 5–7 kg. Interestingly, similar to mice *(18)*, CNTF's effect appears to persist beyond discontinuation of the medication.

These preliminary findings required confirmation in large prospective clinical trials *(17)*. Thus, a phase III trial for Axokine began in 2001, and approx 2000 patients were enrolled. After 1 yr of treatment, the placebo-controlled study of 1467 Axokine-treated subjects and 501 placebo-treated subjects demonstrated that obese subjects treated with Axokine lost more weight than those who received placebo (25.1 vs 17.6%) and experienced a greater average weight loss than those receiving placebo (6.2 vs 2.6 lb). Although the phase III study met its primary end points and many individuals achieved a medically meaningful weight loss, the average weight loss was limited by the development of antibodies, beginning after about 3 mo of Axokine treatment in almost two-thirds of subjects *(19)*. Thus, the future for Axokine as a potential antiobesity medication remains unknown.

NPY, AGOUTI-RELATED PROTEIN, AND MELANIN-CONCENTRATING HORMONE RECEPTOR ANTAGONISTS

NPY is the most potent orexigenic agent known in humans, exerting its physiological effects through a series of NPY receptor subtypes (Y_1, Y_2, Y_4, Y_5, and Y_6) that are members of the G protein-coupled receptor (GPCR) family. NPY Y_1 and NPY Y_5 are the receptor subtypes that are most likely responsible for centrally mediated NPY-induced feeding responses, and NPY Y_5 receptor antagonists have been shown to be effective in reducing food intake in various animal models of feeding *(20)*. For this reason, it is thought that NPY receptor–specific ligands may have value in several therapeutic areas including the treatment of obesity *(21)*. New hydrazide derivatives were described as antagonist compounds of the NPY Y_5 receptor, characterized by their selectivity on the Y_5 receptor owing to their nonaffinity for the receptor subtype Y_1 *(22,23)*. Their potential use in human obesity remains to be proved. In addition, agouti-related protein receptor antagonists and melanin-concentrating hormone receptor antagonists are in various stages of development, but because these neuropeptides have pleiotropic effects, altering their hypothalamic levels or activity to produce weight loss may prove to be a challenge.

MELANOCORTIN RECEPTOR AGONISTS

Converging lines of evidence, including genetic, physiological, and pharmacological data obtained in rodents and humans, support a role for melanocortin receptor 3 (MC3R) and melanocortin receptor 4 (MC4R) in the regulation of energy homeostasis (see Chapter 5). The possible therapeutic role of melanocortin receptor agonists and antagonists in the treatment of obesity and eating disorders, respectively, is an active area of clinical research *(24)*. Intranasal treatment with an MC4R agonist, α-melanocyte-stimulating hormone/$ACTH_{4-10}$, reduced body weight in lean subjects by 0.79 kg over 6 wk *(25)*, but did not alter body weight in two obese persons with proopiomelanocortin deficiency *(26)*. Thus, the results of larger, randomized trials of MC4R agonists are greatly anticipated. MC3R agonists may also result in some weight loss, but most importantly, improve metabolism through a more beneficial partitioning of nutrients, and dual MC4R/MC3R agonists may reduce body weight and improve metabolic comorbidities.

CNS Agents That Affect Neurotransmitters or Neural Ion Channels

ANTIDEPRESSANTS

Obesity is known to be associated with psychopathology, with depression and anxiety the most commonly reported, especially in binge-eating individuals *(27)*. A recent study concluded that, in general, obese people are at increased risk of depression *(28)*. Thus, the use of antidepressants could be justified in many cases. Drugs that are currently being used for the treatment of mood disorders and are associated with weight loss and, therefore, are possible candidates for the treatment of obesity, include (1) selective serotonin reuptake inhibitors (SSRIs) such as fluoxetine, sertraline, fluvoxamine, and citalopram; (2) the serotonin-noradrenaline reuptake inhibitor venlafaxine; and (3) the noradrenaline and dopamine reuptake inhibitor bupropion. Centrally acting antiobesity drugs, such as D-fenfluramine and sibutramine, act in part by increasing dopamine, norepinephrine, or serotonin receptor signaling to decrease food intake *(29)*. Although future serotonin agonists could have a significant therapeutic potential, this class of medications is being approached with extreme caution owing to the cardiopulmonary toxicity associated with the previously approved 5-hydroxytryptamine-releasing agent D-fenfluramine *(30)*.

Selective Serotonin Reuptake Inhibitors. The mechanism underlying the effect of SSRIs on weight is most likely by increasing the synaptic level of the serotonin and by indirectly activating serotonin receptors implicated in appetite regulation. Other proposed mechanisms are inhibition of NPY release and activation of the appetite suppressant pathway via the corticotropin-releasing factor. Fluoxetine (Sarafem® or Prozac®: 10, 20, and

40 mg and a weekly formula capsule of 90 mg containing enteric-coated granules) is the best studied SSRI in obesity. Short-term studies with fluoxetin in obesity reported a weight loss rate significantly higher than in the placebo group, but long-term trials of fluoxetine in obesity have raised doubts about the long-term efficiency of this drug in obese subjects without an underlying psychiatric condition. In a 52-wk, multicenter placebo-controlled trial of fluoxetine (60 mg) including 458 nondepressed obese patients without depression, the difference in weight loss between the groups was significant at wk 20, but not at wk 52 *(31)*. The same investigators, however, reported a significant weight loss in patients with bulimia nervosa in a long-term study *(32)*. In conclusion, specific subgroups of obese patients may benefit form fluoxetine treatment (fluoxetine is approved by the Food and Drug Administration [FDA] for the treatment of bulimia nervosa) *(33)*. Sertraline (Zoloft®: 200 mg), fluvoxamine (Luvox®: 25, 50, 100 mg) and citalopram (Celexa®: 40–60 mg) in the field of obesity were evaluated only in small clinical trials. Sertraline reduced weight significantly compared with placebo, but the long-term effectiveness remains doubtful, because it failed to prevent the rebound weight gain and/or to maintain the weight loss after its discontinuation *(34)*. The weight loss with fluvoxamine or citalopram in separate 12-wk studies tended to be greater in the treatment group than in the placebo group, but was not significantly different *(35,36)*. By contrast, all the aforementioned drugs were effective in reducing binge-eating frequency and BMI in patients with binge-eating disorders *(33,37–39)*.

Serotonin-Noradrenaline Reuptake Inhibitors. Venlafaxine (Effexor®: 25, 37.5, 50 mg; Effexor XL®: 150 mg) acts via the same mechanism as sibutramine, i.e., by inhibiting the reuptake of serotonin and norepinephrine. Its potential as a weight loss agent was evaluated only in a small case series of 35 obese patients who were binge eaters. The drug was effective in reducing the frequency of binge eating and decreased body weight *(40)*, but further studies are needed to elucidate fully its role in the therapeutic armamentarium.

Noradrenaline and Dopamine Reuptake Inhibitors. Bupropion (Wellbutrin® or Zyban®: 100, 150, 200 mg), a drug that is currently approved for treatment of depression and smoking cessation, acts by blocking the reuptake of noradrenaline and dopamine, but without affecting serotonin reuptake. It has recently been shown to produce a 6.2% weight loss, compared with 1.6% in the placebo group, in a short-term trial (8–12 wk) in overweight subjects *(41)*. In a long-term (24–48 wk) randomized, controlled trial (300–400 mg of bupropion vs placebo) in 327 obese patients, bupropion was associated with a significant reduction in weight in a dose-dependent manner and also resulted in maintenance of the weight loss at wk 48 *(42)*.

ANTIEPILEPTIC DRUGS

Among the new antiseizure agents, zonisamide and topiramate, which have been associated with weight loss, are now being tested as promising drugs for the treatment of obesity.

Zonisamide (Zonegran®: 100 mg). Zonisamide, which is, FDA approved for adults with epilepsy, was initially found to be associated with weight loss in patients with epilepsy, with weight loss an adverse effect, in clinical trials of seizure treatment *(43)*. Therefore, its weight loss effect was subsequently tested in obese subjects (see discussion on clinical trials). The primary mechanism of action appears to be on sodium and calcium channels, by blocking repetitive-firing voltage-sensitive Na channels, and reducing voltage-dependent T-type Ca^{2+} currents, consequently stabilizing neuronal membranes and suppressing neuronal hypersynchronization. Because of its chemical structure (similar to that of acetazolamide), it also has a weak inhibiting effect on the enzyme carbonic anhydrase. Its dual mechanism of action makes it a drug for epilepsy that is resistant to other antiepileptic drugs. In vivo, however, zonisamide has also been shown to have serotoninergic and dopaminergic properties, and these effects on the brain may explain, at least in part, its weight loss properties *(33)*. Its pharmacokinetic profile is favorable for clinical use: the drug is rapidly absorbed, food has no effect on bioavailability, it is not bound to plasma proteins, it has a long half-life (63–69 h in healthy volunteers), it does not induce its own metabolism, nor does it induce liver enzymes. It is excreted primarily in urine as the parent drug and as a glucuronide metabolite; zonisamide renal clearance decreases with decreased renal function *(44)*. Contraindications are hypersensitivity to sulfonamides or zonisamide, and adverse effects at the usual antiepileptic dosage include cognitive CNS-related adverse effects (fatigue, somnolence), psychiatric symptoms such as depression and psychosis (2.2%), psychomotor slowing (difficulties with concentration and speech or language problems, difficulties in word finding), and kidney stones (4%). Precautions should be taken in patients with hepatic and renal diseases.

Regarding clinical trials in obesity, in a 16-wk long randomized, double-blind, placebo-controlled phase II trial of 60 obese subjects on a hypocaloric diet (500 kcal/d less than a weight maintaining diet), it was found that administration of zonisamide (100–600 mg/d) resulted in at least 5% weight loss compared with 1% with placebo, and a single-blind extension of the same trial for another 16 wk resulted in even more weight loss (9.4 vs 1.8%) *(45)*. In addition, zonisamide (100–600 mg/d) in the treatment of obese subjects with binge-eating disorder reduced binge-eating frequency and body weight. Fifteen outpatients with binge-eating disorder as defined in *Diagnostic and Statistical Manual of Mental Disorders*, 4th ed. were enrolled for a 12 wk, open-label prospective study (but only eight completed the study). Although the drug was well tolerated, one patient developed a serious renal event, nephrolithiasis with pyelonephritis *(46)*. Furthermore, zonisamide (Zonegran: 100–600 mg/d) in conjunction with a reduced-calorie diet (deficit of 500 kcal/d) resulted in a mean weight loss of 9.2 kg compared with diet alone (the placebo group lost 1.5 kg) in a randomized placebo-controlled study (92% obese women, only five men enrolled) for 32 wk. This regimen was well tolerated. This study also measured the improvement in quality of life, by the Impact of Weight on Quality of Life (IWQOL) questionnaire, and concluded that health, work, mobility, and activities of daily living were all significantly improved in the zonisamide group at both 16 and 32 wk. Ten patients in the zonisamide group reported fatigue vs one patient in the placebo group. Otherwise, no adverse effects were reported differentially between the groups *(47)*. In conclusion, zonisamide is a promising drug for weight reduction, but further larger trials will be needed to determine the overall safety, efficacy, and cost-effectiveness of this compound.

Topiramate (Topamax®: 25-, 50-, 100-, and 200-mg Tablets and 15- and 25-mg Sprinkle Capsules). Another antiepileptic drug, approved for use as an adjunctive therapy for the treatment of partial onset seizures in adults *(48)*, topiramate has also been shown to decrease appetite and body weight in patients with epilepsy *(49,50)* and to improve metabolic parameters associated with weight loss in patients with bipolar disorder *(51,52)*. Its antiseizure effect is probably mainly exerted through blocking voltage-dependent sodium channels and augmenting the activity of the neurotransmitter γ-aminobutyrate (γ-aminobutyric acid [GABA]) at some subtypes of the GABA-A receptor. The drug also antagonizes the kainate subtype of the glutamate receptor and inhibits the carbonic anhydrase enzyme, particularly isozymes II and IV. These latter effects have been proposed as possible mechanisms involved in weight reduction and reduced appetite (53). In addition, topiramate proved to have insulin-sensitizing properties and a favorable effect on plasma glucose levels. Recent experiments utilizing euglycemic hyperinsulinemic clamp studies in treated and untreated insulin-resistant Zucker Diabetic Fatty (ZDF) rats as well as lean insulin-sensitive animals revealed increased in vivo insulin sensitivity in treated ZDF rats. A 30–40% increase in the glucose infusion rate, a 40% increase in the ability of insulin to suppress hepatic glucose output, and increased free fatty acid (FFAs) suppression from 40 to 75% were observed in treated animals. In adipose tissue, topiramate enhances insulin suppression of lipolysis. Ex vivo, a marked increase in insulin-stimulated glucose transport was observed in isolated adipocytes but not in isolated soleus muscle. In conclusion, it appears that treatment with topiramate leads to insulin sensitization, an effect that is exerted predominantly through adipose tissue. The mechanism by which topiramate exerts insulin-sensitizing effects is independent of peroxisome proliferator-activated receptor γ (PPARγ): studies on direct PPARγ binding and transactivation assays revealed no activity of the compound on the PPARγ receptor (54).

Regarding pharmacokinetic profile, topiramate has a relative bioavailability of 80%, which is not affected by food, and a peak of plasma concentrations occurring at approx 2 h following a 400-mg oral dose. Topiramate is only 13–17% bound to human plasma proteins, and the mean plasma elimination half-life is 21 h after single or multiple doses. Topiramate is primarily eliminated unchanged in the urine. Side effects most commonly reported in an epileptic population were somnolence, dizziness, ataxia, psychomotor slowing, speech disorders, memory difficulties, paresthesia, and diplopia. Several serious effects need to be noted: metabolic acidosis can be caused by renal bicarbonate loss owing to the inhibitory effect of topiramate on carbonic anhydrase, and acute myopia syndrome with secondary glaucoma and occurrence of kidney stones (1.5%) have been reported in patients receiving topiramate (55).

A growing literature shows the effectiveness of topiramate in binge-eating disorders (33). A randomized, placebo-controlled trial of 61 obese patients with binge eating showed a mean weight reduction of 5.9 kg in the treatment group (on a median topiramate dose of 212 mg/d; range: 50–600) vs 1.2 kg in the placebo group after wk 14. Topiramate was also associated with significantly greater reductions in binge frequency (topiramate: 94%; placebo: 46%) and a reduction in diastolic blood pressure (BP). The most common reasons for discontinuing topiramate in this trial were headache and paresthesias (56). In addition, a 6-mo randomized, placebo-controlled, dose-ranging trial of 385 nondiabetic obese subjects without comorbid psychiatric conditions (57) divided into five treatment groups (placebo and topiramate at 64, 96, 192, or 384 mg/d) reported a mean weight loss in the groups of 2.6, 5.0, 4.8, 6.3, and 6.3% respectively. Twenty-one percent of patients taking topiramate withdrew because of adverse events that were dose related; most commonly reported were paresthesia (36–50%) and memory difficulties (11–28%). A multicenter, double-blind, placebo-controlled study (1289 subjects) investigating three doses of topiramate (96, 192, and 256 mg/d) was designed as a long-term study (up to 2 yr on the assigned dose). Weight loss was observed for up to 60 wk and subjects in the placebo group lost 1.7% of their baseline body weight, while subjects in the topiramate treatment groups (96, 192, and 256 mg/d) lost 7.0, 9.1, and 9.7%, respectively. Weight loss was accompanied by significant improvements in

BP, glucose, and insulin (58). The study was terminated prematurely, however, owing to an increased frequency of side effects, the most frequent ones observed during the titration phase and related to the central or peripheral nervous system. Side effects included paresthesia, difficulty with concentration/attention, depression, difficulty with memory, language problems, nervousness, and psychomotor slowing. The sponsor ended the study early in order to develop a new controlled-release formulation with the potential to enhance tolerability and simplify dosing in this patient population.

ENDOCANNABINOIDS

Clues to the possible normal roles of endocannabinoids first came from the documentation of effects of marijuana (cannabis smokers often experience extreme hunger pangs, which cannabis smokers refer to as "the munchies") and marijuana-derived exogenous cannabinoids, which have a stimulating effect on eating (59). Experimental evidence has demonstrated that endocannabinoids (anandamide and 2-arahidonoyl glycerol), acting via the cannabinoid receptor type 1 (CB1), regulate energy homeostasis through central orexigenic as well as peripheral lipogenic mechanisms (60). Rimonabant (originally SR141716, Acomplia: 5–20 mg, not yet approved in the United States), a specific CB1 antagonsit and also a neurokin 3 antagonist, is a promising compound for the treatment of obesity and metabolic syndrome. In addition, rimonabant may prove to be useful for smoking cessation, because it reduces nicotine-seeking behavior induced by reexposure to nicotine-associated stimuli and prevents relapse to smoking in ex-smokers (61). Initial relatively small phase I–II studies using rimonabant in obese humans led to a dose-dependent weight loss of up to 4 kg over 16 wk with only minor GI side effects (1). Phase III trials involving more than 6000 obese subjects are now ongoing in both the United States and Europe. According to preliminary results of the Rimonabant in Obesity–North America, trial, the largest and the longest rimonabant study (3040 adult patients randomized to rimonabant or placebo for 2 yr), reported at the American Heart Association 2004 Scientific Session, daily treatment with 20 mg of rimonabant was associated with a significant reduction in weight (62.5% of subjects lost >5% of their body weight, and 33% >10% of body weight) and waist circumference and improvements in high-density lipoprotein cholesterol levels (increase by 24.5% in the treatment group compared with 13.8% for the placebo group), triglycerides levels (decrease by 9.9% vs 1.6% for placebo) and insulin sensitivity. The drug was very well tolerated without major side effects (62). Researchers await the release of more safety data, including dropout rates and weight rebound after treatment, from the 2-yr trial, which is anticipated in 2005 (63).

GI-Neural Pathway Agents

GHRELIN

Ghrelin, a peptide produced by the enterochromaffin cells in the mucosa of the stomach fundus, besides being a potent growth hormone (GH) secretagogue, is the only orexigenic gut-derived peptide. Systemic administration of ghrelin (0.2–25.6 pmol/ [kg·min]) for up to 270 min to achieve two- to threefold higher levels than baseline resulted in increased GH, appetite scores (64), food intake (by almost 30% at a free-choice buffet meal), as well as glucose levels in uncontrolled, nonrandomized studies in lean subjects (65). Although initial animal studies on a ghrelin receptor antagonist demonstrate weight loss with preservation of lean body mass (66), results from ongoing trials in humans have not yet been published. Finally, it has also been proposed that ghrelin antagonists may prove to be particularly effective in patients with Prader-Willi syndrome, who have significantly higher ghrelin concentrations than equally obese control subjects. This remains to be seen as well.

PEPTIDE YY

Peptide YY (PYY) is another peptide secreted by the enterochromaffin cells of the small and large bowel. Although it has structural homology with NPY, in contrast to NPY, PYY inhibits food intake and decreases gastric motility. In double-blind, placebo-controlled, crossover interventional studies, PYY infusions (2 nmol/m^2) for 90 min resulted in significant appetite suppression with decreased hunger scores, a 30% decrease in short-term energy intake, and a significant decrease in the 24-h energy intake in both lean and obese subjects (67,68), indicating that replacement doses to normalize PYY levels in obese subjects may be adequate to suppress appetite and decrease energy intake. These findings make intranasal PYY, which is currently in phase I–II clinical trials, a potentially promising treatment for obesity, but needs to be evaluated further.

GLUCAGON-LIKE PEPTIDE-1 AND DIPEPTIDYL PEPTIDASE IV INHIBITORS

Glucagon-like peptide-1 (GLP-1) is another peptide secreted by the enterochromaffin cells in the small and large intestine in response to nutrients (primarily products of carbohydrates and to a lesser degree by fat hydrolysis). GLP-1 circulates in the bloodstream as an amide (GLP-1 7–36) to augment meal-stimulated insulin secretion (an effect that is glucose dependent) and to inhibit glucagon release, gastric emptying, and food intake. It has also been reported to improve β-cell function by increasing key gene expression involved in insulin secretion, to reduce β-cell apoptosis, and to have an insulin-sensitizing effect. It is inactivated in plasma by dipeptidyl peptidase IV (DPP-IV), an enzyme that is widespread, but mainly distributed in the endothelium of capillaries. Over half of the secreted GLP-1 is inactivated by DPP-IV at its own production sites (69). GLP-1 exerts its effects via GLP-1 receptors, which are mainly present in the nucleus tractus solitarius in the brain stem and in the hypothalamic arcuate nucleus, but are also found in the periphery (pancreas, lung, kidney, heart, GI tract) (70). Intravenous GLP-1 infusions (50 pmol/[kg·hr]) for 240 min significantly increased satiety and sense of fullness and decreased short-term energy intake by 12% in an early phase, placebo-controlled, randomized, blinded, crossover study in healthy, normal-weight humans (71). Therefore, therapeutic strategies exploiting GLP-1 in the area of obesity and diabetes are currently focusing on two directions: (1) the development of potent analogs of GLP-1 (receptor agonists) and (2) the use of selective inhibitors of DPP-IV to prevent in vivo degradation and enhance levels of intact biologically active peptides (72).

Enzyme-Resistant GLP-1 Analogs. Compounds similar to GLP-1 were first isolated from the lizard venom of Heloderma species, including *H. horridum* and *H. suspectum*, which are native to several American states. Lizard venom contains a number of highly bioactive peptides including the peptides exendin-3 and exendin-4. These peptides were named exendin because they were isolated from an exocrine gland and were subsequently shown to have endocrine actions (73). Oxyntomodulin, a 37 amino acid peptide that contains the 29 amino acid sequence of glucagon followed by an 8 amino acid carboxy-terminal extension, also known as exendin-9, is another molecule that may act by activating the GLP-1 receptor. A single infusion of oxyntomodulin suppresses appetite and reduces food intake in humans over a 12-h period (74). Exendin-4, a 39 amino acid peptide, initially isolated from the Gila monster salivary gland, is a GLP-1 agonist that is resistant to DPP-IV because of the penultimate NH_2-terminal glycine, instead of alanine (72). In healthy humans, acute iv infusion of exendin-4 reduces both fasting and postprandial glucose levels (75). Exenatide, a synthetic exendin-4, has now reached phase III of clinical development. When given alone in patients with type 2 diabetes, it acutely reduces fasting glucose, and when given twice daily over 5 d before breakfast and dinner, it reduces postprandial glucose (76). When given in combination with sulfonylureas over 30 wk in a multicenter (100 sites in the United States), randomized, triple-blind, placebo-controlled trial in 337 patients, exenatide (5–10 µg subcutaneously twice daily before breakfast and dinner) significantly reduced HbA1c level and weight in patients with type 2 diabetes, who had failed sulfonylurea therapy (maximally effective doses). The drug was well tolerated (the most frequent adverse effects were GI in nature, such as nausea (5% in the 10-g group vs 2% in the placebo group), vomiting, diarrhea, or constipation, and decreased in incidence after wk 8 of treatment. Mild to moderate cases of hypoglycemia were also reported (77). Exenatide mirrors the effects of GLP-1, which include glucose-dependent stimulation of insulin secretion, suppression of glucagon secretion, reduction of appetite, and delay of food absorption. A long-acting release formulation of Exenatide (Exenatide LAR) is in the early stages of development (78). Another GLP-1 analog resistant to DPP-IV and with a longer half-time, suitable for once daily administration, liraglutide, resulted in improved glycemic control after 12 wk of administration in a randomized, double-blind, placebo-controlled trial in patients with type 2 diabetes and also had a trend toward weight reduction (79). These findings suggest that GLP-1 receptor agonists may have a potential role in the treatment of type 2 diabetes and obesity.

DPP-IV Inhibitors. DPP-IV has an important role in the rapid degradation of at least two of the hormones released during food ingestion: GLP-1 and glucose-dependent insulinotropic polypeptide (formerly known as gastric inhibitory polypeptide). Inhibition of this enzyme is thought to increase levels of the active forms of both incretin hormones and, therefore, to increase insulin release in a glucose-dependent manner after a meal (80). Preclinical studies with DPP-IV inhibitors have demonstrated that increasing levels of endogenously released incretins, such as GLP-1, stabilize energy intake and improve insulin secretion, glucose tolerance, hypertriglyceridemia and FFA levels (81,82). In human studies, initial administration of a short-acting inhibitor, and then a long-term study (4–12 wk of once daily treatment) with LAF237, which has now reached phase III clinical development (83,84), proved that fasting and postprandial glucose levels as well as HbA1c decreased significantly compared with placebo, without any effect on weight balance. Although there are a few concerns about potential side effects (inhibition of the enzyme DPP-IV, which is also responsible for degradation of other peptides including vasoactive intestinal peptide, NPY, GH-releasing hormone, GLP-2, and PYY, and possible interference with T-cell activation and immune function), DPP-IV inhibitors remain a promising new drug category for treatment of type 2 diabetes given their biochemical structure and the potential for administration via the oral route (72).

BOMBESIN

Bombesin, originally purified from the skin of a European frog, *Bombina bombina*, and the two mammalian bombesin-like peptides (gastrin-releasing peptide [GRP] and neuromedin B) have a wide range of functions (i.e., promotion of cell growth; regulation of body temperature; and release of gastrin, CCK, and pancreatic polypeptide), but the most pronounced effect is that of modulating feeding behavior. Feeding suppression is mediated via G protein-coupled receptors (GPCRs) (neuromedin via the BB_1 receptor and GRP via the BB_2 receptor) and is at least in part independent of CCK (85). The BB_3 receptors, also known as BRS-3, have no endogenous ligands. The BRS-3 pathway seems to be more important in feeding behavior, because BRS-deficient mice exhibit moderate obesity caused by increased food intake and decreased energy expenditure, as well as hypertension and diabetes (86,87), whereas BB_1- (neuromedin receptor) or BB_2- (GRP receptor) deficient mice exhibit normal feeding behavior and do not become obese (88,89). A small early phase, double-blind, placebo-controlled, crossover study of 12 nonobese humans showed that administration of a relatively high dose of iv bombesin (1.33 and 4 ng/[kg·min]) for approx 13 min suppressed spontaneous food intake in response to test meal without affecting meal duration and other than for a sensation of sickness there were no overt side effects (90). Specific ligands for BRS-3 have been studied and have enhanced selectivity for the human orphan receptor BRS-3 (91–93). Thus, specific ligands for BRS-3 represent a new potential anorectic antiobesity medication, but their potential use in humans remains to be shown in the future.

CHOLECYSTOKININ

Intravenous administration of CCK (2.25 μg) for 10 min reduced food intake by 40% and enhanced the sense of satiety in a small early phase, blinded, placebo-controlled, crossover study with 12 nonobese subjects (94). Results of more advanced clinical trials with CCK or CCK receptor agonists are greatly anticipated (66).

AMYLIN

Amylin, a 37 amino acid peptide secreted by pancreatic β-cells in response to a meal, with the same diurnal variation as insulin, exerts its effects via specific receptors in the CNS (area postrema but also nucleus accumbens and dorsal raphe). Amylin complements insulin action by suppressing postprandial glucagon release, slows gastric emptying, and attenuates feeding behavior, consequently facilitating weight loss. An amylin analog (pramlintide) with a more favorable and stable formula has been developed for sc administration and has reached late-stage clinical development as an adjunct treatment to insulin in type 1 and type 2 insulin-dependent diabetics. In 1-yr-long clinical trials for type 1 and type 2 diabetics, as adjunct to insulin, administration of pramlintide (3 to 4 X 60 μg before meals) helped normalize fluctuations in glucose level by slowing gastric emptying and suppressing glucagon secretion during the prandial/postprandial period. It also improved glycemic control by decreasing significantly HbA1c and body weight. This medication caused no significant hypoglycemia, and the most common side effect reported was nausea, which is dose dependent and decreases over time (95).

Agents That May Increase Resting Metabolic Rate

β3-Adrenergic receptors are expressed mainly in adipose tissue and play an important role in lipolysis and thermogenesis. Activation of these receptors suppresses leptin expression and production, as well as food intake, by a mechanism that is independent of leptin (96). Chronic administration of β3-adrenergic receptor agonists to obese rodents reduces the size of adipocytes and results in weight loss. However, acute administration of the drugs induces remarkable insulin secretion, the mechanism of which is still unclear *(97).* Several β3-adrenergic receptor agonists are in various stages of development as antiobese or antidiabetic agents. The first study to show the acute effect of β3-adrenergic receptor agonists (L-796568 in a single dose of 1000 mg) in humans *(98)* confirmed the increased lipolysis and energy expenditure in overweight men. The chronic effects, however, have not yet been studied in obese humans, although the chronic administration of another β3-adrenergic receptor agonist (FR-149175) had favorable effects on energy expenditure in rats (Zucker fatty rats): the thermogenic effect was not attenuated by chronic exposure to agonists, and chronic treatment with FR-149175 caused a decrease in both body weight gain and white fat pad weight at doses that induced lipolysis in acute treatment (1 and 3.2 mg/kg by mouth) *(99).*

Other Diverse Agents

Other agents, including corticotropin-releasing hormone agonists, brain-derived neurotrophic factor/TrKB receptor, urocortin and corticotrophin-releasing hormone and their receptors, galanin, phytostanol analogs, functional oils, P57, amylase inhibitors, GH fragments, synthetic analogs of dehydroepiandrosterone sulfate, antagonists of adipocyte 11β-hydroxysteroid dehydrogenase type 1 activity, inhibitors of fatty acid synthesis, carboxypeptidase inhibitors, indanones/indanols, aminosterols, and other GI lipase inhibitors (ATL962), as well as several other potential targets for the development of new obesity treatments, are also under intensive investigation, but a detailed discussion of these targets is beyond the scope of this review.

REFERENCES

1. Vastag B. Experimental drugs take aim at obesity. JAMA 2003;289(14):1763, 1764.
2. Thearle M, Aronne LJ. Obesity and pharmacologic therapy. Endocrinol Metab Clin North Am 2003;32(4):1005–1024.
3. Knowler WC, Barrett-Connor E, Fowler SE, et al. Reduction in the incidence of type 2 diabetes with lifestyle intervention or metformin. N Engl J Med 2002;346(6):393–403.
4. Padwal R, Li SK, Lau DC. Long-term pharmacotherapy for overweight and obesity: a systematic review and meta-analysis of randomized controlled trials. Int J Obes Relat Metab Disord 2003;27(12):1437–1446.
5. Bays HE. Current and investigational antiobesity agents and obesity therapeutic treatment targets. Obes Res 2004;12(8):1197–1211.
6. Farooqi IS, Matarese G, Lord GM, et al. Beneficial effects of leptin on obesity, T cell hyporesponsiveness, and neuroendocrine/metabolic dysfunction of human congenital leptin deficiency. J Clin Invest 2002;110(8):1093–1103.
7. Oral EA, Simha V, Ruiz E, et al. Leptin-replacement therapy for lipodystrophy. N Engl J Med 2002;346(8):570–578.
8. Heymsfield SB, Greenberg AS, Fujioka K, et al. Recombinant leptin for weight loss in obese and lean adults: a randomized, controlled, dose-escalation trial. JAMA 1999;282(16):1568–1575.
9. Bjorbaek C, Elmquist JK, Frantz JD, Shoelson SE, Flier JS. Identification of SOCS-3 as a potential mediator of central leptin resistance. Mol Cell 1998;1(4):619–625.
10. Chan JL, Heist K, DePaoli AM, Veldhuis JD, Mantzoros CS. The role of falling leptin levels in the neuroendocrine and metabolic adaptation to short-term starvation in healthy men. J Clin Invest 2003;111(9):1409–1421.
11. Welt CK, Chan JL, Bullen J, et al. Recombinant human leptin in women with hypothalamic amenorrhea. N Engl J Med 2004;351(10):987–997.
12. Sendtner M, Carroll P, Holtmann B, Hughes RA, Thoenen H. Ciliary neurotrophic factor. J Neurobiol 1994;25(11):1436–1453.
13. ALS CNTF Treatment Study Group. A double-blind placebo-controlled clinical trial of subcutaneous recombinant human ciliary neurotrophic factor (rHCNTF) in amyotrophic lateral sclerosis. Neurology 1996;46(5):1244–1249.

14. Xu B, Dube MG, Kalra PS, et al. Anorectic effects of the cytokine, ciliary neurotropic factor, are mediated by hypothalamic neuropeptide Y: comparison with leptin. Endocrinology 1998;139(2): 466–473.

15. Gloaguen I, Costa P, Demartis A, et al. Ciliary neurotrophic factor corrects obesity and diabetes associated with leptin deficiency and resistance. Proc Natl Acad Sci USA 1997;94(12):6456–6461.

16. Lambert PD, Anderson KD, Sleeman MW, et al. Ciliary neurotrophic factor activates leptin-like pathways and reduces body fat, without cachexia or rebound weight gain, even in leptin-resistant obesity. Proc Natl Acad Sci USA 2001;98(8):4652–4657.

17. Ettinger MP, Littlejohn TW, Schwartz SL, et al. Recombinant variant of ciliary neurotrophic factor for weight loss in obese adults: a randomized, dose-ranging study. JAMA 2003;289(14):1826–1832.

18. Bluher S, Moschos S, Bullen J Jr, et al. Ciliary neurotrophic factorAx15 alters energy homeostasis, decreases body weight, and improves metabolic control in diet-induced obese and UCP1-DTA mice. Diabetes 2004;53(11):2787–2796.

19. Regeneron Announces Results of Phase III Obesity Study. Regeneron Pharmaceuticals, Tarrytown, New York, (Nasdaq:REGN). http://regn.com/investor/press_detail.asp?v_c_id=169(3.31.2003) Accessed Oct. 23, 2004.

20. Kordik CP, Luo C, Zanoni BC, et al. Pyrazolecarboxamide human neuropeptide Y5 receptor ligands with in vivo antifeedant activity. Bioorg Med Chem Lett 2001;11(17):2287–2290.

21. Silva AP, Cavadas C, Grouzmann E. Neuropeptide Y and its receptors as potential therapeutic drug targets. Clin Chim Acta 2002;326(1–2):3–25.

22. Galiano S, Erviti O, Perez S, et al. Synthesis of new thiophene and benzo[b]thiophene hydrazide derivatives as human NPY Y(5) antagonists. Bioorg Med Chem Lett 2004;14(3):597–599.

23. Juanenea L, Galiano S, Erviti O, et al. Synthesis and evaluation of new hydrazide derivatives as neuropeptide Y Y5 receptor antagonists for the treatment of obesity. Bioorg Med Chem 2004;12(17): 4717–4723.

24. MacNeil DJ, Howard AD, Guan X, et al. The role of melanocortins in body weight regulation: opportunities for the treatment of obesity. Eur J Pharmacol 2002;450(1):93–109.

25. Fehm HL, Smolnik R, Kern W, McGregor GP, Bickel U, Born J. The melanocortin melanocyte-stimulating hormone/adrenocorticotropin(4–10) decreases body fat in humans. J Clin Endocrinol Metab 2001;86(3):1144–1148.

26. Krude H, Biebermann H, Schnabel D, et al. Obesity due to proopiomelanocortin deficiency: three new cases and treatment trials with thyroid hormone and ACTH4–10. J Clin Endocrinol Metab 2003;88(10):4633–4640.

27. Telch CF, Agras WS. Obesity, binge eating and psychopathology: are they related? Int J Eat Disord 1994;15(1):53–61.

28. Roberts RE, Kaplan GA, Shema SJ, Strawbridge WJ. Are the obese at greater risk for depression? Am J Epidemiol 2000;152(2):163–170.

29. Schwartz MW, Woods SC, Porte D Jr, Seeley RJ, Baskin DG. Central nervous system control of food intake. Nature 2000;404(6778):661–671.

30. Heisler LK, Cowley MA, Kishi T, et al. Central serotonin and melanocortin pathways regulating energy homeostasis. Ann NY Acad Sci 2003;994:169–174.

31. Goldstein DJ, Rampey AH Jr, Enas GG, Potvin JH, Fludzinski LA, Levine LR. Fluoxetine: a randomized clinical trial in the treatment of obesity. Int J Obes Relat Metab Disord 1994;18(3):129–135.

32. Goldstein DJ, Wilson MG, Thompson VL, Potvin JH, Rampey AH Jr. Long-term fluoxetine treatment of bulimia nervosa. Fluoxetine Bulimia Nervosa Research Group. Br J Psychiatry 1995;166(5): 660–666.

33. Appolinario JC, Bueno JR, Coutinho W. Psychotropic drugs in the treatment of obesity: what promise? CNS Drugs 2004;18(10):629–651.

34. Wadden TA, Bartlett SJ, Foster GD, et al. Sertraline and relapse prevention training following treatment by very-low-calorie diet: a controlled clinical trial. Obes Res 1995;3(6):549–557.

35. Abell CA, Farquhar DL, Galloway SM, Steven F, Philip AE, Munro JF. Placebo controlled doubleblind trial of fluvoxamine maleate in the obese. J Psychosom Res 1986;30(2):143–146.

36. Szkudlarek J, Elsborg L. Treatment of severe obesity with a highly selective serotonin re-uptake inhibitor as a supplement to a low calorie diet. Int J Obes Relat Metab Disord 1993;17(12):681–683.

37. McElroy SL, Hudson JI, Malhotra S, Welge JA, Nelson EB, Keck PE Jr. Citalopram in the treatment of binge-eating disorder: a placebo-controlled trial. J Clin Psychiatry 2003;64(7):807–813.

38. Hudson JI, McElroy SL, Raymond NC, et al. Fluvoxamine in the treatment of binge-eating disorder: a multicenter placebo-controlled, double-blind trial. Am J Psychiatry 1998;155(12):1756–1762.

39. McElroy SL, Casuto LS, Nelson EB, et al. Placebo-controlled trial of sertraline in the treatment of binge eating disorder. Am J Psychiatry 2000;157(6):1004–1006.

40. Malhotra S, King KH, Welge JA, Brusman-Lovins L, McElroy SL. Venlafaxine treatment of binge-eating disorder associated with obesity: a series of 35 patients. J Clin Psychiatry 2002;63(9):802–806.

41. Gadde KM, Parker CB, Maner LG, et al. Bupropion for weight loss: an investigation of efficacy and tolerability in overweight and obese women. Obes Res 2001;9(9):544–551.

42. Anderson JW, Greenway FL, Fujioka K, Gadde KM, McKenney J, O'Neil PM. Bupropion SR enhances weight loss: a 48-week double-blind, placebo- controlled trial. Obes Res 2002;10(7): 633–641.

43. Oommen KJ, Mathews S. Zonisamide: a new antiepileptic drug. Clin Neuropharmacol 1999;22(4): 192–200.

44. Leppik IE. Zonisamide: chemistry, mechanism of action, and pharmacokinetics. Seizure 2004; 13(Suppl 1):S5–S9.

45. Gadde KM, Franciscy DM, Wagner HR, Krishnan KR. Zonisamide for weight loss in obese adults: a randomized controlled trial. JAMA 2003;289(14):1820–1825.

46. McElroy SL, Kotwal R, Hudson JI, Nelson EB, Keck PE. Zonisamide in the treatment of binge-eating disorder: an open-label, prospective trial. J Clin Psychiatry 2004;65(1):50–56.

47. Kim CS. Zonisamide effective for weight loss in women. J Fam Pract 2003;52(8):600, 601.

48. Privitera MD. Topiramate: a new antiepileptic drug. Ann Pharmacother 1997;31(10):1164–1173.

49. Rosenfeldt WE, Schaefer PA, Pace K. Weight loss patterns with topiramate therapy. Epilepsia 1997;38(Suppl 3):58 (Abst).

50. Norton J, Potter D, Edwards K. Sustained weight loss associated with topiramate. Epilepsia 1997;38(Suppl 3):60 (Abst).

51. Chengappa KN, Rathore D, Levine J, et al. Topiramate as add-on treatment for patients with bipolar mania. Bipolar Disord 1999;1(1):42–53.

52. Chengappa KN, Levine J, Rathore D, et al. Long-term effects of topiramate on bipolar mood instability, weight change and glycemic control: a case-series. Eur Psychiatry 2001;16(3):186–190.

53. Richard D, Ferland J, Lalonde J, Samson P, Deshaies Y. Influence of topiramate in the regulation of energy balance. Nutrition 2000;16(10):961–966.

54. Wilkes JJ, Nelson E, Osborne M, Demarest KT, Olefsky JM. Topiramate is an insulin sensitizing compound in vivo with direct effects on adipocytes in female ZDF rats. Am J Physiol Endocrinol Metab 2005;288(3):E617–E624.

55. TOPAMAX (topiramate). Clinical pharmacology. RxList Web site. The internet drug index. Accessed October 26, 2004. www.rxlist.com/cgi/generic2/topiram_cp.htm.

56. McElroy SL, Arnold LM, Shapira NA, et al. Topiramate in the treatment of binge eating disorder associated with obesity: a randomized, placebo-controlled trial. Am J Psychiatry 2003;160(2): 255–261.

57. Bray GA, Hollander P, Klein S, et al. A 6-month randomized, placebo-controlled, dose-ranging trial of topiramate for weight loss in obesity. Obes Res 2003;11(6):722–733.

58. Wilding J, Van Gaal L, Rissanen A, Vercruysse F, Fitchet M. A randomized double-blind placebo-controlled study of the long-term efficacy and safety of topiramate in the treatment of obese subjects. Int J Obes Relat Metab Disord 2004;28(11):1399–1410.

59. Kirkham TC. Endogenous cannabinoids: a new target in the treatment of obesity. Am J Physiol Regul Integr Comp Physiol 2003;284(2):R343, R344.

60. Cota D, Marsicano G, Tschop M, et al. The endogenous cannabinoid system affects energy balance via central orexigenic drive and peripheral lipogenesis. J Clin Invest 2003;112(3):423–431.

61. Le Foll B, Goldberg SR. Rimonabant, a CB1 antagonist, blocks nicotine-conditioned place preferences. Neuroreport 2004;15(13):2139–2143.

62. Peck P. Rimonabant maintains both weight and waist reductions at 2 years. Medscape Medical News. Accessed November 10, 2004. www.medscape.com/viewarticle/493514.

63. Acomplia (Rimonabant)—Investigational Agent for the Management of Obesity. drugdevelopment-technology.com: the website for the drug development industry. Accessed November 30, 2004. www.drugdevelopment-technology.com/projects/rimonabant/.

64. Wren AM, Seal LJ, Cohen MA, et al. Ghrelin enhances appetite and increases food intake in humans. J Clin Endocrinol Metab 2001;86(12):5992–5995.

65. Broglio F, Arvat E, Benso A, et al. Ghrelin, a natural GH secretagogue produced by the stomach, induces hyperglycemia and reduces insulin secretion in humans. J Clin Endocrinol Metab 2001;86(10):5083–5086.

66. Tartaglia LA, Moxham CM. New molecular targets for the treatment of obesity. In: Caro JF, ed. Obesity. www.endotext.org/obesity/obesity21/obesityframe21.htm; Accessed Aug. 19, 2003.

67. Batterham RL, Cowley MA, Small CJ, et al. Gut hormone PYY(3-36) physiologically inhibits food intake. Nature 2002;418(6898):650–654.

68. Batterham RL, Cohen MA, Ellis SM, et al. Inhibition of food intake in obese subjects by peptide YY3-36. N Engl J Med 2003;349(10):941–948.

69. Hansen L, Deacon CF, Orskov C, Holst JJ. Glucagon-like peptide-1-(7–36)amide is transformed to glucagon-like peptide-1-(9–36)amide by dipeptidyl peptidase IV in the capillaries supplying the L cells of the porcine intestine. Endocrinology 1999;140(11):5356–5363.

70. Gutzwiller JP, Degen L, Heuss L, Beglinger C. Glucagon-like peptide 1 (GLP-1) and eating. Physiol Behav 2004;82(1):17–19.

71. Flint A, Raben A, Astrup A, Holst JJ. Glucagon-like peptide 1 promotes satiety and suppresses energy intake in humans. J Clin Invest 1998;101(3):515–520.

72. Deacon CF. Therapeutic strategies based on glucagon-like peptide 1. Diabetes 2004;53(9):2181–2189.

73. Eng J, Andrews PC, Kleinman WA, Singh L, Raufman JP. Purification and structure of exendin-3, a new pancreatic secretagogue isolated from Heloderma horridum venom. J Biol Chem 1990;265(33): 20,259–20,262.

74. Cohen MA, Ellis SM, Le Roux CW, et al. Oxyntomodulin suppresses appetite and reduces food intake in humans. J Clin Endocrinol Metab 2003;88(10):4696–4701.

75. Edwards CM, Stanley SA, Davis R, et al. Exendin-4 reduces fasting and postprandial glucose and decreases energy intake in healthy volunteers. Am J Physiol Endocrinol Metab 2001;281(1):E155–E161.

76. Kolterman OG, Buse JB, Fineman MS, et al. Synthetic exendin-4 (exenatide) significantly reduces postprandial and fasting plasma glucose in subjects with type 2 diabetes. J Clin Endocrinol Metab 2003;88(7):3082–3089.

77. Buse JB, Henry RR, Han J, Kim DD, Fineman MS, Baron AD. Effects of exenatide (exendin-4) on glycemic control over 30 weeks in sulfonylurea-treated patients with type 2 diabetes. Diabetes Care 2004;27(11):2628–2635.

78. Exenatide—Investigational Agent for Type 2 Diabetes. drugdevelopment-technology.com: the website for the drug development industry. Accessed November 30, 2004. www.drugdevelopment-technology.com/projects/exenatide/.

79. Madsbad S, Schmitz O, Ranstam J, Jakobsen G, Matthews DR. Improved glycemic control with no weight increase in patients with type 2 diabetes after once-daily treatment with the long-acting glucagon-like peptide 1 analog liraglutide (NN2211): a 12-week, double-blind, randomized, controlled trial. Diabetes Care 2004;27(6):1335–1342.

80. Deacon CF, Ahren B, Holst JJ. Inhibitors of dipeptidyl peptidase IV: a novel approach for the prevention and treatment of Type 2 diabetes? Expert Opin Investig Drugs 2004;13(9):1091–1102.

81. Pederson RA, White HA, Schlenzig D, Pauly RP, McIntosh CH, Demuth HU. Improved glucose tolerance in Zucker fatty rats by oral administration of the dipeptidyl peptidase IV inhibitor isoleucine thiazolidide. Diabetes 1998;47(8):1253–1258.

82. Sudre B, Broqua P, White RB, et al. Chronic inhibition of circulating dipeptidyl peptidase IV by FE 999011 delays the occurrence of diabetes in male zucker diabetic fatty rats. Diabetes 2002;51(5): 1461–1469.

83. Ahren B, Landin-Olsson M, Jansson PA, Svensson M, Holmes D, Schweizer A. Inhibition of dipeptidyl peptidase-4 reduces glycemia, sustains insulin levels, and reduces glucagon levels in type 2 diabetes. J Clin Endocrinol Metab 2004;89(5):2078–2084.

84. Pratley R, Galbreath E. Twelve-week monotherapy with the DPP-4 inhibitor, LAF237 improves glycemic control in patients with type 2 diabetes. Diabetes 2004;53(Suppl 2):A83.

85. Yamada K, Wada E, Santo-Yamada Y, Wada K. Bombesin and its family of peptides: prospects for the treatment of obesity. Eur J Pharmacol 2002;440(2–3):281–290.

86. Ohki-Hamazaki H, Watase K, Yamamoto K, et al. Mice lacking bombesin receptor subtype-3 develop metabolic defects and obesity. Nature 1997;390(6656):165–169.

87. Yamada K, Wada E, Wada K. Bombesin-like peptides: studies on food intake and social behaviour with receptor knock-out mice. Ann Med 2000;32(8):519–529.

88. Ohki-Hamazaki H, Sakai Y, Kamata K, et al. Functional properties of two bombesin-like peptide receptors revealed by the analysis of mice lacking neuromedin B receptor. J Neurosci 1999;19(3):948–954.

89. Wada E, Watase K, Yamada K, et al. Generation and characterization of mice lacking gastrin-releasing peptide receptor. Biochem Biophys Res Commun 1997;239(1):28–33.

90. Muurahainen NE, Kissileff HR, Pi-Sunyer FX. Intravenous infusion of bombesin reduces food intake in humans. Am J Physiol 1993;264(2 Pt 2):R350–R354.

91. Weber D, Berger C, Heinrich T, Eickelmann P, Antel J, Kessler H. Systematic optimization of a lead-structure identities for a selective short peptide agonist for the human orphan receptor BRS-3. J Pept Sci 2002;8(8):461–475.

92. Weber D, Berger C, Eickelmann P, Antel J, Kessler H. Design of selective peptidomimetic agonists for the human orphan receptor BRS-3. J Med Chem 2003;46(10):1918–1930.

93. Mantey SA, Coy DH, Entsuah LK, Jensen RT. Development of bombesin analogs with conformationally restricted amino acid substitutions with enhanced selectivity for the orphan receptor human bombesin receptor subtype 3. J Pharmacol Exp Ther 2004;310(3):1161–1170.

94. Muurahainen N, Kissileff HR, Derogatis AJ, Pi-Sunyer FX. Effects of cholecystokinin-octapeptide (CCK-8) on food intake and gastric emptying in man. Physiol Behav 1988;44(4–5):645–649.

95. Kruger DF, Gloster MA. Pramlintide for the treatment of insulin-requiring diabetes mellitus: rationale and review of clinical data. Drugs 2004;64(13):1419–1432.

96. Mantzoros CS, Qu D, Frederich RC, et al. Activation of beta(3) adrenergic receptors suppresses leptin expression and mediates a leptin-independent inhibition of food intake in mice. Diabetes 1996;45(7):909–914.

97. Sakura H, Togashi M, Iwamoto Y. [Beta 3-adrenergic receptor agonists as anti-obese and anti-diabetic drugs]. Nippon Rinsho 2002;60(1):123–129.

98. van Baak MA, Hul GB, Toubro S, et al. Acute effect of L-796568, a novel beta 3-adrenergic receptor agonist, on energy expenditure in obese men. Clin Pharmacol Ther 2002;71(4):272–279.

99. Hatakeyama Y, Sakata Y, Takakura S, Manda T, Mutoh S. Acute and chronic effects of FR-149175, a beta 3-adrenergic receptor agonist, on energy expenditure in Zucker fatty rats. Am J Physiol Regul Integr Comp Physiol 2004;287(2):R336–R341.

Appendix

Resources

Violeta Stoyneva, BS
and Christos S. Mantzoros, MD, DSc

INTRODUCTION

Obesity and diabetes are both chronic diseases that affect every aspect of a person's life. Secondary to medical treatment, education is the single most important tool for their management. Education is also of critical importance in raising public awareness, and it can help curb the global epidemic of these related conditions.

Following is a list of government agencies and voluntary associations that provide information and resources related to obesity and diabetes.

DIABETES ORGANIZATIONS

American Association of Diabetes Educators (AADE)
100 West Monroe, Suite 400
Chicago, IL 60603
Tel.: 800-338-3633 or 312-424-2426
Fax: 312-424-2427
Diabetes Educator Access Line: 800-TEAMUP4 (800-832-6874)
E-mail: aade@aadenet.org
Web site: www.diabeteseducator.org

American Diabetes Association (ADA)
1701 North Beauregard Street
Alexandria, VA 22311
Tel.: 800-DIABETES (800-342-2383)
Fax: 703-549-6995
E-mail: askada@diabetes.org
Web site: www.diabetes.org

From: *Contemporary Diabetes: Obesity and Diabetes*
Edited by: C. S. Mantzoros © Humana Press Inc., Totowa, NJ

American Podiatric Medical Association (APMA)
9312 Old Georgetown Road
Bethesda, MD 20814-1621
Foot Care Information Center: 800-FOOT-CARE (800-366-8227)
Tel.: 301-581-9200
Fax: 301-530-2752
E-mail: askapma@apma.org
Web site: www.apma.org

American Porphyria Foundation (APF)
PO Box 22712
Houston, TX 77227
Tel.: 713-266-9617
Fax: 713-840-9552
E-mail: porphyrus@aol.com
Web site: www.porphyriafoundation.com

Centers for Disease Control and Prevention
National Center for Chronic Disease Prevention and Health Promotion
Division of Diabetes Translation
PO Box 8728
Silver Spring, MD 20910
Tel.: 877-CDC-DIAB (877-232-3422)
Fax: 301-562-1050
E-mail: diabetes@cdc.gov
Web site: www.cdc.gov/diabetes

Diabetes Action Research & Education Foundation
426 C Street, NE
Washington, DC 20002
Tel.: 202-333-4520
E-mail: daref@diabetesaction.org
Web site: www.diabetesaction.org

Diabetes Exercise and Sports Association (DESA)
8001 Montcastle Drive
Nashville, TN 37221
Tel.: 800-898-4322
Fax: 602-433-9331
E-mail: desa@diabetes-exercise.org
Web site: www.diabetes-exercise.org/index.asp

Diabetes Institutes Foundation (DIF)
855 W. Brambleton Avenue
Norfolk, VA 23510
Tel.: 866-DIF-CURE or 757-446-8420
Fax: 757-446-8429
E-mail: difcure@aol.com
Web site: www.dif.org

Indian Health Service (IHS)
Division of Diabetes Treatment and Prevention
5300 Homestead Road, NE
Albuquerque, NM 87110
Tel.: 505-248-4182
Fax: 505-248-4188
E-mail: diabetesprogram@mail.ihs.gov
Web site: www.ihs.gov/medicalprograms/diabetes

International Diabetes Federation (IDF)
Avenue Emile De Mot 19-B-1000
Brussels, Belgium
Tel.: +32-2-538 55 11
Fax: +32-2-538 51 14
E-mail: info@idf.org
Web site: www.idf.org/home/

Joslin Diabetes Center
One Joslin Place
Boston, MA 02215
Tel.: 800-JOSLIN-1 (800-567-5461) or 617-732-2400
Web site: www.joslin.org

Juvenile Diabetes Research Foundation International (JDRF)
120 Wall Street
New York, NY 10005-4001
Tel.: 800-533-CURE (800-533-2873)
Fax: 212-785-9595
E-mail: info@jdrf.org
Web site: www.jdf.org

National Certification Board for Diabetes Educators (NCBDE)
330 East Algonquin Road, Suite #4
Arlington Heights, IL 60005
Tel.: 847-228-9795
Fax: 847-228-8469
Phone requests for exam applications: 913-541-0400
E-mail: info@ncbde.org
Web site: www.ncbde.org

National Diabetes Education Program (NDEP)
One Diabetes Way
Bethesda, MD 20814-9692
Tel.: 800-438-5383
E-mail: ndep@info.nih.gov
Web site: http://ndep.nih.gov

National Diabetes Information Clearinghouse (NDIC)
1 Information Way
Bethesda, MD 20892-3560
Tel.: 800-860-8747
Fax: 703-738-4929
E-mail: ndic@info.niddk.nih.gov
Web site: www.diabetes.niddk.nih.gov

Hepatitis Foundation International (HFI)
504 Blick Drive
Silver Spring, MD 20904-2901
Tel.: 800-891-0707 or 301-622-4200
Fax: 301-622-4702
E-mail: hfi@comcast.net
Web site: www.hepfi.org

National Eye Institute (NEI)
National Eye Health Education Program (NEHEP)
2020 Vision Place
Bethesda, MD 20892-3655
Tel.: 800-869-2020 (for health professionals only) or 301-496-5248
Fax: 301-402-1065
E-mail: 2020@nei.nih.gov
Web site: www.nei.nih.gov

National Institute of Diabetes and Digestive and Kidney Diseases
31 Center Drive, MSC-2560
Building 31, Room 9A-04
Bethesda, MD 20892-2560
Tel.: 301-496-3583 or 301-496-5877
Fax: 301-496-7422 or 301-402-2125
E-mail: dkwebmaster@extra.nid.nih.gov
Web site: www.niddk.nih.gov

National Kidney and Urologic Diseases Information Clearinghouse (NKUDIC)
3 Information Way
Bethesda, MD 20892-3580
Tel.: 800-891-5390
Fax: 703-738-4929
E-mail: nkudic@info.niddk.nih.gov
Web site: www.kidney.niddk.nih.gov or www.urologic.niddk.nih.gov

National Kidney Foundation (NKF)
30 East 33rd Street
New York, NY 10016
Tel.: 800-622-9010 or 212-889-2210
Fax: 212-689-9261 or 212-779-0068
E-mail: info@kidney.org
Web site: www.kidney.org

National Institute of Dental and Craniofacial Research
Bethesda, MD 20892-2190
Tel.: 301-496-4281
E-mail: nidcrinfo@mail.nih.gov
Web site: www.nidcr.nih.gov

Pedorthic Footwear Association (PFA)
7150 Columbia Gateway Drive, Suite G
Columbia, MD 21046-1151
Tel.: 410-381-7278 or 800-673-8447
Fax: 410-381-1167
E-mail: info@pedorthics.org
Web site: www.pedorthics.org

United Network for Organ Sharing (UNOS)
PO Box 2484
Richmond, VA 23218
Tel.: 804-782-4800
E-mail: askunos@unos.org
Web site: www.unos.org

OBESITY ORGANIZATIONS

Academy for Eating Disorders (AED)
60 Revere Drive, Suite 500
Northbrook, IL 60062
Tel.: 847-498-4274
Fax: 847-480-9282
E-mail: aed@aedweb.org
Web site: www.aedweb.org/index.cfm

American Gastroenterological Association (AGA)
4930 Del Ray Avenue
Bethesda, MD 20814
Tel.: 301-654-2055
Fax: 301-654-5920
Web site: www.gastro.org

American Obesity Association (AOA)
1250 24th Street, NW
Suite 300
Washington, DC 20037
Tel.: 202-776-7711
Fax: 202-776-7712
Web site: www.obesity.org

American Sleep Apnea Association (ASAA)
1424 K Street NW, Suite 302
Washington, DC 20005
Tel.: 202-293-3650
Fax: 202-293-3656
E-mail: asaa@sleepapnea.org
Web site: www.sleepapnea.org

American Society for Bariatric Surgery (ASBS)
100 SW 75th Street, Suite 201
Gainesville, FL 32607
Tel.: 352-331-4900
Fax: 352-331-4975
E-mail: info@asbs.org
Web site: www.asbs.org

American Society of Abdominal Surgeons (ASAS)
1 East Emerson Street
Melrose, MA 02176
Tel.: 781-665-6102
Fax: 781-665-4127
E-mail: office@abdominalsurg.org
Web site: www.abdominalsurg.org

American Society of Bariatric Physicians (ASBP)
2821 S. Parker Road, Suite 625,
Aurora, CO 80014
Tel.: 303-770-2526
Fax: 303-779-4834
E-mail: info@asbp.org
Web site: www.asbp.org

Cyclic Vomiting Syndrome Association (CVSA)
CVSA USA/Canada
3585 Cedar Hill Road, NW
Canal Winchester, OH 43110
Tel.: 614-837-2586
Fax: 614-837-2586
E-mail: waitesd@cvsaonline.org
Web site: www.cvsaonline.org

Digestive Disease National Coalition (DDNC)
507 Capitol Court NE, Suite 200
Washington, DC 20002
Tel.: 202-544-7497
Fax: 202-546-7105
E-mail: ronanoe@hmcw.org
Web site: www.ddnc.org

Gastro-Intestinal Research Foundation (GIRF)
70 East Lake Street, Suite 1015
Chicago, IL 60601-5907
Tel.: 312-332-1350
Fax: 312-332-4757
E-mail: girf@earthlink.net
Web site: www.girf.org

International Association for the Study of Obesity (IASO)
231 North Gower Street
London NW1 2NS
United Kingdom
Tel.: +44 (0) 20 7691 1900
Fax: +44 (0) 20 7387 6033
E-mail: inquiries@iaso.org or obesity@iotf.org
Web site: www.iaso.org or www.iotf.org

International Foundation for Functional Gastrointestinal Disorders (IFFGD)
PO Box 170864
Milwaukee, WI 53217-8076
Tel.: 888-964-2001 or 414-964-1799
Fax: 414-964-7176
E-mail: iffgd@iffgd.org
Web site: www.iffgd.org

National Association to Advance Fat Acceptance (NAAFA)
PO Box 188620
Sacramento, CA 95818
Tel.: 916-558-6880
Fax: 916-558-6881
E-mail: naafa@naafa.org
Web site: http://naafa.org

National Digestive Diseases Information Clearinghouse (NDDIC)
2 Information Way
Bethesda, MD 20892-3570
Tel.: 800-891-5389
Fax: 703-738-4929
E-mail: nddic@info.niddk.nih.gov
Web site: www.digestive.niddk.nih.gov

National Eating Disorders Association (NEDA)
603 Stewart Street, Suite 803
Seattle, WA 98101
Tel.: 800-931-2237 or 206-382-3587
E-mail: info@nationaleatingdisorders.org
Web site: www.nationaleatingdisorders.org

North American Association for the Study of Obesity (NAASO)
8630 Fenton Street, Suite 918
Silver Spring, MD 20910
Tel.: 301-563-6526
Fax: 301-563-6595
Web site: www.naaso.org

Overeaters Anonymous (OA)
World Service Office
PO Box 44020
Rio Rancho, NM 87174-4020
Tel.: 505-891-2664
E-mail: info@oa.org
Web site: www.oa.org

Pediatric/Adolescent Gastroesophageal Reflux Association (PAGER)
PO Box 486
Buckeystown, MD 21717
Tel.: 301-601-9541
Fax: 630-982-6418
E-mail: gergroup@aol.com
Web site: www.reflux.org

President's Council on Physical Fitness and Sports
Department W
200 Independence Avenue, SW Room 738-H
Washington, DC 20201-0004
Tel.: 202-690-9000
Fax: 202-690-5211
Web site: www.fitness.gov

Shape Up America!
12154 Darnestown Road, Suite 607
North Potomac, MD 20878
Tel.: 240-715-3900
Fax: 240-632-1075
E-mail: info@shapeup.org
Web site: www.shapeup.org

The Society for Surgery of the Alimentary Tract (SSAT)
900 Cummings Center, Suite 221-U
Beverly, MA 01915
Tel.: 978-927-8330
Fax: 978-524-8890
E-mail: ssat@prri.com
Web site: www.ssat.com

Society of American Gastrointestinal and Endoscopic Surgeons (SAGES)
11300 West Olympic Boulevard, Suite 600
Los Angeles, CA 90064
Tel.: 310-437-0544
Fax: 310-437-0585
Web site: www.sages.org

Weight-control Information Network (WIN)
National Institute of Diabetes and Digestive and Kidney Diseases
1 WIN Way
Bethesda, MD 20892-3665
Tel.: 877-946-4627
Fax: 202-828-1028
E-mail: win@info.niddk.nih.gov
Web site: http://win.niddk.nih.gov/index.htm

ORGANIZATIONS OF COMMON INTEREST

American Academy of Pediatrics (AAP)
141 Northwest Point Boulevard
Elk Grove Village, IL 60007-1098
Tel.: 847-434-4000 or 888-227-1770
E-mail: csc@aap.org
Web site: www.aap.org

American Association of Clinical Endocrinologists (AACE)
1000 Riverside Avenue, Suite 205
Jacksonville, FL 32204
Tel.: 904-353-7878
Fax: 904-353-8185
E-mail: info@aace.com
Web site: www.aace.com

American Dietetic Association (ADA)
120 South Riverside Plaza, Suite 2000
Chicago, IL 60606-6995
Tel.: 800-366-1655
Fax: 312-899-4739
E-mail: hotline@eatright.org
Web site: www.eatright.org/public/

American Heart Association
7272 Greenville Avenue
Dallas, TX 75231-4596
Tel.: 800-AHA-USA1 (800-242-8721) or 214-706-1220
Fax: 214-706-1341
Web site: www.americanheart.org

American Institute for Cancer Research (AICR)
1759 R Street, NW
Washington, DC 20009
Tel.: 800-843-8114 or 202-323-7744
Fax: 202-328-7226
E-mail: aicrweb@aicr.org
Web site: www.aicr.org

American Liver Foundation (ALF)
75 Maiden Lane, Suite 603
New York, NY 10038-4810
Tel.: 800-GO-LIVER (800-465-4837), 888-4HEP-USA
    (888-443-7872), or 212-668-1000
Fax: 212-483-8179
E-mail: info@liverfoundation.org
Web site: www.liverfoundation.org

American Society for Parenteral and Enteral Nutrition (ASPEN)
8630 Fenton Street, Suite 412
Silver Spring, MD 20910
Tel.: 800-727-4567 or 301-587-6315
Fax: 301-587-2365
E-mail: aspen@nutr.org
Web site: www.nutritioncare.org

Center for Nutrition Policy and Promotion (CNPP)
3101 Park Center Drive, Room 1034
Alexandria, VA 22302-1594
Tel.: 703-305-7600
Fax: 703-305-3400
E-mail: john.webster@cnpp.usda.gov
Web site: www.usda.gov/cnpp/

Dietary Guidelines for Americans
U.S. Department of Agriculture and U.S. Department of Health
    and Human Services
Web site: www.health.gov/dietaryguidelines

The Endocrine Society
4350 East West Highway, Suite 500
Bethesda, MD 20814-4426
Tel.: 301-941-0200
Fax: 301-941-0259
E-mail: societyservices@endo-society.org
Web site: www.endo-society.org

Food and Nutrition Information Center (FNIC)
USDA/ARS/National Agricultural Library
10301 Baltimore Avenue, Room 105

Beltsville, MD 20705-2351
Tel.: 301-504-5719; TTY: 301-504-6856
Fax: 301-504-6409
E-mail: fnic@nal.usda.gov
Web site: www.nal.usda.gov/fnic

National Cancer Institute (NCI)
Public Inquiries Office
6116 Executive Boulevard, Room 3036A
Bethesda, MD 20892-8322
Tel.: 800-4-CANCER (800-422-6237); TTY: 800-332-8615
E-mail: cancergovstaff@mail.nih.gov
Web site: www.cancer.gov

National Center on Sleep Disorders Research
National Heart, Lung, and Blood Institute
6705 Rockledge Drive, Suite 6022
Bethesda, MD 20892-7993
Tel.: 301-435-0199
Fax: 301-480-3451
E-mail: ncsdr@nih.gov
Web site: www.nhlbi.nih.gov/sleep

National Heart, Lung, and Blood Institute (NHLBI)
Education Programs Information Center
PO Box 30105
Bethesda, MD 20824-0105
Tel.: 301-592-8573; TTY: 240-629-3255
Fax: 240-629-3246
E-mail: nhlbiinfo@nhlbi.nih.gov
Web site: www.nhlbi.nih.gov

National Institute on Aging (NIA)
Information Center
PO Box 8057
Gaithersburg, MD 20898
Tel.: 800-222-2225; TTY: 800-222-4225
E-mail: niaic@jbs1.com
Web site: www.nia.nih.gov

**North American Society for Pediatric Gastroenterology, Hepatology
   and Nutrition (NASPGHAN)**
PO Box 6
Flourtown, PA 19031
Tel.: 215-233-0808
Fax: 215-233-3918
E-mail: naspghan@naspghan.org
Web site: www.naspghan.org

U.S. Department of Agriculture (USDA)
1400 Independence Avenue, SW
Washington, DC 20250
Tel.: 800-727-9540 or 202-720-2791
Web site: www.usda.gov/wps/portal/usdahome

U.S. Food and Drug Administration (FDA)
Office of Consumer Affairs
5600 Fishers Lane
Rockville, MD 20857
Tel.: 888-INFO-FDA (888-463-6332) and 888-SAFE-FOOD
    (888-723-3366) (Food Information Line)
Fax: 301-443-9767
Web site: www.fda.gov

U.S. Government's Food Safety Web Site
www.foodsafety.gov

INDEX